A Clinician's Guide to Respiratory Diseases

A Clinician's Guide to Respiratory Diseases

Editor: Stephen Rogers

AMERICAN
MEDICAL PUBLISHERS
www.americanmedicalpublishers.com

AMERICAN
MEDICAL PUBLISHERS
www.americanmedicalpublishers.com

Cataloging-in-Publication Data

A clinician's guide to respiratory diseases / edited by Stephen Rogers.
p. cm.
Includes bibliographical references and index.
ISBN 978-1-63927-847-3
1. Respiratory organs--Diseases. 2. Respiratory organs--Diseases--Diagnosis.
3. Respiratory organs--Diseases--Treatment. 4. Respiratory infections.
5. Respiratory insufficiency. 6. Respiratory allergy. I. Rogers, Stephen.
RC731 .C55 2023
616.2--dc23

American Medical Publishers,
41 Flatbush Avenue,
1st Floor, New York,
NY 11217, USA

ISBN 978-1-63927-847-3 (Hardback)

Contents

Preface

This book aims to highlight the current researches and provides a platform to further the scope of innovations in this area. This book is a product of the combined efforts of many researchers and scientists, after going through thorough studies and analysis from different parts of the world. The objective of this book is to provide the readers with the latest information of the field.

Respiratory diseases are a group of diseases that affect the lungs and other parts of the human respiratory system. These diseases can be classified into three types, namely, airway diseases, lung tissue disease and lung circulation diseases. The main cause of respiratory diseases is air pollution, smoking tobacco, or breathing asbestos and radon. Airway diseases are conditions that affect airways carrying oxygen and other gases into and out of the lungs. Some common airway diseases are bronchiectasis, asthma and chronic obstructive pulmonary disease (COPD). Asthma is a major chronic respiratory disease that causes difficulty in breathing. Some common symptoms of asthma include wheezing, coughing and tightness in the chest. The diseases that affect the structure of the lung tissue are called lung tissue diseases. They are caused by scarring or inflammation of the tissues which restrict the lungs from expanding properly. This book is a practical guide to respiratory diseases. It includes some of the vital pieces of work being conducted across the world, on various topics related to these diseases. This book includes contributions of experts and doctors which will provide innovative insights into respiratory diseases.

I would like to express my sincere thanks to the authors for their dedicated efforts in the completion of this book. I acknowledge the efforts of the publisher for providing constant support. Lastly, I would like to thank my family for their support in all academic endeavors.

Editor

1

A Rare Case of Hypersensitivity Pneumonitis due to Florida Red Tide

Raju Reddy,[1] Nupur Verma,[2] and Tan-Lucien Mohammed[2]

[1]*Division of Pulmonary, Critical Care and Sleep Medicine, Department of Internal Medicine, University of Florida, 1600 SW Archer Rd, P.O. Box 100225, Gainesville, FL, USA*
[2]*Department of Radiology, University of Florida, 1600 SW Archer Rd, P.O. Box 100374, Gainesville, FL, USA*

Correspondence should be addressed to Raju Reddy; raju.reddy@medicine.ufl.edu

Academic Editor: Javier de Miguel-Díez

Florida red tides occur annually due to proliferation of the marine dinoflagellate *Karenia brevis*, which produces neurotoxins known as brevotoxins. Inhalational exposure to brevotoxins usually results in upper airway symptoms only. Rarely does exposure lead to lower respiratory tract symptoms as in our case. We report a case of a 50-year-old man who presented with a 4-week history of dyspnea after exposure to the red tide. Computed tomography (CT) of the chest showed diffuse bilateral ground glass opacities and interstitial thickening. Bronchoalveolar lavage cultures and cytology were negative. The patient was started on steroids. Over the next few weeks, the patient's symptoms resolved. Repeat CT chest showed complete resolution of the ground glass opacities. Steroids were then tapered. Most patients who are exposed to algal blooms have self-limiting symptoms. Patients with asthma are particularly susceptible to worsening respiratory symptoms after exposure to brevotoxin aerosols. This case highlights that, in rare cases, exposure to red tide can results in severe lower respiratory tract symptoms.

1. Case Presentation

A 50-year-old man with a history of hypertension, 30-pack year tobacco history and pulmonary embolism 12 years prior to admission presented with a 4-week history of progressively worsening dyspnea. His symptoms began with a dry cough, mild dyspnea and fevers. He was given a course of levofloxacin and azithromycin. While his cough and fevers resolved, his dyspnea continued to worsen. These symptoms began after he was exposed to the Florida red tide. Four weeks earlier, the patient reported going to the beach for a swim. Unfortunately, he swam into a large area of red tide (Figure 1). Florida red tides occur due to high concentrations of algal blooms, particularly *Karenia brevis (K. brevis)* which gives the water a red discoloration (Figure 2). Immediately after the exposure, the patient began to have symptoms. He denied any recent travel, illicit drug use and occupational exposures. He also denied receiving any blood transfusions recently. He worked as a nurse.

On initial examination, the patient was profoundly hypoxic requiring FiO2 0.8 to maintain an appropriate oxygen saturation via high flow nasal canula. He was ill appearing and was in mild respiratory distress. The remainder of the examination was significant for bibasilar crackles and absence of pedal edema. Initial labs were significant for white blood cell count at 28 x 10^3 cells/μL with neutrophilia and absence of eosinophilia. Other significant labs included elevated brain natriuretic peptide 440 pg/mL (normal < 100 pg/mL) and normal procalcitonin 0.22 ng/mL (normal < 0.5 ng/mL) levels. The patient was started on broad spectrum antibiotics.

Computed tomography (CT) of the chest showed a lower predominant ground-glass attenuation, along with small cysts and smooth interlobular septal thickening (Figures 3(a) and 3(b)). There were no centrilobular nodules. A bronchoscopy was performed on the day of admission. The patient was not a candidate for a transbronchial biopsy due to high oxygen requirements. Bronchoalveolar lavage (BAL) fluid analysis showed 88% macrocytes and 10% lymphocytes. The patient was continued on anti-bacterial therapy while further work-up continued. Despite a weeklong course of board spectrum antibiotics, he continued to have high oxygen requirements. At this point, differential diagnosis included acute hypersensitivity pneumonitis (HP) due to red-tide exposure, respiratory bronchiolitis associated interstitial

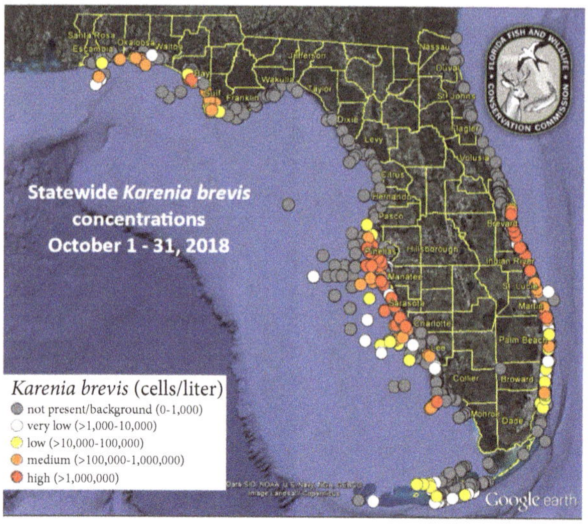

FIGURE 1: Concentrations of *Karenia brevis* during exposure. Image source: Florida Fish and Wildlife Conservation Commission.

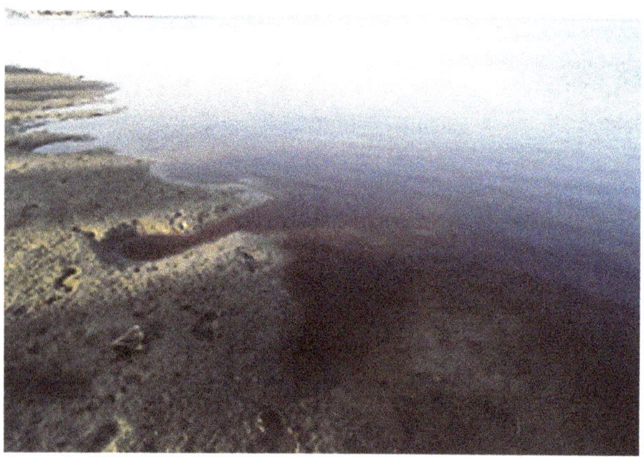

FIGURE 2: *Karenia brevis* proliferation. Source: Florida Fish and Wildlife Commission.

lung disease (RB-ILD), desquamative interstitial pneumonia (DIP) and acute respiratory distress syndrome (ARDS). The remainder of the BAL fluid analysis was negative for bacterial and fungal cultures, viral studies including influenza and cytology noted no organisms or malignant cells. Other negative findings included an autoimmune work-up for connective tissue disease including an extended myositis panel and hypersensitivity panel.

Since the cultures were negative, the patient was started on Prednisone 1 mg/kg daily with a diagnosis of HP due to red tide exposure. While RB-ILD and DIP remained in consideration, the patient had a clear temporal association of symptom onset after an inhalational exposure. Furthermore, the patient had not smoked for the last 4 weeks prior to presentation at our institution. Despite being off cigarettes, his dyspnea continued to worsen. Of note, BAL findings in patients with RB-ILD or DIP are typically macrocyte predominant similar to our patient, whereas in HP, BAL findings are lymphocytic predominant. However, smokers with HP may not have a marked BAL lymphocytosis compared to non-smokers [1]. In addition, up to two-thirds of patients with RB-ILD or DIP improve once they quit smoking [2]. In cases where they do not improve with quitting smoking, corticosteroids provide only marginal benefit [3]. Our patient however noted a dramatic improvement with steroids. Together, the initial symptom onset after exposure, persistence of symptoms despite quitting smoking and improvement with steroids, suggested that the patient developed an acute case of HP following exposure to the red tide. CT chest obtained 8 weeks after initial presentation showed significant improvement of the ground glass attenuation and interstitial thickening (Figures 3(c) and 3(d)). The patient was gradually weaned off steroids over the next 4 weeks. While most cases of red tide exposure lead to upper airway symptoms only, this case highlights that patients may also develop lower airway symptoms.

2. Discussion

Florida red tides occur due to proliferation of the toxic dinoflagellate, *K. brevis*. *K. brevis* is a unicellular organism found widely in the Gulf of Mexico [4]. It produces PbTx-2 and PbTx-3, the major brevotoxins that are responsible for both neurologic symptoms if ingested and upper airway symptoms if inhaled [5, 6]. The tide peaks in late summer to early fall and can last from days to months. The longest documented red tide bloom lasted for 30 months from 1994 to 1997 [7]. The current red tide bloom began in October 2017, peaked from July 2018 to October 2018 and ended in March 2019 [8]. Our patient was exposed to red tide during a period of high concentration (Figure 1). While the annual number of cases of brevotoxin exposure is unknown, studies show an increase in emergency room visits for respiratory symptoms during peak periods [9]. Kirkpatrick *et al.* found a 19% increase in rates of pneumonia diagnoses during a red tide period compared to a non-red tide period.

Typically, exposure to brevotoxins results in upper airway symptoms only. This is because average size of the aerosolized toxin is 8-9μ whereas particles need be less than 5μ to enter the lower respiratory tract [10]. In one study of 27 healthy individuals exposed to low level brevotoxins, 35% developed throat irritation, 53% developed cough, and 23% developed nasal congestion whereas on days with higher levels of brevotoxins, 54% developed throat irritation, 77% developed cough and 23% developed nasal congestion [11]. In addition, study participants had a slight reduction in peak expiratory flows and forced expiratory volume-1 (FEV1) on exposed days compared to unexposed days but no reduction in their exercise capacity. Other studies have found a direct correlation between symptoms and exposure burden with higher levels of toxin in the air leading to lower respiratory tract involvement [12]. Our patient likely developed lower respiratory tract symptoms because he had a heavy exposure burden. He was exposed to not only the aerosolized toxin on the beach but also brevotoxins in the water while swimming. *K. brevis* is easily lysed and thus releases toxin in to the water. Of note, the brevotoxin is stored in clams and oysters

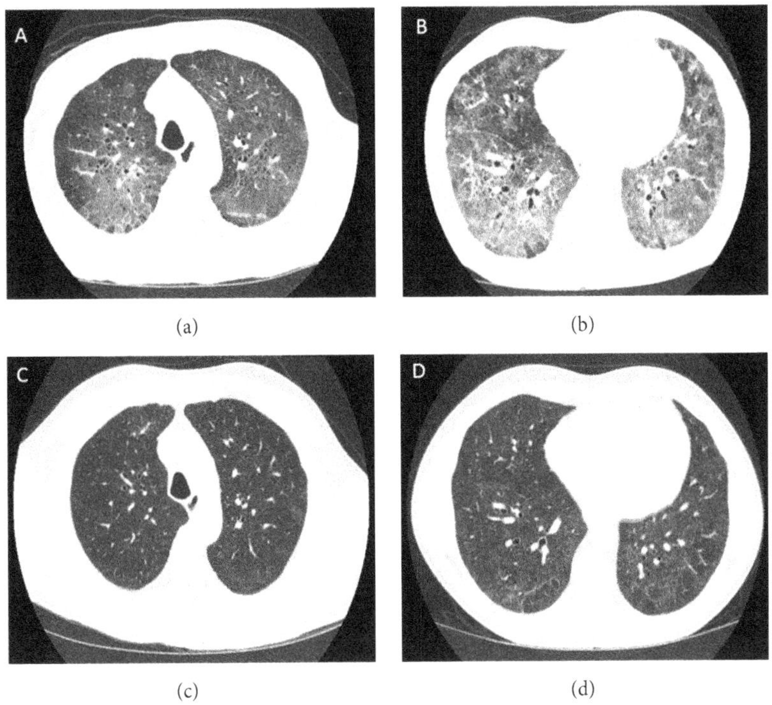

FIGURE 3: (a) and (b) At the time of presentation, axial computed tomography of the chest images show upper lobe predominant ground glass attenuation, mild interlobular septal thickening and small cysts. (c) and (d) Eight weeks following treatment, axial computed tomography of the chest images shows near complete resolution of ground-glass attenuation, interlobular septal thickening and cysts.

which accounts for the neurotoxic poisoning in people who consume contaminated shellfish.

Of particular concern is exposure of brevotoxin in uncontrolled asthmatics. In a study of 97 patients with self-reported asthma, there was significant reduction in FEV1 after only 1 hour of exposure to the aerosolized toxin [13]. These findings were particularly more prominent in patients who used their inhalers more frequently. In another study of 125 asthmatics, 38 patients were more reactive to the toxin. These patients had larger reductions in FEV1 following exposure [14]. In addition, prior to enrollment, these patients were using asthma medications more frequently and were more likely to have been hospitalized for respiratory symptoms in the last 12 months. Together, these findings suggest that patients who have uncontrolled asthma may be more susceptible to developing respiratory symptoms following exposure to the brevotoxin.

Exposure to the inhaled toxin results in mass cell degranulation and histamine release resulting in elevated levels of inflammatory cytokines such as interleukin-6 which may account for the respiratory symptoms [12]. From a public health standpoint, preventing exposure to the toxin is critical. Humans can be exposed through food, water and air [15]. The brevotoxin is odorless, tasteless and heat stable [15]. During periods of algal bloom, the public and particularly asthmatics must be counseled to stay indoors since the aerosolized toxin can travel up to 2 miles inland depending on the wind conditions [16]. Therefore, asthmatic patients living inland should remain aware of potential exposure in the right conditions. Other measures to minimize exposure include wearing a paper surgical mask to decrease exposure [5, 16].

This case highlights the respiratory pathology associated with red tide exposure. The majority of cases are limited to upper respiratory tract infection. However, with a large exposure burden, the lower respiratory tract can be involved as was our case.

References

[1] Y. Lacasse, M. Selman, U. Costabel et al., "Clinical diagnosis of hypersensitivity pneumonitis," *American Journal of Respiratory and Critical Care Medicine*, vol. 168, no. 8, pp. 952–958, 2003.

[2] S. A. Yousem, T. V. Colby, and E. A. Gaensler, "Respiratory bronchiolitis-associated interstitial lung disease and its relationship to desquamative interstitial pneumonia," *Mayo Clinic Proceedings*, vol. 64, no. 11, pp. 1373–1380, 1989.

[3] J. H. Ryu, J. L. Myers, S. A. Capizzi, W. W. Douglas, R. Vassallo, and P. A. Decker, "Desquamative interstitial pneumonia and respiratory bronchiolitis- associated interstitial lung disease," *CHEST*, vol. 127, no. 1, pp. 178–184, 2005.

[4] F. M. Dolah, "Marine algal toxins: origins, health effects, and their increased occurrence," *Environmental Health Perspectives*, vol. 108, no. 1, pp. 133–141, 2000.

[5] L. E. Fleming, B. Kirkpatrick, L. C. Backer et al., "Review of Florida red tide and human health effects," *Harmful Algae*, vol. 10, no. 2, pp. 224–233, 2011.

[6] Y. S. Cheng, Y. Zhou, C. M. Irvin et al., "Characterization of marine aerosol for assessment of human exposure to brevetoxins," *Environmental Health Perspectives*, vol. 113, no. 5, pp. 638–643, 2005.

[7] "Florida fish and wildlife conservation commission," https://myfwc.com/research/redtide/monitoring/database/.

[8] "Florida fish and wildlife commission," https://www.flickr.com/photos/myfwc/sets/72157635398013168/with/40785861763/.

[9] B. Kirkpatrick, L. E. Fleming, L. C. Backer et al., "HARMFUL emergency room respiratory diagnoses admissions," *Water*, vol. 5, no. 5, pp. 526–533, 2006.

[10] Y. S. Cheng, J. D. McDonald, D. Kracko et al., "Concentration and particle size of airborne toxic algae (brevetoxin) derived from ocean red tide events," *Environmental Science & Technology*, vol. 39, no. 10, pp. 3443–3449, 2005.

[11] L. C. Backer, B. Kirkpatrick, L. E. Fleming et al., "Occupational exposure to aerosolized brevetoxins during florida red tide events: effects on a healthy worker population," *Environmental Health Perspectives*, vol. 113, no. 5, pp. 644–649, 2005.

[12] L. C. Backer, L. E. Fleming, A. Rowan et al., "Recreational exposure to aerosolized brevetoxins during Florida red tide events," *Harmful Algae*, vol. 2, no. 1, pp. 19–28, 2003.

[13] L. E. Fleming, B. Kirkpatrick, L. C. Backer et al., "Aerosolized red-tide toxins (brevetoxins) and asthma," *CHEST*, vol. 131, no. 1, pp. 187–194, 2007.

[14] J. A. Bean, L. E. Fleming, B. Kirkpatrick et al., "Florida red tide toxins (brevetoxins) and longitudinal respiratory effects in asthmatics," *Harmful Algae*, vol. 10, no. 6, pp. 744–748, 2011.

[15] G. M. Hallegraeff, D. M. Anderson, A. D. Cembella, and H. O. Enevoldsen, *Manual on Harmful Marine Microalgae*, NESCO, 2003, https://unesdoc.unesco.org/ark:/48223/pf0000131711.

[16] B. Kirkpatrick, R. Pierce, Y. S. Cheng et al., "Inland transport of aerosolized Florida red tide toxins," *Harmful Algae*, vol. 9, no. 2, pp. 186–189, 2010.

2

Asthma Symptoms in Bakeries at Parakou, Benin

Serge Ade,[1,2] Mênonli Adjobimey,[3,4] Gildas Agodokpessi,[3,4] Marie Sylvie Kouassi,[1] Fabien A. Gounongbe,[1] Ibrahim Cisse,[1] and Spero H. R. Hounkpatin[1]

[1]*Faculty of Medicine, University of Parakou, Parakou, Benin*
[2]*International Union Against Tuberculosis and Lung Diseases, Paris, France*
[3]*Faculty of Health Sciences, University of Abomey-Calavi, Cotonou, Benin*
[4]*National and Teaching Hospital of Respiratory Diseases, Cotonou, Benin*

Correspondence should be addressed to Serge Ade; adeserg@yahoo.fr

Academic Editor: Nicole S. L. Goh

Background and Objectives. There is a dearth of information on asthma among bakers in low-income settings. The objectives of this study were to determine (i) the prevalence of asthma symptoms, (ii) factors associated with probable occupational asthma (OA), and (iii) work habits that might lead to a dusty workplace environment, Parakou, Benin. *Materials and Methods.* This was a mixed methods (cross-sectional quantitative and qualitative) study carried out between March and September 2018. *Results.* Of 210 employees/apprentices in 26 bakeries, 190 (91.48%) were included in the study: median age was 25.50 (IQR = 22 – 32) years, 157 (82.63%) were aged <40 years, and the male-to-female ratio was 26.14. Of these, 111 (58.42%) worked in a salted bread and 79 (41.58%) in a sweet bread bakery. An asthma history was reported by 3.68%. Symptoms consistent with asthma, work-related asthma, OA, and work-aggravated asthma were found in 13.68%, 12.63%, 10%, and 2.63%, respectively. Asthma confirmation was obtained in 15.79% of bakers with probable OA and in 23.08% of all bakers with suspected asthma. A history of allergic rhinoconjunctivitis was associated with probable OA (aOR = 106; 95%CI = 17.79 – 2093; $p < 0.001$). Of the 24 bakers with probable work-related asthma, 3 (12.50%) were prescribed a short-acting beta2-agonist and 2 (8.33%) an inhaled corticosteroid. No worker had had a systematically planned annual medical visit; some habits at work were identified as leading to flour and dust suspension at the workplace. *Conclusion.* Clinical manifestations of OA were common among bakers in Parakou and were associated with allergic rhinoconjunctivitis. There is a need to improve technical preventive measures and treatment, as well as to institute systematic medical visits for these workers.

1. Introduction

The baker's profession is well known to be strongly associated with occupational asthma (OA) worldwide, including in low- and middle-income countries (LMICs) [1–3]. Numerous allergens in a bakery may induce sensitization and allergic reactions. Particles that are derived from wheat, rye, and oats are reported to be highly allergenic. Wheat, the most common flour used for bread making, contains more than forty allergens, with water-soluble globulins and albumins thought to be the most allergenic. Baker's yeast, fungal alpha-amylase, improvers such as lecithin, soy flour, additives such as malted products, and contaminants that include storage mites and moulds are also sources of sensitization in bakeries [1, 4, 5].

The prevalence of asthma symptoms appears to be high among bakers. In a study carried out in France on artisanal bakery employees, the prevalence of asthma symptoms was nearly 17% [6]. Work-related asthma (WRA) is estimated to affect 5 to 10% of bakers [4], and this includes OA and worked-aggravated asthma (WAA). OA occurs in workers with no previous asthma whose first symptoms are initiated by exposure to agents at work. WAA is characterised by a worsening of symptoms of asthma in a worker with previously known asthma before any exposure to the work-related agents [7]. In a study conducted in Cape Town, the prevalence of OA was 13% and that of WAA was 3% [8].

In LMICs, similar to other OAs, baker's asthma is either underdiagnsoed or diagnosed late [3], due to several reasons that include lack of knowledge about disease symptoms and fear of job loss [1, 3]. This has harmful consequences not only for the individual but also for the whole family and systematic medical visits for workers are often missed [3]. Furthermore, recommended diagnostic tools such as specific bronchial challenges or immunological testing to specific allergens present in the workplace [7] are often not available. With challenges in implementing medical and technical preventive measures in these countries, we hypothesize that the burden of OA and WAA may be frequent among bakers despite the low number of studies in the literature from these settings, especially from sub-Saharan Africa.

The objectives of this preliminary study were to determine the prevalence of asthma manifestations, factors assocciasted with OA, and work habits that promote increased dust in the workplace among bakers in Parakou city in Benin.

2. Materials and Methods

2.1. Study Design. This was a mixed cross-sectional quantitative and qualitative study using data that were prospectively collected between March and September 2018.

2.2. Setting. The study was carried out in salted and sweet bread bakeries in Parakou, a city located in the north-central part of Benin with a population of 255,478 in 2013 [9]. Theoretically, Parakou has 37 bakeries, 17 produce salted and 20 produce sweet bread. However, only 11 (64.71%) salted and 15 (75%) sweet bread bakeries were really functional and these were all visited. In Parakou, similar to the rest of the country, baker's asthma is recognised as an occupational disease by Table no. 72 of the list of occupational diseases (unpublished data).

2.3. Study Population. All employees and apprentice bakers who gave their formal consent were included in the study. For those under 18 years of age, informed consent from a parent (or guardian) was obtained prior to the survey.

2.4. Data Collection and Principal Variables. For each individual worker included in the study, information was anonymously collected on demographic characteristics, comorbidities, type of bakery worked in, duration in the profession, position in the company, and presence of asthma symptoms. Bakers were then examined; and in those who reported asthma symptoms, their onset or aggravation during working hours at the bakery and their improvement during holidays were investigated. Bakers were then examined using spirometry with Spirodoc® (serial number: SN A23-0W.00398), followed by reversibility testing after inhalation through a chamber of salbutamol 400 μg dosage. The tests were performed by a well-trained medical student according to American Thoracic Society (ATS) and European Respiratory Society (ERS) guidelines [10]. Results were interpreted by an experienced pulmonologist and in line with ATS and ERS guidelines [11].

In addition, workers' habits in their respective positions in the bakery were observed during manufacturing of the bread in order to identify any practices that might promote flour dusting in the bakery. All this information was recorded in a data documentation form filled out by the investigator.

2.5. Diagnostic Criteria

(1) *Asthma Symptoms.* Asthma symptoms considered in this study included the four cardinal symptoms of the disease, namely, dyspnoea, wheezing, coughing, and chest tightness [12]

(2) *Reversible Obstructive Pulmonary Disorder.* This was defined by comparing the individual ratio of forced expiratory volume in one second (FEV1) and vital capacity (VC) to the lower limit of normal; and significant reversibility was diagnosed by an increase in FEV1 $\geq$ 12% and 200 ml in absolute values. The extrapolations that have been proposed to derive African standards were used to determine theoretical values [10, 11]

(3) *Confirmed Asthma.* The diagnosis was made in a symptomatic worker with a reversible obstructive disorder [12]

(4) *History of Asthma.* Any worker who reported having asthma symptoms in the past or was diagnosed with asthma by a medical doctor or was taking asthma medication before starting work at the bakery

(5) *Probable OA.* A worker who reported (a) never having had asthma symptoms before starting baking; (b) triggering of symptoms during working hours; and (c) improvement in symptoms while on holiday [7]

(6) *Probable WAA.* A worker who reported (i) a history of asthma before starting work at bakery; (ii) worsening of symptoms during work hours at bakery; and (iii) improvement while on holiday [7]

(7) *Probable Work-Related Asthma (WRA).* Association of OA and WAA manifestations [7]

(8) *Probable Asthma in Bakery.* Association of WRA and nonwork-related asthma

(9) *Allergic Rhinitis.* The diagnosis was based on symptoms and referred to repeated symptoms of sneezing, rhinorrhea, nasal pruritus, and a blocked nose triggered by some factors and without evidence for any respiratory infection [13]

2.6. Statistical Analysis. The data were entered into the Epi-Data Entry client software v2.0.7.7.22 (EpiData Association, Odense, Denmark). Data were analyzed using software R version 3.6.0. Percentages were calculated to describe qualitative variables, medians (and interquartile range (IQR)) for quantitative variables. Factors associated with probable OA were investigated by univariate analysis and then multivariate analysis using multiple logistic regression. All exposure factors with a p value ≤ 0.10 on univariate analysis were included in the multivariate analysis. The crude and adjusted odds ratios, their 95% confidence interval (95% CI), and the p values were determined. Levels of significance were set at 5%.

Table 1: Characteristics of workers investigated in bakeries at Parakou, Benin, March–September 2018.

	Number	(%)
Gender		
Males	183	(96.32)
Females	7	(3.68)
Age		
Median age (year)	25.50	
Interquartile range (year)	22-32	
Range (year)	13-66	
Tobacco status		
Nonsmoker	181	(95.26)
Current smoker	8	(4.21)
Ex-smoker	1	(0.53)
Allergic rhinitis	36	(18.95)
Allergic conjunctivitis	28	(14.74)
Eczema	11	(5.79)
Family atopy	10	(5.26)
Type of bakery		
Salted bread bakery	111	(58.42)
Sweet bread bakery	79	(41.58)
Duration of bakery working		
Median (year)	5	
Interquartile range (year)	1–11.5	
Range (year)	0.1-44	
Position at the time of the survey in the bakery		
Shaper/laminator	94	(49.47)
Kneader	51	(26.84)
Oven baker	29	(15.26)
Cashier	13	(6.84)
Cleaner	3	(1.58)
Total	190	

2.7. *Ethical Considerations.* The study was approved by the Local Ethics Committee for Biomedical Research of the University of Parakou, Benin.

3. Results

3.1. *Characteristics of Bakers and Prevalence of Asthma Symptoms and of Confirmed Asthma.* Overall, of the 210 employees or apprentices that were identified in the 26 bakeries, 190 (91.48%) consented to participate in the survey. The median age was 25.50 ($IQR = 22 - 32$) years, 157 (82.63%) were aged less than 40 years, and the male-to-female ratio was 26.14. Of these bakers, 111 (58.42%) worked in a salted bread and 79 (41.58%) in a sweet bread bakery, with a median duration of working in the bakery being 5 ($IQR = 1 - 11.5$) years. There were 94 (49.47%) who were employed in priority as processors/laminators (Table 1).

The prevalence of a history of asthma was 3.68%. The prevalence of probable WRA was 12.63%. More specifically, the prevalence of probable OA and WAA was 10% and 2.63%, respectively. Of the 24 bakers with probable WRA, 3 (12.50%) were prescribed a short-acting beta$_2$-agonist and 2 (8.33%) an inhaled corticosteroid. The prevalence of probable asthma in bakeries was 13.68% (Tables 2 and 3). The prevalence of confirmed asthma was 15.79% among workers with probable OA and 23.08% among all bakers with probable WRA (Table 4).

Table 2: Prevalence of asthma symptoms and evolution during working hours of bakers at Parakou, Benin, March–September 2018.

	Number	(%)
Asthma symptoms		
Dyspnea		
Absent	166	(87.37)
Only during working hours	19	(10)
Already present but worsened during working hours	5	(2.63)
Wheezing		
Absent	186	(97.89)
Only during working hours	2	(1.05)
Already present but worsened during working hours	2	(1.05)
Cough		
Absent	176	(92.63)
Only during working hours	9	(4.74)
Already present but worsened during working hours	5	(2.63)
Chest tightness		
Absent	180	(94.74)
Only during working hours	7	(3.68)
Already present but worsened during working hours	3	(1.58)

Table 3: Prevalence of asthma symptoms, of work-related and nonwork-related asthma symptoms in bakeries at Parakou, Benin, March–September 2018.

	Bakers with asthma symptoms	%
History of asthma	7	(3.68)
Bakers with asthma symptoms or history of asthma	26	(13.68)
Probable work-related asthma	24	(12.63)
Probable occupational asthma	19	(10)
Probable work-aggravated asthma	5	(2.63)
Probable non work-related asthma	2	(1.05)
Total	190	

3.2. *Characteristics and Factors Associated with Probable OA.* The median age of workers with probable OA was 24 ($IQR = 20 - 30$) years. They were all males. In 5 (26.32%) workers, respiratory symptoms were preceded by nasal and ocular symptoms. Three workers (15.79%) had bilateral wheezing during pulmonary auscultation at the time of the survey. Ten (52.63%) workers were shapers/rolling mill

Table 4: Spirometry results of bakers with asthma symptoms or an history of asthma at Parakou, Benin, March–September 2018.

	Total	Spirometry done	OVD* reversible (%[$])
Bakers with asthma symptoms or history of asthma	26	26	6 (23.08)
Probable work-related asthma	24	24	5 (20.83)
Probable occupational asthma	19	19	3 (15.79)
Probable work-aggravated asthma	5	5	2 (40)
Probable nonwork-related asthma	2	2	1 (50)

* OVD = obstructive ventilatory disorder. [$]Denominator = number of spirometry performed.

Table 5: Factors associated with probable occupational asthma, after univariate and multiple logistic regression analysis among bakers at Parakou, Benin, March–September 2018.

	n/N	%	Bivariate analysis			Multivariate analysis	
			cOR	P value	aOR	IC 95% aOR	P value
Age			0.98	0.567			
Sex				0.992			
Female	0/7	(0)	1				
Male	19/179	(10.61)	$5.10.10^{6}$				
Family asthma				0.982			
No	18/176	(10.23)	1				
Yes	1/10	(10)	0.98				
Allergic rhinoconjunctivitis				<0.001			
No	1/144	(0.69)	1				
Yes	18/42	(42.86)	$1.07.10^{2}$		106	17.79 - 2093	<0.001
Eczema				<0.001			
No	13/175	(7.43)	1				
Yes	6/11	(54.55)	14.95		2.14	0.51 - 9.50	0.300
Smoking				0.240			
No	17/177	(9.60)	1				
Yes	2/9	(22.22)	2.69				
Type of bakery				0.067			
Sweet bread bakery	4/77	(5.19)	1		1		
Salted bread bakery	15/109	(13.76)	2.91		0.60	0.12 - 2.95	0.519
Duration of bakery working			0.98	0.534			

cOR = crude odds ratio; aOR = adjusted odds ratio; 95% CI = 95% confidence interval.

operators, 6 (31.58%) were oven bakers, and 3 (15.79%) were kneaders. The median duration of working in a bakery was 4 (IQR = 1 – 13) years and range 48 days to 20 years. At univariate analysis, an association between OA and factors such as age, sex, history of family asthma, allergic rhinoconjonctivis, eczema, smoking, type of bakery, and duration of bakery working was sought. The position was not included among the potential risk factors since this was not specific to a designated worker. They usually have a frequent turnover between the different positions. After multiple logistic regression, a history of allergic rhinoconjunctivitis was associated with probable OA (aOR = $1.06.10^{2}$; 95%CI = 17.79 – 2093; $p < 0.001$), after adjustment for eczema and type of bakery (Table 5).

3.3. Annual Medical Check-Up and Work Habits Assessment. None of the workers who were interviewed had, to date, systematically planned any annual medical visits for the checking of asthma symptoms combined with respiratory measurements such as peak flow or spirometry. No personal protective equipment was used by workers and no specific ventilation system was in place.

Additionally, there were some habits and behaviours favouring the suspension of flour and dust in the air, mainly occuring during the mixing process. Of the 26 bakeries that were visited, the emptying of the flour bag was not done gently in two (8%). In 12 bakeries, water was not poured into the mixer before the flour. In salted bread bakeries, the flour was spilled into the mixer before the ice cubes. At the end of the emptying of the bag into the mixer, the officer tapped it to make sure that all the flour was poured. The flour that was not yet completely immersed in the water lifted up as soon as the mixer was started. The baker became sprinkled with flour several times:

during the emptying of the mixer tank, on the dough pieces before the division, the planks, the work surface during shaping, the shovel, and the breads before baking. Sweeping and cleaning were not done in a wet environment, resulting thereby once again in flour and dust suspension.

4. Discussion

The objectives of this study were to determine the prevalence of clinical asthma manifestations, factors associated with symptoms suggestive of OA and work habits and behaviours that might promote increased dust in the workplace among bakers in Parakou city, a sub-Saharan African setting. One of the strengths of the study was the recruitment of almost all the bakers who worked in this town, with the inclusion of more than nine tenths of them in the study. In addition, data on the different variables were prospectively collected, reducing thereby missing information-related bias. The main limitation of the study was the inability to confirm the diagnosis of baker's asthma. As mentioned above, specific bronchial challenge testing and investigation of the sensitization to allergens present in the occupational environment could not be carried out in our routine working conditions, due to the weakness of our technical platforms. We tried to perform serial measurements of peak expiratory flow during both working days and holidays to confirm the diagnosis of OA [7]. Unfortunately, this was found time-consuming by the bakers, who were mostly daily workers and were paid proportionally to their achievement at work. Moreover, the study did not receive any funding to motivate them by providing some incentives. Despite these limitations, the study showed some interesting findings.

The high male predominance among the workers who were investigated has been reported in other studies [14]. Workers were also relatively young, with a median age of 25.50 years and over 80% aged less than 40 years. Older workers may have stopped working earlier, due to the occurrence of occupational diseases including OA. It was not possible, in this study, to investigate the real reasons why each former worker stopped working at bakery.

The prevalence of asthma symptoms among bakers in Parakou was 13.68%, slightly lower than that found by Gillet in 2015 in France, 17% [6]. However, the proportion found was much higher than that reported in the general population in this city, 3.6% [15]. The prevalence was comparable to that reported by Sigari et al. from Sanandaj, Iran, in 2006, at 13% [14]. The prevalence of probable OA and WAA was 10% and 2.63%, respectively. The same trend was reported by Baatjies et al. in a study carried out in Cape Town between 2003 and 2004. These authors found 13% and 3%, respectively, for OA and WAA. In their study, in addition to clinical manifestations, the diagnosis was made using nonspecific bronchial hyperreactivity and skin testing for wheat, rye, barley, maize, *Lepidoglyphus destructor* (a storage mite), fungal amylase, and/or specific IgE isolation [8].

Respiratory symptoms among bakers are frequent according to many studies conducted in developed countries [16]. Bakers and confectioners are those most commonly affected by OA in France, with an annual incidence of 683 cases per million workers [17]. In Norway and the United Kingdom, exposure to grain and flour dust is reported to be the second leading cause of OA [4, 18, 19]. Over the period 1992-1997, the incidence of asthma among bakers in the United Kingdom was estimated at 951 cases per million people per year [19]. In Norway, the incidence of baker's asthma was 2.4 and 1 case per 1000 person-years, respectively, for men and women [18]. Worse, the number of asthma cases among bakers was thought to have increased in recent years [4], probably due to a better appropriation of symptoms and diagnostic tools.

In our setting, the true proportion of bakers with WRA or OA may be even higher than that reported in this study, since some employees, fearing to lose their job, may not have declared their symptoms, contributing to an underestimation of the disease. Additionally, some bakers are not administratively declared and therefore cannot be correctly followed-up. Another possible cause that may contribute to underestimating this prevalence is lack of recognition of asthma symptoms by some bakers.

Considering the challenges in achieving serial measurements of peak expiratory flow, a flow-volume curve with reversibility was performed in all symptomatic workers or those with a previous history of asthma. The diagnosis of asthma was confirmed among 15.79% of workers suspected of having OA and among 23.08% of all bakers with probable asthma. The absence of obstructive disorder between attacks was not surprising and has also been previously reported by others [12, 20].

After logistic regression, rhinoconjunctivitis was associated with OA after having adjusted for other factors. Several authors had highlighted the role of atopy in promoting the occurrence of OA [1]. Baker's asthma is preceded by allergic rhinitis, as it is often the case with sensitization to high molecular weight agents [1, 8, 16]. Adequate treatment of this comorbidity is strongly recommended; otherwise, it may worsen asthma symptoms and prevent the control of the disease [7, 16]. New workers who already have allergic diseases should be better informed on the high risk of developing asthma in bakeries, especially if preventive measures are not implemented. Such patients also require special attention during follow-up visits.

Finally, assessment of workers' habits revealed many behaviours that promote increased dust at the workplace during the many stages of bread making. There is need for urgent implementation of relevant technical prevention measures in these bakeries. Taking into account local resources, this may include delicately placing flour bags, not tapping the bag, and using a mixer at a slow speed until the flour is mixed into the liquid ingredients. Cleaning of floors and work surfaces after their humidification should also be advocated. Additionally, although this was not investigated in our study, we recommend the introduction of an effective ventilation system to reduce the air concentration of particles. Storing flour in the right conditions of temperature and humidity that inhibit the growth of microorganisms can be recommended. Other actions would include use of personal protective equipment such as masks. Flour exposure limit values are proposed in some countries [21, 22]. Training of exposed workers is essential for behavioural change, and according to some authors, this could effectively reduce dust in the workplace by 54% [9]. Finally, medical follow-up visits with regular measurement of respiratory volume and air flow must be instituted in every bakery, a unique way to ensure early, total, and definitive eviction. In the same way, it is urgent to improve treatment among symptomatic patients, since the proportion of those undergoing treatment was low before the survey.

5. Conclusion

Clinical manifestations of OA were common among bakers in Parakou, and they were associated with allergic rhinoconjunctivitis. Many of the behaviours during bread making promoted increased dust by flour, and these should be corrected by strengthening technical prevention measures. Finally, we advocate for systematic annual follow-up visits of workers in this sector.

Disclosure

The funders had no role in study design, data collection and analysis, decision to publish, or preparation of the paper.

Acknowledgments

The authors thank all the bakers who participated to this work. Serge Ade is a Union Operational Research Fellow. He is part-time financially supported by the International Union against Tuberculosis and Lung Disease (The Union), Paris, France, through an Operational Research Fellowshisp. Funding was from an anonymous donor and the Department for International Development, UK.

References

[1] J. Ameille, A. Larbanois, A. Descatha, and O. Vandenplas, "Epidemiology and etiologic agents of occupational asthma," *Revue des Maladies Respiratoires*, vol. 23, no. 6, pp. 726–740, 2006.

[2] G. Krüll, P. Gianella, P. Soccal, and J. A. Pralong, "Occupational asthma," *Revue Médicale Suisse*, vol. 12, no. 539, pp. 1972–1975, 2016.

[3] M. F. Jeebhay and S. Quirce, "Occupational asthma in the developing and industrialised world: a review," *International Journal of Tuberculosis and Lung Disease*, vol. 11, no. 2, pp. 122–133, 2007.

[4] S. Quirce and A. Diaz-perales, "Diagnosis and management of grain-induced asthma," *Allergy, Asthma & Immunology Research*, vol. 5, no. 6, pp. 348–356, 2013.

[5] A. Stobnicka and R. L. Górny, "Exposure to flour dust in the occupational environment," *International Journal of Occupational Safety and Ergonomics*, vol. 21, no. 3, pp. 241–249, 2015.

[6] P. Gillet, "Prevalence of respiratory allergies in bakeries," *Archives des Maladies Porfessionnelles et de l'Environnement*, vol. 76, no. 5, pp. 478–484, 2015.

[7] X. Baur, T. Sigsgaard, T. B. Aasen et al., "Guidelines for the management of work-related asthma," *European Respiratory Journal*, vol. 39, no. 3, pp. 529–545, 2012.

[8] R. Baatjies, A. L. Lopata, I. Sander et al., "Determinants of asthma phenotypes in supermarket bakery workers," *European Respiratory Journal*, vol. 34, no. 4, pp. 825–833, 2009.

[9] R. Baatjies, T. Meijster, D. Heederik, I. Sander, and M. F. Jeebhay, "Effectiveness of interventions to reduce flour dust exposures in supermarket bakeries in South Africa," *Occupational and Environmental Medicine*, vol. 71, no. 12, pp. 811–818, 2014.

[10] Global Initiative for Asthma, "Pocket guide for asthma management (for adults and children other than 5 years) Updated 2019," http://www.ginaasthma.org.

[11] M. R. Miller, J. Hankinson, V. Brusasco et al., "Standardisation of spirometry," *European Respiratory Journal*, vol. 26, no. 2, pp. 319–338, 2005.

[12] R. Pellegrino, G. Viegi, V. Brusasco et al., "Interpretative strategies for lung function tests," *European Respiratory Journal*, vol. 26, no. 5, pp. 948–968, 2005.

[13] World Allergy Organization (WAO), *WAO White Book on Allergy (Update: 2013)*, p. 248, 2013, http://www.worldallergy.org/UserFiles/file/WhiteBook2-2013-v8.pdf.

[14] N. Sigari, E. Rahimi, K. Yazdanpanah, and A. Sharifian, "Prevalence of asthma and rhinitis in bakery workers in the city of Sanandaj, Iran," *Iran Journal of Allergy, Asthma and Immunology*, vol. 6, no. 4, pp. 215–218, 2007.

[15] S. Ade, M. C. Flatin, A. C. Dovonou et al., "Prevalence of bronchial asthma symptoms associated with allergic rhinitis manifestations in Parakou, Benin," *Journal of Functional Ventilation and Pulmonology*, vol. 8, no. 24, pp. 24–28, 2017.

[16] N. Rosenberg, "Allergie respiratoire du boulanger," *Documents pour le médecin du travail*, vol. 90-TR-29, pp. 189–196, 2002.

[17] J. Ameille, G. Pauli, A. Calastreng-Crinquand et al., "Reported incidence of occupational asthma in France, 1996–99: the ONAP programme," *Occupational and Environmental Medicine*, vol. 60, no. 2, pp. 136–141, 2003.

[18] H. L. Leira, U. Bratt, and S. Slastad, "Notified cases of occupational asthma in Norway: exposure and consequences for health and income," *American Journal of Industrial Medicine*, vol. 48, no. 5, pp. 359–364, 2005.

[19] J. C. McDonald, H. L. Keynes, and S. K. Meredith, "Reported incidence of occupational asthma in the United Kingdom, 1989-97," *Occupational and Environmental Medicine*, vol. 57, no. 12, pp. 823–829, 2000.

[20] V. P. Luks, K. L. Vandemheen, and S. D. Aaron, "Confirmation of asthma in an era of overdiagnosis," *European Respiratory Journal*, vol. 36, no. 2, pp. 255–260, 2010.

[21] P. Cullinan, D. Lowson, M. J. Nieuwenhuijsen et al., "Work related symptoms, sensitisation, and estimated exposure in workers not previously exposed to flour," *Occupational and Environmental Medicine*, vol. 51, no. 9, pp. 579–583, 1994.

[22] R. Houba, G. Doekes, and D. Heederik, "Occupational respiratory allergy in bakery workers: a review of the literature," *American Journal of Industrial Medicine*, vol. 34, no. 6, pp. 529–546, 1998.

3

Cicatricial Organizing Pneumonia with Dendriform Pulmonary Ossification: An Unusual Cause for a Recurrent Pneumothorax

Mnahi Bin Saeedan,[1] Carol Farver,[2] Atul C. Mehta ,[3] and Ruchi Yadav [1]

[1]*Section of Thoracic Imaging, Imaging Institute, Cleveland Clinic, Cleveland, OH, USA*
[2]*Department of Pathology, University of Michigan, Ann Arbor, MI, USA*
[3]*Department of Pulmonary and Critical Care Medicine, Cleveland Clinic, Cleveland, OH, USA*

Correspondence should be addressed to Ruchi Yadav; YADAVR@ccf.org

Academic Editor: Tun-Chieh Chen

Cicatricial organizing pneumonia is an uncommon form of organizing pneumonia, which may manifest as persisting linear opacities on computerized tomography (CT) scan mimicking a fibrosing interstitial pneumonia. It may also manifest with pulmonary ossification, which is a metaplastic bone formation within the lung tissue. The latter presentation could be either nodular or dendriform, both secondary to underlying lung disease and rarely idiopathic. Dendriform pulmonary ossification (DPO) has rarely been described as a cause of spontaneous pneumothorax. We present a case of a 55-year-old male with history of recurrent pneumothoraces and worsening dyspnea on exertion. A CT of the chest revealed progressive bilateral sub-pleural and peribronchovascular reticular opacities associated with densely ossified branching and nodular opacities. Video-assisted thoracoscopic biopsy of the lung demonstrated cicatricial organizing pneumonia with areas of marked diffuse DPO. The case highlights that dendriform pulmonary ossification arising from cicatricial organizing pneumonia should be considered in the differential diagnosis of recurrent pneumonias among patients with lower lobe sub-pleural reticular opacities. The case highlights that dendriform pulmonary ossification rarely can cause spontaneous pneumothorax and can be associated with cicatricial organizing pneumonia and reticular opacities on imaging.

1. Introduction

Organizing pneumonia (OP) is characterized by the presence of organizing fibromyxoid proliferations within the lumens of respiratory bronchioles and alveolar ducts. Peripheral and /or peribronchiolar consolidations are the most frequent findings of OP on a computerized tomography (CT) scan. These opacities could be migratory in nature. OP is often steroid-responsive and reversible with total resolution of radiological opacities, but occasionally may recur [1, 2].

Cicatricial OP (OPc) is a newly described entity in the pathology literature [3, 4] and distinguished from conventional OP by formation of irreversible dense fibrous bands and small nodules in the background of conventional OP [4]. The reported CT findings of OPc are variable and range from typical imaging findings of OP to lower lobes predominant peribronchovascular and subpleural reticular opacities with or without pulmonary ossification [4]. The latter is characterized by metaplastic ossification in the lung and is classified into nodular (NPO) and dendriform (DPO) subtypes [5]. Dendriform pulmonary ossification is usually described in association with chronic lung disease including usual interstitial pneumonia (UIP) [5, 6] although it can be seen in isolation [7, 8]. Dendriform pulmonary ossification presenting with spontaneous pneumothorax has been reported in a few occasions [9–14] but rarely with OPc [4]. We report a case of cicatricial organizing pneumonia with DPO who presented with recurrent pneumothorax. The clinical, radiological and pathological findings as well as the pulmonary functions have been described.

2. Case Report

A 55 year-old, nonsmoker male presented with a recurrent large left pneumothorax requiring a chest tube placement. He had a same side pneumothorax three and six years earlier, also requiring a chest tube placement. The patient also reported

Table 1: Pulmonary function test over several years.

	FEV1		FVC		FEV1/FVC %	DLco	
	Value	Predicted %	Value	Predicted %		Value	Predicted %
2019	2.22	55%	3.01	57%	74	N/A	N/A
2017	2.62	69%	3.77	76%	70	20.74	68%
2015	2.96	76%	4.11	82%	72	24.76	80%
2014	3.15	81%	4.16	82%	76	24.76	80%
2013	3.41	87%	4.47	88%	76	23.61	76%
2012	3.39	85%	4.50	88%	75	32.39	103%

FVC: forced vital capacity, FEV1: forced expiratory volume in 1 second, DLCO: diffusing capacity of the lung for carbon monoxide (ml/min/mmHg), N/A: not available.

dyspnea on exertion with stairs and inclines, which had progressed over last three years along with a dry cough.

He had a remote exposure to quails while training hunting dogs. He was known to have hypertension and suffered with symptoms of gastroesophageal reflux disorder (GERD). His physical examination was unremarkable. A review of his pulmonary function revealed gradual decline in his FEV1, FVC and diffusion capacity over the past seven years (Table 1).

Review of serial chest CT imaging revealed progressive bilateral sub-pleural and peribronchovascular branching dense opacities suggestive of DPO (Figure 1). He underwent VATS wedge resection of the left upper and lower lobes, which confirmed foci of dendriform ossification consisting of islands of ossifying fibrosis (Figure 2). In addition, there were scattered foci of OP, which, in some areas, had a more hyalinizing/cicatricial type morphology consistent with OPc. Many of the foci of DPO were associated with the OPc and showed transitions from conventional OP to OPc to the DPO (Figure 3). Dendriform pulmonary ossification foci were present in the subpleural region and occasionally adjacent to the visceral pleura (Figure 4). Given these imaging and pathological findings, the patient was diagnosed with DPO with cicatricial OP as the likely cause of his dyspnea, recurrent spontaneous pneumothoraces, and progressive restrictive impairment of lung function. Since there is no established medical treatment, his treatment plan was monitoring his symptoms and lung function and considering lung transplantation in case of progression.

3. Discussion

Organizing pneumonia is usually steroid-responsive and pathologically characterized by presence of loose fibromyxoid plugs within the lumens of the respiratory bronchioles and alveolar ducts [1, 2]. Cicatricial OP is distinguished from conventional OP by formation of irreversible dense fibrous bands and small nodules in a background of small or large foci of conventional OP [4]. In OPc, fibromyxoid plugs as seen in OP may be seen transitioning to more hyalinizing fibrous band/nodule of cicatricial OP and into foci of ossification on imaging as well as on pathology [4]. In our case, foci of DPO consisting of islands of ossifying fibrosis were present throughout both the left upper and lower lobes. In addition, there were scattered foci of hyalinizing/cicatricial type organizing pneumonia [4], representing a more chronic form of organizing pneumonia. Isolated focal plugs of hyalinized intra-alveolar tissue can be incidentally seen on in lobar resections for unrelated primary indications and should not confused with OPc. OPc tends to show bilateral and diffuse or patchy distribution on imaging [3, 4]. Fibrosing OP is a different from OPc, though it is not clearly determined what this pattern may represent. It may be form of disease where the fibrous tissues cause expansion of the alveolar septal interstitium such as in late organizing stages of diffuse alveolar damage or fibrotic forms of nonspecific interstitial pneumonia (NSIP) [3].

On CT, conventional OP presents as patchy bilateral peribronchial and subpleural consolidations [15–19], which may be migratory [20]. The classic "atoll" [20] or the "reverse halo" sign [18] is only seen in 20% cases manifesting as ground glass opacities with surrounding crescentic or ring-shaped consolidation [21] Perilobular opacities bordering the periphery of the secondary pulmonary nodules are observed [16, 19, 22] in more than half of OP cases. Manifestations of OPc include ground glass opacities, often associated with consolidations [15] and 1–10 mm nodular opacities with consolidation [16, 17]. Less common imaging features are subpleural or peribronchial irregular reticular opacities with areas of consolidation [15, 16, 19] and large nodules or mass-like consolidation [23]. Only 40% of the reported OPc cases show typical imaging appearance and other cases show variable nonspecific imaging findings including peribronchial and peripheral reticular opacities with or without evidence of pulmonary ossification [4]. Reticular opacities on CT imaging are seen in cicatricial OP cases where fibrous bands and nodules are the predominant feature on pathology with minor conventional OP. Presence of branching high densities on CT is suggestive of dendriform pulmonary ossification.

Pulmonary ossification is a metaplastic process where mature bone is present in the alveolar interstitium and/or alveolar spaces. Pulmonary ossification is classified into DPO and NPO. NPO is usually a localized process of lamellar bone and can occur in the setting of chronic congestion as seen in mitral valve stenosis. Unlike DPO, NPO usually does not contain bone marrow (fat or hematopoietic cells) [5]. On CT, NPO manifests as lower lobe predominant small, often highly attenuating, centrilobular nodules that may coalesce [24]. In DPO,

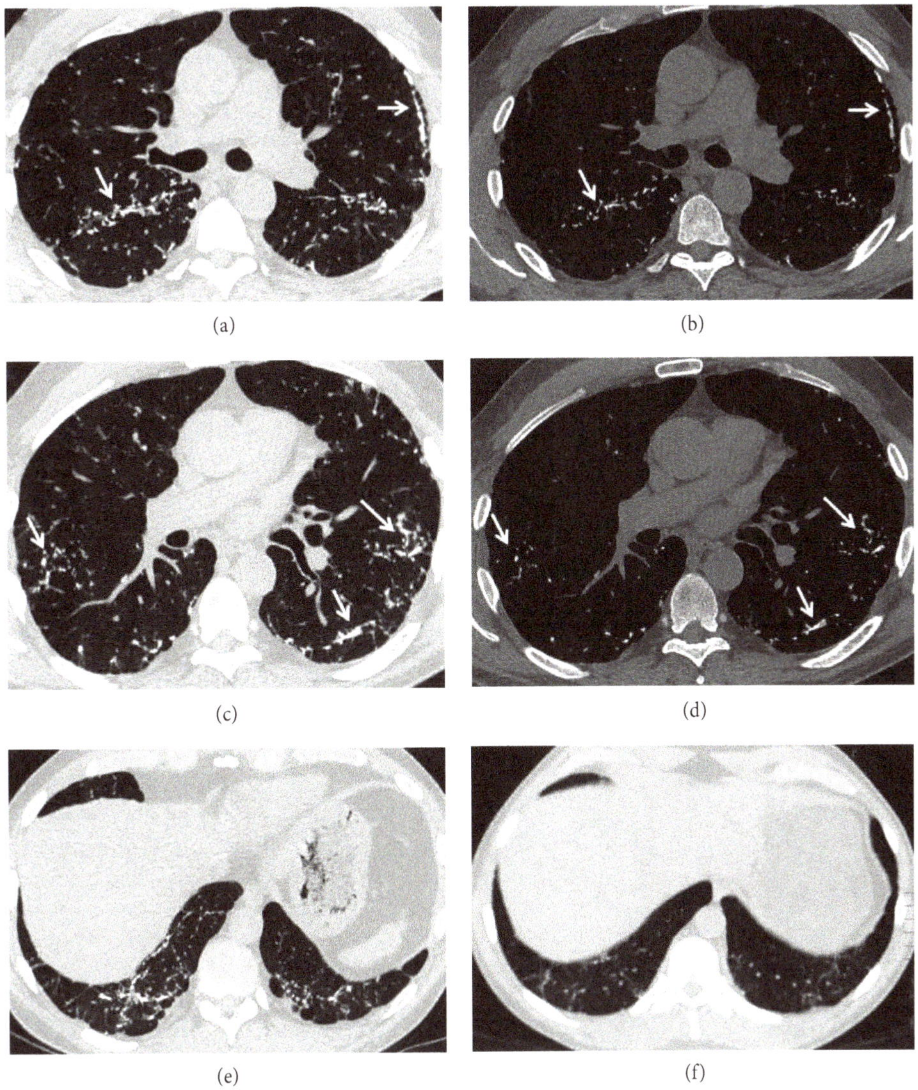

FIGURE 1: Axial chest CT images using lung (a), (c) and bone (b), (d) windows show bilateral branching dense nodular opacities (arrows) with mild associated reticulation. Some of the nodule are high in attenuation and almost iso-dense to ribs on bone windows. Axial images using lung widow (e), (f) at the level of lung bases were obtained 5 years apart and show evidence of progression.

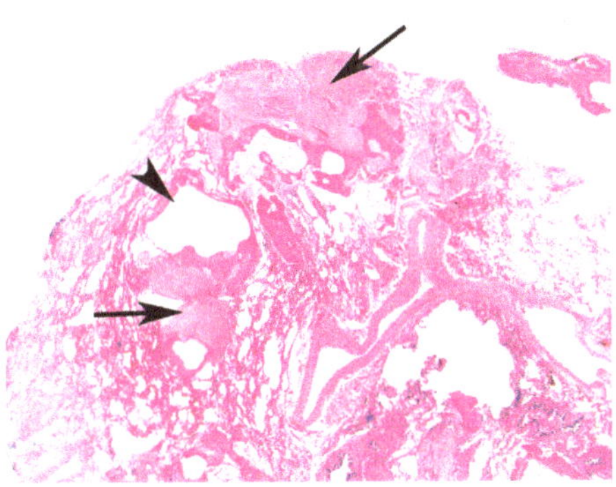

FIGURE 2: Large area of subpleural diffuse pulmonary ossification revealing lamellar bone with a more complicated pattern and areas of marrow elements including fat (arrowhead). Adjacent areas of cicatricial OP (arrows) are present (Hematoxylin and eosin; 12.5x).

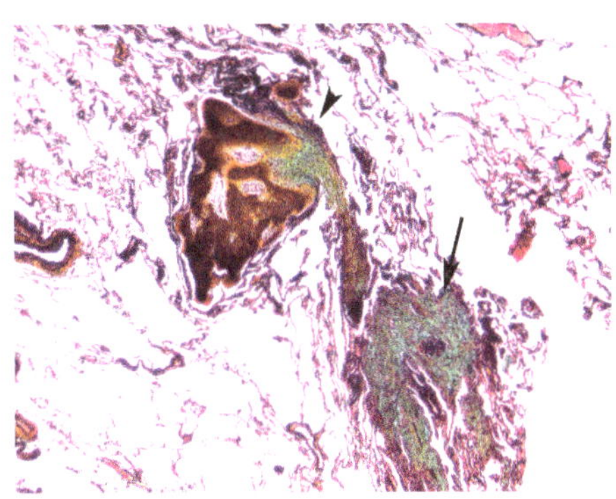

FIGURE 3: Areas of OP (arrow) with adjacent foci of cicatricial OP transitioning to DPO (arrowhead) (Movat stain; 20x).

Table 2: Differential diagnosis of pulmonary calcifications and ossifications.*

Calcifications	
Dystrophic: calcifications in diseased lung	(1) Infections: granulomatous infection such as histoplasmosis and tuberculosis and viral infections such as varicella (2) Granulomatous noninfectious disease: sarcoidosis (3) Occupational lung disease: silicosis, coal workers' pneumoconiosis (4) Metabolic lung diseases: amyloidosis, pulmonary alveolar microlithiasis
Metastatic: calcifications in normal lung	(1) Hypercalcemia in the setting of chronic renal failure, other causes of primary hyperparathyroidism, Paget's disease, parathyroid carcinoma or multiple myeloma
Calcified metastasis	(1) Metastases such as mucinous carcinoma, chondrosarcoma and synovial sarcoma
Ossifications	
NPO	In patients with chronic venous congestion such as long standing mitral stenosis
DPO	In patients with interstitial fibrosis
Bone forming neoplasms	Osteogenic sarcoma metastasis

*Modified from reference [8]. NPO: nodular pulmonary ossification, DPO: dendriform pulmonary ossification.

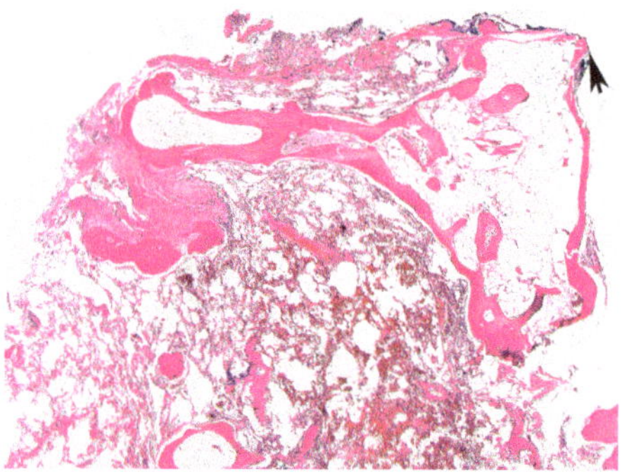

Figure 4: Focal areas of DPO in the subpleura with areas that appeared to extend through the pleura (arrow) (Hematoxylin and eosin; 40x).

more complicated tubular branching lamellar bone is seen, usually with marrow elements that can be seen in the alveolar space and expanding into alveolar septae [5]. DPO is commonly seen in the setting of chronic lung disease, UIP in particular [5, 6]. It has been described with cicatricial OP [4], and can be seen in isolation [7, 8].

DPO manifests on CT as small (several millimeters in diameter) nodules, which are seen predominantly in the peripheral interstitium (interlobular septa, subpleural and perifissural spaces). These nodules form contiguous and branching pattern resembling tree branches. In most instances these nodules are of high attenuation, reflecting the underlying ossification. The detection of small high-attenuation foci is improved using thin slices and maximum-intensity-projection images. DPO has tendency to affect lower lobes and posterior aspect of upper lobes. Association with recurrent aspiration and DPO has been suggested [7]. The presented patient had a history of GERD, which may be associated with recurrent episodes of aspiration. Pulmonary calcifications are commonly encountered on chest imaging and can be seen in several entities (Table 2) [8]. Distinction between pulmonary calcifications and ossification on imaging is not always possible. However, the distribution and the branching pattern are characteristic of DPO [7].

Spontaneous pneumothorax has been reported in several cases of DPO [9–14] including one case with cicatricial OP and DPO [4]. This case with cicatricial OP and DPO reported by Churg et al. [4] is likely the same case was reported by Tsai et al. [10]. In our case, foci of DPO were present in the subpleural areas, presumably causing recurrent pneumothoraces. It has been suggested that a subpleural sharp bony spicule may cause the pneumothorax by puncturing the visceral pleura [10, 13, 14]. None of the reported cases nor our case has other causes to explain the pneumothoraces, such as cystic or bullous lung disease, trauma, or bronchopleural fistula.

The case we present showed evidence of radiographic progression and worsening restrictive pattern on PFT over several years. The reported cases of cicatricial OP by Churg and his colleagues [4] have been suggested to be stable. However, almost half of those reported by Yousem [3] had persistent or progressive disease at a median of 110 months of follow-up. This may suggest that cicatricial OP is a spectrum and cases with minor conventional OP and predominant dense organization with fibrous bands and nodules may persist or even progress.

In summary, we present a case of cicatricial OP with DPO presenting with recurrent pneumothoraces and slow progressive pulmonary physiologic restrictive impairment. Cicatricial OP should be considered in the differential diagnosis of peribronchial or subpleural reticular opacities with DPO. Radiologists and clinicians alike should be aware of this newly described entity as distinct from other classical fibrosing processes, its potential association with DPO, and the presumed association between subpleural DPO and spontaneous pneumothorax.

Acknowledgments

(1) Respiratory Institute, Cleveland Clinic, Cleveland, Ohio; (2) Imaging Institute, Cleveland Clinic, Cleveland, Ohio; (3) Pathology and Laboratory Medicine Institute, Cleveland Clinic, Cleveland, Ohio.

References

[1] J. F. Cordier, V. Cottin, R. Lazor, and F. Thivolet-Bejui, "Many faces of bronchiolitis and organizing pneumonia," *Seminars in Respiratory and Critical Care Medicine*, vol. 37, no. 3, pp. 421–440, 2016.

[2] V. Cottin and J. F. Cordier, "Cryptogenic organizing pneumonia," *Seminars in Respiratory and Critical Care Medicine*, vol. 33, no. 5, pp. 462–475, 2012.

[3] S. A. Yousem, "Cicatricial variant of cryptogenic organizing pneumonia," *Human Pathology*, vol. 64, pp. 76–82, 2017.

[4] A. Churg, J. L. Wright, and A. Bilawich, "Cicatricial organising pneumonia mimicking a fibrosing interstitial pneumonia," *Histopathology*, vol. 72, no. 5, pp. 846–854, 2018.

[5] J. F. Lara, J. F. Catroppo, D. U. Kim, and D. da Costa, "Dendriform pulmonary ossification, a form of diffuse pulmonary ossification: report of a 26-year autopsy experience," *Archives of Pathology and Laboratory Medicine*, vol. 129, no. 3, pp. 348–353, 2005.

[6] T. S. Kim, J. Han, M. P. Chung, M. J. Chung, and Y. S. Choi, "Disseminated dendriform pulmonary ossification associated with usual interstitial pneumonia: incidence and thin-section CT-pathologic correlation," *European Radiology*, vol. 15, no. 8, pp. 1581–1585, 2005.

[7] J. F. Gruden, D. B. Green, A. C. Legasto, E. A. Jensen, and P. M. Panse, "Dendriform pulmonary ossification in the absence of usual interstitial pneumonia: CT features and possible association with recurrent acid aspiration," *AJR American Journal of Roentgenology*, vol. 209, no. 6, pp. 1209–1215, 2017.

[8] L. Jamjoom, M. Meziane, and R. D. Renapurkar, "Dendriform pulmonary ossification: report of two cases," *Indian Journal of Radiology and Imaging*, vol. 23, no. 1, pp. 15–18, 2013.

[9] H. Matsuo, T. Handa, M. Tsuchiya et al., "Progressive restrictive ventilatory impairment in idiopathic diffuse pulmonary ossification," *Internal Medicine*, vol. 57, no. 11, pp. 1631–1636, 2018.

[10] A. P. Tsai, J. C. English, D. Murphy, and D. D. Sin, "Recurrent pneumothorax related to diffuse dendriform pulmonary ossification in genetically predisposed individual," *Respirology Case Report*, vol. 5, no. 2, p. e00211, 2016, eCollection 2017 Mar.

[11] N. T. Harvey, S. Heraganhally, V. Au, D. Ellis, S. Klebe, and D. W. Henderson, "Idiopathic diffuse dendriform pulmonary ossification in a dental technician," *Pathology*, vol. 44, no. 4, pp. 363–365, 2012.

[12] A. Azuma, H. Miyamoto, T. Enomoto, J. Usuki, and S. Kudoh, "Familial clustering of dendriform pulmonary ossification," *Sarcoidosis Vasculitis and Diffuse Lung Disease*, vol. 20, no. 2, pp. 152–154, 2003.

[13] J. Abe, H. Oura, H. Niikawa, H. Yaegashi, and T. Kondo, "Dendriform pulmonary ossification: unusual cause of spontaneous pneumothorax," *Thorax*, vol. 69, no. 1, pp. 97–98, 2014.

[14] T. Kato, K. Ishikawa, M. Kadoya, K. Okamoto, and M. Kaji, "Spontaneous pneumothorax in a patient with dendriform pulmonary ossification: report of a case," *Surgery Today*, vol. 42, no. 9, pp. 903–908, 2012.

[15] L. M. Bouchardy, J. E. Kuhlman, W. C. Ball, R. H. Hruban, F. B. Askin, and S. S. Siegelman, "CT findings in bronchiolitis obliterans organizing pneumonia (BOOP) with radiographic, clinical and histologic correlation," *Journal of Computer Assisted Tomography*, vol. 17, no. 3, pp. 352–357, 1993.

[16] K. S. Lee, P. Kullnig, T. E. Hartman, and N. L. Müller, "Cryptogenic organizing pneumonia: CT findings in 43 patients," *American Journal of Roentgenology*, vol. 162, no. 3, pp. 543–546, 1994.

[17] N. L. Muller, C. A. Staples, and R. R. Miller, "Bronchiolitis obliterans orga-nizing pneumonia: CT features in 14 patients," *American Journal of Roentgenology*, vol. 154, no. 5, pp. 983–987, 1990.

[18] S. J. Kim, K. S. Lee, Y. H. Ryu et al., "Reversed halo sign on high-reso-lution CT of cryptogenic organizing pneumonia: diagnostic implications," *American Journal of Roentgenology*, vol. 180, no. 5, pp. 1251–1254, 2003.

[19] M. Ujita, E. A. Renzoni, S. Veeraraghavan, A. U. Wells, and D. M. Hansell, "Organizing pneumonia: perilobular pattern at thin-section CT," *Radiology*, vol. 232, no. 3, pp. 757–761, 2004.

[20] M. Zompatori, V. Poletti, G. Battista, and M. Diegoli, "Bronchiolitis obliterans with organizing pneumonia (BOOP), presenting as a ring-shaped opacity at HRCT (the atoll sign): a case report," *La Radiologia medica*, vol. 97, pp. 308–310, 1999.

[21] A. E. Voloudaki, D. E. Bouros, M. E. Froudarakis, G. E. Datseris, E. G. Apostolaki, and N. C. Gourtsoyiannis, "Crescentic and ring-shaped opacities: CT features in two cases of bronchiolitis obliterans organizing pneumonia (BOOP)," *Acta Radiologica*, vol. 37, no. 6, pp. 889–892, 1996.

[22] M. A. Spiteri, P. Klenerman, M. N. Sheppard, S. Padley, T. J. K. Clark, and A. Newman-Taylor, "Seasonal crypto-genic organising pneumonia with biochemical cholestasis: a new clinical entity," *The Lancet*, vol. 340, no. 8814, pp. 281–284, 1992.

[23] M. Akira, S. Yamamoto, and M. Sakatani, "Bronchiolitis obliterans organizing pneumonia manifesting as multiple large nodules or masses," *American Journal of Roentgenology*, vol. 170, no. 2, pp. 291–29, 1998.

[24] K. Woolley and P. Stark, "Pulmonary parenchymal manifestations of mitral valve disease," *Radiographics*, vol. 19, no. 4, pp. 965–972, 1999.

4

Solitary Pulmonary Nodule: A Diagnostic Dilemma

Pardeep Masuta [1] and Ioana Amzuta [2]

[1]*Pulmonary & Critical Care, SUNY Upstate Medical University, Syracuse, USA*
[2]*Assistant Professor of Medicine, Pulmonary & Critical Care, SUNY Upstate Medical University, Syracuse, USA*

Correspondence should be addressed to Pardeep Masuta; masutap@upstate.edu

Academic Editor: Shih-Yi Lee

This case describes a woman with a history of tobacco abuse who presented with a dry cough and was found to have an enlarging, 4 cm right upper lobe nodule without lymphadenopathy on CT imaging of the chest. Initial biopsies of the nodule suggested follicular lymphoma, but after obtaining more tissue, the pathology was negative for malignancy and instead showed necrotizing pneumonia. She proceeded to have negative infectious serology and cultures. She had negative rheumatological testing including MPO ANCA, PR-3 ANCA, and rheumatoid factor. She did not have renal failure, hemoptysis, weight loss, arthralgia, or upper airway inflammation. She ultimately underwent a right upper lobectomy, as the nodule was enlarging on repeat imaging. The pathology of the lung showed necrotizing granulomas with giant cells and fibrosis, but lacked active vasculitis or palisading histiocytes, further obscuring the diagnosis. She was conservatively managed with intranasal steroids, cough suppressants and antihistamines given her lack of severe symptoms. The diagnosis was most consistent with granulomatosis with polyangiitis (GPA) presenting as a solitary pulmonary nodule with pathology reflecting a mild degree of disease activity. The patient may manifest further signs of the disease while being monitored clinically.

1. Introduction

Granulomatosis with polyangiitis (GPA) is an inflammatory condition that causes a severe, systemic, necrotizing vasculitis. The most common manifestations include constitutional symptoms such as fevers, malaise, and weight loss; respiratory tract symptoms such as hemoptysis, epistaxis and pulmonary nodules; and progressive renal failure with hematuria. The initial presentation varies significantly between patients, and this can make the diagnosis particularly difficult as the symptoms can resemble other diseases such as eosinophilic granulomatosis with polyangiitis (EGPA), microscopic polyangiitis (MPA), infections, and malignancies.

2. Case Presentation

A 66-year-old female with a distant 15 pack year smoking history presented to the pulmonary clinic for evaluation of a 4 cm right upper lobe mass found on a CT thorax. She had a dry cough with occasional fatigue and night sweats that began about a year earlier. She denied recent travel, weight loss, hemoptysis, epistaxis, wheezing, joint pain, hematuria, peripheral edema, orthopnea, easy bruising or alopecia. Her vitals and physical exam were within normal limits on room air.

She had been treated as an outpatient for presumed community acquired pneumonia when her symptoms first began. Follow up chest X-ray showed a persistent opacity in the right upper lobe and a CT scan showed a large, spiculated 4 cm right upper lobe mass (Figure 1). It was hypermetabolic with an SUV of 19 on PET CT (Figure 2). Her pulmonary function tests revealed a moderate reduction in diffusion capacity without obstruction or restriction. Her FEV1/FVC ratio was 71%. FVC was 90% of predicted at 2.94 L. FEV1 was 83% of predicted at 2.08 L. Her TLC was 94% of predicted at 4.77 L and vital capacity was 90% of predicted at 2.94 L. Her DLCO was 54% of predicted at 12.8.

She underwent a bronchoscopy and EBUS guided needle aspiration of the mass. Pathology revealed a population of CD10 positive lymphocytes suggestive of follicular lymphoma.

A CT guided biopsy was performed to obtain additional tissue for histological and genetic testing. It surprisingly

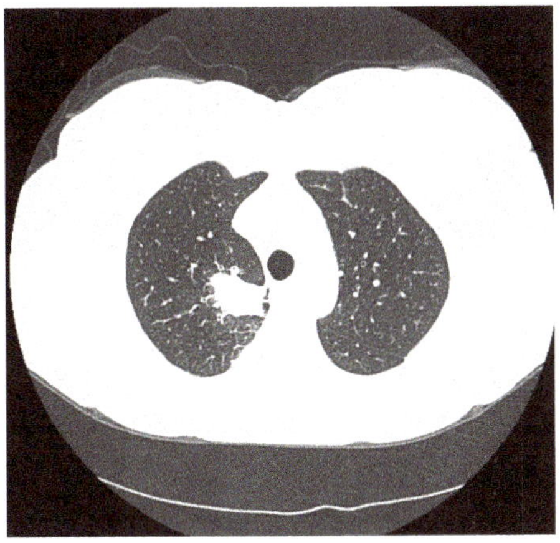

FIGURE 1: CT scan of the thorax showing a large right upper lobe spiculated nodule.

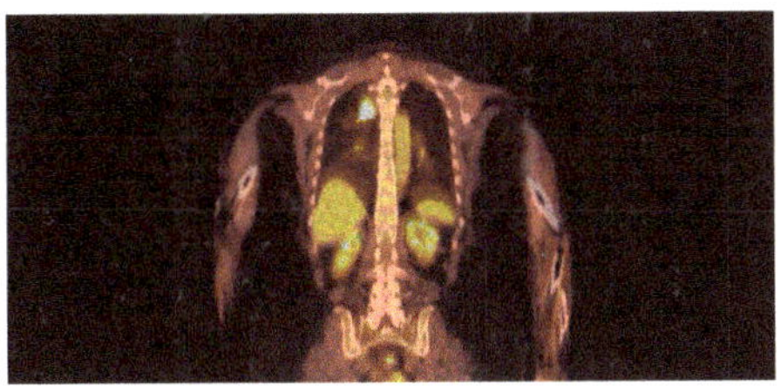

FIGURE 2: PET CT showing a hypermetabolic right upper lobe nodule.

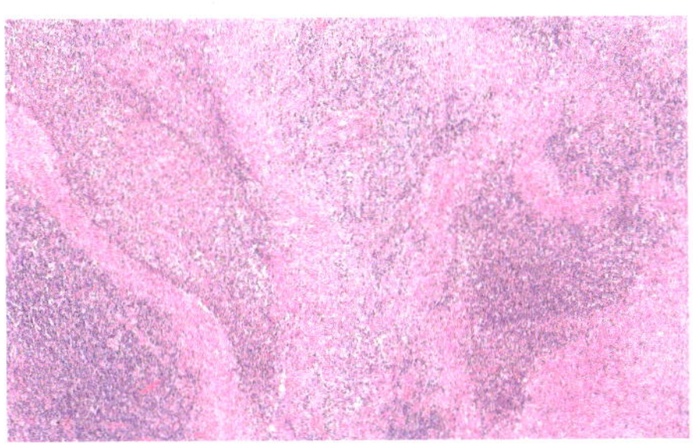

FIGURE 3: High power histopathology of lung showing necrotizing inflammation.

turned out to be negative for lymphoma but instead showed necrotizing pneumonia. There were areas of necrosis with surrounding fibrosis. Neoplastic cells were not identified (Figures 3 and 4). AFB cultures and fungal cultures were negative. Quantiferon, aspergillus galactomannan, histoplasma, blastomyces and coccidioides antibodies were also negative. ANCA serology including MPO (<9 u/mL) and PR3 (<3.5 u/mL) testing was negative. Rheumatoid factor, C3 and C4 were also negative. Her ANA speckled pattern was 250. Her urinalysis had 3+ protein with a normal protein/creatinine ratio. There were no casts. Her BMP and CBC were within normal limits without eosinophilia.

The patient's cough persisted despite conservative treatment with intranasal steroids, cough suppression, and antihistamines. ENT evaluation with nasopharyngolaryngoscopy (NPL) did not reveal upper airway inflammation or ulceration.

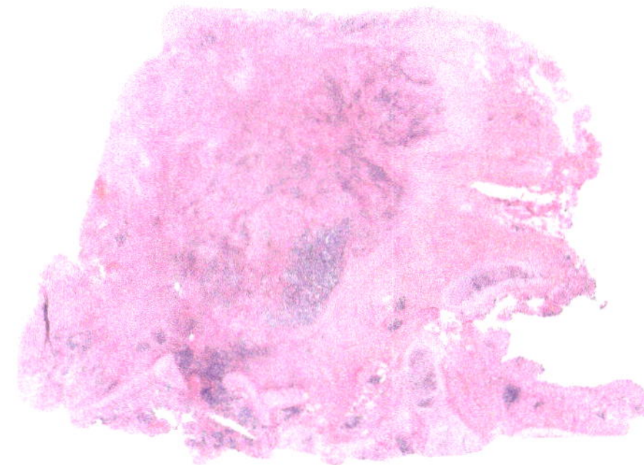

FIGURE 4: Low power histopathology of lung showing necrotizing inflammation.

A repeat CT scan of the thorax showed that the mass was enlarging.

A video assisted thoracoscopy (VAT) with right upper lobectomy was performed. It revealed a right upper lung mass with multiple adhesions to the pleura. The pathology revealed necrotizing granulomas with eosinophils and giant cells. There were no malignant cells, active vasculitis, or organisms found.

The favored diagnosis was granulomatosis with polyangiitis (GPA).

3. Discussion

Granulomatosis with polyangiitis is often associated with a positive cytoplasmic ANCA and manifests with constitutional symptoms, upper/lower respiratory tract symptoms, and renal symptoms [1–5].

Diagnosis can be difficult as the spectrum of disease varies greatly between people. Without treatment, the disease can cause multi-organ destruction. Patients can have fever, myalgia, and weight loss for months without signs of organ involvement [1]. Upper airway symptoms such as epistaxis, recurrent sinusitis, or saddle-nose deformity can be helpful to differentiate it from other forms of vasculitis such as microscopic polyangiitis (MPA) [1–3]. Up to 90 percent of patients with GPA have some form of upper respiratory involvement compared with 35 percent of those with MPA [4]. 25 percent of patients can have pulmonary involvement which can cause cough, stridor, wheezing, or hemoptysis from alveolar hemorrhage. Renal involvement is common in GPA, presenting as hematuria and progressive renal failure. Active glomerulonephritis is usually demonstrated in up to 85 percent of patients within the first two years of disease onset [5]. Diagnosis is achieved by demonstrating this constellation of symptoms along with imaging, immunological, and histological findings.

ANCA testing should be performed on any adult patient presenting with symptoms suspicious for vasculitis, but the absence of ANCA does not exclude the diagnosis of GPA. Approximately 90 percent of patients with GPA or MPA are ANCA positive [6]. PR3-ANCA is positive in 80–90 percent of GPA patients with the remainder being MPO-ANCA. The disease activity can correlate with the degree of positivity of PR3-ANCA at the time of sampling. Less than 10% of patients with active, generalized GPA will have negative ANCA titers. In respiratory limited subsets, up to 40 percent of patients may be ANCA negative while up to 80 percent of patients with renal-limited vasculitis are actually positive for MPO-ANCA [6–8].

A hypermetabolic, solitary, and spiculated nodule can be malignant (e.g., adenocarcinoma, small cell carcinoma or metastatic), infectious (e.g., tuberculosis, histoplasmosis or cryptococcosis), or inflammatory in nature. Common causes of inflammatory nodules include sarcoidosis, rheumatoid nodules and vasculitides such as GPA.

Sarcoidosis is a common inflammatory condition that usually affects young and middle aged patients between 20 and 40. It can involve multiple organ systems, but affects the lungs in 90% of cases. It most commonly presents with mediastinal lymphadenopathy and bilateral reticular opacities on chest X-ray imaging. Nodular sarcoid is a rare pulmonary manifestation of sarcoidosis. Sarcoid nodules usually present as bilateral, multiple opacities occupying the perihilar or peripheral lung zones on a chest CT. These lesions may be accompanied by mediastinal lymphadenopathy and galaxy sign (small satellite nodules that border the periphery of larger nodules) [3]. This patient did not have significant lymphadenopathy, systemic symptoms, or other pulmonary nodules.

Rheumatoid nodules are one of the most common pulmonary manifestations of rheumatoid arthritis [9]. They usually do not cause pulmonary symptoms despite being about 1–3 cm in size. They can cavitate on very rare occasions. During that time, they may be prone to becoming infected, increasing the risk for pneumonia and lung abscesses. Other common pulmonary manifestations of rheumatoid arthritis include interstitial lung disease and pleural disease. These patients can have other symptoms of rheumatoid arthritis such as peripheral polyarthritis and joint destruction. Treatment includes controlling the underlying rheumatoid arthritis with NSAIDS and immunomodulatory therapy [9, 10].

Although the most common imaging abnormality in patients with GPA is multiple, bilateral pulmonary nodules, there is significant variability [6, 11–13]. Findings include bronchial wall thickening, effusions, consolidations, and ground glass opacities [11–13]. These can be localized or diffused; with or without adenopathy. Nodules can vary anywhere from 3 mm to over 30 mm and from solid to cavitating. These are often hypermetabolic on 18F-fluorodeoxyglucose PET/CT, making it difficult to differentiate between malignancy, pneumonia or noninfectious inflammatory conditions [6, 12, 13].

The diagnosis of GPA should be confirmed by a biopsy of the suspected site of active disease whenever possible. The most commonly affected sites are the kidneys followed by the lungs. The usual findings in either site are necrotizing granulomatosis, seen as foci of necrosis and granulomas with palisading histiocytes (with the long axis perpendicular to the necrotic center) and vasculitis [7, 11, 14, 15]. Renal biopsy findings usually parallel the severity of the patient's disease on clinical presentation [7, 8]. Findings can show mild focal and segmental glomerulonephritis in patients with asymptomatic hematuria to diffuse, crescentic glomerulonephritis and necrosis in patients with renal failure. Arteritis and granulomas are occasionally seen [7, 8]. This patient had very mild symptoms and did not have any signs of renal failure; therefore, a renal biopsy was not performed. The pulmonary lesions in GPA are usually firm, hemorrhagic, yellowish-gray nodules with an average size of 2.4 cm on gross inspection [8, 15]. There may be central necrosis which is noncaseating and friable. Transmural infiltration of blood vessels with inflammatory cells can be noted on microscopy. In patients presenting with alveolar hemorrhage, pulmonary capillaritis is a key finding [15]. The most abundant infiltrating inflammatory cells include neutrophils, lymphocytes, and multinucleated giant cells. There may be occasional eosinophil infiltration seen, but it is usually without peripheral eosinophilia. Small areas of organizing pneumonia with microabscesses could also be noted [15]. Negative stains and cultures are needed to rule out infectious etiologies such as tuberculosis or histoplasmosis.

The lack of classical symptoms, negative ANCA serology, and no active vasculitis on histology complicated the diagnosis in this patient. This likely represented a mild degree of disease activity; evidenced by her relative lack of extrapulmonary symptoms [11]. She may develop further signs of the disease going forward. This patient demonstrates a rare case of GPA manifesting as a solitary pulmonary nodule and the importance of maintaining a broad differential based on clinical and imaging findings for this potentially life threatening disease.

References

[1] C. Comarmond and P. Cacoub, "Granulomatosis with polyangiitis (Wegener): clinical aspects and treatment," *Autoimmunity Reviews*, vol. 13, no. 11, pp. 1121–1125, 2014.

[2] C. Jean-François, D. Valeyre, L. Guillevin, R. Loire, and B. Jeanne-Marie, *Pulmonary Wegener's Granulomatosis. CHEST*, vol. 97, no. 4, pp. 906–912, 1990.

[3] J. Mostafa, D. Farrokh, and N. Mohammadpanah, "Multiple bilateral pulmonary nodules masquerading as pulmonary metastasis; a case of nodular sarcoidosis," *Electronic Physician*, vol. 8, no. 8, pp. 2802–2806, 2016.

[4] P. Seo and J. H. Stone, "The antineutrophil cytoplasmic antibody-associated vasculitides," *The American Journal of Medicine*, vol. 117, p. 39, 2004.

[5] G. S. Hoffman, G. S. Kerr, R. Y. Leavitt et al., "Wegener granulomatosis: an analysis of 158 patients," *Annals of Internal Medicine*, vol. 116, no. 6, pp. 488–498, 1992.

[6] G. S. Hoffman and U. Specks, "Antineutrophil cytoplasmic antibodies," *Arthritis Rheumatology*, vol. 41, no. 9, pp. 1521–1537, 1998.

[7] P. M. K. Lutalo and D. P. D'Cruz, "Diagnosis and classification of granulomatosis with polyangiitis (aka Wegener's granulomatosis)," *Journal of Autoimmunity*, vol. 48–49, pp. 94–98, 2014.

[8] C. O. Savage, C. G. Winearls, D. J. Evans, A. J. Rees, and C. M. Lockwood, "Microscopic polyarteritis: presentation, pathology and prognosis," *An International Journal of Medicine*, vol. 56, no. 467, 1985.

[9] B. Russell, S. Mohan, R. Chahal, S. Carette, and C. Pagnoux, "Prognostic significance of cavitary lung nodules in granulomatosis with polyangiitis (Wegener's): a clinical imaging

study of 225 patients," *Arthritis Care & Research*, vol. 70, no. 7, pp. 1082–1089, 2018.

[10] T. E. King Jr., E. J. Kim, and B. W. Kinder, "Connective tissue diseases," in *Interstitial Lung Disease*, M. I. Schwarz and T. E. King Jr., Eds., 689 pages, People's Medical Publishing House-USA, Shelton, CT, 5th edition, 2011.

[11] E. J. Mark, D. B. Flieder, and O. Matsubara, "Treated Wegener's granulomatosis: distinctive pathological findings in the lungs of 20 patients and what they tell us about the natural history of the disease," *Human Pathology*, vol. 28, no. 4, pp. 450–458, 1997.

[12] G. Luis, O. de la Ajuria-Illarramendi, C. Puente-Bujidos et al., "PET/CT findings of granulomatosis with polyangiitis presenting as a solitary pulmonary nodule and mimicking lung cancer," *Journal of Clinical Rheumatology*, 2019.

[13] K. Lee, T. Kim, K. Fujimoto et al., "Thoracic manifestation of Wegener's granulomatosis: CT findings in 30 patients," *European Radiology*, vol. 13, no. 1, pp. 43–51, 2003.

[14] A. Masiak, Z. Zdrojewski, R. Pęksa et al., "The usefulness of histopathological examinations of nonrenal biopsies in the diagnosis of granulomatosis with polyangiitis," *Reumatologia*, vol. 55, no. 5, pp. 230–236, 2017.

[15] S. A. Yousem, "Wegener's granulomatosis," in *Thurlbeck's Pathology of the Lung*, A. M. Churg, J. L. Myers, H. D. Tazelaar, and J. L. Wright, Eds., p. 371, Thieme, New York, 3rd edition, 2005.

5

Sputum Smear Positive Pulmonary Tuberculosis Diagnostic Dropout Rate in Public Health Facilities, Addis Ababa, Ethiopia

Daniel Melese Desalegn,[1,2] Kumera Terfa Kitila,[1,2] Boja Dufera Taddese,[1,2] Tinsae Kidanemariam Hailu,[2] Tariku Takle Dinku,[1,2] Kassahun Demisse Asferie,[1,2] Hanna Mekonnen Balcha,[1,2] Chalachew Sisay Gebeyehu,[1,2] and Girmay Medhin[3]

[1]*Ethiopian Public Health Institute (EPHI), Addis Ababa, Ethiopia*
[2]*Addis Ababa Public Health Research and Emergency Management Core Process, Addis Ababa City Administration Health Bureau, Addis Ababa, Ethiopia*
[3]*Aklilu Lemma Institute of Pathobiology Addis Ababa University, Addis Ababa, Ethiopia*

Correspondence should be addressed to Daniel Melese Desalegn; danimelese2013@gmail.com

Academic Editor: Kazuyoshi Kuwano

Background. Prolonged laboratory diagnostic process of tuberculosis can lead to failure to complete the diagnosis and increase dropout rate of smear positive pulmonary tuberculosis (PTB) cases. This implies such dropout patients without completing diagnosis are critical as infected individuals remain untreated in the community, providing more opportunities for transmission of the disease and adversely affecting the epidemic. The aim of this research is to determine the level of smear positive PTB diagnosis dropout rate of spot-morning-spot sputum microscopy diagnosis method in public health facilities, in Addis Ababa, Ethiopia. *Methods.* Retrospective review of patient documents in 13 public health facilities' TB laboratory in Addis Ababa was conducted from October 2011 to March 2016. Data was computerized using Epi-info software and analysed using SPSS version 20.0 software. Descriptive numerical summaries were used to present the findings. Association between the dropout rate and demographic variables was assessed by Chi-square (X^2). Bivariate model using Odds Ratio (OR) with a 95% Confidence Interval (CI) was calculated. P-Value less than 0.05 was taken as statistically significant. *Results.* Of 41,884 presumptive TB patients registered during the 53 months for laboratory investigation, 5.9% were positive for the first spot sputum smear microscopy. Among these positive cases, 142 (5.8%) and 298 (12.1%) did not come back to the laboratory to submitted early morning and second spot sputum specimens, respectively. The diagnostic dropout for morning sputum specimen in hospitals was 5.6% (58/1039) and in health centres was 5.9% (84/1424). However, higher proportion of dropout for second spot sputum specimen in hospitals was 16.4% (170/1039), compared to the health centres, 8.9% (128/1424). Diagnostic dropout of sputum smear microscopy had no significant association with sociodemographic variable (P value >0.05), while it had significant association with facility type (P value <0.05). *Conclusion.* In this study smear positive pulmonary tuberculosis diagnostic dropout rate was high compared to WHO reported for the new strategy shift implying the importance of shifting to same-day approach. Hence, shifting from conventional to same day is crucial to minimize the TB diagnostic dropout rate in the study area and other similar settings. Further research is needed/recommended in the local setting to compare the yield and dropout rates between same-day and conventional sputum smear microscopy approach.

1. Background

Sputum smear microscopy diagnosis is one of the key pillars of strategies for tuberculosis control. Unfortunately, the smear positivity depends on time of sputum collection, the number specimens to be examined, and the load of bacilli in specimen [1]. As a result, TB control program recommended spot-morning-spot (SMS) to increase the positivity yields of sputum smears examine. However, it may be costly and inconvenient for patients who have to make multiple visits to health facilities to submit three sputum specimens over several days [2–4]. This approach can prolong the diagnostic process of TB suspected individuals, which may lead to dropout of TB patients from diagnostic paths [1].

Smear positive PTB diagnostic dropout cases are more common in TB prevalent setting. Studies conducted in Africa at different setting showing 6 to 38% TB cases failed (dropped out) from diagnostic pathway (loss to follow-up during diagnostic period) [2]. Systematic review and meta-analysis has shown that patients assigned to same-day diagnosis were more likely to submit both specimens (dropout= 2%) than patients screened conventionally (dropout=5.8%) [4]. Hence, to minimize the dropout, WHO has recently recommended a reduction in the number of specimens examined from three to two in settings with appropriate external quality assurance systems of smear microscopy being in place and good-quality microscopy results have been documented [4, 5]. Operational research is needed to ensure the quality assurance based on the country-specific evidence in terms of accuracy, diagnostic dropout rate, and external quality assurance systems of smear microscopy before switching to same-day diagnosis. However, the strength of quality assurance system is questionable and TB diagnostic dropout is unknown in our setting. Therefore, this study was designed to determine the level of smear positive PTB diagnostic dropout rate of spot-morning-spot (SMS) sputum microscopy diagnosing method in public health facilities in Addis Ababa, Ethiopia, with the potential to generalize the findings to the whole country and beyond.

2. Methods

2.1. Study Design and Setting. Retrospective patient record review was conducted in Addis Ababa city covering the period from October 2011 to March 2016. Addis Ababa city Administration has a population of 3,384,569, with annual growth rate of 3.8% [6]. Health care facility expansion has improved physical access to health services with an emphasis on primary health care units, resulting in potential health service coverage of Addis Ababa to an estimated 100%. The city has 47 hospitals, 204 higher, 226 medium, 143 lower private clinics, and 100 public health centres [7]. Regarding TB diagnostic services, at the time of this assessment, all private hospitals, higher clinics, and all public health facilities were providing TB diagnostic and treatment services.

2.2. Study Subjects. Thirteen health facilities' laboratories (10 health centres and 3 hospital laboratories) providing tuberculosis diagnostic and treatment service and those which have records of Ziehl-Neelsen (ZN) stained smear microscopy resulting from October 2011 to March 2016 were included in the current study. Individual patients data documented in the TB record book of these laboratories were used as study subjects.

2.3. Data Sources and Sampling. Health institutions were selected using simple random sampling with the plan of obtaining three hospitals from six public hospitals and ten health centres (one from each subcity). The health facilities' sputum smear microscopy records, from a period of 2011 to 2016, were used as data source. Status of the record was assessed during reviews of records.

2.4. Inclusion and Exclusion Criteria. All PTB cases having complete records in the laboratory, from the years 2011 to 2016, were included. However, follow-up case, any form of TB other than PTB, TB laboratory results performed by other than ZN technique, and incomplete records were excluded from analysis.

2.5. Data Management and Statistical Analysis. The collected data were checked for completeness and consistency and computerized using Epi-info software. The data were coded and analysed using SPSS version 20.0 (SPSS Inc., Chicago, USA) software. Descriptive numerical summaries were used to present the findings of sociodemographic characteristics and trends of pulmonary tuberculosis diagnostic dropout rate. Association between the dropout rate and demographic variables was assessed by Chi-square (X^2). Bivariate model using Odds Ratio (OR) with a 95% Confidence Interval (CI) was calculated after excluding missing data to identify factors associated with the smear positive PTB diagnostic dropout rate. P-value less than 0.05 was taken as statistically significant.

2.6. Data Quality Assurances. Before extracting data from records, data collectors were adequately trained and they were instructed to check the completeness of each data before submission. Quality of data collection process was supervised and monitored by the principal investigator.

2.7. Operational Definition. Diagnosis dropout: it is defined as the patient does not turn back to submit the morning and/or the second spot sputum specimens, while their first sputum examination is positive.

Conventional (two-day) sputum microscopy diagnostic approach: TB suspect patient to give three sputum specimens (SMS) within two consecutive days to diagnosis TB.

Same-day sputum microscopy diagnostic approach: a new sputum microscopy diagnosis algorithm requires a TB suspect patient to give two sputum specimens (SS) within the same day to diagnosis TB.

3. Result

3.1. Sociodemographic Characteristics. During the target period 41,884 presumptive TB patients were registered for sputum smear microscopy examination in the study health facilities. Among these patients 2,463 were positive for the first spot sputum samples. Of these first spot positive TB cases, 1,291(52.4%) were males, 70(2.8%) were below the age of 15 years, and 594(24.1%) were above 35 years. Records were incomplete for 194(7.8%) on patients age and 95(3.9%) on patient sex [Table 1].

3.2. Diagnostic Dropout Rate of Smear Positive PTB. Of 41,884 presumptive TB cases recorded in the laboratory registration book in the period from the year 2011-2016, 2,463(5.9%) were

TABLE 1: Socio demographic characteristics of Smears positive PTB diagnostic dropout rate at public health facilities in Addis Ababa, Ethiopia, from 2011-2016.

Variables		Number	Percent
Age group in year	<15	70	2.8
	15-18	170	6.9
	19-35	1435	58.3
	36-55	456	18.5
	>55 y	138	5.6
	Data missing	194	7.9
	Total	*2463*	*100*
Sex	Male	1291	52.4
	Female	1077	43.7
	Data missing	95	3.9
	Total	*2463*	*100*

smear positive for the first spot sputum samples. Among 2,463 first spot smear positive TB cases, 142 (5.8%) and 298(12.1%) did not get back (dropout) to submit morning and second spot sputum specimen, respectively. Overall sputum smear positive diagnosis dropout rate was 17.9% (440/2463); no patients had dropped out for both sputum (the morning and the second pot). The diagnostic dropout rate for morning sputum positive specimen in hospitals was 5.6% (58/1,039) and in health centres was 5.9% (84/1,424). However, higher proportion of dropout rate for second spot sputum positive specimen in hospitals was 16.4% (170/1,039) compared to the health centres, 9.0% (128/1,424). Percentage dropout for morning positive specimen was 5.7% (4/70) in the younger age group (i.e., below the age of 15 years) and 5.6% (33/594) in the older age group (i.e., above 35 years of age). Similarly, percentage dropout for second spot positive specimen was 7.1% (5/70) in the younger age group and 12.8% (76/594) in the older age group. Diagnostic dropout rate for morning positive specimen was 72/1,291(5.6%) among males and 60/1,077(5.6%) among females. The dropout rate for second spot positive specimen was 154/1,291(11.9%) among males and 126/1,077(11.7%) among females [Table 2].

3.3. Trends of Diagnostic Dropout Rate of Smear Positive PTB. Among 142 TB diagnostic dropouts for morning specimen, 31/540(5.7%), 35/491(7.1%), 24/440(5.4%), 26/434(6.0%), 17/348(4.9%), and 9/210(4.3%) were in the years 2011, 2012, 2013, 2014, 2015, and 2016, respectively. Whereas among 298 TB diagnostic dropouts for second spot, 73/540(13.5%), 66/491(13.4%), 45/440(10.2%), 59/434(13.6%), 37/348(9.6%), and 18/210(8.6%) were in the years 2011, 2012, 2013, 2014, 2015, and 2016, respectively [Figure 1].

In mono-variate analysis, the trends of diagnostic dropout of sputum smear microscopy had no significant changes among the years from 2011 to 2016 (P value >0.05), even though the number of patients diagnostic dropout becomes slightly decreasing to the year 2016 (Table 3).

3.4. Factors Affecting Sputum Smear Positive PTB Diagnostic Dropout. In this study diagnostic dropout of sputum smear microscopy had no statistically significant association with sociodemographic variables (P value >0.05), while diagnostic dropout had significant association with facility type (P value < 0.05) (Table 4).

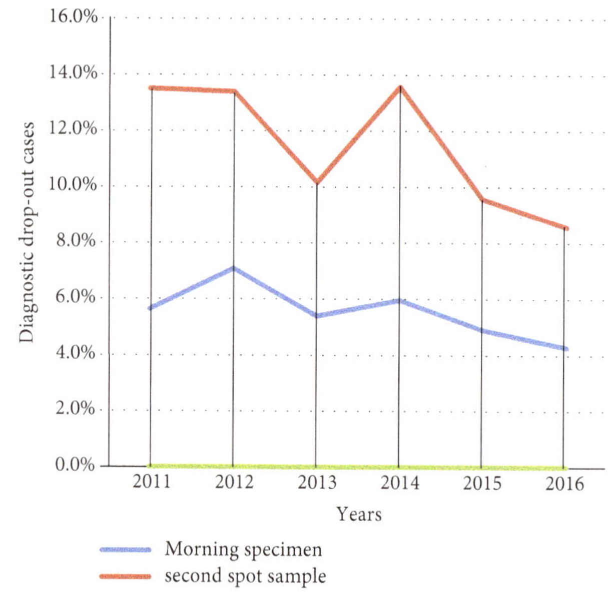

FIGURE 1: Trends of sputum smears positive pulmonary tuberculosis diagnostic dropout rate from 2011-2016.

4. Discussion

From the total presumptive TB cases registered for sputum smear microscopy diagnosis, the positivity rate for first spot specimens was 5.9%. Among these first spot positive cases, 17.9% did not come back to the laboratory to submit second and/or third specimens on the next day visit. The diagnostic dropout rate in Addis Ababa was higher than the number that WHO reported. The higher dropout rate was associated with the second sputum spot collection and related to hospital services in comparison to health centres. The diagnostic dropout rate was increased by ages but not significantly.

In the current study smear positivity rate was lower than the previous report of 14.2% in Metehara Sugar Factory Hospital, 9.2% in South East Ethiopia, and 10.4% in North Gondar Zone [8–10]. However, it was comparable to the 6.1% reported previously in Mwanza, Tanzania [11]. Similar studies indicated that sputum positivity rate depended on different factors including patients' factors, sputum sample quality, and laboratory diagnostic capacity [12, 13]. Improving TB diagnostic capacity, staining quality, sample collection, and adherence to the national TB laboratory standards is crucial to increase smear positivity [12, 13].

Diagnostic dropout rate for second spot sputum specimen in the current study was higher than 5.8% reported by WHO for new strategy shift, 5% reported in Pakistan, and 10.2% reported in Botswana [4, 14, 15]. It was comparable to the finding of 13% reported in Chennai of India [16]. It was lower than studies which reported 52.0% in South Africa, 37.6% in Lilongwe of Malawi, and 38.0% in Ghana [17–19].

TABLE 2: Mono-variate analysis the association between dropout rate and age, sex, health facility and period of registration of sputum smear positive PTB at public health facilities in Addis Ababa, Ethiopia, from 2011-2016.

Independent variables	First sputum AFB positive	Not submit the morning spot(a)				Not submit the 2nd spot (b)				Not submit the morning or the 2nd spots (a+b)				p -values
		n	%	OR	95%CI	n	%	OR	95%CI	n	%	OR	95%CI	
Total	*2463*	*142*	*5.8%*			*298*	*12.1%*			*440*	*17.9%*			
Age in year														
< 15yr.	70	4	5.7%	1.03	0.35-3.00	5	7.1%	0.52	0.20-1.34	9	12.9%	0.66	0.32-1.36	0.236
15 - 35yr.	1605	90	5.6%	1.01	0.69-1.49	182	11.3%	0.87	0.65-1.16	272	16.9%	0.91	0.71-1.16	
> 35yr.	594	33	5.6%	1		76	12.8%	1		109	18.4%	1		
Missing	194	15	7.7%			35	18.0%			50	25.8%			
Sex														
Male	1291	72	5.6%	1		154	11.9%	1		226	17.5%	1		
Female	1077	60	5.6%	1	0.7-1.42	126	11.7%	0.98	0.76-1.26	186	17.3%	0.98	0.79-1.22	
Missing	95	10	10.5%			18	18.9%			28	29.5%			
Health facilities														
Hospital	1039	58	5.6%	0.94	0.62-1.33	170	16.4%	1.98	1.55-2.53	228	21.9%	1.61	1.31-1.98	<0.001*
Health Center	1424	84	5.9%	1		128	9.0%	1		212	14.9%	1		
Year of sputum submission														
2011	540	31	5.7%	1		73	13.5%	1		104	19.3%	1		
2012	491	25	7.1%	1.26	0.76-2.08	66	13.4%	0.99	0.69-1.42	101	20.6%	1.09	0.80-1.47	
2013	440	24	5.5%	0.95	0.55-1.64	45	10.2%	0.73	0.49-1.08	69	15.7%	0.78	0.56-1.09	
2014	434	26	6.0%	1.05	0.61-1.79	59	13.6%	1.01	0.70-1.46	85	19.6%	1.02	0.74-1.41	0. 362
2015	348	17	4.9%	0.84	0.46-1.55	37	10.6%	0.80	0.50-1.09	54	15.5%	0.79	0.57-1.09	
2016	210	9	4.3%	0.73	0.34-1.57	18	8.6%	0.81	0.51-1.09	27	12.9%	0.83	0.61-1.31	

Key: * statistically significant, *P<0.00.*

TABLE 3: Mono-variate analysis the association between dropout and registration of sputum submission period at public health facilities in Addis Ababa, Ethiopia, from 2011-2016.

Independent variables	First AFB positive	Not submit the morning spot(a)				Not submit the 2nd spot (b)				Not submit the morning or the 2nd spots (a+b)				p -value
		n	%	OR	95%CI	n	%	OR	95%CI	n	%	OR	95%CI	
Total	*2463*	*142*	*5.8%*			*298*	*12.1%*			*440*	*17.9%*			
Year of sputum submission														
2011-2013	1471	90	6.1%	1		184	12.5%	1		274	18.6%	1		0.229
2014-2016	992	52	5.2%	0.85	0.61-1.21	59	5.9%	0.91	0.71-1.17	166	11.2%	0.88	0.71-1.09	

The difference might be due to health-system-related factors including delays in getting the results of sputum smears microscopy diagnosis and tracing mechanism of dropout cases. Patient related factors including understanding the nature of the disease, its severity, and potential benefits of early diagnosis and treatment initiation might vary among different countries. In addition, the way health workers treat patients (handling systems) might be as factors for TB diagnostic dropout. This clearly indicates that, besides shifting from conventional to same-day TB diagnostic approach, there is need to work on different factors to minimize diagnostic dropout rate in the study area and others similar setting.

In this study diagnostic dropout rate for second spot sputum specimen in hospital was high as compared to the health centres. Studies conducted in Botswana and South Africa have also reported high dropout rate in hospital [15, 20]. The possible reasons for this can be that customers might perceive that hospital has better services which might cause additional workload in hospitals, resulting in long waiting time, delays in receiving results, and patients' dissatisfaction which might contribute to increasing dropout in hospital. In

Table 4: Determinants on sputum smears positive pulmonary tuberculosis diagnostic dropout rate in public health facilities, in Addis Ababa, Ethiopia; from 2011 to 2016.

Variables	Drop out of diagnostic			Crude Odds		P-value
	Yes	No	%Yes	Ratio	95%CI	
Age groups (years)						
<15	9	61	12.9%	1		
15-35	272	1333	16.9%	1.32	0.71-2.45	0.380
35+	109	485	18.4%	1.43	0.76-2.69	0.258
Sex						
Male	226	1065	17.5%	1		
Female	186	891	17.3%	0.99	0.83-1.18	0.881
Facilities						
Hospital	228	811	21.9%	1		
Health Center	212	1212	14.9%	0.62	0.51-0.77	<0.001*

*Statistically high significant, P<0.005.

addition, accessibility of health centres might contribute to the difference. The health centres coverage in Addis Ababa is near 100% and easily accessible and does not incur much cost for patients to summit second and third specimens on the next day visit, which might reduce dropout in health centres.

In this study diagnostic dropout rate in the age ranges of 15-35 years was lower than 39.2% reported from Vietnam among age group of 15–34 years [21]. The diagnostic dropout rate for second spot specimen among male was lower compared to the study which reported 70.5% in Vietnam [21]. In this study diagnostic dropout rate was higher among males compared to females. Study of Vietnam and South India also reported high drop out among male than female [21, 22]. These findings point toward the need to further study age and sex differences in TB diagnostic dropout rate in order to inform age and sex specific diagnostic defaulter prevention.

5. Strengths and Limitations of the Study

This is a study based on a very large size retrospective patient's record review to determine the conventional sputum smears microscopy diagnostic dropout rate. The result may be used as an input for the national TB control program by providing reliable and accurate conclusions implying the importance of shifting to same-day approach. However, the findings are not without limitations. Results are dependent only on the record review, despite some demography data which was incomplete in the laboratory log books. In addition this study was conducted only in public health facilities and hence does not necessarily illustrate the situation in private health situations.

6. Conclusion and Recommendations

In this study smears positive PTB diagnostic dropout rate of conventional sputum microscopy was highly compared to WHO reported for the new strategy shift implying the importance of shifting to same-day approach. The results from this investigation reinforce the importance that patients should promptly seek the appropriate medical attention following onset of TB symptoms. This study indicated that a high number of presumptive TB cases failed to submit morning and second spot specimen for laboratory investigation; as a result, a high number of active TB cases were untreated and might be potential source of TB transmission to the community, resulting in potential TB transmission to their close contacts, including those caring for the sick person at the later stages of the disease and with the ever increasing threat of MDR and XDR-TB as well as HIV. Hence, shifting from conventional to same-day sputum microscopy is crucial to minimize the TB diagnostic dropout rate in the study area and others similar setting. Research is needed in the local setting to compare the yield and dropout rates between same-day and conventional sputum smear microscopy approach.

Abbreviations

AFB: Acid Fast Bacillus (or Bacilli)
EQA: External quality assessment
SMS: Spot-morning-spot
TB: Tuberculosis
PTB: Pulmonary tuberculosis
WHO: World Health Organization
ZN: Ziehl-Neelsen stain.

Authors' Contributions

Daniel Melese Desalegn designed the study, developed the proposal, and led data collection, analysis, and writing up the result. Kumera Terfa Kitila and Girmay Medhin critically review and made progressive suggestions from the design to final writing up of the result. All of the authors were participated in data collection, analysis, and interpretation critically evaluated and approved the manuscript.

Acknowledgments

The authors would like to thank Addis Ababa City Administration Health Bureau and respective health facilities for their cooperation. Our thanks also extend to data collectors and supervisors for their cooperation during the study period.

References

[1] S. Rao, "Sputum smear microscopy in DOTS: are three samples necessary? An analysis and its implications in tuberculosis control," *Lung India*, vol. 26, no. 1, pp. 3-4, 2009.

[2] P. MacPherson, R. M. G. J. Houben, J. R. Glynn, E. L. Corbett, and K. Kranzer, "Pre-treatment loss to follow-up in tuberculosis patients in low- and lower-middle-income countries and high-burden countries: a systematic review and meta-analysis," *Bulletin of the World Health Organization*, vol. 92, no. 2, pp. 126–138, 2014.

[3] N. Neharkar and A. Nagaokar, "Health profile of DOTS-registered tuberculosis cases in a tertiary care hospital," *International Journal of Medical Science and Public Health*, vol. 4, no. 7, p. 910, 2015.

[4] World Health Organization, "Same-day diagnosis of tuberculosis by microscopy. Policy statement," WHO/HTM/TB/2011, 2011, http://whqlibdoc.who.int/publications/2011/9789241501606_eng.pdf.

[5] WHO, "Proposed reduction of number of smears for the diagnosis of pulmonary TB. Background document," Geneva, Switzerland, 2007, http://www.who.int/tb/laboratory/reduction_of_smears.pdf.

[6] Central statistical agency of Ethiopia (CSA), "Summary and Statistical Report of the 2007 Population and Housing Census Results," Addis Ababa, Ethiopia, 2008, http://www.ethiopianreview.com/pdf/001/Cen 2007.

[7] Addis Ababa Health bureau, "Operational manual for regional HIV/AIDS care and treatment catchment team activities," Addis Ababa, Ethiopia, 2011.

[8] A. Yohanes, S. Abera, and S. Ali, "Smear positive pulmonary tuberculosis among suspected patients attending metehara sugar factory hospital; eastern Ethiopia," *African Health Sciences*, vol. 12, no. 3, pp. 325–330, 2012.

[9] B. Tulu, N. Dida, Y. Kassa, and B. Taye, "Smear positive pulmonary tuberculosis and its risk factors among tuberculosis suspect in South East Ethiopia; a hospital based cross-sectional study," *BMC Research Notes*, vol. 7, p. 285, 2014.

[10] B. Moges, B. Amare, F. Asfaw et al., "Prevalence of smear positive pulmonary tuberculosis among prisoners in North Gondar Zone Prison, northwest Ethiopia," *BMC Infectious Diseases*, vol. 12, article no. 352, 2012.

[11] J. Seni, B. R. Kidenya, E. Obassy et al., "Low sputum smear positive tuberculosis among pulmonary tuberculosis suspects in a tertiary hospital in Mwanza, Tanzania," *Tanzania Journal of Health Research*, vol. 14, no. 2, pp. 115–120, 2012.

[12] D. M. Desalegn, K. T. Kitila, H. M. Balcha et al., "Misdiagnosis of pulmonary tuberculosis and associated factors in peripheral laboratories: a retrospective study, Addis Ababa, Ethiopia," *BMC Research Notes*, vol. 11, no. 1, p. 291, 2018.

[13] M. A. Asemahagn and G. Amsalu, "Determinants of sputum smear positivity among tuberculosis suspected patients in Bahir Dar City, Northwest Ethiopia," *Annals of Medical and Health Science Research*, vol. 8, pp. 111–117, 2018.

[14] M. S. Khan, S. Khan, and P. Godfrey-Faussett, "Default during TB diagnosis: quantifying the problem," *Tropical Medicine & International Health*, vol. 14, no. 12, pp. 1437–1441, 2009.

[15] T. L. Creek, S. Lockman, T. A. Kenyon, M. Makhoa, N. Chimidza, T. Moeti et al., "Completeness and timeliness of treatment initiation after laboratory diagnosis of tuberculosis in Gaborone, Botswana," *International Journal of Tuberculosis and Lung Disease*, vol. 4, no. 6, pp. 956-951, 2000.

[16] V. Chandrasekaran, R. Ramachandran, J. Cunningham, R. Balasubramaniun, A. Thomas et al., "Factors leading to tuberculosis diagnostic dropout and delayed treatment initiation in Chennai, India," *International Journal of Tuberculosis and Lung Disease*, vol. 9, p. 172, 2005.

[17] E. Botha, S. den Boon, K. A. Lawrence, H. Reuter, S. Verver, C. J. Lombard et al., "From suspect to patient: tuberculosis diagnosis and treatment initiation in health facilities in South Africa," *International Journal of Tuberculosis and Lung Disease*, vol. 12, pp. 936–941, 2008.

[18] J. Kemp, S. B. Squire, I. K. Nyirenda, and F. M. L. Salaniponi, "Is tuberculosis diagnosis a barrier to care?" *Transactions of the Royal Society of Tropical Medicine and Hygiene*, vol. 90, p. 472, 1996.

[19] F. K. Afutu, R. Zachariah, S. G. Hinderaker et al., "High initial default in patients with smear-positive pulmonary tuberculosis at a regional hospital in Accra, Ghana," *Transactions of the Royal Society of Tropical Medicine and Hygiene*, vol. 106, no. 8, pp. 511–513, 2012.

[20] E. Botha, S. Den Boon, S. Verver, R. Dunbar, K. A. Lawrence et al., "Initial default from tuberculosis treatment: how often does it happen and what are the reasons?" *International Journal of Tuberculosis and Lung Disease*, vol. 12, pp. 820–823, 2008.

[21] T. N. Buu, K. Lönnroth, and H. T. Quy, "Initial defaulting in the National Tuberculosis Programme in Ho Chi Minh City, Vietnam: a survey of extent, reasons and alternative actions taken following default," *The International Journal of Tuberculosis and Lung Disease*, vol. 7, no. 8, pp. 735–741, 2003.

[22] P. G. Gopi, V. Chandrasekaran, R. Subramani, and P. R. Narayanan, "Failure to initiate treatment for tuberculosis patients diagnosed in a community survey and at health facilities under a DOTS programme in a district of South India," *Indian Journal of Tuberculosis*, vol. 52, pp. 153–156, 2005.

6

Neutrophil Oxidized-Modified Proteins and Neutrophil Extracellular Traps in Patients with Community-Acquired Pneumonia

Vilen Molotov-Luchanskiy,[1] Altynbek Nukhuly,[2] Larissa Muravlyova,[1] Ryszhan Bakirova,[1] Aruna Kossybayeva,[1] Dmitry Klyuyev,[1] Ludmila Demidchik,[1] and Irina Beinikova[1]

[1]"Karaganda Medical University" Non-commercial Joint-Stock Company, Kazakhstan
[2]Pavlodar State Pedagogical University, Kazakhstan

Correspondence should be addressed to Ryszhan Bakirova; bakir15@mail.ru

Academic Editor: Kazuyoshi Kuwano

Background and Objectives. Community-acquired pneumonia (CAP) has a high mortality rate among adult patients throughout the world. The highest mortality is registered in the older age group with a steady increase in the number of cases of morbidity among persons of working age. Neutrophils are one of the most urgent areas of research, since their condition largely determines the development and outcome of acute pneumonia. We study the indices of oxidative stress and oxidized-modified proteins of neutrophils in CAP patients, depending on the degree of severity, and also compare the detection frequency of neutrophil extracellular traps in the progression of pneumonia. *Materials and Methods.* 51 patients with CAP were divided into 2 groups depending on the severity of the pathological process. The first group (I) consisted of 32 patients with moderate severity of pneumonia. The second group (II) consisted of 19 patients with severe pneumonia. The third group (III), the comparison group, consisted of 14 CAP patients with chronic obstructive pulmonary disease (COPD). The control group consisted of 19 volunteers. *Results.* Statistically significant increase in the level of carbonyl derivatives (CD) in patients of all study groups relative to the control group was revealed. In the group of patients with moderate severity and severe pneumonia, also in CAP patients with COPD, the level of CD exceeded the control group. There was no statistically significant difference in the level of advanced oxidation protein products (AOPP) and myeloperoxidase (MPO) in blood neutrophils between the studied groups. *Conclusion.* Results indicate an oxidative imbalance in neutrophils and contribute to the worsening of the course of the disease.

1. Introduction

Throughout the world remains a high mortality rate among adult patients with community-acquired pneumonia (CAP). The highest mortality is registered in the older age group with a steady increase in the number of cases of morbidity among persons of working age [1, 2]. The mechanisms of CAP development are diverse and depend both on the etiology of the pathogen and the pathways of penetration into the lungs [3]. The study of changes in the functional and metabolic status of neutrophils is one of the most urgent areas of research, since their condition largely determines the development and outcome of acute pneumonia [4]. Neutrophils are the most numerous group of cells of white blood, the main task of which is the destruction of pathogenic bacteria. It is known that the activation of neutrophils, generation of reactive oxygen species (ROS), and secretion of granules with antimicrobial proteins play a major role in eliminating pathogenic microorganisms. At the same time, the long-term activity of granulocytes makes a significant contribution to the damage of lung tissue, contributing to an unfavorable outcome of pneumonia [5].

Thus, neutrophils play a dual role: on the one hand, they perform a protective function; on the other, they are potential mediators of tissue damage. A sufficient number of studies have been devoted to the study of indices of oxidative stress in the blood to assess the severity of the pathological process, but the number of studies of indices of oxidative stress of neutrophils in CAP patients with chronic obstructive pulmonary disease (COPD) and patients with CAP depending on the degree of disease severity is limited [6, 7]. In this aspect, the study of neutrophils and their functional and metabolic status is one of the most urgent and promising tasks, since their condition largely determines the development and outcomes of the disease.

The work is aimed at studying the indices of oxidative stress and oxidized-modified proteins of neutrophils in CAP patients, depending on the degree of severity and CAP patients with COPD, also comparing the detection frequency of neutrophil extracellular traps in the progression of pneumonia.

To achieve the purpose of the study, an oxidative modification of the neutrophil proteins was evaluated by the level of carbonyl derivatives (CD) and advanced oxidation protein products (AOPP) as a result of oxidative damage of proteins in the cell; also, the activity of the neutrophil enzyme—myeloperoxidase (MPO)—and the presence of neutrophil extracellular traps were studied. All the studied parameters were determined in CAP patients, depending on the severity of the disease (in the acute stage) and compared with the control group of conditionally healthy donors and the comparison group. As a comparison group, the CAP patients with COPD were used.

2. Materials and Methods

The study was conducted from the year 2015 to 2016 on the basis of laboratory of the Department of Biochemistry in common with medical institutions, where the diagnosis and collection of blood were conducted for this study. The study included 51 patients diagnosed with community-acquired pneumonia and 14 patients with secondary home pneumonia on a background of COPD of moderate severity and type 2 respiratory failure. At the time of the study, more than 90% of the patients refrained from smoking for two days or more. Prior to the study, informed consent was obtained from all patients and healthy individuals for participation in the study; also, the study was approved by the Ethics Committee of the Karaganda Medical University.

Depending on the severity of the pathological process, CAP patients were divided into 2 groups. The first group (I) consisted of 32 patients with moderate severity pneumonia and type 2 respiratory failure at the age of 27 to 49 years. The second group (II) consisted of patients with severe pneumonia and type 2–3 respiratory failure—19 people aged 21 to 63 years. The third group (III), the comparison group, consisted of 14 CAP patients with COPD in the age range from 32 to 73 years. The control group consisted of 19 nonsmoking, conditionally healthy volunteers without clinical, laboratory, and functional signs of inflammation of the same age range as the patient's groups.

The criteria for inclusion in the study are as follows: community-acquired pneumonia confirmed by the laboratory, instrumental and physical methods, secondary home pneumonia on a background of COPD, age of patients from 18 to 73 years, absence of acute infectious-inflammatory processes of other organs during the study, prolonged (more than 2 weeks) course of pneumonia, and the absence of concomitant pathology of the endocrine system in the stage of decompensation. The exclusion criteria for the study were noninfectious infiltrative lung lesions, such as infarct pneumonia, neoplasms, pulmonary tuberculosis, parasitic invasions, and bronchiectasis.

CAP was diagnosed on the basis of the presence of a pulmonary infiltrate, verified X-ray, and clinical picture (cough with hard-to-separate mucopurulent sputum, chest pain, shortness of breath of mixed character, body temperature up to 38°C). Tachypnea was recorded in the absolute majority of patients. In the CBC, an increase in erythrocyte sedimentation rate, leukocytosis, a shift of the leukocyte formula to the left, and lymphopenia were observed. A bacteriological study of sputum revealed that pneumococci had an etiological role in the development of pneumonia in 79.6% of patients.

After the collection of blood, the upper layer of cells containing leukocytes was collected. The present erythrocytes were destroyed with 0.83% ammonium chloride solution. To wash leukocytes, a phosphate buffer was used. The number of neutrophils was standardized to 1 million in 1 ml of medium. The viability of neutrophils in the test with 0.5% trypan blue was 80%.

The content of carbonyl derivatives (CD) in the neutrophils was determined in the reaction with 2,4-dinitrophenylhydrazine by the method of Levine et al. [8, 9]. The optical density of formed dinitrophenylhydrazones was recorded spectrophotometrically at 370 nm. The AOPP was prepared in vitro as described by Witko-Sarsat et al. [9]. 81% of PBS solution was added to neutrophils in a ratio of 1 : 5, then 200 μl of 15% glacial acetic acid. Immediately at the time of measurement, 100 μl of a 1.16 M KI solution was added, and the absorbance was measured at 340 nm. The activity of myeloperoxidase (MPO) of neutrophils was determined by the method described by Dolgushin et al. [10] which is based on the ability of the enzyme to catalyze the oxidation of indigo carmine with hydrogen peroxide (unit of measure—mcd/l). Detection of neutrophil extracellular traps (NETs) was carried out according to the method described by Dolgushin [10]. The results were expressed in percentage of the number of neutrophils in the field of view. The staining of blood smears was performed according to the May-Grunwald method.

2.1. Statistical Analyses. The comparison of the parameters between study groups, due to nonnormal distributions, was carried out using the Kruskal–Wallis analysis of variances (ANOVA) and median test (the differences were considered reliable at significance level $p < 0.05$) and correlation analysis, using Spearman correlation, to determine the relationship between the activity of MPO and the level of AOPP.

3. Results

When studying oxidized-modified proteins in blood neutrophils, a statistically significant increase in the level of CD in

Table 1: The content of oxidized-modified proteins of neutrophils in study groups.

Study groups	CD (nmol/10^6 cells)			AOPP (μmol/10^6 cells)		
	Median	Lower quartile	Upper quartile	Median	Lower quartile	Upper quartile
Moderate severity pneumonia ($n = 32$)	0.286*	0.230*	0.429*	0.041	0.031	0.113
Severe pneumonia ($n = 19$)	0.312*	0.251*	0.407*	0.058	0.024	0.108
Secondary home pneumonia on a background of COPD ($n = 14$)	0.494*	0.294*	0.580*	0.029	0.019	0.042
Control ($n = 19$)	0.165	0.147	0.286	0.045	0.032	0.057

CD: carbonyl derivatives; AOPP: advanced oxidation protein products; COPD: chronic obstructive pulmonary disease. *Reliability of differences with the control, $p < 0.05$.

patients of all study groups relative to the values of the control group ($p < 0.05$) was revealed (Table 1). According to the received data, there were no statistically significant differences in the content of CD depending on the degree of CAP severity, and no significant differences were found with the comparison group. However, we can note the tendency to increase the level of CD in CAP patients with COPD compared to the other studied groups.

Thus, in the group of patients with moderate severity and severe pneumonia, the level of CD was, on average, exceeded than that of the control group by 73% and 89%, respectively, with a maximum value of 1.02 nmol/106 cells in these groups. At the same time, in CAP patients with COPD, the level of CD was 2.9 times higher relative to the values of the control group. In all groups of patients, there were no values below the control.

In this case, we recorded the presence of two clusters of CD in all groups of patients, both CAP and CAP with COPD. The first cluster is the values of the CD of neutrophils that corresponded to those of the control group. The second cluster is the values of CD of neutrophils that exceeded the values of the control group. The investigated groups of patients differed only in the degree of expression of one or another cluster. This suggests that, despite the burden of the disease, there are patients with a normal level of CD that was also shown by us in earlier studies. Perhaps, this is due to the different functional state of neutrophils.

There was no statistically significant difference in the level of AOPP in blood neutrophils between the studied groups. It can only be noted that for patients with moderate severity and severe pneumonia, there is a tendency for an increase in the AOPP level, while for CAP patients with COPD a tendency for decrease relative to the control group (Table 1).

When studying the activity of neutrophil MPO, according to our data, there was no statistically significant difference between the study groups (Figure 1). In our opinion, this may be due to the fact that the activity of the enzyme depends on the etiology of the disease, since it has been shown that the development of pneumonia from influenza infection reduces MPO activity. Thus, in the work of the authors Nagoev and Betsucova, it was shown that the more severity of influenza-associated pneumonia, the greater inhibition of MPO activity of neutrophils was [11]. According to other data, weighting the course of pneumonia significantly increases the activity of myeloperoxidase [12]. In our study, pneumococci were the dominating etiologic factor in the development of pneumonia, and in 20.4% of the cases, pneumonia was preceded by acute respiratory viral infection and influenza. Therefore, the activity of MPO requires further study depending on the etiology of pneumonia. The percentage ratio of NETs is shown in Figure 2.

The following Figure 2 was revealed in the percentage ratio of NETs among the surveyed groups. In the group of CAP patients with moderate severity, NETs were detected in an amount of 3 to 31 pcs. per 100 neutrophils in 25% of the patients. In group II, NETs were detected in the quantitative range from 1 to 8 pcs. per 100 neutrophils in 52.63% of patients. In the group of patients with pneumonia on the background of COPD, NETs were detected in an amount from 2 to 6 pcs. per 100 neutrophils in 42.86% of the patients. In the control group, neutrophil extracellular traps were absent.

4. Discussion

The results we obtained indicate an increase in the activity of oxidative stress and the intensity of formation of oxidized-modified proteins, since CD and AOPP are indicators of the production of free radicals. With the development of inflammation, increased production of ROS by neutrophils in combination with an imbalance of the antioxidant defense system is a condition for the development of oxidative stress [12]. Oxidative stress, in turn, contributes to the damage of cellular structures in inflammatory lung diseases, where the metabolic activity of neutrophils is not limited by the oxygen content [13]. We detected a statistically significant increase in the content of CD and a trend towards an increase in the AOPP level in neutrophils in CAP patients of both moderate and severe severity. The phenomenon of accumulation of modified proteins can be explained by a decrease in the redox potential in cells and a violation of the processes of their proteolytic degradation. In CAP patients with COPD, a tendency towards a decrease in the content of AOPP relative to control with a statistically significant increase in the CD level was detected. The content of AOPP in cells is associated with MPO activity, since it is believed that the hypochlorous acid produced by the enzyme directly participates in the

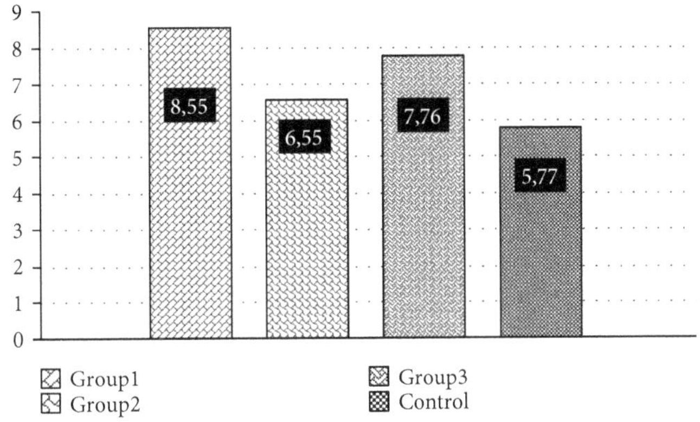

FIGURE 1: Myeloperoxidase activity in the neutrophils of the patient study groups.

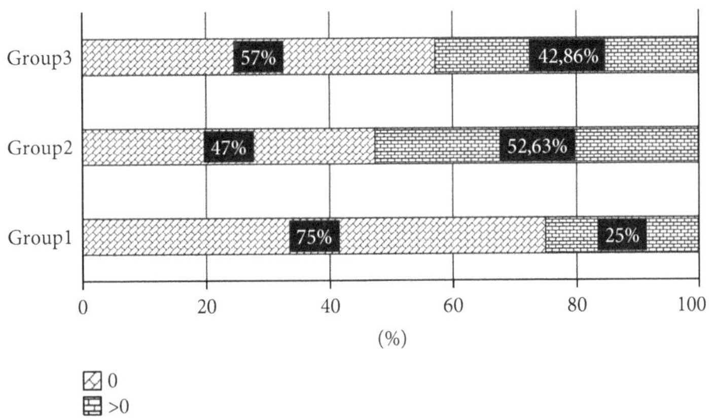

FIGURE 2: The percentage of patients with different amounts of NET's (per 100 neutrophils).

formation of AOPP. In our opinion, in patients with secondary home pneumonia on a background of COPD, the type of oxidative modification of proteins associated with carbonylation predominates, while another type of oxidative modification of proteins, associated with the action of chlorine-containing oxidants and MPO activity, is weakened, which is accompanied by a decrease in AOPP. Neutrophil extracellular traps were found in the blood of patients in the study groups. They were not detected in all patients and their number varied. Thus, with an average severity of pneumonia, the number of traps reached 31 per 100 neutrophils in 25% of patients; in severe pneumonia and pneumonia in COPD, the percentage of patients with NETs increased, but the number of traps did not exceed 8 per 100 neutrophils.

5. Conclusion

The appearance of NETs in the blood of patients, in our opinion, is an unfavorable factor, since, in the formation of NETs, extracellular network-like structures containing DNA and histones are formed. It is known that extracellular histones induce cell damage and provoke the formation of thrombin [14, 15]. Thus, the results that we have revealed indicate an oxidative imbalance in neutrophils, which undoubtedly affects the state of the pulmonary parenchyma and contributes to the worsening of the course of the disease.

Disclosure

The funders had no role in study design, data collection and analysis, decision to publish, or preparation of the paper.

Authors' Contributions

R.B. and L.M. are responsible for writing the manuscript and study design. R.B., A.K., L.D., D.K., I. B., and A.N. are responsible for the sample collection and data. L.M. and V.M.-L. are responsible for the data analysis. D.K., I.B., A.N., A.K., and L.D. are responsible for the statistical analysis. L.M., V.M.-L., and R.B. are responsible for the participants in the discussion. L.M., V.M.-L., and R.B. are responsible for the validation and supervision. All authors have read and agreed to the published version of the manuscript.

References

[1] W. I. Sligl, D. T. Eurich, T. J. Marrie, and S. R. Majumdar, "Age still matters: prognosticating short- and long-term mortality for critically ill patients with pneumonia," *Critical Care Medicine*, vol. 38, no. 11, pp. 2126–2132, 2010.

[2] T. Welte, A. Torres, and D. Nathwani, "Clinical and economic burden of community-acquired pneumonia among adults in Europe," *Thorax*, vol. 67, no. 1, pp. 71–79, 2011.

[3] A. Capelastegui, P. P. España, A. Bilbao et al., "Etiology of community-acquired pneumonia in a population-based study: link between etiology and patients characteristics, process-of-care, clinical evolution and outcomes," *BMC Infectious Diseases*, vol. 12, no. 1, p. 134, 2012.

[4] X. Zhou, Q. Dai, and X. Huang, "Neutrophils in acute lung injury," *Frontiers in Bioscience*, vol. 17, no. 7, pp. 2278–2283, 2012.

[5] J. Bordon, S. Aliberti, R. Fernandez-Botran et al., "Understanding the roles of cytokines and neutrophil activity and neutrophil apoptosis in the protective versus deleterious inflammatory response in pneumonia," *International Journal of Infectious Diseases*, vol. 17, no. 2, pp. e76–e83, 2013.

[6] L. Muravlyova, V. Molotov–Luchankiy, R. Bakirova, D. Klyuyev, L. Demidchik, and V. Lee, "Characteristic of the oxidative stress in blood of patients in dependence of community-acquired pneumonia severity," *Open Access Macedonian Journal of Medical Sciences*, vol. 4, no. 1, pp. 122–127, 2016.

[7] L. A. Demidchik, V. V. Lee, L. Y. Muravlyova et al., "Oxidative metabolism of neutrophils in patients with community-acquired pneumonia," *Current Issues in Pharmacy and Medical Sciences*, vol. 29, no. 1, pp. 5–7, 2016.

[8] R. L. Levine, D. Garland, C. N. Oliver et al., "[49] Determination of carbonyl content in oxidatively modified proteins," *Methods in Enzymology*, vol. 186, pp. 464–478, 1990.

[9] V. Witko-Sarsat, M. Friedlander, C. Capeillère-Blandin et al., "Advanced oxidation protein products as a novel marker of oxidative stress in uremia," *Kidney International*, vol. 49, no. 5, pp. 1304–1313, 1996.

[10] I. I. Dolgushin, J. S. Andreeva, and A. J. Savochkina, *Neytrofil'nyye vnekletochnyye lovushki i metody otsenki funktsional'nogo statusa neytrofilov*, RAMS Publishing House, Moscow, 2009.

[11] B. S. Nagoev and A. M. Betsucova, "Change of activity of indicator of functional and metabolic activity of leucocytes at influenza and postinfluenza pneumonia," *Byulleten' novykh meditsinskikh tekhnologiy*, vol. 18, no. 4, pp. 85-86, 2011.

[12] E. A. Stepovaia, G. V. Petina, T. V. Zhavoronok et al., "Functional properties and oxidative modification of neutrophil and plasma proteins in community-acquired pneumonia," *Klinicheskaya laboratornaya diagnostika*, vol. 3, pp. 18–21, 2010.

[13] Y. V. Prutkina, N. N. Tsybikov, and N. Y. Isakova, "Role of cytotoxic substances of neutrophils and Clara cell protein in development of acute respiratory distress syndrome at virus pneumonia," *Bulletin of physiology and pathology*, vol. 43, pp. 56–60, 2012.

[14] T. A. Fuchs, U. Abed, C. Goosmann et al., "Novel cell death program leads to neutrophil extracellular traps," *Journal of Cell Biology*, vol. 176, no. 2, pp. 231–241, 2007.

[15] F. Semeraro, C. T. Ammollo, J. H. Morrissey et al., "Extracellular histones promote thrombin generation through platelet-dependent mechanisms: involvement of platelet TLR2 and TLR4," *Blood*, vol. 118, no. 7, pp. 1952–1961, 2011.

7

Acute Respiratory Distress Syndrome due to *Mycoplasma pneumoniae* Misinterpreted as *SARS-CoV-2* Infection

Carlos Metz,[1] Torben Rixecker,[1] Sebastian Mang,[1] André Becker,[1] Alexander Maßmann,[2] Sören L. Becker,[3] Cihan Papan,[3] Barbara Gärtner,[3] Frederik Seiler,[1] Guy Danziger,[1] Robert Bals,[1] and Philipp M. Lepper[1]

[1]*Department of Pneumology, Allergology and Critical Care Medicine, Saarland University, Homburg/Saar, Germany*
[2]*Department for Diagnostic and Interventional Radiology, Saarland University Medical Center, Homburg/Saar, Germany*
[3]*Center for Infectious Diseases, Institute of Medical Microbiology and Hygiene, Saarland University, Homburg/Saar, Germany*

Correspondence should be addressed to Philipp M. Lepper; philipp.lepper@uks.eu

Academic Editor: Antonio Corrado

Background. In 2020, a novel coronavirus caused a global pandemic with a clinical picture termed COVID-19, accounting for numerous cases of ARDS. However, there are still other infectious causes of ARDS that should be considered, especially as the majority of these pathogens are specifically treatable. *Case Presentation.* We present the case of a 36-year-old gentleman who was admitted to the hospital with flu-like symptoms, after completing a half-marathon one week before admission. As infection with SARS-CoV-2 was suspected based on radiologic imaging, the hypoxemic patient was immediately transferred to the ICU, where he developed ARDS. Empiric antimicrobial chemotherapy was initiated, the patient deteriorated further, therapy was changed, and the patient was transferred to a tertiary care ARDS center. As cold agglutinins were present, the hypothesis of an infection with SARS-CoV-2 was then questioned. Bronchoscopic sampling revealed *Mycoplasma (M.) pneumoniae.* When antimicrobial chemotherapy was adjusted, the patient recovered quickly. *Conclusion.* Usually, *M. pneumoniae* causes mild disease. When antimicrobial chemotherapy was adjusted, the patient recovered quickly. The case underlines the importance to adhere to established treatment guidelines, scrutinize treatment modalities, and not to forget other potential causes of severe pneumonia or ARDS.

1. Introduction

A novel coronavirus, SARS-CoV-2, caused a global pandemic with a clinical picture termed COVID-19 and accounted for numerous cases of ARDS in early 2020 [1]. To date, there is no convincing evidence for a specific medical therapy for SARS-CoV-2. Most European hospitals prepared for a surge of these patients. COVID-19 leads to a systemic disease primarily affecting the lung. Approximately 15–42% of COVID-19 patients develop ARDS (CARDS) [1–3]. However, there are still other infectious causes of ARDS that should be considered, especially, as the majority of these pathogens are specifically treatable. The case presented here describes a severe infection with *M. pneumoniae* leading to ARDS in an adult, complicated by a delay in diagnosis and effective therapy as COVID-19 was suspected.

2. Case Presentation

On the 14th of March 2020, a 36-year-old gentleman presented at the emergency unit of a nearby hospital with fever, dry cough, and head and limb aches that started three days earlier. In good physical condition and otherwise healthy, he had completed a half-marathon the week before, but on admission to another hospital, he presented with reduced general condition and shortness of breath. Physical examination revealed crackles in the right upper lobe upon auscultation.

Medical, family, and psychosocial history was completely unremarkable.

As SARS-CoV-2 was suspected, he was immediately admitted to the ICU. He received microbiological and virological sampling as well as chest X-ray and thoracic CT. A calculated antimicrobial chemotherapy with piperacillin/tazobactam (3×4.5 g/d i.v.) and clarithromycin (2×500 mg/d i.v.) was started. Polymerase chain reaction (PCR) for SARS-CoV-2 was negative, as were the results for influenza, *Mycobacterium tuberculosis*, and *Legionella* spp. After 2 days, the antimicrobial regimen was changed to meropenem (3×1.0 g/d i.v.), linezolid (2×600 mg/d i.v.), and fosfomycin (3 g/d i.v.) due to persistently elevated inflammatory parameters and further clinical deterioration. The assumption of the patient having COVID-19 was maintained. Imaging of the lungs revealed a diffuse interstitial reticular pattern, multilobular patchy ground-glass opacification, and consolidation of the right upper lobe.

After a week on high-flow oxygen, he deteriorated and was intubated at an oxygenation index (P_aO_2/F_iO_2 ratio) of 130. Despite proning, he deteriorated further (hypercapnia with respiratory acidosis and hypoxemia with a P_aO_2/F_iO_2 ratio 108), needing higher doses of vasopressors, and our hospital's extracorporeal membrane oxygenation (ECMO) team was called on the 22nd of March 2020 to transfer the patient. The patient was reported as having COVID-19 and moderate ARDS with respiratory acidosis.

The ECMO team set out to transfer the patient under COVID-19 personal protective equipment (PPE). In the external hospital, after reviewing the laboratory and imaging findings, as well as the ventilator settings, the team leader decided against implanting an ECMO on site, and the patient was transferred under COVID-19 precautionary measures. Bronchoscopy with bronchoalveolar lavage (BAL) was performed for microbiological sampling and to further elucidate the hypothesis of an infection with SARS-CoV-2. Additionally, a naso- and oropharyngeal swab for SARS-CoV-2 was obtained.

Chest radiographs were reviewed, and a new chest X-ray was made (Figure 1). Imaging showed mainly right-sided pneumonia, not typical for COVID-19, and the hypothesis of COVID-19 was abandoned. Antimicrobial therapy was changed, as atypical pneumonia was suspected. Meropenem (then given continuously i.v., monitored by determination of serum levels) was continued for a total of 7 days, and clarithromycin (2×500 mg/d) was added to the antimicrobial regime again (Table 1). Remarkably, for a young and otherwise healthy individual, the patient had elevated bilirubin and LDH levels, with diminished haptoglobin and macrocytic hyperregenerative anemia (hemoglobin 5.3 g/dL at a $s_{cv}O_2$ of 67%) on admission, demonstrating hemolysis. Coombs' test revealed cold agglutinins the same day.

Microbiological results from a BAL (March 22nd) were negative for *SARS-CoV-2*, *Pneumocystis jirovecii*, *Bordetella pertussis* and *B. parapertussis*, *Chlamydophila pneumoniae*, *Haemophilus influenzae*, *Legionella pneumophila*, *Moraxella catarrhalis*, and *Streptococcus pneumoniae*; however, the patient tested positive for *Mycoplasma (M.) pneumoniae*. Thus, a diagnosis of mycoplasma-related ARDS with cold agglutinin disease was made. The patient was in total substituted with 4 units of packed red blood cells and received only warm infusions. Ventilator support was deescalated soon after change of the antimicrobial regimen, and the patient was extubated on March 25th receiving noninvasive ventilator support for 4 more days with supplementary oxygen up to 40%. Meropenem was continued for a total of 7 days, and clarithromycin (2×500 mg/d) was added to the antimicrobial regime again (Table 1). Hemolysis improved quickly under the antibiotic regime. The patient was discharged from the ICU on March 30th and was discharged home without supplementary oxygen on April 6th. He had no health-related complaints in a telephone interview conducted on June 18th.

3. Discussion

Under the impression of a seemingly predominant microorganism at the time of admission, a clinical diagnosis was established that was questionable according to radiologic evidence. Additionally, inappropriate management of the pulmonary infection might have favored clinical deterioration. Initial antimicrobial therapy was changed early empirically to a regimen that was much less effective for the causative microorganism, despite a microbiological workup. The initial therapy was performed according to current guidelines [4]. The change was meant to extend the spectrum; instead, it missed the causative organism. Furthermore, at the time antimicrobial therapy was changed, treatment failure was not proven.

M. pneumoniae is a common cause of community-acquired pneumonia, particularly in children and young adults [5]. *M. pneumoniae* is a very small bacterium without a peptidoglycan cell wall. It is a common cause of tracheobronchitis and atypical pneumonia mainly because of its adherence to respiratory cells. Infection of host cells occurs through special adhesins and an elongated polar attachment organelle [6]. Usually, the pneumonia caused by *M. pneumoniae* is mild and characterized by a dry cough or self-limiting pneumonia [7]. The rates of ICU admission ranged between 10% and 16%. With an intense epidemiological background of COVID-19 as a cause of respiratory disease leading to a surge of ICU admissions in many countries, the proper diagnosis of treatable causes for ARDS is highly important. Therefore, microbiological testing from respiratory material (bronchial aspirate) using adequate test methods, such as loop-mediated isothermal amplification (LAMP) [8] or quenching probe (QProbe) [9] methods for *M. pneumoniae* diagnosis, is highly important, especially as macrolide resistance rates are increasing in *M. pneumoniae* [10].

Severe ARDS and fatal outcomes due to *M. pneumoniae* are rare and may be the result of unclear clinical features, delayed diagnosis, inappropriate respiratory support, and/or insufficient initial treatment. If additional diagnostic measures are not confirming the suspected pathogen, alternative explanations need to be evaluated. This is especially important if a treatable cause is present, as in the case presented here. However, concomitant cold agglutinin disease is frequently described in the context of *M. pneumoniae* and

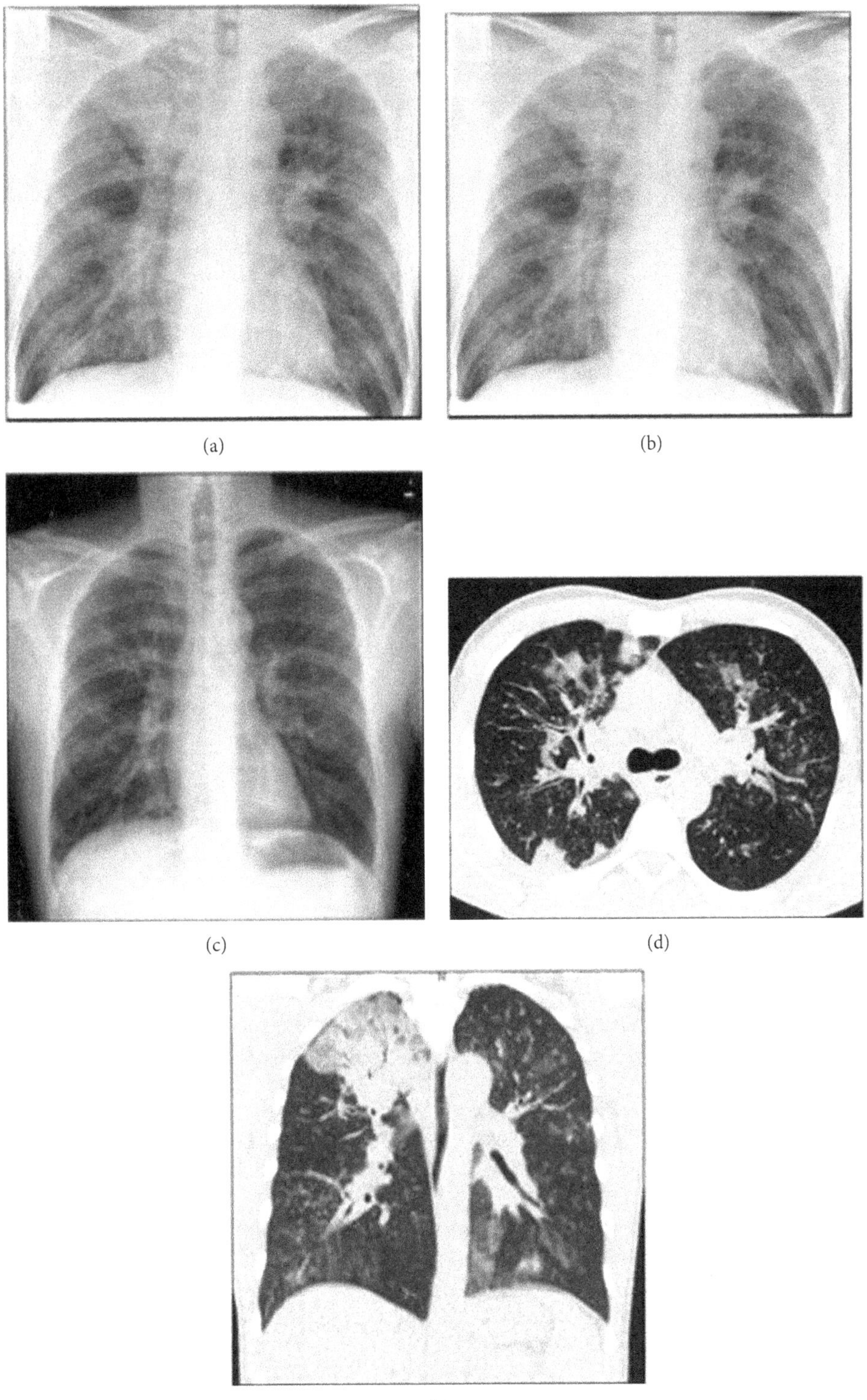

FIGURE 1: (a) Chest radiograph on the day of admission (March 14, 2020) to an external hospital shows consolidation predominantly in the right upper lobe, vague ill-defined opacities in the right lower lobe and left hilar region, and a diffuse interstitial pattern combined with bronchial wall thickening. (b) Chest X-ray on the day of admission to a tertiary care hospital depicts progressive pneumonia characterized by diffuse reticular and nodular patterns (March 22). (c) Chest X-ray shortly after discharge from the ICU (April 2) shows almost complete regression of previous infiltrations. The patient did not need supplementary oxygen at that time. (d, e) Computed tomography of the chest on March 16th confirms consolidation of the right upper lobe and reveals multifocal, patchy consolidations, ill-defined airspace infiltrates, and ground-glass opacifications. Additional centrilobular nodular appearance and thickening of the bronchovascular structures are present.

Table 1: Patient characteristics and laboratory parameters at various time points during infection with *M. pneumoniae*.

Parameter				
Gender		Male		
Age (years)		36		
Height (cm)		190		
Weight (kg)		90		
Body mass index (kg/m^2)		24.9		
Antimicrobial therapy (therapy started on the 14th of March, the patient transferred on the 22nd of March)				
Piperacillin/tazobactam		14.03-18.03		
Meropenem		18.03-24.03		
Linezolid		17.03-22.03		
Fosfomycin		17.03-22.03		
Clarithromycin		14.03-16.03 and 22.03–03.04		
Laboratory findings		*Date*		
	22nd of March	*2nd of April*	*6th of April*	*Normal values*
LDH (IU/L)	993	532	512	0–262
CRP (mg/L)	216	13	4.8	0.0-5.0
Bilirubin (mg/dL)	1.4	0.5	0.4	<1.2
Haptoglobin	<5	n.a.	n.a.	>5
Creatinine (mg/dL)	1.03	0.68	0.76	0.70–1.20
Sodium (mmol/L)	148	140	141	135–145
Potassium (mmol/L)	5.4	4.2	5.6	3.5–5.1
Hemoglobin (g/dL)	5.3	7.7	9.0	14.0–18.0
WBC (G/L)	16.8	6.6	7.6	3.9–10.2
Thrombocytes (T/μL)	351	559	568	140–400
Fibrinogen (g/L)	354	369	420	180–400
Interleukin 6 (pg/mL)	51.5	n.a.	n.a.	<7
D-dimers (mg/L)	12.6	n.a.	n.a.	<0.50

n.a.: not available.

usually develops upon generation of polyclonal IgM antibodies directed against I antigens on RBCs. Hemolysis can be severe but is usually self-limiting, while corticosteroids are reported to be barely effective [11].

If severe pneumonia caused by *M. pneumoniae* should be treated with corticosteroids in general remains unclear. While positive effects have been shown in children, there is a lack of prospective studies defining the appropriate dose and duration of steroid administration in fulminant ARDS with *M. pneumoniae* in adults [12].

Antibiotic therapy of *M. pneumoniae* requires agents such as macrolides or fluoroquinolones that do not target the bacterial cell wall and have good intracellular penetration. In our patient, macrolide therapy was started according to guidelines for severe pneumonia but was stopped after 2 days, and the regimen was unintentionally changed to a less effective one. These decisions might have been driven by the assumption that the patient might have an infection with SARS-CoV-2.

The gold standard for the detection of COVID-19 in symptomatic individuals is the detection of viral RNA in naso- or oropharyngeal swabs by reverse-transcriptase polymerase chain reaction (rtPCR) that can be false negative [13].

Radiologic findings alone are often not reliable for differentiating pneumonia. Moreover, coinfection with other bronchopulmonary pathogens is not uncommon. In general, radiographic findings should be used along with clinical and laboratory data to narrow the differential diagnosis. Currently, there is a threat of misinterpreting clinical pictures and lung imaging as SARS-CoV-2-induced disease. It has been suggested only recently that low-dose CT might be of equal sensitivity and specificity as rtPCR testing of nasopharyngeal swabs [14]. However, multiple infectious diseases might produce similar pictures in pulmonary imaging modalities.

At the time, the patient in the present case acquired the infection leading to ARDS, and the prevalence of COVID-19 in Germany, especially in the Federal State of Saarland, was low (2,078 confirmed cases in Germany on March [12]). In contrast, awareness of COVID-19 was high-flying.

If the prevalence of a specific infectious agent is predominant, it is very likely that the radiologic picture in fact happens to be the at the time frequently encountered infectious agent. However, the effective performance of CT for COVID-19 detection critically depends on the pretest probability for the occurrence of a disease, which in turn influences positive and negative predictive values (PPV and NPV). If the prevalence of a disease is truly low, the PPV for the disease will be low. If caregivers overestimate PPV, they might come to the wrong conclusion if no gold standard for the diagnosis of a disease exists or is accepted.

In the present case, treating physicians unintentionally created an unfavorable situation for the patient urged by erroneous assumptions. Unfortunately, the well-intentioned putative escalation of antimicrobial therapy was less effective for the causative organism.

4. Conclusion

The case presented here underlines the importance of adhering to established treatment guidelines, scrutinizing treatment modalities, and not forgetting other potential causes of severe pneumonia or ARDS to ensure that critically ill patients are safeguarded from common infections even in times ruled by a predominant pathogen.

Abbreviations

ARDS: Acute respiratory distress syndrome
CAD: Cold agglutinin disease
ECMO: Extracorporeal membrane oxygenation
NPV: Negative predictive value
PPE: Personal protective equipment
PPV: Positive predictive value.

Consent

Written informed consent was obtained from the patient for publication of this case report and any accompanying images.

Disclosure

A preprint of this report has been uploaded to ResearchSquare (DOI: 10.21203/rs.3.rs-78362/v1). The funders had no role with regard to this study in the design of the study and collection, analysis, and interpretation of data or in writing the manuscript.

Authors' Contributions

C.M., T.R., F.S., S.M., A.B., A.M., S.L.B., C.P., G.D., R.B., and P.M.L. contributed to the collection, review, and/or analysis of the data; C.M. and P.M.L. drafted the manuscript; T.R., A.B., S.M., F.S., S.S., A.M., S.L.B., C.P., B.G., G.D., and R.B. revised the manuscript for important intellectual content. All authors have seen and approved the final version of the manuscript.

Acknowledgments

COVID-19 research at the University Hospital of Saarland is funded by the Federal State of Saarland, Saarland University, and Dr. Rolf M. Schwiete Foundation.

References

[1] G. Grasselli, A. Zangrillo, A. Zanella et al., "Baseline characteristics and outcomes of 1591 patients infected with SARS-CoV-2 admitted to ICUs of the Lombardy region, Italy," *JAMA*, vol. 323, no. 16, pp. 1574–1581, 2020.

[2] Y. Wang, X. Lu, Y. Li et al., "Clinical course and outcomes of 344 intensive care patients with COVID-19," *American Journal of Respiratory and Critical Care Medicine*, vol. 201, no. 11, pp. 1430–1434, 2020.

[3] X. Yang, Y. Yu, J. Xu et al., "Clinical course and outcomes of critically ill patients with SARS-CoV-2 pneumonia in Wuhan, China: a single-centered, retrospective, observational study," *The Lancet Respiratory Medicine*, vol. 8, no. 5, pp. 475–481, 2020.

[4] S. Ewig, G. Höffken, W. Kern et al., "Behandlung von erwachsenen Patienten mit ambulant erworbener Pneumonie und Prävention - Update 2016," *Pneumologie*, vol. 70, no. 3, pp. 151–200, 2016.

[5] M. W. Boettcher, O. Baetz, and J. Kramer, "Seroprevalence and season variation of Chlamydia pneumoniae and *Mycoplasma pneumoniae* infection in Germany," *Clinical Microbiology and Infection*, vol. 16, p. S6667, 2010.

[6] H. C. Krivan, L. D. Olson, M. F. Barile, V. Ginsburg, and D. D. Roberts, "Adhesion of *Mycoplasma pneumoniae* to sulfated glycolipids and inhibition by dextran sulfate," *The Journal of Biological Chemistry*, vol. 264, no. 16, pp. 9283–9288, 1989.

[7] K. Izumikawa, "Clinical features of severe or fatal *Mycoplasma pneumoniae* pneumonia," *Frontiers in Microbiology*, vol. 7, p. 800, 2016.

[8] T. Notomi, H. Okayama, H. Masubuchi et al., "Loop-mediated isothermal amplification of DNA," *Nucleic Acids Research*, vol. 28, no. 12, article E63, pp. 63e–663, 2000.

[9] S. Kurata, T. Kanagawa, K. Yamada et al., "Fluorescent quenching-based quantitative detection of specific DNA/RNA using a BODIPY((R)) FL-labeled probe or primer," *Nucleic Acids Research*, vol. 29, no. 6, article E34, pp. 34e–334, 2001.

[10] T. Kakiuchi, I. Miyata, R. Kimura et al., "Clinical evaluation of a novel point-of-care assay to detect *Mycoplasma pneumoniae* and associated macrolide resistant mutations," *Journal of Clinical Microbiology*, 2021.

[11] P. L. Swiecicki, L. T. Hegerova, and M. A. Gertz, "Cold agglutinin disease," *Blood*, vol. 122, no. 7, pp. 1114–1121, 2013.

[12] K. Izumikawa, K. Izumikawa, T. Takazono et al., "Clinical features, risk factors and treatment of fulminant *Mycoplasma pneumoniae* pneumonia: a review of the Japanese literature," *Journal of Infection and Chemotherapy*, vol. 20, no. 3, pp. 181–185, 2014.

[13] S. Woloshin, N. Patel, and A. S. Kesselheim, "False negative tests for SARS-CoV-2 infection-challenges and implications," *The New England Journal of Medicine*, vol. 383, no. 6, article e38, 2020.

[14] M. Schulze-Hagen, C. Hübel, M. Meier-Schroers et al., "Low-dose chest CT for the diagnosis of COVID-19," *Deutsches Ärzteblatt International*, vol. 117, no. 22-23, pp. 389–395, 2020.

8

Primary Pulmonary Malignant Melanoma Found While Evaluating New Onset Cough

Fernando Figueroa Rodriguez[1] **Ahsan Uddin,**[2] **and Justine Nasr**[1]

[1]*Department of Internal Medicine, Beaumont Health, Royal Oak, MI, USA*
[2]*Department of Internal Medicine-Pediatrics, Beaumont Health, Royal Oak, MI, USA*

Correspondence should be addressed to Fernando Figueroa Rodriguez; fernando.figueroarodriguez@beaumont.org

Academic Editor: Luis Borderías

Malignant melanoma is a nonepithelial neoplasm of melanocytes. It is tremendously rare for this condition to primarily involve the respiratory tract, accounting only for 0.01% of the lung malignancies. It often presents as a solitary nodule provoking mass effect and/or obstructive symptom. It most commonly affects patients 50 years old and older, with no gender predilection. Complete surgical excision is the treatment of choice; nevertheless, chemotherapy or radiation might be necessary depending on tumor location and/or metastasis status. Recently, biochemotherapy and immunotherapy have emerged as promising treatment modalities. We present a case of Primary Pulmonary Malignant Melanoma (PPMM) in a 76-year-old male with no previous personal or family history of cancer who presented with new onset nonproductive cough. We also present an analysis with high yield points summarizing clinical features, diagnostic workup, and management of PPMM. Finally, we post a table summarizing all the cases ever reported in English literature.

1. Introduction

There are approximately 41,000 melanoma-related deaths in the world yearly and 16,000 new diagnoses every year; nevertheless there are only 41 cases of PPMM reported in the literature since 1916 [1]. Malignant melanoma of the respiratory tract: this malignancy is easily confused with more conventional neoplasms [2]. Its presentation in the pulmonary system can often be asymptomatic or minimally symptomatic leading to a delay in identification and treatment so that many cases are identified at later stages with 67.5% of cases being metastatic at diagnosis. Prognosis is often quite poor and death within six months is the most common outcome. Our case report seeks to add to the literature for this rare and unusual presentation of melanoma of the pulmonary tract of an otherwise low risk patient.

2. Case Presentation

A 76-year-old nonsmoker male with history of Obstructive Sleep Apnea presented for elective a Left Knee Total Arthroplasty. Next day, after a successful intervention the patient developed a nonproductive continuous cough. A Chest X-Ray (CXR) was obtained and showed a nodular, irregular opacity in the right lung (Figure 1). Computerized Tomography (CT) of the Chest followed and demonstrated a 3.2x2x4.3 cm mass in the superior segment of the right lower lobe as well as a 1.6 cm subcarinal lymph node (Figure 2). A Positron Emission Tomography (PET) Scan revealed activity in the right lower lobe on both early and delayed imaging (Figure 3). No other focal abnormalities were seen in the rest of the body. A core biopsy of the right lower lobe revealed an invasive, poorly differentiated, malignant melanoma (Box 1 and Figure 4). He was instructed to follow with pulmonary medicine after discharge and two months later, he underwent elective bronchoscopic wedge resection of the right lower lobe with lymph node dissection and biopsies, as well as biopsies of multiple structures in the respiratory tract. Ultimately, he was diagnosed with 3.7 cm malignant melanoma with negative margins and no evidence of metastasis; thus, no chemotherapy or radiation was indicated (Box 2). Serial

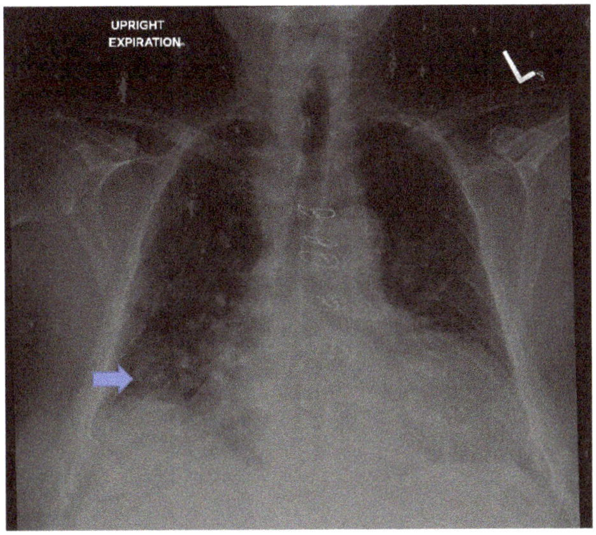

Figure 1: CXR upright-expiration. Arrow: right lower lobe irregular mass like opacity, no evidence of pneumothorax, effusion, or consolidation.

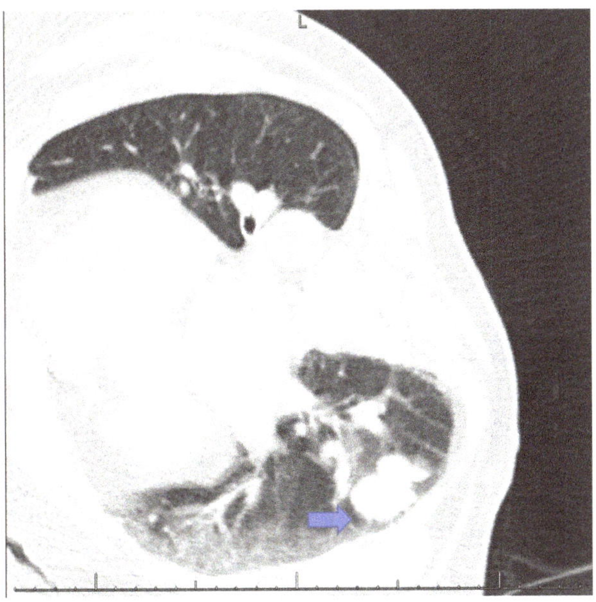

Figure 2: Chest CT. Arrow: 3.2x2x4.3 cm mass in the superior segment of the right lower lobe.

Repeat CXR and CT scans have shown stable postoperative changes but no signs of recurrence. To date, three years and eight months after diagnosis, the patient continues to follow with his pulmonologist and oncologist every 6 months for surveillance visits; no recurrence has been documented so far.

3. Discussion

Malignant melanoma of the skin and mucosae is routinely described as a dark, irregular, and asymmetric lesion, which in its most common form leads to a straight forward diagnosis. In the respiratory tract, this malignancy is easily confused

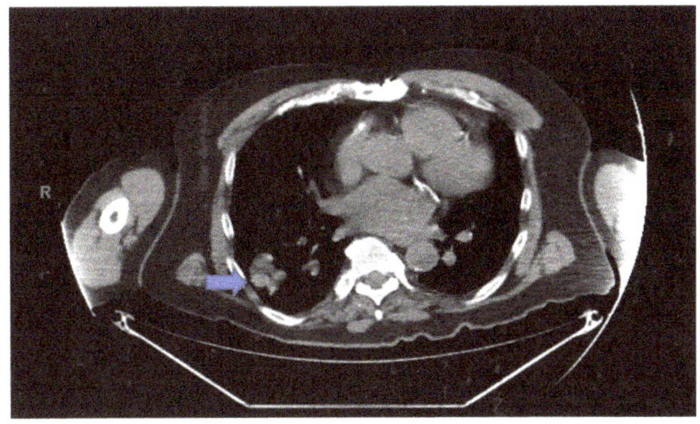

Figure 3: PET scan. Arrow: moderate to intensely increased metabolic activity in the right lower lobe mass (max SUV 8.4 initially increasing to 15.5 on delayed images), without evidence of other focal abnormalities.

with more conventional neoplasms [2]. Although there are no identified risk factors, the incidence of Primary Pulmonary Malignant Melanoma in nonsmokers is exceptionally rare. To date, there are only two cases described in the literature [1]. Our patient is a lifelong nonsmoker.

Due to its endobronchial location, PPMM frequently manifest with symptoms of cough, hemoptysis, dull chest pain, obstructive symptoms such as pneumonia, lobar collapse, or atelectasis. Symptoms of fatigue, malaise, and nighttime diaphoresis and signs of weight loss or lymphadenopathy might accompany the clinical picture as well. In 20-30% of the cases, it will be incidentally found on imaging [2]. Our patient had nonproductive cough as the only presenting symptom.

Pathogenesis is poorly understood; the most accepted theory involves melanocytes migration along with the primordial tubular respiratory tract during embryogenesis which are also present in the esophagus and pharynx. It has also been proposed that neuroendocrine precursor cells have the potential to undergo melanocytic differentiation [43]; finally, the last theory is spontaneous regression of malignant melanoma, which is defined by the complete disappearance of melanocytic neoplastic cells, that is, a primary dermal lesion that generates disseminated disease and then disappears, leading to misclassifying the neoplasm as primary, when it is truly secondary or metastatic [2]. Unfortunately, none of these theories have been fully accepted.

The definitive diagnosis of PPMM is achieved via clinical, radiological, and pathological findings. There are 6 proposed criteria for diagnosis [43].

(1) Junctional changes (nesting) of melanocytes beneath the bronchial epithelium.

(2) Invasion of bronchial epithelium by melanoma cells.

(3) Obvious melanoma cells by immunohistochemical staining.

(4) Solitary lung tumor, with pathology consistent with a primary tumor.

(5) Absence of a cutaneous, mucous membrane, or ocular melanoma.

```
SPECIMEN (S): OTHER, SURGICAL BIOPSY, RIGHT LOWER LOBE LUNG MASS
DIAGNOSIS:
                    * * * ALERT * * * ALERT * * * ALERT * * *
LUNG, RIGHT LOWER LOBE CORE BIOPSY
- - - INVASIVE POORLY DIFFERENTIATED MALIGNANT NEOPLASM (SEE COMENT)
COMMENT:
The sections show lung parenchyma which is infiltrated by a very
poorly differentiated malignant neoplasm composed of single cells
and small infiltrative nests with large, hyperchromatic nuclei
and scant cytoplasm. The background milieu consists of fibrosis,
hemosiderin-laden macrophages and a dense lymphoid infiltrate.
The tumor cells are positive for S100 and SOX-10. The primary
diagnostic differential for this pattern of staining is melanoma.
IMMUNOHISTOCHEMISTRY AND IMMUNOFLUORESCENCE RESULTS
S100: Positive - - - - - SOX-10 Positive
HMB45: Very Focal Positive - - - - - MART-1: Very focal positive
MITF: Very Focal Positive
AE13: Negative - - - - - Polytypic Keratin: Negative
CK20: Negative - - - - - CDX2: Negative
```

Box 1: Biopsy report.

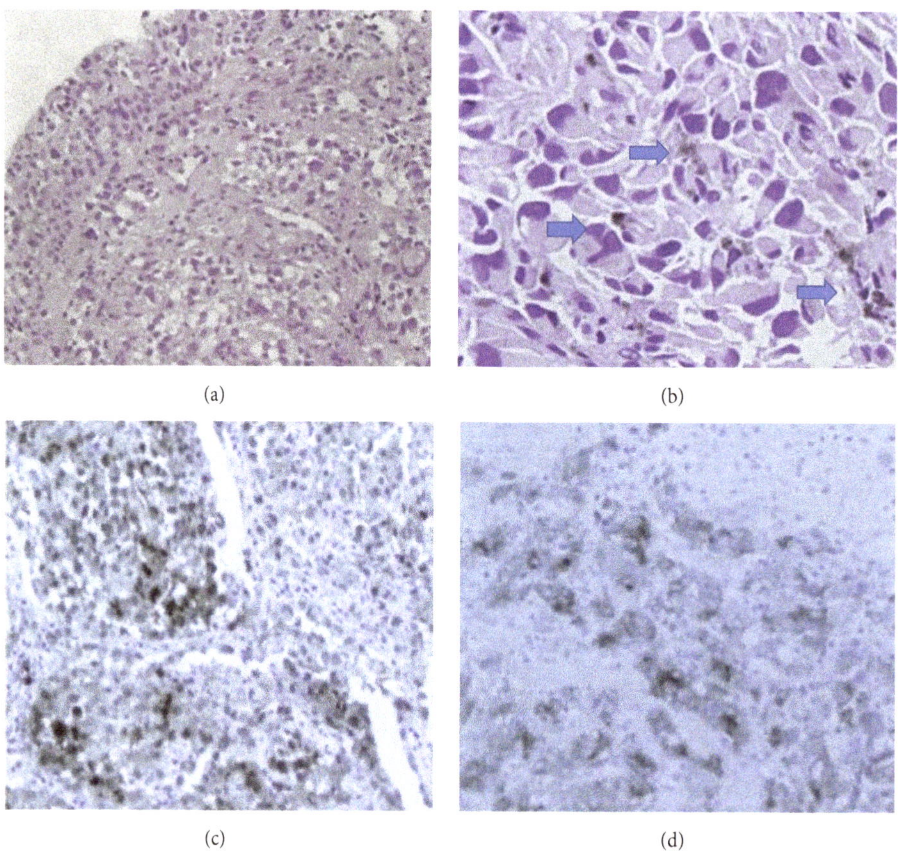

FIGURE 4: H&E stain ((a) 200x; (b) 400x) with tumor cells located under bronchial mucosa composed of epithelioid tumor cells with large amounts of acid cytoplasm and prominent nuclei. Mitotic figures are easily found. Note dark brown pigment in tumor cells (Arrows). Immunohistochemically, tumor cells were positive for S-100 and HBM 45 ((c) and (d)), amongst others.

```
SPECIMEN (S): A. LYMPH NODE BIOPSY, RIGHT LOWER LOBE PULMONARY ARTERYL;
B. SOFT TISSUE BIOPSY, PARATRACHEAL FAT PAD; C. LUNG LOBECTOMY, RIGHT LOWER LOBE.
DIAGNOSIS:
                         * * * ALERT * * * ALERT * * * ALERT * * *
A. RIGHT LOWER LOBE PULMONARY ARTERY LYMPHG NODE, EXCISION.
- - - ANTRACOSIS. NO EVIDENCE OF METASTATIC NEOPLASM (0/1)
B. PARATRACHEAL FAT PAD, EXCISION
- - - NORMAL ADIPOSE TISSUE. NO LYMPH NODES DETECTED
C. LUNG (RIGHT LOWER LOBE), LOBECTOMY
- - - PLEOMORPHIC, MALIGNANT MELANOTIC SPINDLE AND EPITHELIOID CELL
NEOPLASM. MAXIMUM LINEAR DIMENSION OF NEOPLASM: 3.7 CM. NO
EVIDENCE OF PLEURAL INVASION. BRONCHIAL SURGICAL MARGIN IS NEGATIVE
D. PERIBRONCHIAL LYMPH NODES, THREE, EXCISION
- - - ANTRACOSIS. NO EVIDENCE OF METASTATIC NEOPLASM (0/3)
```

Box 2: Bronchoscopy and second biopsy report.

(6) Absence of any other detectable tumor at the time of diagnosis.

The main differential diagnoses to consider are melanocytic carcinoid tumor, melanotic paraganglioma, melanotic schwannoma, and pulmonary metastasis of a malignant melanoma. These tumors can often be excluded by a complete history and physical exam but most importantly, by histopathological and immunohistochemical staining, that is, melanoma cells that stain for S-100 and HMB-45, and possibly by electron microscopy) [39].

Treatment of choice is surgical resection with lymph node dissection; the goal is to obtain negative margins (lobectomy or pneumonectomy). Interferon a-2b is frequently offered to mucosal melanoma patients but has not been formally evaluated in this patient population. Similarly, radiation has no clear role [1]. Biochemotherapy which consists of combination of chemotherapy and immunotherapy has been historically an acceptable choice after taking into consideration the tolerability [44].

Vemurafenib was approved by the Food and Drug Administration (FDA) in 2011 as it blocks the serine/threonine kinase BRAF protein which is found in up to 50% of the melanomas [45]. Dabrafenib was approved approval in 2013 [46], which does act against another subtype of protein (BRAF-V600K and E). In the same year, Trametinib, the first Mitogen Activated Protein Kinase inhibitor, was approved and were used in combination with BRAF inhibitors with excellent results (remission within weeks) although resistance to therapy commonly arises after a median of 6 months. Recently immunotherapy with programmed death-1 (PD-1) checkpoint inhibitors like nivolumab and pembrolizumab has been approved by the FDA for the treatment of metastatic cutaneous melanoma [47]. Palliative radiation therapy is utilized when bulky metastatic disease is present. The above medications were developed for mucosal and cutaneous melanoma but may have an increasing role in the management of PPMM

Per current literature review, if detected and treated in early stages (1 and 2) survival rates range from 60 to 85% at 5 years, whereas stages 3 and 4 range from 15 to 25% only. Late recurrence is uncommon with a reported incidence of 2.4%. Our patient was determined to be at stage 1 at the time of diagnosis; he has survived for almost 4 years and continues to be in remission [48].

4. Literature Review

There are approximately 41,000 melanoma-related deaths in the world yearly and 16,000 new diagnoses every year; nevertheless there are only 41 cases of PPMM reported in the literature since 1916 (see Table 1) [1]. Prognosis is often quite poor and death within six months is the most common outcome.

Given the broad period in which these cases were published, as well as new advances in diagnostic and therapeutic technology, conclusions regarding treatment modalities or the variables that impact survival and mortality are precluded. There are only a few facts that can be stated upon review of the cases above:

(i) Gender distribution was fairly equal with 52% of the patients being males and 48% females.

(ii) The median age at time of diagnosis was 59.1 years (29 to 90).

(iii) The average tumor size was 4.6 cm (1.0 to 10 cm).

(iv) 67.5% of the patients had metastasis at the time of diagnosis. The most common sites were contralateral lung, liver, brain, and bones as detailed above.

5. Conclusion

With this case report and literature review we aim to add critical data to the current medical literature regarding this highly unusual and rare disease. Reliable data regarding clinical presentation, diagnosis, and potential treatments of PPMM is becoming more available to health care workers making this a promising era in the identification and management of this condition, specifically with the establishment of unequivocal diagnostic criteria and the advent of new treatment modalities. Additionally, our findings of disseminated

TABLE 1

Case	Age, Gender	Tumor Size (cm)	Surgery	Adjuvant	Metastasis	Outcome
1 [3]	40 F	2.0	None	None	Not Reported	Died 8 months after diagnosis
2 [4]	48 F	5.0	Pneumonectomy	None	Not Reported	Died after surgery
3 [5]	45 M	2.0	Pneumonectomy	None	Contralateral Lung	Died 6 months after diagnosis
4 [6]	71 M	3.5	Lobectomy	None	None	Alive after 10 years
5 [7]	60 F	4.5	Pneumonectomy	None	None	Alive after 11 years
6 [8]	61 F	10	Segmental Resection	None	Contralateral Lung, Brain	Died 7 months after surgery
7 [9]	40 F	5.0	Lobectomy	None	Not Reported	Not Reported
8 [10]	56 M	4.0	Lobectomy	None	Contralateral Lung, Brain, Liver	Died 14 months after surgery
9 [11]	40 M	2.5	Pneumonectomy	None	None	Alive after 3 years
10 [12]	62 F	Not Reported	Thoracotomy	Radiation	Liver, Eye	Died 4 months after surgery
11 [13]	70 F	Not Reported	None	Radiation	Liver, Ribs, Lymph Nodes	Died 9 weeks after diagnosis
12 [14]	47 M	Not Reported	None	None	None	Died shortly after diagnosis
13 [15]	29 F	5.0	Lobectomy	Chemotherapy	Contralateral Lung, Liver, Heart, Bone	Died 1 month after surgery
14 [16]	80 M	1.5	Excisional Biopsy	Radiation	Contralateral Lung	Died 5.5 months after diagnosis
15 [17]	56 M	4.0	Pneumonectomy	Chemotherapy	Contralateral Lung, Heart	Died 1 month after surgery
16 [18]	42 F	6.0	Lobectomy	None	None	Alive 2.5 year after surgery
17 [19]	58 M	5.0	Lobectomy	None	None	Alive 18 months after surgery
18 [20]	62 M	1.0	Lobectomy	None	Heart, Lymph Nodes	Died 2 months after surgery
19 [21]	30 F	3.0	Lobectomy	None	Contralateral Lung, Heart, Brain	Died 5 months after surgery
20 [22]	90 M	6.0	None	None	Not Reported	Died at the time of diagnosis
21 [23]	59 M	8.0	Lobectomy	Alfa-Interferon	None	Alive 30 months after surgery
22 [24]	41 F	Not Reported	Pneumonectomy	Alfa-Interferon	None	Alive 18 months after surgery
23 [25]	74 M	8.0	Lobectomy	Chemotherapy	None	Died 10 months after surgery
24 [26]	68 F	5.0	Lobectomy	Alfa-Interferon	None	Alive 6 years after surgery
25 [27]	89 M	4.5	Lobectomy	None	None	Alive 5 years after surgery
26 [28]	58 M	2.8	Lobectomy	Dacarbazine	Contralateral Lung	Died 6 months after surgery
27 [29]	69 F	4.0	Lobectomy	Darbazine	Contralateral Lung, Liver, Brain, Skin	Died 6 months after surgery
28 [30]	52 F	2.0 - 2.4	None	Dacarbazine	Brain	Died 4 months after surgery
29 [31]	65 F	6.0	None	Darbazine	None	Alive 6 months after surgery
30 [32]	68 M	5.0	Pneumonectomy	Dacarbazine, Vincristine, Nimustine	Contralateral Lung	Died 2 months after diagnosis
31 [33]	62 F	5.0	None	Dacarbazine	Thoracic Vertebrae, Pleura	Alive 12 months after diagnosis
32 [34]	56 M	3.2	Pneumonectomy	Radiation	Cervical Spine	Alive 6 months after diagnosis
33 [35]	60 M	4.5	Pneumonectomy	Alfa-Interferon	None	Alive 18 months aftr surgery
34 [36]	58 F	9.0	None	None	None	Died 2 months after diagnosis
35 [37]	69 F	6.0	Lobectomy	Dacarbazine	None	Died 6 months after surgery
36 [38]	63 M	5.0	None	None	None	Died 2 months after diagnosis
37 [39]	82 F	8.0	None	None	None	Died 3 months after diagnosis

TABLE 1: Continued.

Case	Age, Gender	Tumor Size (cm)	Surgery	Adjuvant	Metastasis	Outcome
38 [40]	55 M	3.0	None	Dacarbazine, Alfa-Interferon	Skin, Brain	Died 3 months after diagnosis
39 [41]	69 M	5.0	None	None	Brain, Thoracic Vertebrae	Died 3 months after diagnosis
40 [42]	60 M	3.0	None	None	Lymph Nodes	Died 2 months after diagnosis
41 [1]	56 F	Not Reported	None	Dacarbazine, Alfa - Interferon, Ipilimumab	Brain	Died 5 months after diagnosis

disease and prompt surgical intervention being the strongest factors influencing survival are perfectly exemplified by our case report. At this time randomized studies are univariably defiant as with any rare disorder.

References

[1] C. Kyriakopoulos and G. Zarkavelis, "Primary pulmonary malignant melanoma: report of an important entity and literature review," *Case Reports in Oncological Medicine*, vol. 2017, Article ID 8654326, 9 pages, 2017.

[2] H. Khosravi, A. L. Akabane, A. Alloo, R. M. Nazarian, and G. M. Boland, "Metastatic melanoma with spontaneous complete regression of a thick primary lesion," *JAAD Case Reports*, vol. 2, no. 6, pp. 439–441, 2016.

[3] O. F. Kunkel and E. Torrey, "Report of a case of primary melanotic sarcoma of lung presenting difficulties in differentiating from tuberculosis," *New York State Journal of Medicine*, vol. 16, pp. 198–201, 1916.

[4] G. A. Carlucci and R. C. Schleussner, "Primary (?) melanoma of the lung: a case report," *The Journal of Thoracic and Cardiovascular Surgery*, vol. 11, pp. 643–649, 1941-1942.

[5] R. Salm, "A primary malignant melanoma of the bronchus," *The Journal of Pathology*, vol. 85, pp. 121–126, 1963.

[6] R. J. Reed III and E. M. Kent, "Solitary pulmonary melanomas: two case reports," *The Journal of Thoracic and Cardiovascular Surgery*, vol. 48, pp. 226–231, 1964.

[7] J. D. Reid and V. T. Mehta, "Melanoma of the lower respiratory tract," *Cancer*, vol. 19, no. 5, pp. 627–631, 1966.

[8] O. A. Jensen and J. Egedorf, "Primary malignant melanoma of the lung," *Scandinavian journal of respiratory diseases*, vol. 48, no. 2, pp. 127–135, 1967.

[9] M. S. Allen and E. C. Drash, "Primary melanoma of the lung," *Cancer*, vol. 21, no. 1, pp. 154–159, 1968.

[10] C. F. Taboada, J. D. McMurray, R. A. Jordan, and W. D. Seybold, "Primary melanoma of the lung," *Chest*, vol. 62, no. 5, pp. 629–631, 1972.

[11] Z. Weshler, A. Sulkes, J. Kopolovitch, A. Leviatan, and E. Shifrin, "Bronchial malignant melanoma," *Journal of Surgical Oncology*, vol. 15, no. 3, pp. 243–248, 1980.

[12] A. J. Robertson, D. J. M. Sinclair, P. P. Sutton, and W. Guthrie, "Primary melanocarcinoma of the lower respiratory tract," *Thorax*, vol. 35, no. 2, pp. 158-159, 1980.

[13] G. N. Gephardt, "Malignant melanoma of the bronchus," *Human Pathology*, vol. 12, no. 7, pp. 671–673, 1981.

[14] P. H. B. Carstens, J. G. Kuhns, and C. Ghazi, "Primary malignant melanomas of the lung and adrenal," *Human Pathology*, vol. 15, no. 10, pp. 910–914, 1984.

[15] P. Cagle, M. L. Mace, D. M. Judge, R. B. Teague, R. K. Wilson, and S. D. Greenberg, "Pulmonary melanoma. Primary vs metastatic," *CHEST*, vol. 85, no. 1, pp. 125-126, 1984.

[16] S. L. Demeter, C. Fuenning, and J. B. Miller, "Primary malignant melanoma of the lower respiratory tract: endoscopic identification," *Cleveland Clinic Journal of Medicine*, vol. 54, no. 4, pp. 305–308, 1987.

[17] A. A. Alghanem, J. Mehan, and A. A. Hassan, "Primary malignant melanoma of the lung," *Journal of Surgical Oncology*, vol. 34, no. 2, pp. 109–112, 1987.

[18] F. Santos, L. M. Entrenas, F. Sebastian et al., "Primary bronchopulmonary malignant melanoma: case report," *Scandinavian Cardiovascular Journal*, vol. 21, no. 2, pp. 187–189, 1987.

[19] S. P. Bagwell, S. D. Flynn, P. M. Cox, and J. A. Davison, "Primary malignant melanoma of the lung," *American Review of Respiratory Disease*, vol. 139, no. 6, pp. 1543–1547, 1989.

[20] G. Bertola, B. Pasquotti, S. Morassut, S. Massarut, R. Sigon, and C. Rossi, "Primary lung melanoma," *Italian Journal of Surgical Sciences*, vol. 19, no. 2, pp. 187–189, 1989.

[21] D. Ost, C. Joseph, H. Sogoloff, and G. Menezes, "Primary pulmonary melanoma: case report and literature review," *Mayo Clinic Proceedings*, vol. 74, no. 1, pp. 62–66, 1999.

[22] N. B. Erdal, Z. Karakurt, I. Pandul, and C. Tahaoğlu, "A case report: primary pulmonary melanoma," *Turkish Respiratory Journal*, vol. 1, no. 1, pp. 72–74, 2000.

[23] A. Dountsis, C. Zisis, E. Karagianni, and J. Dahabreh, "Primary malignant melanoma of the lung: a case report," *World Journal of Surgical Oncology*, vol. 1, article 26, 2003.

[24] V. S. Reddy, J. Mykytenko, L. I. Giltman, and K. A. Mansour, "Primary malignant melanoma of the lung: review of literature and report of a case," *The American Surgeon*, vol. 73, no. 3, pp. 287–289, 2007.

[25] B. Zuckermann, M. Papiashvilli, and I. Bar, "Primary pulmonary malignant melanoma of right upper lobe of lung," *Israel Medical Association Journal*, vol. 13, no. 7, pp. 440-441, 2011.

[26] E. Seitelman, P. Donenfeld, K. Kay, K. Takabe, S. Andaz, and S. Fox, "Successful treatment of primary pulmonary melanoma," *Journal of Thoracic Disease*, vol. 3, no. 3, pp. 207-208, 2011.

[27] S. Neri, T. Komatsu, J. Kitamura, K. Otsuka, N. Katakami, and Y. Takahashi, "Malignant melanoma of the lung: report of two cases," *Annals of Thoracic and Cardiovascular Surgery*, vol. 17, no. 2, pp. 170–173, 2011.

[28] L. Gong, X. Liu, W. Zhang et al., "Primary pulmonary malignant melanoma: a clinicopathologic study of two cases," *Diagnostic Pathology*, vol. 7, no. 1, article 123, 2012.

[29] A. Ouarssani, F. Atoini, R. Reda, F. A. Lhou, and M. I. Rguibi, "Malignant melanoma of the lung: a case report," *Pan African Medical Journal*, vol. 11, article 68, 2012.

[30] C. L. Dos Santos, L. R. Fernandes, M. Meruje, and F. Barata, "Primary pulmonary melanoma: the unexpected tumor," *BMJ Case Reports*, 2013.

[31] K. Kamaleshwaran, S. Natarajan, J. Parthiban, S. Mehta, K. Radhakrishnan, and A. Shinto, "Rare case of extradural spinal metastasis from primary lung malignant melanoma detected with fluorine-18 fluorodeoxyglucose-positron emission tomography/computed tomography," *Indian Journal of Nuclear Medicine*, vol. 29, no. 1, pp. 57-58, 2014.

[32] X. Zhang, Y. Wang, and J. Du, "Primary malignant melanoma of left lower lobe of lung: a case report and review of the literature," *Oncology Letters*, vol. 10, no. 1, pp. 528–530, 2015.

[33] A. Gupta, D. Bhattacharya, S. Jain, and J. C. Suri, "Primary malignant melanoma of the lung: case report and literature review," *The Indian Journal of Chest Diseases & Allied Sciences*, vol. 57, no. 3, pp. 181–184, 2015.

[34] K. Postrzech-Adamczyk, M. Chabowski, B. Głuszczyk-Ferenc et al., "Malignant melanoma of the lung: case series," *Kardiochirurgia i Torakochirurgia Polska*, vol. 12, no. 1, pp. 72–76, 2015.

[35] K. Hwang, K. Hwang, J. Jung et al., "Primary pulmonary malignant melanoma: an unexpected tumor," *Tuberculosis and Respiratory Diseases*, vol. 78, no. 3, pp. 272–275, 2015.

[36] A. Filippini, F. Zorzi, C. Bna', A. Arnaboldi, and T. Sabatini, "Dark sputum: an atypical presentation of primary pulmonary malignant melanoma," *Respiratory Medicine Case Reports*, vol. 15, pp. 118–120, 2015.

[37] S. R. Kim, H.-Y. Yoon, G. Y. Jin, Y. H. Choe, S. Y. Park, and Y. C. Lee, "Pulmonary malignant melanoma with distant metastasis assessed by positron emission tomography-computed tomography," *Thoracic Cancer*, vol. 7, no. 4, pp. 503–507, 2016.

[38] Y. Feng, J. Zhao, Q. Yang et al., "Pulmonary melanoma and "crazy paving" patterns in chest images: a case report and literature review," *BMC Cancer*, vol. 16, no. 1, article 592, 2016.

[39] R. Maeda, N. Isowa, H. Onuma, H. Miura, H. Tokuyasu, and Y. Kawasaki, "Primary malignant melanoma of the lung with rapid progression," *General Thoracic and Cardiovascular Surgery*, vol. 57, no. 12, pp. 671–674, 2009.

[40] K. Singh, M. C. Sharma, D. Jain, and R. Kumar, "Melanotic medullary carcinoma of thyroid—report of a rare case with brief review of literature," *Diagnostic Pathology*, vol. 3, no. 1, article no. 2, 2008.

[41] K. Iihara, K. Yamaguchi, Y. Fujioka, and S. Uno, "Pigmented neuroendocrine tumor of the lung, showing neuromelanin," *Pathology International*, vol. 52, no. 11, pp. 734–739, 2002.

[42] R. P. Petersen, S. I. Hanish, J. C. Haney et al., "Improved survival with pulmonary metastasectomy: an analysis of 1720 patients with pulmonary metastatic melanoma," *The Journal of Thoracic and Cardiovascular Surgery*, vol. 133, no. 1, pp. 104.e2–110.e2, 2007.

[43] D. Apostolos and C. Zisis, "Primary malignant melanoma of the lung: a case report," *World Journal of Surgical Oncology*, vol. 1, no. 26, 2003.

[44] R. Dummer, A. Hauschild, N. Lindenblatt, G. Pentheroudakis, and U. Keilholz, "Cutaneous melanoma: ESMO clinical practice guidelines for diagnosis, treatment and follow-up," *Annals of Oncology*, vol. 26, supplement 5, pp. v126–v132, 2015.

[45] G. V. Long, A. M. Menzies, A. M. Nagrial et al., "Prognostic and clinicopathologic associations of oncogenic BRAF in metastatic melanoma," *Journal of Clinical Oncology*, vol. 29, no. 10, pp. 1239–1246, 2011.

[46] P. A. Ascierto, D. Minor, A. Ribas et al., "Phase II trial (BREAK-2) of the BRAF inhibitor dabrafenib (GSK2118436) in patients with metastatic melanoma," *Journal of Clinical Oncology*, vol. 31, no. 26, pp. 3205–3211, 2013.

[47] S. Yun, N. D. Vincelette, M. R. Green, A. E. Wahner Hendrickson, and I. Abraham, "Targeting immune checkpoints in unresectable metastatic cutaneous melanoma: a systematic review and meta-analysis of anti-CTLA-4 and anti-PD-1 agents trials," *Cancer Medicine*, vol. 5, no. 7, pp. 1481–1491, 2016.

[48] S. Ugurel, J. Röhmel, P. A. Ascierto et al., "Survival of patients with advanced metastatic melanoma: the impact of novel therapies," *European Journal of Cancer*, vol. 53, pp. 125–134, 2016.

9

Outcomes of a Clinical Pathway for Pleural Disease Management: "Pleural Pathway"

Srinivas R. Mummadi and Peter Y. Hahn

Department of Pulmonary and Critical Care Medicine, Metro Health-University of Michigan Health, Suite 220, 2122 Health Dr. SW, Wyoming, MI 49519, USA

Correspondence should be addressed to Srinivas R. Mummadi; m.srinivasreddy@gmail.com

Academic Editor: Charlie Strange

Background and Objectives. Clinical pathways are evidence based multidisciplinary team approaches to optimize patient care. Pleural diseases are common and accounted for 3.4 billion US $ in 2014 US inpatient aggregate charges (HCUPnet data). An institutional clinical pathway ("pleural pathway") was implemented in conjunction with a dedicated pleural service. Design, implementation, and outcomes of the pleural pathway (from August 1, 2014, to July 31, 2015) in comparison to a previous era (from August 1, 2013, to July 31, 2014) are described. *Methods.* Tuality Healthcare is a 215-bed community healthcare system in Hillsboro, OR, USA. With the objective of standardizing pleural disease care, locally adapted British Thoracic Society guidelines and a centralized pleural service were implemented in the *"pathway"* era. System-wide consensus regarding institutional guidelines for care of pleural disease was achieved. Preimplementation activities included training, acquisition of ultrasound equipment, and system-wide education. An audit database was set up with the intent of prospective audits. An administrative database was used for harvesting outcomes data and comparing them with the *"prior to pathway"* era. *Results.* 54 unique consults were performed. A total of 55 ultrasound examinations and 60 pleural procedures were performed. All-cause inpatient pleural admissions were lower in the "pathway" era ($n = 9$) compared to the "prior to pathway" era ($n = 17$). Gains in average case charges (21,737$ versus 18,818.2$/case) and average length of stay (3.65 versus 2.78 days/case) were seen in the "pathway" era. *Conclusion.* A "pleural pathway" and a centralized pleural service are associated with reduction in case charges, inpatient admissions, and length of stay for pleural conditions.

1. Introduction

Clinical pathways have been described as evidence based multidisciplinary team approaches to optimize patient care for a presenting clinical diagnosis [1, 2]. Salutary effects on patient outcomes, length of stay, and hospital costs have been observed with implementation of clinical pathways [3]. Pleural diseases are common and accounted for 3.4 billion US $ in 2014 US inpatient aggregate charges ("National Bill" as estimated by HCUPnet, a query system based on Healthcare Cost and Utilization Project [HCUP] data) [4]. Due to wide variation in practice styles for managing initial manifestations of pleural disease [5, 6], an institutional clinical pathway ("pleural pathway") adapted from the British Thoracic Society (BTS) pleural disease guidelines [7–11] was implemented in conjunction with a dedicated pleural service [12, 13]. We hypothesized that improved inpatient outcomes (lower average length of stay, charges, and admissions) would have resulted due to the implementation of a pleural pathway. A narrative on the design, implementation, and outcomes of the pleural pathway in comparison to the prior era is provided in this manuscript. Some of the results of this study were previously reported in the form of an abstract [14].

2. Methods

2.1. Design. A descriptive observational study design was used for studying outcomes of a clinical pathway and a centralized pleural disease service in a community healthcare system.

2.2. Setting. Tuality Healthcare (An Oregon Health & Science University [Portland, OR] partner) is a 215-bed healthcare system in Hillsboro, OR, USA. It is comprised of two hospitals and additional outpatient treatment facilities. Outpatient and inpatient consultative services for pulmonary disease are provided by pulmonary consultants and thoracic surgeons with procedural support from radiology. Pleural disease management prior to the introduction of the pleural pathway was provided using the following modalities:

(1) Large spontaneous pneumothoraces: emergency room (ER) insertion of large bore chest tubes (>14 F) was followed by inpatient admission and general/thoracic surgery consultation.

(2) Unilateral pleural effusions presenting with mediastinal shift were admitted to the hospital. Stable unilateral pleural effusions were aspirated in the scheduled outpatient radiology setting and followed by the referring physician.

(3) Non-ultrasound-guided management of pleural diseases was carried out in the pulmonary clinic.

(4) Prolonged air leaks (secondary spontaneous pneumothorax, postoperative) were managed with watchful waiting and if needed via surgical intervention by thoracic surgery.

(5) Fibrinolytics (tPA + DNase) were not used in management of empyema.

In May 2014, an institutional need was felt for standardizing pleural disease care in response to observed institutional variation in pleural care and low performance on a publicly reportable healthcare quality measure (Patient Safety Indicator # 6 measuring rates of iatrogenic pneumothorax). In response to the need, locally adapted BTS 2010 pleural guidelines [7–11] were devised by the author (SM). Two thoracic ultrasound and pleural procedures, trained pulmonary physicians, and a nurse practitioner constituted the pleural service. Key deviations from the BTS guidelines included using noncontrast CT scan for further diagnostic imaging of an aspirated unilateral pleural effusion, narrow bore (8 F) chest tube and Heimlich valve insertion for outpatient management of primary spontaneous pneumothorax, and use of intrabronchial valves for prolonged air leaks (see Supplementary Materials (available here)). When indicated, pleuroscopic examination and parietal pleural biopsies were performed by a pulmonary physician aided by an anesthesiologist administered moderate sedation. Overnight hospital observation was performed after pleuroscopy procedure. Gravity assisted thoracentesis drainage was adopted institutionally.

A system-wide consensus was generated via multidisciplinary efforts across diverse division meetings (Emergency Department, Pulmonary & Hospital Medicine, General & Thoracic Surgery, Interventional Radiology, Primary Care) over a span of 3 months. Approvals for institutional guidelines emphasizing patient safety (ultrasound assistance for pleural procedures in the nonradiology setting [15, 16], nurse driven "pleural checklists" [17]) and turnaround time (inpatient pleural consults answered within 24 hours; 72 hours for outpatients palliated in the ER and assured follow-up in the pulmonary clinic for discharged patients) were sought and buy-in was secured from all the stakeholders. Algorithms for management of unilateral pleural effusions (exudative, transudative, malignant, hemothorax, empyema) and spontaneous pneumothoraces (8 F chest tube coupled with a self-contained Heimlich valve apparatus as the primary modality) were approved and disseminated throughout the institution. Shift towards ambulatory care of unilateral pleural effusions was promoted to primary care teams in monthly primary care administrative meetings. Admission avoidance was stated as an intended benefit. In preparation, pleural supply carts (narrow bore chest tubes [8 F], medium bore chest tubes [14 F], Heimlich valves, thoracentesis kits) were designed and standardized across multiple locations (pulmonary clinic, ER, and the intensive care unit). Ultrasound machines with high and low frequency probes were already available in the ER and intensive care unit. Pulmonary clinic acquired a new low frequency probe and shared the existing ultrasound machine/high frequency probe with endocrinology clinic. In addition, minimally invasive interventions for prolonged air leaks (bronchoscopic insertion of IBV® valves) were promoted institutionally. Funding support was obtained from the hospital and aided by building a business case centered on cost effectiveness of coordinated pleural care, usage of ultrasound, and potential to improve upon the publicly reported quality measures. Preimplementation system-wide education [7] (didactic lectures, simulated and supervised practice of chest tube care, fibrinolytic installation) was completed for all the nursing units involved in the care of pleural disease patients before the "go-live" date.

Outpatient and inpatient pleural consults were channelled via a "pleural pathway" with the pleural consultative service as the cornerstone starting on August 1, 2014.

An audit database (Microsoft Excel, Redmond, Washington, USA) was set up with the intent of prospective audits and capturing data about patients seen through this pathway. Database management support was provided by a trained medical assistant. A one-year audit was performed by comparing outcomes data from the "pathway" era (from August 1, 2014, to July 31, 2015) with a "prior to pathway" era (from August 1, 2013, to July 31, 2014). Outcomes data such as number, type of diagnostic and therapeutic procedures, ultrasound examinations performed, and adverse events were restricted to pleural pathway patients and housed in the audit database.

Data for average case charge (US $), average length of stay (LOS) in days, and number of inpatient admissions in both eras were extracted utilizing the visual analytic tools of a subscription service focusing on care variation (Crimson Clinical Advantage Continuum of Care, Release CCC.2016.09. Isaac Newton, Washington, DC, USA). These data are derived from coding and billing records of the institution and are restricted to inpatients. The following diagnosis-related group (DRG) codes [18] were used to define pleural diseases during the analysis: 187 (pleural effusion *with* complication or comorbidity [CC]), 188 (pleural effusion *without* complication or comorbidity [CC] and major complication or comorbidity [MCC]), 199 (pneumothorax *with* MCC), 200 (pneumothorax *with* CC), and 201 (pneumothorax *without* CC and MCC). Examples of conditions that define major comorbidity (MCC)/comorbidity (CC) are provided in footnotes of Table 2.

Information regarding annual number of inpatient admissions and ER visits was obtained from the Department of Finance's comparative statistics detail report. An exemption for institutional review board's review and need for individual consent was granted by Western IRB (submission tracking number 1-900642-1).

3. Results

Hospital recorded 3,549 inpatient admissions in the "prior to pathway" era and 3,154 inpatient admissions in the "pathway" era. Emergency room (ER) recorded 31,232 visits in the "prior to pathway" era and 32,688 visits in the "pathway" era.

Audit findings during the pathway era are described in Table 1. 54 unique pleural consults spanning over ER, inpatient and outpatient domains, were provided during the pathway era. All the consults were performed as stated in the institutional guidelines (i.e., inpatient pleural consults answered within 24 hours; 72 hours for outpatients palliated in the ER and assured follow-up in the pulmonary clinic for discharged patients). There was no documented follow-up for 7 consultations due to patients' preferences. Complications recorded in the audit are as follows: pain during fluid drainage phase of thoracentesis (n = 5), iatrogenic pneumothoraces (n = 2), chest drain dislodgement (n = 3). One case of subcutaneous emphysema was recorded in the audit. Additional information regarding complications is provided in Table 1.

Outcomes data for pleural conditions are presented in Table 2. Overall, all-cause pleural inpatient admissions were lower in the pathway era (17 in the "prior to pathway" era versus 9 in the "pathway" era). This was accompanied by lower average case charges (21,737 versus 18,818.2$) and lower average length of stay (3.65 versus 2.78 days).

While pleural effusion with significant comorbid conditions saw a decrease in charges, there was no observed decrease in LOS and inpatient admissions. Pleural effusion with no associated comorbidities saw an increase in case charges with no change in LOS.

Pneumothorax irrespective of associated comorbidity saw a decrease in the number of inpatient admissions, length of stay, and average case charges.

4. Discussion

This study is the first in North America describing a dedicated ambulatory/inpatient pleural clinical pathway and associated gains in the efficiency domain of healthcare quality [19]. Recent developments in advancing the diagnosis and management of pleural disease call for a redesigned care model in tune with the modern definition of healthcare quality [19]. Emergency admissions for pleural effusions are recognized as a contributor to the inefficiency of healthcare [20] and are a target for admission avoidance in the UK [13]. Outpatient treatment of primary spontaneous pneumothoraces using an 8 F narrow bore chest tube and Heimlich valve has been shown to be safe and cost effective [21, 22]. Intrapleural t-PA and DNase have been shown to improve the drainage, length of stay, and the frequency of surgical intervention in empyema. Indwelling pleural catheters have replaced repeated thoracentesis as the primary modality for management of malignant pleural effusions [23, 24]. Despite the recognition of pleural medicine as a distinct subspecialty, a recent audit in the UK found that only 21% of facilities (serving 33 million patients) incorporated a specialist pleural disease clinic [25]. Changes in institutional practice guidelines augmented by education [26] and audit have been shown to positively impact the outcomes in pleural disease [27].

In our analysis, charges for pleural effusion care increased and were offset by a reduction in pneumothorax charges. In 1996, a small randomized trial found similar savings with a narrow bore chest tube insertion and ambulatory management of spontaneous pneumothorax patients (cost savings of 5660 US$/patient and savings of 5 bed days per case) [28]. While definite attribution is difficult, it is likely that the usage of moderate sedation and overnight in-hospital observation for pleuroscopy cases (performed for undiagnosed exudative pleural effusions) have played a role in the increase of pleural effusion costs. Recently a multicenter experience reported local anesthetic pleuroscopy with the same day discharge as safe, effective, and efficient suggesting further room for cost savings [29].

Resources are needed for a functional pleural pathway including training, acquisition of ultrasound machines, and associated probes housed in nonradiology settings. However, it is likely that such investment yields returns by enhancing timely and safe care [30]. Delay in acquiring outpatient ultrasound scans due to radiology scheduling load contributes to costs of 24,890 US $ per annum [30]. A non-ultrasound-guided thoracentesis complicated by a pneumothorax increases the cost of hospitalization by $ 2,801 and increases the length of stay by 1.5 days [31]. Costs for iatrogenic pneumothorax escalate once the patient is hospitalized [32]. It is essential that physician champions utilize such data in their funding requests to the senior leadership. An important component of this pathway was the role of ER physicians adopting the institutional guidelines for the management of unilateral pleural effusions and spontaneous pneumothoraces in achieving the goals of this pathway [33]. This is a crucial factor in determining the success of a pleural pathway.

Complications observed in our series deserve further attention. 7.3% of inserted drains fell out in a recent British audit highlighting the need for improvement in securement strategies [25]. 14% (3/21 insertions) of chest drains dislodged in our audit suggesting that it is an important area for further quality improvement.

There are several methodological limitations to our study. Administrative databases were used for cost effectiveness metrics and were restricted to inpatients. Inpatient charges were utilized as surrogate for costs. Information was lacking about outpatient charges including radiology procedures. It is also possible that not all patients presenting with pleural conditions were channelled via the pleural pathway. Audit data

Table 1: Key findings from the audit during the pathway era (from August 1, 2014, to July 31, 2015).

Characteristics	Results
Age at evaluation	63 (56–75)
Median (IQR)—yr.	
Female sex—no. (%)	15 (40.5)
Unique consults*—no.	54
Initial consult location—no. (%)	
Emergency department	12 (22.2)
Outpatient	20 (37)
Inpatient	22 (40.7)
Consults with documented follow up—no. (%)	47 (87)
Ultrasound examinations—no.	55
Primary pleural diagnosis—no.	40
Primary spontaneous pneumothorax	3
Secondary spontaneous pneumothorax	5
Traumatic pneumothorax	4
Noninfectious and nonmalignant exudative effusions	7
Empyema[∂]	3
Paramalignant effusion	4
Malignant pleural effusion	5
Transudate effusions	5
Others (giant bullae, indwelling IPC s/p pleurodesis, normal pleural ultrasound exam)	4
Pleural procedures—no.	60
8 F chest tube insertion[π]	6
14 F chest tube insertion	4
>14 F chest tube insertion[†]	8
Thoracentesis	26
Indwelling pleural catheter (IPC) insertion	3
IPC removal[Ω]	1
Pleuroscopy (with and without pleural biopsy)	3
IBV® valve insertion[ß]	3
VATS assisted bleb resection[Δ]	3
Surgical decortication	3
Complications—no.	14
Pain during fluid drainage	5
Iatrogenic pneumothorax[¶]	2
ER evaluation due to patient concerns[$]	2
Chest drain dislodgement[‡]	3
IPC track metastasis	1
Subcutaneous emphysema	1

*8 patients had more than one unique consult due to recurrent disease on the same or contralateral side. There were 37 unique patients in the audit. [∂]These patients received initial fibrinolytic treatment (tPA + DNase). [π]8 F tube with an inbuilt Heimlich valve apparatus. [†]Two insertions were in the setting of secondary spontaneous pneumothoraces with acute respiratory failure and one insertion to palliate a concurrent large pleural effusion and an iatrogenic pneumothorax. Five insertions were in the postoperative setting; [Ω]Removed in the ER (after pleurodesis confirmation) in the context of a Health Information Exchange alert about multiple area ER visits for a "nonfunctional catheter." [ß]IBV Valve (Spiration, Redmond, WA, USA) is a unidirectional valve that blocks air entry distally and is inserted via a bronchoscopic procedure. In our series, all of them were inserted in prolonged air leaks due to secondary spontaneous pneumothoraces. [Δ]Video assisted thoracoscopy. [¶]One of the episodes required an ambulatory 8 F chest tube. 2nd episode required hospital admission due to lack of credible follow-up. [$]Emergency room evaluation related to patient concerned about serosanguinous discharge into the ambulatory 8 F chest tube. [‡]None of the dislodged chest tubes required reinsertion.

TABLE 2: Outcomes data for inpatient pleural care (DRG codes) during the two eras: "prior to pathway" versus "pathway."

Pleural condition	Inpatient admissions in prior to pathway era	Inpatient admissions during pathway era	Average LOS in prior to pathway era (days)	Average LOS during pathway era (days)	Average case charges in prior to pathway era ($)	Average case charges during pathway era ($)
Pleural effusion with MCC[¥] & CC[∞]	4	3	3.00	3.00	22,884.7	17,092
Pleural effusion without MCC[¥] & CC[∞]	3	3	2.67	2.67	12,874.3	24,081.6
Pneumothorax with MCC[¥]	3	0	5.67	0	36,637.3	0
Pneumothorax with CC[∞]	5	2	2.80	3.00	18,706.6	14,277.5
Pneumothorax without CC[∞] & MCC[¥]	2	1	5.50	2.00	17,967	11,563
Overall pleural conditions	17	9	3.65	2.78	21,737	18,818.2

[¥]MCC: major complications/comorbid conditions such as congestive heart failure, stroke, coma, acute MI, HIV, acute respiratory failure, and cardiac arrest.
[∞]CC: complications/comorbid conditions such as angina, delirium, dementia, anemia, cachexia, and COPD with exacerbation.

were not available on patients outside the pathway during the study period. A cost benefit analysis incorporating input costs was not performed. Lack of propensity matching and an interrupted-time series design impacts the validity of these findings. We acknowledge that our series has a relatively small sample size and is based on a retrospective and limited time frame of observation. Lack of control cohorts in the baseline and the intervention period is a significant limitation. However, no prior attempts exist in reporting improvements in processes/outcomes after implementation of coordinated pleural care. We believe our study should be viewed as an attempt in stimulating further research in this field.

In conclusion, we report the evolution of a clinical pathway and a centralized pleural service for the care of pleural disease in a community healthcare system. Lower case charges and length of stay were observed for inpatient pleural conditions, largely mediated by strides in pneumothorax management. However, these findings need further study.

Additional Points

Summary at a Glance. A descriptive narrative of a clinical pathway for pleural disease is the focus of this manuscript. Administrative data (charges, length of stay) were examined in *"before"* and *"during"* clinical pathway eras. Our study offers a real-life model of efficient pleural disease care.

References

[1] J. Cheah, "Development and implementation of a clinical pathway programme in an acute care general hospital in Singapore," *International Journal for Quality in Health Care*, vol. 12, no. 5, pp. 403–412, 2000.

[2] L. Kinsman, T. Rotter, E. James, P. Snow, and J. Willis, "What is a clinical pathway? Development of a definition to inform the debate," *BMC Medicine*, vol. 8, no. 1, 2010.

[3] T. Rotter, L. Kinsman, E. James et al., "Clinical pathways: effects on professional practice, patient outcomes, length of stay and hospital costs," *The Cochrane Database of Systematic Reviews*, vol. 3, Article ID CD006632, 2010.

[4] HCUPnet, *Healthcare Cost and Utilization Project (HCUP)*, Agency for Healthcare Research and Quality, Rockville, MD, USA, 2014, http://hcupnet.ahrq.gov/.

[5] T. L. R. Medicine, "Pleural medicine-rethinking practice to improve patient care," *The Lancet Respiratory medicine*, vol. 3, no. 7, p. 497, 2015.

[6] H. Elsayed, W. Kent, J. McShane, R. Page, and M. Shackcloth, "Treatment of pneumothoraces at a tertiary centre: Are we following the current guidelines?" *Interactive CardioVascular and Thoracic Surgery*, vol. 12, no. 3, pp. 430–433, 2011.

[7] T. Havelock, R. Teoh, D. Laws, and F. Gleeson, "Pleural procedures and thoracic ultrasound: British Thoracic Society Pleural Disease Guideline 2010," *Thorax*, vol. 65, supplement 2, pp. i61–i76, 2010.

[8] A. MacDuff, A. Arnold, and J. Harvey, "Management of spontaneous pneumothorax: British Thoracic Society pleural disease guideline 2010," *Thorax*, vol. 65, no. 2, pp. ii18–ii31, 2010.

[9] H. E. Davies, R. J. O. Davies, and C. W. H. Davies, "Management of pleural infection in adults: British Thoracic Society Pleural Disease Guideline 2010," *Thorax*, vol. 65, supplement 2, pp. ii41–ii53, 2010.

[10] M. E. Roberts, E. Neville, R. G. Berrisford, G. Antunes, and N. J. Ali, "Management of a malignant pleural effusion: British Thoracic Society pleural disease guideline 2010," *Thorax*, vol. 65, no. 2, pp. ii32–ii40, 2010.

[11] C. Hooper, Y. C. G. Lee, and N. Maskell, "Investigation of a unilateral pleural effusion in adults: British Thoracic Society

pleural disease guideline 2010," *Thorax*, vol. 65, supplement 2, pp. ii4–ii17, 2010.

[12] C. E. Hooper, Y. C. G. Lee, and N. A. Maskell, "Setting up a specialist pleural disease service," *Respirology*, vol. 15, no. 7, pp. 1028–1036, 2010.

[13] R. L. Young, R. Bhatnagar, A. R. L. Medford, and N. A. Maskell, "Evaluation of an ambulatory pleural service: Costs and benefits," *British Journal of Hospital Medicine*, vol. 76, no. 10, p. 608, 2015.

[14] S. R. Mummadi, L. Bettencourt, and P. Y. Hahn, "Outcomes Of A Dedicated Pleural Service In A Healthcare System," *American Journal of Respiratory and Critical Care Medicine*, vol. 193, 2016.

[15] A. Perazzo, P. Gatto, C. Barlascini, M. Ferrari-Bravo, and A. Nicolini, "Can ultrasound guidance reduce the risk of pneumothorax following thoracentesis?" *Jornal Brasileiro de Pneumologia*, vol. 40, no. 1, pp. 6–12, 2014.

[16] P. A. Patel, F. R. Ernst, and C. L. Gunnarsson, "Ultrasonography guidance reduces complications and costs associated with thoracentesis procedures," *Journal of Clinical Ultrasound*, vol. 40, no. 3, pp. 135–141, 2012.

[17] K. C. See, K. Jamil, A. P. Chua, J. Phua, K. L. Khoo, and T. K. Lim, "Effect of a pleural checklist on patient safety in the ultrasound era," *Respirology*, vol. 18, no. 3, pp. 534–539, 2013.

[18] R. B. Fetter, Y. Shin, J. L. Freeman, R. F. Averill, and J. D. Thompson, "Case mix definition by diagnosis-related groups," *Medical Care*, vol. 18, 2, pp. 1–53, 1980.

[19] Institute of Medicine Committee on Quality of Health Care in America, *Crossing the Quality Chasm: A New Health System for the 21st Century*, National Academies Press, Washington, DC, USA, 2001, Copyright by the National Academy of Sciences. All rights reserved.

[20] M. Botana Rial, V. L. Fernández, C. R. Represas, A. P. Sanmartín, V. del Campo Pérez, and A. Fernández-Villar, "Cost-Effectiveness Study of the Diagnosis of Pleural Effusion in Chest Diseases Outpatient Clinic," *Arch Bronconeumol*, vol. 46, no. 9, pp. 473–478, 2010.

[21] T. Tsuchiya and A. Sano, "Outpatient Treatment of Pneumothorax with a Thoracic Vent: Economic Benefit," *Respiration*, vol. 90, no. 1, pp. 33–39, 2015.

[22] S. M. Lai and A. K. Tee, "Outpatient treatment of primary spontaneous pneumothorax using a small-bore chest drain with a Heimlich valve: the experience of a Singapore emergency department," *European Journal of Emergency Medicine*, vol. 19, no. 6, pp. 400–404, 2012.

[23] M. Shafiq, K. D. Frick, H. Lee, L. Yarmus, and D. J. Feller-Kopman, "Management of Malignant Pleural Effusion: A Cost-Utility Analysis," *Journal of bronchology interventional pulmonology*, vol. 22, no. 3, pp. 215–225, 2015.

[24] R. C. Boshuizen, S. Onderwater, S. J. A. Burgers, and M. M. Van Den Heuvel, "The use of indwelling pleural catheters for the management of malignant pleural effusion - Direct costs in a dutch hospital," *Respiration*, vol. 86, no. 3, pp. 224–228, 2013.

[25] C. Hooper and N. Maskell, "British Thoracic Society national pleural procedures audit 2010," *Thorax*, vol. 66, no. 7, pp. 636-637, 2011.

[26] D. R. Duncan, T. I. Morgenthaler, J. H. Ryu, and C. E. Daniels, "Reducing iatrogenic risk in thoracentesis: Establishing best practice via experiential training in a zero-risk environment," *Chest*, vol. 135, no. 5, pp. 1315–1320, 2009.

[27] K. Cantwell, S. Burgess, I. Patrick et al., "Improvement in the prehospital recognition of tension pneumothorax: The effect of a change to paramedic guidelines and education," *Injury*, vol. 45, no. 1, pp. 71–76, 2014.

[28] M. Roeggla, G. Roeggla, M. Muellner, A. Wagner, and A. N. Laggner, "The cost of treatment of spontaneous pneumothorax with the thoracic vent compared with conventional thoracic drainage," *Chest*, vol. 110, no. 1, p. 303, 1996.

[29] I. Psallidas, J. P. Corcoran, J. Fallon et al., "Provision of Day-Case Local Anesthetic Thoracoscopy: A Multicenter Review of Practice," *Chest*, vol. 151, no. 2, pp. 511-512, 2017.

[30] K. Bateman, D. Downey, and T. Teare, "Thoracic ultrasound for pleural effusion: Delays and cost associated with departmental scanning," *Respiratory Medicine*, vol. 104, no. 4, pp. 612–614, 2010.

[31] C. J. Mercaldi and S. F. Lanes, "Ultrasound guidance decreases complications and improves the cost of care among patients undergoing thoracentesis and paracentesis," *Chest*, vol. 143, no. 2, pp. 532–538, 2013.

[32] H. G. Colt and T. Matsuo, "Hospital charges attributable to bronchoscopy-related complications in outpatients," *Respiration*, vol. 68, no. 1, pp. 67–72, 2001.

[33] E. Weldon and J. Williams, "Pleural Disease in the Emergency Department," *Emergency Medicine Clinics of North America*, vol. 30, no. 2, pp. 475–499, 2012.

10

Positive Retrospective SARS-CoV-2 Testing in a Case of Acute Respiratory Distress Syndrome of Unknown Etiology

A. Burkett,[1] S. McElwee,[2] C. Margaroli,[3] P. Bajpai,[1] A. Elkholy,[1] U. Manne,[1] K. Wille,[3] and P. Benson[1]

[1]*Department of Pathology, Division of Anatomic Pathology, University of Alabama at Birmingham, Birmingham, Alabama, USA*
[2]*Department of Medicine, Division of Cardiovascular Disease, University of Alabama at Birmingham, Birmingham, Alabama, USA*
[3]*Department of Medicine, Division of Pulmonary, Allergy & Critical Care Medicine, University of Alabama at Birmingham, Birmingham, Alabama, USA*

Correspondence should be addressed to P. Benson; pvbenson@uabmc.edu

Academic Editor: Tun-Chieh Chen

In order to elucidate the cause of acute respiratory distress syndrome of unknown etiology in a pre-pandemic patient, molecular techniques were used for detection of SARS-CoV-2. We used a SARS-CoV-2 nucleocapsid protein immunofluorescence stain to retrospectively identify an individual with diffuse alveolar damage on autopsy histology who had negative respiratory virus panel results in February, 2020, in Birmingham, Alabama. In situ hybridization for SARS-CoV-2 RNA revealed evidence of widespread multiorgan SARS-CoV-2 infection. This death antecedes the first reported death of a State of Alabama resident diagnosed with SARS-CoV-2 by 26 days.

1. Introduction

Though the initial outbreak was described in Wuhan, China, with subsequent spread to the United States by January 2020, it has been assumed that the infection emerged months prior to being recognized by the World Health Organization [1]. The first case of COVID-19 in Alabama was reported on March 12, 2020 [2]. Prior to this report, the first reported death of an Alabama resident with COVID-19 occurred on March 25, 2020 [3]. To determine the cause of acute respiratory distress syndrome (ARDS), molecular techniques for the detection of SARS-CoV-2 were used on autopsy tissue.

2. Case Report

A 79-year-old male with hypertensive cardiovascular disease, heart failure, hyperlipidemia, and diabetes type 2 presented from an outside hospital on February 9, 2020, with acute chest pain and dyspnea. CT angiogram (CTA) showed a Type B dissection and ascending aortic aneurysm. He was transferred to our tertiary care hospital. Work-up revealed metabolic derangement, cardiomegaly with trace pericardial effusion, pleural effusions, and diffuse ground glass opacities suggestive of pulmonary edema. His hospital course was complicated by difficulties maintaining his oxygen saturation, requiring high flow nasal cannula; CTA on February 16 demonstrated the Type B aortic dissection was suggestive of pulmonary embolism and showed ground glass attenuation of the bilateral aerated lung fields and consolidation of the left lower lobe (Figure 1(a)). The patient was advanced to BiPAP without improvement and was transferred to the cardiopulmonary critical care unit for hypoxic respiratory failure, requiring intubation on February 24, 2020. A bronchoscopy confirmed ARDS. A respiratory viral panel was negative for Influenza A (subtype H1, H3 and 2009 H1N1), Influenza B, RSV A and B, Parainfluenza 1, 2, 3, and 4, Human Metapneumovirus, Human Rhinovirus/Enterovirus, Adenovirus, and Coronavirus. On February 25,

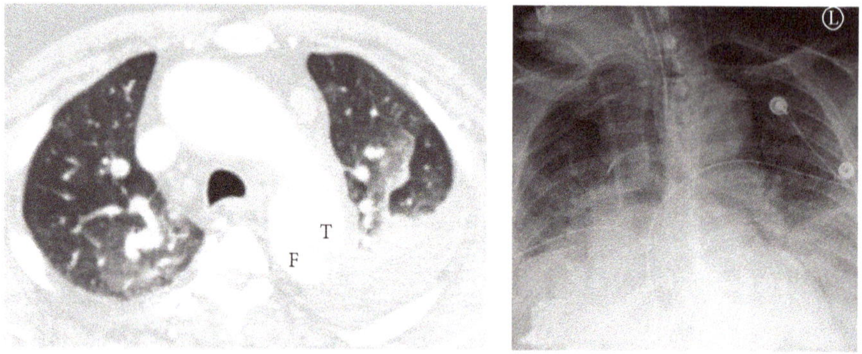

(a) (b)

Figure 1: (a) CTA of chest (February 16, 2020) with Type B aortic dissection (T: true lumen; F: false lumen). (b) Chest X-ray (February 28, 2020) with bilateral pulmonary opacities and pleural effusions.

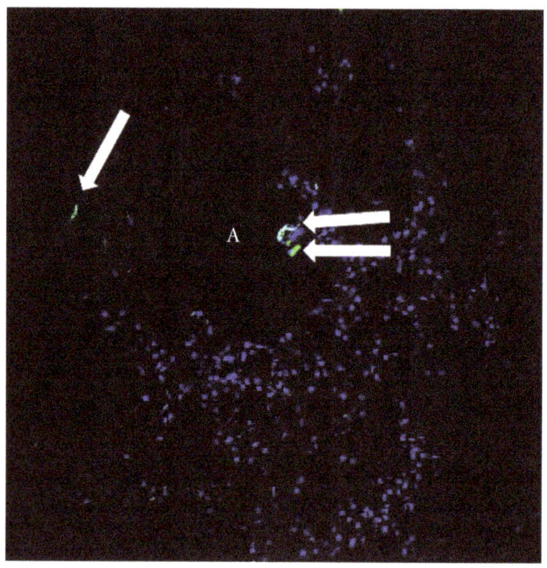

Figure 2: SARS-CoV-2 nucleocapsid protein immunofluorescence in lung. Arrows indicate green positive signal. A = alveolar space. Blue = DAPI nuclear stain.

the patient had PEA arrest, but return of spontaneous circulation was achieved with chest compressions. Chest X-ray on February 28, 2020, showed bilateral pulmonary opacities and pleural effusions (Figure 1(b)). He continued to be unable to maintain oxygen saturation despite intubation and aggressive fluid removal. Death occurred on February 28, 2020.

Written consent for autopsy was obtained from the next of kin including consent for diagnostic, research, and education use; however, no written consent has been obtained from the patient as there is no identifiable patient data included in this case report. Autopsy performed March 2, 2020, showed signs of hypertensive and atherosclerotic cardiovascular disease with severe cardiomegaly (650 g) and four chamber dilatation, nephrosclerosis, and diffuse hypertensive vascular changes within the brain. There was dilation of the aortic root and a Type B aortic dissection extending from the left subclavian artery without rupture. The lungs showed significant bilateral consolidation (combined lung weight of 1970 g) and pulmonary edema without evidence of a pulmonary thromboembolism. Lung histology showed diffuse intra-alveolar hemorrhage and fibrin, with numerous areas showing organizing fibrinous exudates with macrophages and occasional activated type II pneumocytes. Chronic bronchitis and emphysema were present. Immunofluorescence for SARS-CoV-2 nucleocapsid protein was focally positive on one lung section (Figure 2). In situ hybridization (ISH) for SARS-CoV-2 RNA was performed using RNA scope technology (Bio-Techne Corp., Minneapolis, MN). Two RNA probes were used, one for the sense strand of SARS-CoV-2 RNA (turquoise signal) and one for the antisense strand of SARS-CoV-2 RNA (red signal). ISH showed SARS-CoV-2 in the lungs, myocardium, liver, kidneys, and brain (Figures 3 and 4). Both ISH probes showed varying degrees of intensity. The lungs, heart, and brain showed predominantly red signal indicating replicating

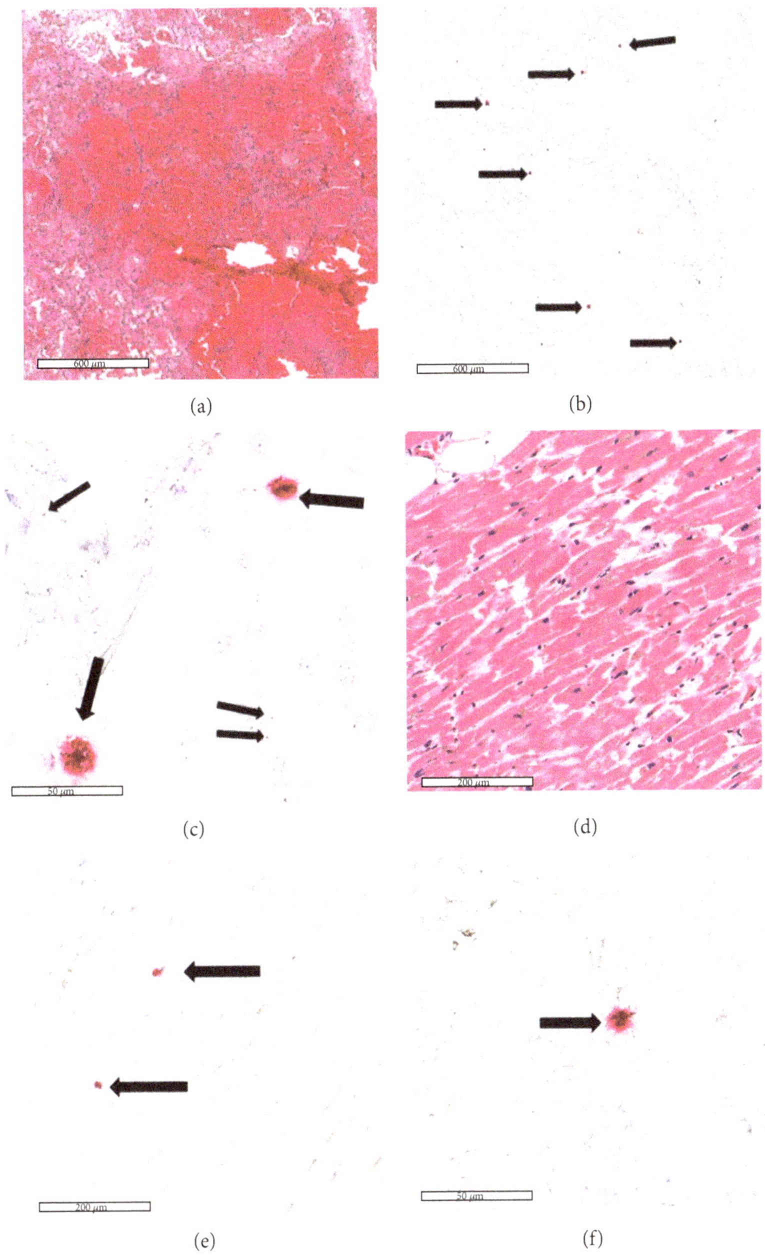

FIGURE 3: (a) Lung H&E 4x (scale bar: 600 μm) with diffuse alveolar hemorrhage and alveolar fibrin. (b) SARS-CoV-2 ISH 4x (scale bar: 50 μm). (c) SARS CoV-2 ISH 40x (scale bar: 50 μm). (d) Heart H&E 20x E: Heart SARS-CoV-2 ISH 20x (scale bar: 200 μm). (f) Heart SARS CoV-2 ISH 40x (scale bar: 50 μm). Black arrows: positive antisense SA RS-CoV-2 RNA probe red signal.

virus. Sections of the liver and kidney showed areas of turquoise signal indicating nonreplicating virus in addition to red replicating virus signal (Figure 4). Replicating virus signal was present in the ependymal lining cells and in the parenchyma of the midbrain (Figure 4(c)).

3. Discussion

Two reports used molecular techniques to show no earlier emergence of COVID-19 in California, USA [4], and Basel, Switzerland [5]. A more recent report successfully identified SARS-CoV-2 in a Canadian renal transplant patient whose death occurred on February 10, 2020 [6]. The case presented here is the first to retrospectively identify a case of lethal SARS-CoV-2 infection with clinical ARDS which predates the first recognized SARS-CoV-2-related death in Alabama by 26 days. Although earlier cases were later detected, the Center for Disease Control reported the first COVID-19 death in Washington State on February 29, 2020, one day later than the case we report here [7]. While the identification of a case demonstrates an earlier communal spread of the SARS-CoV-2 virus, additional retrospective studies are essential in determining the earliest regional and national transmission of the virus. The SARS-CoV-2 RNA ISH showed widespread involvement of multiple organs as would be expected in viremia.

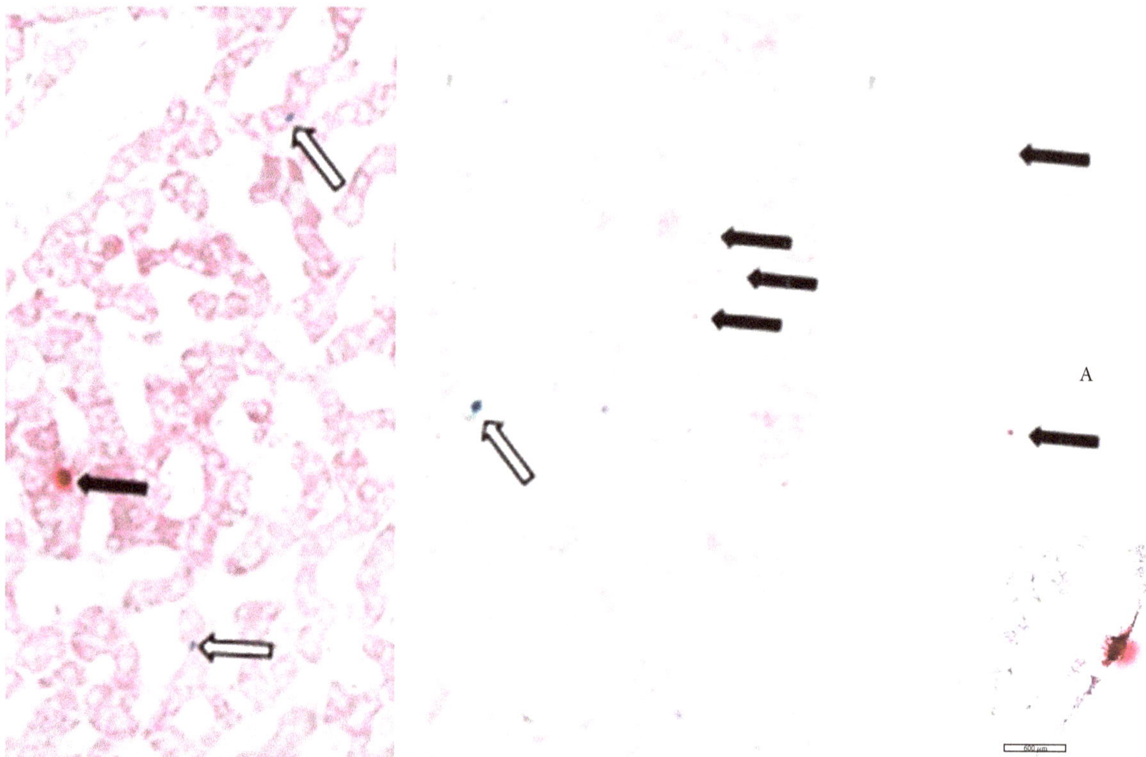

(a) (b) (c)

FIGURE 4: SARS-CoV-2 ISH of the liver (a) and kidney (b) (40x: scale bar, 60 μm) and midbrain (c) (2x: scale bar, 600 μm) and inset 40x (scale bar, 50 μm). A: cerebral aqueduct. Black arrows: red signal (antisense strand RNA-replicating virus). White arrows: turquois signal (sense strand RNA-nonreplicating virus).

4. Conclusion

Our report confirms the presence of SARS-CoV-2 in Alabama 13 days prior to its reported emergence in the state and precedes the first reported SARS-CoV-2 death in Alabama by 26 days. The widespread positive staining for SARS-CoV-2 RNA in the lungs, heart, liver, kidneys, and brain confirmed the disseminated nature of the infection and the cause of the patient's ARDS. Analysis of additional prepandemic autopsy cases may add to the understanding of epidemiology of COVID-19 and provide retrospective answers to clinical questions.

References

[1] M. A. Lauxmann, N. E. Santucci, and A. M. Autrán-Gómez, “The SARS-CoV-2 coronavirus and the COVID-19 outbreak,” *International Brazilian Journal of Urology*, vol. 46, Supplement 1, pp. 6–18, 2020.

[2] https://mynbc15.com/news/local/adph-holds-press-conference-about-covid-19/.

[3] https://www.alabamapublichealth.gov/news/2020/03/25b.html/ .

[4] C. A. Hogan, N. Garamani, M. K. Sahoo, C. Huang, J. Zehnder, and B. A. Pinsky, “Retrospective screening for SARS-CoV-2 RNA in California, USA, late 2019,” *Emerging Infectious Diseases*, vol. 26, no. 10, pp. 2487-2488, 2020.

[5] J. D. Haslbauer, V. Perrina, M. Matter, A. Dellas, M. J. Mihatsch, and A. Tzankov, “Retrospective post-mortem SARS-CoV-2 RT-PCR of autopsies with COVID-19-suggestive pathology supports the absence of lethal community spread in Basel, Switzerland, before February 2020,” *Pathobiology*, vol. 88, no. 1, pp. 95–105, 2021.

[6] E. L. Simms, H. Chung, L. Oberding et al., “Post-mortem molecular investigations of SARS-CoV-2 in an unexpected death of a recent kidney transplant recipient,” *American Journal of Transplantation*, vol. 21, no. 7, pp. 2590–2595, 2021.

[7] https://www.cdc.gov/media/releases/2020/s0229-COVID-19-first-death.html/.

11

Association of Vitamin D Deficiency and Newly Diagnosed Pulmonary Tuberculosis

Vijay Jaimni,[1] Barkur Ananthakrishna Shasty,[1] Sharath P. Madhyastha,[1] Ganesh V. Shetty,[1] Raviraja V. Acharya,[1] Ragini Bekur,[1] and Akhila Doddamani[2]

[1]*Department of Medicine, Kasturba Medical College, Manipal Academy of Higher Education, 576104, Manipal, Karnataka, India*
[2]*Department of Community Medicine, Kasturba Medical College, Manipal Academy of Higher Education, 576104, Manipal, Karnataka, India*

Correspondence should be addressed to Sharath P. Madhyastha; dr.sharathymc@gmail.com

Academic Editor: Kazuyoshi Kuwano

Introduction. Vitamin D has a significant role in host immune defense against Mycobacterium tuberculosis. It has been suggested that pulmonary tuberculosis may be associated with lower levels of vitamin D. Present study was therefore undertaken to identify the association between vitamin D deficiency and pulmonary tuberculosis. *Methods.* A case-control study was conducted in a tertiary care hospital from 2014 to 2016, including 50 adult newly diagnosed sputum positive pulmonary tuberculosis patients as cases and 50 age and sex-matched healthy participants as control groups. All participants in the study group had undergone detailed clinical examination and routine laboratory investigations, including vitamin D, calcium, and sputum for AFB. The clinical characteristics, X-ray findings, sputum AFB, and vitamin D levels were analyzed and compared with data obtained from healthy controls. *Results.* In both groups, the majority were men (88%). BMI was significantly ($<0.0001*$) lower in the tuberculosis group (19.40 (17.20, 22.0) vs. 24.00 (22.50, 25.47)). Serum vitamin D levels were significantly lower ($P = 0.012$) in the tuberculosis group (19 (7.75, 27.25) ng/dl) as compared to the control group (25 (19.75, 32.00) ng/dl). Out of 50 TB patients, 27 (54%) had vitamin D deficiency, while among healthy controls, only 13 (26%) had vitamin D deficiency. Among vitamin D deficient PTB patients, 44% had 3+/hpf AFB in sputum smear examination. *Conclusion.* The prevalence of vitamin D deficiency in pulmonary tuberculosis cases is very high. Hypovitaminosis D was associated with more severe clinical symptoms, higher sputum smear positivity, and extensive lesions in chest radiograph among pulmonary tuberculosis patients.

1. Introduction

Vitamin D or calciferol is a fat-soluble vitamin that has a significant clinical role in calcium homeostasis and bone metabolism. Vitamin D from the skin and diet is metabolized in the liver to 25-hydroxyvitamin D (25(OH)D), which is used to determine the patient's vitamin D status. This 25(OH)D is converted to its active form, 1,25-dihydroxy vitamin D (1,25(OH)2 D) in the kidneys by the enzyme 25-hydroxyvitamin D-1αhydroxylase [1]. Vitamin D has a vital role in host immune defense against *Mycobacterium tuberculosis* (MTB). It has been observed that vitamin D induces antimicrobial peptide cathelicidin which inhibits mycobacterium multiplication in the macrophages [2, 3]. High serum vitamin D concentrations and hypercalcemia have been described in patients with tuberculosis. Activated macrophages in granulomas are the most likely source of the high calcitriol levels [4, 5]. But many studies worldwide have suggested that pulmonary tuberculosis (PTB) is associated with lower levels of vitamin D [6–8]. Also, few studies showed no significant difference between the mean serum calcium and vitamin D level between the PTB patients and the controls [9, 10]. Present study was therefore undertaken to identify the relation between vitamin D levels and PTB.

2. Materials and Methods

The present study was a case-control study carried out in a tertiary care hospital, Manipal, India, from October 2014 to April 2016, which included 100 participants. Participants were split into 2 groups. The first group (study group) comprised 50 newly diagnosed sputum smear-positive PTB patients admitted to general medicine and pulmonary medicine departments. Group 2 (control group) formed 50 age and gender-matched healthy controls enrolled from the general population that included relatives of admitted patients and health care workers with the similar ethnic and socio-economic background as that of the study group. PTB was ruled out in the control group by a thorough history and clinical examination. Approval from the Institutional Ethics Committee (IEC 631/2014) was sought and granted. Written informed consent was taken from all the participants.

2.1. Inclusion Criteria. All patients aged more than 18 years with newly diagnosed sputum smear-positive pulmonary tuberculosis were included in the study group.

2.2. Exclusion Criteria. Participants with self-reported diseases like human immune deficiency (HIV) virus infection, diabetes mellitus, cancer; patients who were on corticosteroids and chemotherapeutic drugs; and patients with extrapulmonary tuberculosis, pregnancy or lactating mothers, sarcoidosis, and parathyroid disorders were excluded. Patients who were on vitamin D, calcium supplements, anticonvulsants, diuretics, or any other drug which interacts with vitamin D and patients with chronic liver or renal disease, malabsorption conditions, gastric, or bowel resection were also excluded from the study.

All participants underwent a detailed medical history and clinical examinations. Routine lab investigations like complete blood count, liver and kidney function tests, blood glucose levels, HIV ELISA, HBsAg and anti-HCV serology, serum calcium, and albumin levels were done in all participants. Chest radiograph and at least two baseline early morning sputum samples were obtained from each patient for acid-fast staining, as per the Revised National Tuberculosis Control Program (RNTCP) guidelines [11].

Serum 25(OH)D level was measured before initiating antitubercular therapy (ATT). Although 1,25(OH)2D is the biologically active form of vitamin D, the ideal marker for vitamin D deficiency is 25(OH)D. Because 25(OH)D is the major circulating form of vitamin D and circulating concentration of 1,25(OH)2D is 1000th the concentration of 25(OH)D. The half-life for 1,25(OH)2D is very less compared to 25(OH)D. Finally, as a person becomes vitamin D deficient and develops secondary hyperparathyroidism, the renal 1-OHase generates more 1,25(OH)2D. Thus, when a patient is vitamin D insufficient, there is often a normal or even elevated blood level of 1,25(OH)2D. Hence, the measurement of 25(OH)D is the only method to determine vitamin D deficiency [12]. As per the Endocrine Society clinical practice guidelines, 25(OH)D levels were divided into three categories [1]. 25(OH)D level $\leq$ 20 ng/ml was considered as deficient, 25(OH)D level 21–29 ng/ml as insufficient, and 25(OH)D level more than 30 ng/ml was considered as optimal. The serum 25(OH)D concentration was measured by electrochemiluminescence immunoassay (ECLIA). The analyzer used was Beckman coulter Access-2, manufactured in California, USA, and the quality control (QC) measures were instituted by BIORAD (both internal and external QC). Analyzer reference range of serum 25(OH)D level is 2.0–167 ng/ml OR 5.0–417 nmol/l. According to WHO definition, "hemoglobin level less than 12 gm/dl in women and less than 13 gm/dl in men is considered as anemic." [13] Hypoalbuminemia was defined as a total serum albumin level less than 3.5 g/dl while hypocalcaemia as corrected serum calcium concentration less than 9 mg/dl [14].

The corrected serum calcium concentration for the albumin levels was calculated using following formula, "Corrected total calcium (mg/dL) = 0.8 x [4 – serum albumin (g/dL)] + Total calcium (mg/dL)." [15]

Based on chest X-ray findings, tuberculosis was categorized into two categories [16–18].

(1) Primary pulmonary tuberculosis (PPT) includes parenchymal disease, typically manifests as dense, homogeneous parenchymal consolidation predominantly in the lower and middle lobe (subpleural sites), lymphadenopathy, and pleural effusion

(2) Progressive pulmonary tuberculosis (PrPT) includes parenchymal disease as patchy consolidation (typically in the upper lobe), cavitatory lesion, miliary tuberculosis, and multiple mediastinal lymphadenopathies

Based on sputum smear findings, tuberculosis was grouped into three categories [2, 19].

(1) +++ per hpf. (3+/high power field)

(2) ++ per hpf

(3) + or scanty per hpf

Patients who were found to have vitamin D deficiency were given a therapeutic dose of vitamin D as per the recommendations [1].

2.3. Statistical Analysis. Data analysis was carried out using the SPSS software 20.0. Results are presented as median and interquartile range (IQR). Continuous variables were analyzed using Mann–Whitney *U* test. Associations between the categorical variables were analyzed by using Fisher's exact test or chi-squared test. The statistical significance was set at $P \leq 0.05$.

3. Results

A total of 100 participants were included in the study, out of whom 50 were newly diagnosed sputum smear-positive PTB and 50 were age and sex-matched healthy controls. In both groups, the majority were men (88%). There was no significant variation in age and sex between the two groups. BMI (body mass index) was significantly ($P < 0.0001$ ∗) lower in the tuberculous group as compared to healthy controls. There was a significantly higher proportion of smokers ($n = 19$ (38%)) among the PTB cases compared to controls ($n = 10$ (20%)). Vitamin D levels were significantly lower in the tuberculosis group (19 (7.75, 27.25)) than in the control group (25 (19.75, 32.00)) (Table 1).

TABLE 1: Determinants of pulmonary tuberculosis.

Variables	Group 1 ($n = 50$) (tuberculosis)	Group 2 ($n = 50$) (control)	P value
BMI (kg/m^2) (median, IQR)	19.40 (17.20, 22.0)	24.00 (22.50, 25.47)	<0.0001*
Serum 25(OH)D (ng/dl) (median, IQR)	19 (7.75, 27.25)	25 (19.75, 32.00)	0.012*
Serum albumin (median, IQR)	3.18 (2.70, 3.70)	4.30 (3.94, 4.50)	<0.0001*
Corrected serum calcium (median, IQR)	9 (8.67, 9.20)	9.20 (8.98, 9.50)	0.18

Mann–Whitney U test, $^*P \leq 0.05$ (statistical significance). BMI: body mass index; 25(OH)D: 25-hydroxyvitamin D.

TABLE 2: Vitamin D levels among pulmonary tuberculosis patients ($N = 50$) and controls ($N = 50$).

Vitamin D levels		Tuberculosis patients n (%)	Healthy controls n (%)	p value
Deficient (< 20 ng/ml)	Present	27 (54%)	13 (26%)	0.004*
	Absent	23 (46%)	37 (74%)	
Insufficient (20-30 ng/ml)	Present	14 (28%)	20 (40%)	0.205
	Absent	36 (72%)	30 (60%)	
Sufficient (> 30 ng/ml)	Present	9 (18%)	17 (34%)	0.068
	Absent	41 (82%)	33 (66%)	

Chi-squared test, $^*P \leq 0.05$ (statistical significance).

TABLE 3: Vitamin D level in primary pulmonary tuberculosis and progressive pulmonary tuberculosis.

Vitamin D levels	Primary pulmonary tuberculosis N (%)	Progressive pulmonary tuberculosis N (%)	p value
Deficient (< 20 ng/ml) ($n = 27$)	7 (25.93%)	20 (74.07%)	0.0009*
Insufficient (20-30 ng/ml) ($n = 14$)	3 (21.43%)	11 (78.57%)	0.007*
Sufficient (> 30 ng/ml) ($n = 9$)	1 (10%)	8 (90%)	0.003*

Fisher's exact test, $^*P \leq 0.05$ (statistical significance).

TABLE 4: Comparison of vitamin D levels with sputum findings in pulmonary tuberculosis.

Vitamin D levels	Sputum smear AFB density 3 + N (%)	2 + N (%)	1 + or scanty N (%)	P value
Deficient (< 20 ng/ml) ($n = 27$)	12 (44%)	11 (41%)	4 (15%)	0.046*
Insufficient (20-30 ng/ml) ($n = 14$)	5 (36%)	6 (42%)	3 (22%)	0.601
Sufficient (> 30 ng/ml) ($n = 9$)	3 (33%)	2 (22%)	4 (44%)	0.873

Fisher's exact test, $^*P \leq 0.05$ (statistical significance).

Out of 50 TB patients, 27 (54%) had vitamin D deficiency, and 18% had sufficient levels. While among healthy controls, only 13 (26%) had deficient vitamin D levels. The difference is statistically significant (p-0.004) (Table 2).

Tuberculosis was categorized into PPt and PrPt based on X-ray findings. In the present study, out of 50 patients with pulmonary tuberculosis, 27 were found to have deficit vitamin D levels; in the deficient category, 7 (26%) had PPt while 20 (74%) had PrPt. Out of 14 patients with insufficient vitamin D levels, 3 (21%) had PPt, while 11 (78%) had PrPt (Table 3).

In the present study, out of 50 patients with pulmonary tuberculosis, 27 had deficient vitamin D levels, out of whom 12 (44%) had 3+ AFB/hpf in sputum smear examination, 11 (41%) had 2+ AFB/hpf, and 4 (15%) had 1+ AFB/hpf (Table 4).

4. Discussion

4.1. Vitamin D Levels in Tubercular Patients and Healthy Controls. Vitamin D, a fat-soluble vitamin, has a vital role in host immunity against *Mycobacterium tuberculosis*. Calcitriol is the biologically active form of vitamin D, which leads to the expression of a peptide called cathelicidin. This cathelicidin is a microbicidal peptide that acts against *Mycobacterium tuberculosis* [3]. It has been illustrated that vitamin D supplementation leads to augmented expression of cathelicidin peptide in the macrophages and thereby boosting innate immunity in patients with tuberculosis [20].

The present study conducted on newly diagnosed sputum positive pulmonary tuberculosis patients and healthy controls showed that the prevalence of vitamin D deficiency was significantly higher in patients with tuberculosis than the healthy group. In the tuberculosis group, 27 (54%) patients were found to have a deficit in vitamin D compared to 13 (26%) in the healthy control groups.

Many studies were done from various continents suggesting vitamin D levels are low in patients with pulmonary tuberculosis [21–24]. A case-control study in Vietnam, which involved 166 TB patients and 219 controls, showed that the prevalence of vitamin D insufficiency was 35.4% in men with tuberculosis compared to 19.5% in controls ($P = 0.01$) [21]. Other studies done on African populations in Guinea-Bissau [22], Asian immigrant population of Gujarati origin, residing in UK [23], and African people living in Melbourne [24] also reported that vitamin D levels were significantly reduced in tuberculosis patients. Even in India, a case-control study done by Sashidharan et al. in Kerala observed very low levels of vitamin D in tuberculosis patients compared to healthy controls [25].

4.2. Clinical Symptoms in Hypovitaminosis D and Tuberculosis. Hypovitaminosis D can present in tuberculosis patients with nonspecific symptoms such as bone and muscle pain, arthralgia, and tiredness. These clinical features are often present in multiple disease entities such as connective tissue diseases, chronic fatigue syndrome, fibromyalgia, or even depression. Hence, the diagnosis may be delayed in many cases [26].

In the present study, 40% of the tuberculosis patients who were found to be vitamin D deficient presented with myalgia and bone pain. 70% of the patients in this group complained of generalized weakness. In the healthy group, 30% of the controls who were deficient in vitamin D levels presented with bone pain and myalgia, and 50% complained of generalized weakness.

Chronic severe vitamin D deficiency in adults may lead to proximal muscle weakness, bone pain, and osteomalacia. Less severe vitamin D inadequacy leads to elevation of PTH (secondary hyperparathyroidism), leading to increased bone demineralization, bone loss, and finally osteoporosis and fracture [27].

4.3. Low Vitamin D Levels and Degree of Sputum Smear Positivity. A cross-sectional study done by Yuvaraj et al. [2] in India, which included 65 sputum AFB positive PTB patients and 65 healthy controls, showed a significant difference in the deficiency of vitamin D with a rise in sputum smear positivity associated with a substantial negative correlation between vitamin D levels and degree of sputum smear positivity. The study concluded that the lower the vitamin D, the higher the MTB bacterial load [2]. In the present study also, we observed a significant negative correlation between vitamin D levels and degree of sputum smear positivity and levels of sputum positivity.

4.4. Low Vitamin D Levels and Chest X-Ray Findings in Tuberculous Patients. In the present study, based on chest X-ray findings, out of the 27 patients with vitamin D deficiency, 74% (20) had progressive pulmonary tuberculosis, and only 25% (7) had primary pulmonary tuberculosis. The patients with deficient vitamin D levels were found to have bilateral and extensive lesions in the radiological evaluation of X-ray chest.

A randomized, double-blinded, multicentric study done by Salahuddin et al. [28] revealed the negative correlation between vitamin D levels and the severity of chest X-ray involvement. They also reported that the correction of vitamin D deficiency accelerated the clinical and radiographic improvement in all patients with tuberculosis [28].

A randomized controlled trial done by Khandelwal et al. [29] included 266 children with intrathoracic tuberculosis found that more than half of subjects had progressive pulmonary TB (56%). The remaining participants belonged to primary pulmonary complex (30.5%) and pleural effusion (13.5%). They have also found that only 9% had sufficient levels of vitamin D [29].

4.5. The Relation between Vitamin D Levels and Severity of Pulmonary Tuberculosis. In our study, the patients with low vitamin D levels had a higher degree of sputum smear positivity and more extensive lesions in chest radiograph suggestive of more severe tuberculosis.

A cross-sectional study by Rathored et al. included 354 MDR-TB stated that MDR-TB patients have significantly lower levels of vitamin D and serum calcium. They also reported that there was delayed smear conversion in patients with vitamin D deficiency [30]. Tuberculosis itself can lead to paradoxical depletion of vitamin D metabolism during therapy, thus linking the severity of the disease [31].

4.6. Limitations of the Study

(1) In the present study, an adequate sample size was not achieved as the survey was time-bound. Hence, it is difficult to generalize the study findings. Further prospective studies with larger sample size are required to understand the relation between vitamin D and tuberculosis

(2) There may be differences in UV exposure among study participants and its possible role in serum vitamin D deficiency

(3) Patients were given a therapeutic dose of vitamin D, and they were not followed up. Further studies are required to study vitamin D's role in the prognosis and outcome of pulmonary tuberculosis

5. Conclusion

In the present study, vitamin D deficiency is highly prevalent among patients with pulmonary tuberculosis compared to healthy individuals. Hypovitaminosis D is associated with more severe clinical symptoms in patients with tuberculosis. Vitamin D deficiency is associated with a higher degree of sputum smear positivity and more extensive lesions in chest radiograph among pulmonary tuberculosis patients.

Acknowledgments

We acknowledge all the participants who were involved in the study and Dr. Alladi Mohan, Professor and Head, Department of Medicine, Sri Venkateswara Institute of Medical Sciences, Tirupati, Andhra Pradesh, India, for his guidance.

References

[1] M. F. Holick, "Vitamin D deficiency," *The New England Journal of Medicine*, vol. 6, pp. 266–281, 2007.

[2] B. Yuvaraj, M. G. Sridhar, S. V. Kumar, and T. Kadhiravan, "Association of serum vitamin D levels with bacterial load in pulmonary tuberculosis patients," *Tuberculosis and Respiratory Diseases*, vol. 79, no. 3, pp. 153–157, 2016.

[3] A. R. Martineau, R. J. Wilkinson, K. A. Wilkinson et al., "A single dose of vitamin D enhances immunity to mycobacteria," *American Journal of Respiratory and Critical Care Medicine*, vol. 176, no. 2, pp. 208–213, 2007.

[4] J. Cadranel, M. Garabedian, B. Milleron, H. Guillozo, G. Akoun, and A. J. Hance, "1,25(OH)2D2 production by T lymphocytes and alveolar macrophages recovered by lavage from normocalcemic patients with tuberculosis," *The Journal of Clinical Investigation*, vol. 85, no. 5, pp. 1588–1593, 1990.

[5] C. C. Shek, A. Natkunam, V. Tsang, C. S. Cockram, and R. Swaminathan, "Incidence, causes and mechanism of hypercalcaemia in a hospital population in Hong Kong," *The Quarterly Journal of Medicine*, vol. 77, no. 3, pp. 1277–1285, 1990.

[6] N. Talat, S. Perry, J. Parsonnet, G. Dawood, and R. Hussain, "Vitamin d deficiency and tuberculosis progression," *Emerging Infectious Diseases*, vol. 16, no. 5, pp. 853–8555, 2010.

[7] M. D. Kearns and V. Tangpricha, "The role of vitamin D in tuberculosis," *Journal of Clinical & Translational Endocrinology*, vol. 1, no. 4, pp. 167–169, 2014.

[8] M. Workineh, B. Mathewos, B. Moges et al., "Vitamin D deficiency among newly diagnosed tuberculosis patients and their household contacts: a comparative cross-sectional study," *Archives of Public Health*, vol. 75, no. 1, p. 25, 2017.

[9] T. T. Tan, B. C. Lee, and B. A. Khalid, "Low incidence of hypercalcaemia in tuberculosis in Malaysia," *The Journal of Tropical Medicine and Hygiene*, vol. 96, no. 6, pp. 349–351, 1993.

[10] F. Keleştimur, M. Güven, M. Ozesmi, and H. Paşaoğlu, "Does tuberculosis really cause hypercalcemia?," *Journal of Endocrinological Investigation*, vol. 19, no. 10, pp. 678–681, 1996.

[11] Central TB Division, Directorate General of Health Services, Ministry of Health and Family Welfare, *TB India 2014: RNTCP Status Report*, Ministry of Health and Family Welfare, New Delhi, India, 2014.

[12] M. F. Holick, "Vitamin D," *Clinical Reviews in Bone and Mineral Metabolism*, vol. 1, no. 3-4, pp. 181–207, 2002.

[13] World Health Organisation, "Worldwide Prevalence of Anaemia 1993-2005," WHO, 2008, https://www.who.int/nutrition/publications/micronutrients/anaemia_iron_deficiency/9789241596657/en/.

[14] M. S. Cooper and N. J. L. Gittoes, "Diagnosis and management of hypocalcaemia," *BMJ*, vol. 336, no. 7656, pp. 1298–1302, 2008.

[15] National Kidney Foundation, "K/DOQI clinical practice guidelines for bone metabolism and disease in chronic kidney disease," *American Journal of Kidney Diseases*, vol. 42, 4 Suppl 3, pp. S1–201, 2003.

[16] J. H. Woodring, H. M. Vandiviere, A. M. Fried, M. L. Dillon, T. D. Williams, and I. G. Melvin, "Update: the radiographic features of pulmonary tuberculosis," *AJR. American Journal of Roentgenology*, vol. 146, no. 3, pp. 497–506, 1986.

[17] M. G. Harisinghani, T. C. McLoud, J. A. Shepard, J. P. Ko, M. M. Shroff, and P. R. Mueller, "Tuberculosis from head to toe," *Radiographics*, vol. 20, no. 2, pp. 449–470, 2000.

[18] J. Burrill, C. J. Williams, G. Bain, G. Conder, A. L. Hine, and R. R. Misra, "Tuberculosis: a radiologic review," *Radiographics*, vol. 27, no. 5, pp. 1255–1273, 2007.

[19] RNTCP, *Tuberculosis Manual*, Government of India, Central Tuberculosis, New Delhi, 2005.

[20] P. T. Liu, S. Stenger, H. Li et al., "Toll-like receptor triggering of a vitamin D-mediated human antimicrobial response," *Science*, vol. 311, no. 5768, pp. 1770–1773, 2006.

[21] L. T. Ho-Pham, N. D. Nguyen, T. T. Nguyen et al., "Association between vitamin D insufficiency and tuberculosis in a Vietnamese population," *BMC Infectious Diseases*, vol. 10, no. 1, p. 306, 2010.

[22] C. Wejse, R. Olesen, P. Rabna et al., "Serum 25-hydroxyvitamin D in a West African population of tuberculosis patients and unmatched healthy controls," *The American Journal of Clinical Nutrition*, vol. 86, no. 5, pp. 1376–1383, 2007.

[23] R. J. Wilkinson, M. Llewelyn, Z. Toossi et al., "Influence of vitamin D deficiency and vitamin D receptor polymorphisms on tuberculosis among Gujarati Asians in west London: a case-control study," *Lancet*, vol. 355, no. 9204, pp. 618–621, 2000.

[24] K. B. Gibney, L. MacGregor, K. Leder et al., "Vitamin D deficiency is associated with tuberculosis and latent tuberculosis infection in immigrants from sub-Saharan Africa," *Clinical Infectious Diseases*, vol. 46, no. 3, pp. 443–446, 2008.

[25] P. K. Sasidharan, E. Rajeev, and V. Vijayakumari, "Tuberculosis and vitamin D deficiency," *The Journal of the Association of Physicians of India*, vol. 50, pp. 554–558, 2002.

[26] M. F. Holick, "High prevalence of vitamin D inadequacy and implications for health," *Mayo Clinic Proceedings*, vol. 81, no. 3, pp. 353–373, 2006.

[27] E. F. Eriksen and H. Glerup, "Vitamin D deficiency and aging: implications for general health and osteoporosis," *Biogerontology*, vol. 3, no. 1/2, pp. 73–77, 2002.

[28] N. Salahuddin, F. Ali, Z. Hasan, N. Rao, M. Aqeel, and F. Mahmood, "Vitamin D accelerates clinical recovery from tuberculosis: results of the SUCCINCT study [supplementary Cholecalciferol in recovery from tuberculosis]. A randomized, placebo-controlled, clinical trial of vitamin D supplementation in patients with pulmonary tuberculosis'," *BMC Infectious Diseases*, vol. 13, p. 22, 2013.

[29] D. Khandelwal, N. Gupta, A. Mukherjee et al., "Vitamin D levels in Indian children with intrathoracic tuberculosis," *The Indian Journal of Medical Research*, vol. 140, no. 4, pp. 531–537, 2014.

[30] J. Rathored, S. K. Sharma, B. Singh et al., "Risk and outcome of multidrug-resistant tuberculosis: vitamin D receptor polymorphisms and serum 25(OH)D," *The International Journal of Tuberculosis and Lung Disease*, vol. 16, no. 11, pp. 1522–1528, 2012.

[31] K. E. Nnoaham and A. Clarke, "Low serum vitamin D levels and tuberculosis: a systematic review and meta-analysis," *International Journal of Epidemiology*, vol. 37, no. 1, pp. 113–119, 2008.

12

Pneumocystis jirovecii Pneumonia in an Immunocompetent Japanese Man

Hiromi Ide,[1] Yoshikazu Yamaji,[2] Kazunori Tobino,[1] Masanobu Okahisa,[1] Kojin Murakami,[1] Yuki Goto,[1] Takuto Sueyasu,[1] Saori Nishizawa,[1] Kohei Yoshimine,[1] Miyuki Munechika,[1] Masafumi Oya,[3] and Yuka Hiraki[3]

[1]*Department of Respiratory Medicine, Iizuka Hospital, Japan*
[2]*Department of Respiratory Medicine and Infectious Disease, Graduate School of Medicine, Yamaguchi University, Japan*
[3]*Department of Pathology, Iizuka Hospital, Japan*

Correspondence should be addressed to Hiromi Ide; ghiromix7@gmail.com

Academic Editor: Akif Turna

We herein report the case of a 37-year-old immunocompetent man who died from *Pneumocystis jirovecii* pneumonia (PCP). He was initially treated for an acute exacerbation of interstitial pneumonia; however, the elevation of the patient's serum (1-3) β-D glucan (BG) level suggested the possibility of PCP and sulfamethoxazole trimethoprim was added. A postmortem pathological examination and retrospective Grocott's methenamine silver (GMS) staining of the bronchoalveolar lavage fluid (BALF), which was obtained on the day of admission, revealed PCP. The present case suggests that it is essential to perform a BG assay and GMS staining of BALF specimens when patients show diffuse ground-glass opacity on chest computed tomography, regardless of their immune status.

1. Introduction

Pneumocystis jirovecii pneumonia (PCP) is a common opportunistic infection in patients with acquired immune deficiency syndrome (AIDS) [1]. In patients with human immunodeficiency virus (HIV), a low CD4+ lymphocyte count (<200 cells/μL) is a risk factor for the development of PCP; underlying malignancies, organ transplantation and immunosuppressive medications are other risk factors. PCP in patients without any of these risk factors is extremely rare [2]. We herein report a case of PCP in an immunocompetent patient.

2. Case Presentation

A 37-year-old Japanese man presented to our hospital with a nonproductive cough of two weeks in duration. He did not have fever or dyspnea. He had a history of right hemiparesis, intellectual disability with pica, and symptomatic epilepsy caused by intracerebral hemorrhage, which occurred at two years of age. He had never smoked or consumed alcoholic beverages.

His initial vital signs were as follows: blood pressure, 105/55 mm Hg; pulse rate, 70 beats/minute; respiratory rate, 18 breaths/min; SpO_2, 93% in room air; body temperature, 36.5°C. There was no lymphadenopathy. Auscultation revealed no chest rales. A cardiovascular examination was normal, and no murmurs, rubs, or gallops were detected. Abdominal and neurological examinations were unremarkable, and the patient had no rash or petechiae. A chest radiograph revealed bilateral diffuse infiltration (Figure 1). Chest computed tomography (CT) revealed bilateral airspace consolidation and ground-glass opacity (Figure 2).

The patient's laboratory test values were as follows: hemoglobin, 14.9 g/dl; white blood cell count, 8,850/mm^3 with a left shift; platelets, 329,000/mm^3; serum aspartate aminotransferase 29 U/L (normal, 0-35 U/l); serum alanine aminotransferase, 31 U/L (normal, 0-35 U/l); serum lactate dehydrogenase, 425 U/L (normal, 119-229 U/l); serum total protein, 5.3 g/dl (normal, 6.5-8 g/dl); serum albumin, 2.1

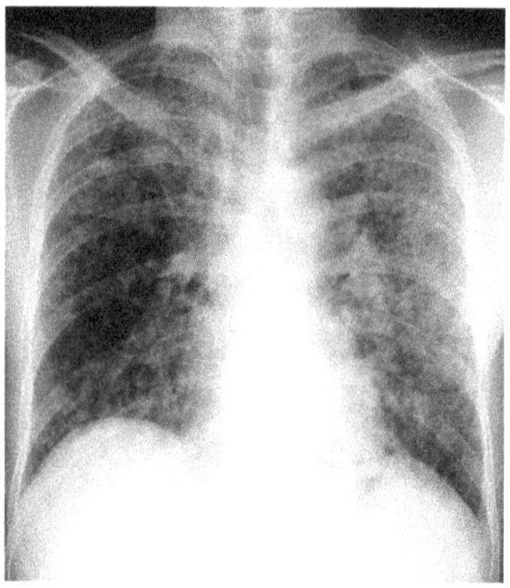

FIGURE 1: A chest radiograph obtained on the day of admission showed bilateral diffuse alveolo-interstitial infiltration, particularly in the left lung.

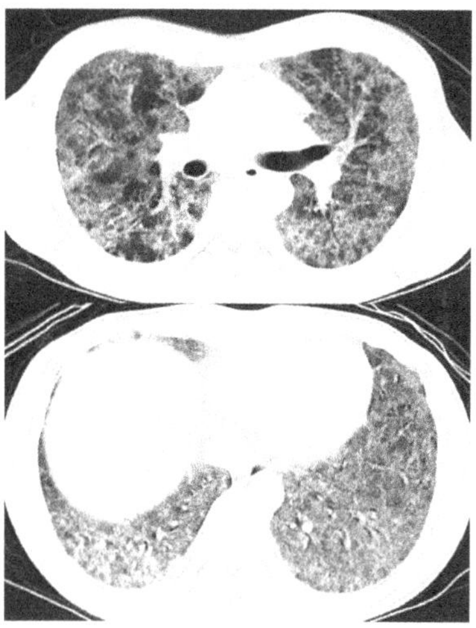

FIGURE 2: Chest computed tomography revealed bilateral airspace consolidation and ground-glass opacity.

g/dl (normal, 4-5 g/dl); serum C-reactive protein, 9.18 mg/dl (normal, < 0.2 mg/dl); serum KL-6, 2940 U/ml (normal, < 500 U/ml); serum surfactant protein D, 173.0 ng/ml (normal, < 109.9 ng/mL); and serum surfactant protein A, 115.0 ng/ml (normal, < 43.8 ng/mL). The patient's serum was negative for rheumatoid factor and antinuclear antibodies. The serum levels of immunoglobulin M, G, and A were within the normal ranges. An electrocardiogram revealed normal findings. An examination of the patient's sputum showed no predominant pathogen and no acid-fast organisms were observed on staining. Two sets of blood cultures were prepared at the time of admission; however, they did not yield any organisms.

The patient underwent a fiberoptic bronchoscopic examination that revealed a normal endobronchial system, and combined bronchoalveolar lavage (BAL)/transbronchial biopsy (TBLB) was performed. BAL fluid (BALF) was obtained from the right middle lobe. The results of the BALF analysis were as follows: histiocytes, 87%; neutrophils, 6%; lymphocytes, 4%; and eosinophils, 3%. Routine cultures of bronchial the washings were negative. The TBLB sample from the right upper lobe revealed alveolar septal thickening due to chronic inflammation, as well as collagen-type fibrosis.

After these examinations, the patient was diagnosed with acute interstitial pneumonia, and intravenous levofloxacin (500 mg) was administered once daily with corticosteroid pulse therapy (methylprednisolone [1000 mg] for three days) followed by prednisolone (1 mg/kg/day). On the 5th day after the initiation of therapy, his respiratory condition worsened and noninvasive positive pressure ventilation was started. His interstitial pneumonia was thought to be getting worse, and cyclophosphamide (500 mg/body) was administered intravenously. On the same day, an additional examination revealed the elevation of the serum (1-3) β-D glucan (BG) level (104.3 pg/ml; normal, <6.0 pg/ml). He was therefore suspected to have fungal infection or PCP, and voriconazole (200 mg, every 12 hours) and sulfamethoxazole trimethoprim (1600 mg and 320 mg, respectively, every 8 hours) were started. An additional HIV antibody test was negative and the serum protein electrophoresis revealed normal findings. Despite the additional antifungal therapy, his respiratory status gradually worsened, and intravenous corticosteroid pulse therapy (methylprednisolone [1000 mg] for three days) and cyclophosphamide therapy (500 mg/body) were each administered a second time, on the 8th and 11th days, respectively, without improvement. The patient died due to respiratory failure on the 12th day.

A postmortem pathological examination of the lung tissue demonstrated that the alveolar spaces were filled with foamy amorphous material composed of abundant numbers of cystic forms of *Pneumocystis jirovecii* and cellular debris, as well as an inflammatory reaction with hyaline membranes (Figure 3). Retrospectively, Grocott's methenamine silver (GMS) staining of the BALF and TBLB samples obtained on the day of admission revealed a small amount of the cystic form of *Pneumocystis jirovecii* (Figure 4). It was therefore thought that PCP had been present on the day of his admission.

3. Discussion

Pneumocystis jirovecii was first described by Chagas in 1909, but it was not shown to cause human disease until 1951. In Europe, an epidemic of PCP occurred in Europe in premature and malnourished children the late 1930s and 1940s. In the 1960s and 1970s, cases of PCP were seen in patients with congenital immune defects, acquired defects secondary to malignancy or its treatment, organ transplantation, and disorders that were treated with corticosteroids or cytotoxic drugs. However, PCP remained a relatively rare condition until 1981, when AIDS was described. Since then there has been a significant increase in the incidence of PCP, which has become the most infectious complication in patients with AIDS.

The risk of PCP is increased 5-fold in in HIV patients with a CD4+ lymphocyte count of ≤200 cells/μL [7]. The other major risk factors for PCP in patients with and without HIV include—but are not limited to—a history of hematological

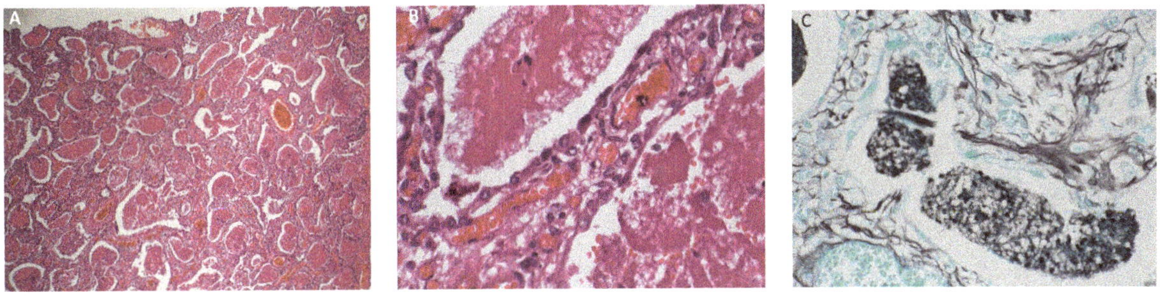

(a) (b) (c)

FIGURE 3: (a) A photomicrograph (original magnification, ×40; hematoxylin-eosin staining) of a section of lung tissue. The section showed homogeneous septal thickening and intra-alveolar eosinophilic exudate. (b) A high-power photomicrograph (original magnification, ×400; hematoxylin-eosin staining) of a section of lung tissue showed thickening of the alveolar septa due to both chronic inflammation and a small amount of collagen. The intra-alveolar spaces were filled with foamy acellular eosinophilic exudate. (c) A high-power photomicrograph (original magnification, ×400; Grocott's methenamine silver staining) of a section of lung tissue. Numerous cysts of *Pneumocystis jirovecii* were observed within the intra-alveolar foamy exudate.

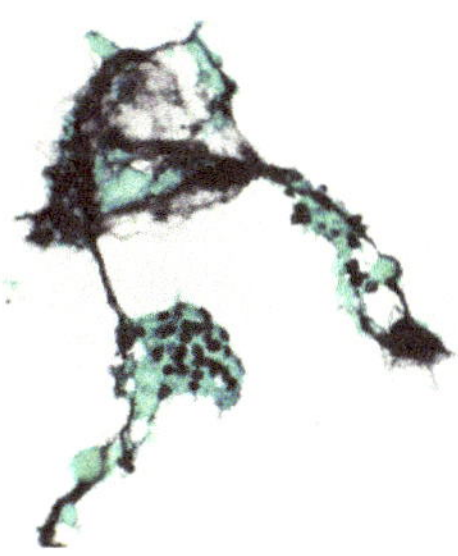

FIGURE 4: Grocott's methenamine silver staining of bronchoalveolar lavage fluid samples obtained on the day of admission revealed a small number of cystic forms of *Pneumocystis jirovecii.*

malignancy, organ transplantation, inflammatory conditions, solid tumors, and the use of immunosuppressive drugs. Moreover the most significant risk factors for PCP in patients without HIV are glucocorticoid use and cellmediated immunity defects, which lead to lung surfactant alterations, thereby predisposing the patient to pneumonia [8].

To the best of our knowledge, there are a few reports of PCP in patients without underlying immunosuppressive diseases (Table 1). In 1993, Cano et al. described five patients who developed PCP without any underlying conditions associated with immunosuppression; in their literature review, they only identified 11 other reported cases [3]. Since then, another three cases of PCP in immunocompetent patients have been reported [4–6]. In Cano's case series, two patients had previous or simultaneous infection by another microorganism (*e.g.*, a viral upper respiratory tract infection or *Mycoplasma pneumoniae*). It was hypothesized that of PCP might develop in patients in whose immunocompetence shows a transitory alteration due to a previous or concomitant infection. In fact, Mycoplasma is reported to lead to the polyclonal activation of B cells and the suppression of T cells, which would explain the appearance of transitory cutaneous anergy [9]. However, the precise mechanisms that lead to the development of PCP remain unclear.

A definitive diagnosis of PCP is made by the visualization of pneumocystis organisms on histopathological staining. The cell wall of the cysts can be visualized with GMS staining. The induction of sputum with hypertonic saline has a diagnostic yield of approximately 60% and should be performed as the initial diagnostic procedure, particularly in patients with AIDS [10]. Sputum induction may be less sensitive in patients without HIV infection because the immunodeficiency caused by HIV infection typically leads to a greater alveolar load of Pneumocystis organisms. Early fiberoptic bronchoscopy is recommended for patients in whom induced sputum is negative or from whom an induced sputum sample cannot be obtained. The diagnostic yield of BAL is >90%, and this may be increased if multiple lobes are sampled [10]. Open-lung biopsy is the most invasive procedure; however, shows very high sensitivity and specificity because it provides the greatest amount of tissue for the diagnosis [11].

We first suspected acute interstitial pneumonia based on the patient's symptoms, the physical examination findings, and the TBLB and CT findings. At first, the patient's BALF was not subjected to GMS staining (which subsequently revealed *Pneumocystis jirovecii* infection) because we considered that it was highly unlikely that *Pneumocystis jirovecii* was the causative organism based on the patient's immune status and past medical history. The high level of BG helped us to make a definitive diagnosis. BG is a cell wall component of all fungi. The serum is typically tested to determine the level of BG for the diagnosis of invasive *Aspergillus*; however, BG is also present in the cell wall in patients with PCP.

PCP is typically associated with high levels of BG. The levels should decline with effective therapy. The potential utility of this assay was illustrated in a retrospective case-control study of 295 patients with suspected PCP. Among these subjects, BALF specimens were observed by microscopy to detect PCP and serum samples were tested for BG [12]. In that study, the BG assay had a sensitivity of 92% and a specificity of 86% for detecting PCP. In our case, the serum BG level was 104.3 pg/ml (normal,

TABLE 1: Review of previously published cases.

Author	Patient demographics	Initial presentation	Initial radiological findings	Means of diagnosis	Outcome
	39-year-old man	Fever and dyspnea	Left pleural effusion and bilateral interstitial infiltrate	GMS staining of TNA specimens	Survive
	30-year-old man	Fever and dyspnea	Diffuse alveolar infiltrate	GMS staining of BALF specimens	Survive
Cano [3]	37-year-old woman	Fever, cough, and malaise	Bilateral alveolointerstitial infiltrate	GMS staining of BALF specimens	Survive
	37-year-old man	Cough and purulent sputum	Bilateral nonhomogeneous alveolar infiltrate	GMS staining of TNA specimens	Survive
	55-year-old man	Fever and chill	Bilateral alveolar infiltrate in the middle and lower fields	GMS staining of BALF specimens	Survive
Koshy [4]	56-year-old man	Cough, dyspnea, and hemoptysis	Bilateral nonhomogenous opacities in the middle and lower zones	GMS staining of induced sputum	Survive
Harris [5]	51-year-old man	None	A right upper lung nodule	Open lung biopsy	Survive
Nejmi [6]	30-year-old woman	Productive cough and dyspnea.	Reticulo-micro-nodular opacities in the right lung	Induced sputum	Survive
Present case	37-year-old man	Non-productive cough	Bilateral diffuse infiltration	GMS staining of BALF specimens	Dead

PCP indicates *Pneumocystis jirovecii* pneumonia; BALF, bronchoalveolar lavage fluid; GMS, Grocott's methenamine silver; TNA, transthoracic needle aspiration; COPD, chronic obstructive pulmonary disease

<6.0 pg/ml); thus, we could consider PCP in the differential diagnosis and began to treat the patient accordingly. After treatment with sulfamethoxazole/trimethoprim, the value was decreased to 33.3 pg/ml, nevertheless we were unable to save the patient. A serum BG assay is helpful in the differential diagnosis for PCP, and should be performed whenever high-resolution chest CT reveals diffuse bilateral ground-glass attenuation, including reticulation, septal thickening and micronodules and air space consolidation in a patient with suspected IP, because healthy individuals can develop PCP, similarly to our case.

In conclusion, we experienced a case of PCP in a patient without any underlying risk factors. It may therefore be necessary to perform a serum BG assay and GMS staining of BALF specimens in patients with diffuse ground-glass opacity, regardless of the patient's immune status.

Abbreviations

BALF: Bronchioloalveolar lavage fluid
CT: Computed tomography
GMS: Grocott's methenamine silver
PCP: Pneumocystic pneumonia
TBLB: Transbronchial lung biopsy.

Consent

Written informed consent was obtained from the patient's family.

Authors' Contributions

All those named as authors have made substantial contributions to the conception and design of the study, acquisition of data, analysis and interpretation of data, drafting the article, or revising it critically for important intellectual content. All authors read and approved the final manuscript. All named authors have read the manuscript and have agreed to submit the paper to Case Reports in Pulmonology in its present form.

References

[1] F. J. Palella Jr., K. M. Delaney, A. C. Moorman et al., "Declining morbidity and mortality among patients with advanced human immunodeficiency virus infection," *The New England Journal of Medicine*, vol. 338, no. 13, pp. 853–860, 1998.

[2] J. L. Jacobs, D. M. Libby, R. A. Winters et al., "A cluster of pneumocystis carinii pneumonia in adults without predisposing illnesses," *The New England Journal of Medicine*, vol. 324, no. 4, pp. 246–250, 1991.

[3] S. Cano, F. Capote, A. Pereira, E. Calderon, and J. Castillo, "Pneumocystis carinii pneumonia in patients without predisposing illnesses: acute episode and follow-up of five cases," *CHEST*, vol. 104, no. 2, pp. 376–381, 1993.

[4] G. Koshy, J. M. Koshy, M. John, and D. Deodhar, "Pneumocystis jirovecii pneumonia in an immunocompetent host," *Annals of Tropical Medicine and Public Health*, vol. 8, no. 4, pp. 122–124, 2015.

[5] K. Harris, R. Maroun, M. Chalhoub, and D. Elsayegh, "Unusual presentation of pneumocystis pneumonia in an immunocompetent patient diagnosed by open lung biopsy," *Heart, Lung and Circulation*, vol. 21, no. 4, pp. 221–224, 2012.

[6] L. Amro, G. Hamzaoui, H. Sajiai, H. Serhane, and A. A. Yazidi, "Pneumocystis jiroveci Pneumonia in an immunocompetent female patient," *Case Reports in Clinical Medicine*, 2014.

[7] W. T. Hughes, "Natural mode of acquisition for de novo infection with pneumocystis carinii," *The Journal of Infectious Diseases*, vol. 145, no. 6, pp. 842–848, 1982.

[8] M. Chabé, E. Dei-Cas, C. Creusy et al., "Immunocompetent hosts as a reservoir of Pneumocystis organisms: Histological and RT-PCR data demonstrate active replication," *European Journal of Clinical Microbiology & Infectious Diseases*, vol. 23, no. 2, pp. 89–97, 2004.

[9] G. H. Cassell and B. C. Cole, "Mycoplasmas as agents of human disease," *The New England Journal of Medicine*, vol. 304, no. 2, pp. 80–89, 1981.

[10] M. Cruciani, P. Marcati, M. Malena, O. Bosco, G. Serpelloni, and C. Mengoli, "Meta-analysis of diagnostic procedures for Pneumocystis carinii pneumonia in HIV-1-infected patients," *European Respiratory Journal*, vol. 20, no. 4, pp. 982–989, 2002.

[11] L. L. Michaelis, G. S. Leight Jr., R. D. Powell Jr., and V. T. DeVita, "Pneumocystis pneumonia: The importance of early open lung biopsy," *Annals of Surgery*, vol. 183, no. 3, pp. 301–306, 1976.

[12] S. Tasaka, N. Hasegawa, S. Kobayashi et al., "Serum indicators for the diagnosis of pneumocystis pneumonia," *CHEST*, vol. 131, no. 4, pp. 1173–1180, 2007.

13

The Impact of COVID-19 on Hospitalised COPD Exacerbations in Malta

Yvette Farrugia, Bernard Paul Spiteri Meilak, Neil Grech, Rachelle Asciak, Liberato Camilleri, Stephen Montefort, and Christopher Zammit

Mater Dei Hospital, Triq id-Donaturi tad-Demm, Msida MSD2090, Malta

Correspondence should be addressed to Yvette Farrugia; yvette.a.farrugia@gov.mt

Academic Editor: Zsofia Lazar

Introduction and Aims. The first COVID-19 case in Malta was confirmed on the 7th of March 2020. This study is aimed at investigating a significant difference between the number of acute exacerbations of chronic obstructive pulmonary disease (AECOPD) admissions and their inpatient outcome at Mater Dei Hospital during the COVID-19 pandemic when compared to the same period in 2019. Furthermore, we aim to determine predictors of mortality in AECOPD inpatients. *Method.* Data was collected retrospectively from electronic hospital records during the periods 1st March until 10th May in 2019 and 2020. *Results.* There was a marked decrease in AECOPD admissions in 2020, with a 54.2% drop in admissions ($n = 119$ in 2020 vs. $n = 259$ in 2019). There was no significant difference in patient demographics or medical comorbidities. In 2020, there was a significantly lower number of patients with AECOPD who received nebulised medications during admission (60.4% in 2020 vs. 84.9% in 2019; $p \leq 0.001$). There were also significantly lower numbers of AECOPD patients admitted in 2020 who received controlled oxygen *via* venturi masks (69.0% in 2020 vs. 84.5% in 2019; $p = 0.006$). There was a significant increase in inpatient mortality in 2020 (19.3% [$n = 23$] and 8.4% [$n = 22$] for 2020 and 2019, respectively, $p = 0.003$). Year was found to be the best predictor of mortality outcome ($p = 0.001$). The lack of use of SABA pre-admission treatment ($p = 0.002$), active malignancy ($p = 0.003$), and increased length of hospital stay ($p = 0.046$) were also found to be predictors of mortality for AECOPD patients; however, these parameters were unchanged between 2019 and 2020 and therefore could not account for the increase in mortality. *Conclusions.* There was a decrease in the number of admissions with AECOPD in 2020 during the COVID-19 pandemic, when compared to 2019. The year 2020 proved to be a significant predictor for inpatient mortality, with a significant increase in mortality in 2020. The decrease in nebuliser and controlled oxygen treatment noted in the study period did not prove to be a significant predictor of mortality when corrected for other variables. Therefore, the difference in mortality cannot be explained with certainty in this retrospective cohort study.

1. Introduction

The World Health Organization (WHO) declared COVID-19 as a worldwide pandemic on the 11th of March 2020. Since the first case detected in Wuhan, Hubei Province of China on 31st December 2019, there have been 150.99 million confirmed cases and 3.17 million deaths registered worldwide as of 1st May 2021 [1]. As a result, people's lives have been impacted dramatically, economic growth grinding to a halt, sending the world into a deep recession [2]. The pandemic has also generated a challenge in the routine care of hospitalised patients. Hospital administrations underwent an overhaul with respect to patient management and treatment protocols, aiming to limit the spread of COVID-19 among patients and healthcare workers.

COVID-19 is propagated by the spread of droplets, particularly by aerosol-generating procedures (AGPs) [3]. A conflict of opinion arose among guidelines, where some favoured the use of nebulisers as it was felt that this treatment should not be classified as an AGP, while others recommended abstaining from nebuliser use. In this context, chronic obstructive pulmonary disease (COPD) patients must be considered as they frequently suffer from acute exacerbations requiring hospital admission for treatment including nebulised bronchodilators. Therefore, patients admitted with an acute exacerbation of COPD (AECOPD) are at risk of being unable to access necessary treatment due to a change in guidelines which could have adverse effects on clinical outcomes [4].

During the pandemic, the first COVID-19 case in Malta was confirmed on the 7th of March 2020, imported from Italy [5]. The first cases of local transmission in Malta were later recorded on the 16th of March 2020. As the COVID-19 pandemic began to affect the Maltese Islands, local guidelines were implemented for inpatients judged to have a high risk of carrying the virus. Until these patients were confirmed to test negative for the SARS-CoV-2 virus, the use of nebulised medications, venturi masks, and non-invasive ventilation (NIV) was limited given the risk of aerosol production. Therefore, this led to the alteration of local treatment guidelines for patients who presented with a deterioration in their pre-existing respiratory condition, primarily asthma and COPD, who are the main subgroup of patients who use these treatment modalities.

During the H1N1 pandemic, a study about social behaviour found that even in the early stages of the pandemic, people in Hong Kong started to avoid going to hospital due to a fear of contracting the virus. This fear stemmed from previous experience during the SARS pandemic [6]. In March of 2020, during the first wave of COVID-19, this phenomenon was also demonstrated in Malta, where there was a significant decline in patients presenting with acute cardiac conditions such as myocardial infarctions. A delay in presentation to the Emergency Department (ED) was demonstrated due to a fear of contracting COVID-19 from within the hospital [7]. Containment measures have also impacted hospitalization rates of strokes [8] and myocardial infarctions [9] in centres abroad. A single-centre study in Germany noted a decrease in AECOPD admissions, and the authors postulated that the reasons were multifactorial. The factors discussed include possible COVID-19 protection with COPD treatment, improvement in air quality secondary to lockdown measures, and reduced face-to-face interaction, altogether contributing towards a reduction in AECOPD admissions [10]. Leung et al. (2020) also noted that data for patients presenting with an AECOPD during this pandemic may be skewed because such patients abstain from presenting to hospital due to fear of exposure to SARS-CoV-2, or may seek help late in the disease course, resulting in delayed management and excess mortality in this subgroup [11]. We hypothesised that the decline and delay in presentation of AECOPD admissions noted in other centres was mirrored locally.

2. Aim

The aim of this study was to establish the impact of COVID-19 pandemic on the number of AECOPD hospital admissions and their inpatient outcome at Mater Dei Hospital, Malta, between 1st March and 10th May 2020, by comparing to the corresponding period in 2019. Furthermore, we aimed to determine predictors of mortality in AECOPD inpatients.

3. Method

This study was a retrospective, observational, cross-sectional study. Data was collected from electronic hospital records. No patients were approached or contacted at any point for the study, and no unique identifying information was collected. The study protocol was approved by the local ethics committee (University of Malta, reference number: FRECMDS_1920_182).

All patients over the age of 18, admitted to Mater Dei Hospital with AECOPD between the 1st of March and 10th of May 2020, were included in this study. The same period from 2019 was used as a control. The diagnosis of an AECOPD was based on the following criteria: change in stable symptoms including increased exertional dyspnoea, chronic cough, and wheeze; the patient's own past medical history and social history, with particular attention to smoking history; imaging; and a response to inhalers and nebulised medications. There were no exclusion criteria. Patients were considered negative for COVID-19 based on results using reverse transcription polymerase chain reaction (RT-PCR).

Assuming a population of 20,000 (4% prevalence of the Maltese population as based on the European Health Interview Survey 2014) and a confidence level of 95%, a sample size of 377 was needed. Statistical analyses were performed using IBM SPSS (SPSS Inc., USA). Variables included gender, locality, medical comorbidities, management modalities used, and inpatient treatment. All variables between the groups were compared using chi-square analysis, Kruskal-Wallis test, and Spearman 2-tailed correlations, accepting a p value ≤ 0.05 as significant. The Fisher exact test was used in cases where sample size was small, such as in the case of non-invasive ventilation use, intensive care admission, and tracheal intubation rate.

To determine predictors of mortality in both cohorts of AECOPD inpatient admissions, a univariate analysis of mortality was carried out using the chi-square test for categorical datasets and independent samples t-test for continuous variables.

The major limitation of the chi-square test and independent samples t-test is that they investigate the relationship between mortality outcome and a single predictor. It is well known that a lone predictor could be rendered a very important contributor in explaining variations in the mortality outcome but would be rendered unimportant in the presence of other predictors. In other words, the suitability of a predictor in a model fit often depends on what other predictors are included with it. To address this limitation, a logistic regression model was fitted to relate mortality outcome (dependent variable) to the predictors of mortality described above. A forward stepwise procedure was used to identify the parsimonious model.

4. Results

A total of 119 and 260 patients were admitted with AECOPD during the period of 1st March to 10th May 2020 and 2019,

Table 1: Demographics and comorbidities of patients hospitalised with AECOPD and COPD pre-admission treatment.

Patient demographics	2019		2020		Chi-square	p value
	n	%	n	%		
Gender—male	199	76.5%	89	74.8%	0.137	0.711
Gender—female	61	23.5%	30	25.2%		
Active smoker (within the last 6 months)	102	54.0%	38	43.7%	2.524	0.112
Comorbidity						
Ischaemic heart disease	80	30.8%	28	23.5%	2.028	0.154
Chronic heart failure	103	39.6%	47	39.5%	0.000	0.986
Hypertension	159	61.1%	78	65.5%	0.879	0.349
Diabetes mellitus	71	27.3%	34	28.6%	0.057	0.812
Asthma	17	6.5%	5	4.2%	0.811	0.368
Cerebrovascular disease	22	8.4%	9	7.6%	0.086	0.770
Peripheral vascular disease	19	7.3%	5	4.2%	1.361	0.243
Pulmonary embolism/deep vein thrombosis	11	4.2%	3	2.5%	0.688	0.407
Active malignancy	27	10.4%	18	15.1%	1.771	0.183
Psychiatric history	44	16.9%	23	19.3%	0.257	0.612
COPD pre-admission treatment						
SABA	179	71.0%	90	78.3%	2.108	0.146
LABA	136	54.0%	57	49.6%	0.614	0.433
SAMA	158	62.7%	77	67.0%	0.622	0.430
LAMA	32	12.7%	21	18.3%	1.977	0.160
ICS	122	48.4%	45	39.1%	2.744	0.098
Home nebulisers	21	8.3%	6	5.2%	1.167	0.280
Home NIV	6	2.4%	3	2.6%	0.014	0.906
Home LTOT	64	25.4%	29	25.0%	0.007	0.935

SABA: short-acting beta-agonist; LABA: long-acting beta-agonist; SAMA: short-acting muscarinic antagonist; LAMA: long-acting muscarinic antagonist; ICS: inhaled corticosteroid use; NIV: non-invasive ventilation; LTOT: long-term oxygen therapy.

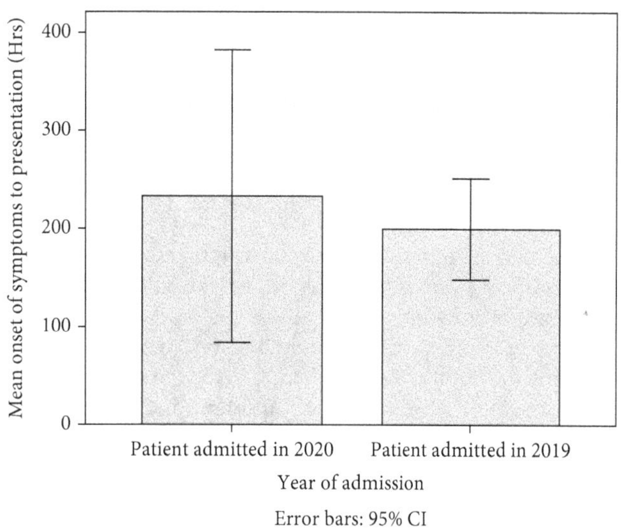

Figure 1: Graph showing the mean time between onsets of symptoms prior to presentation in AECOPD hospitalisations in 2019 compared with 2020.

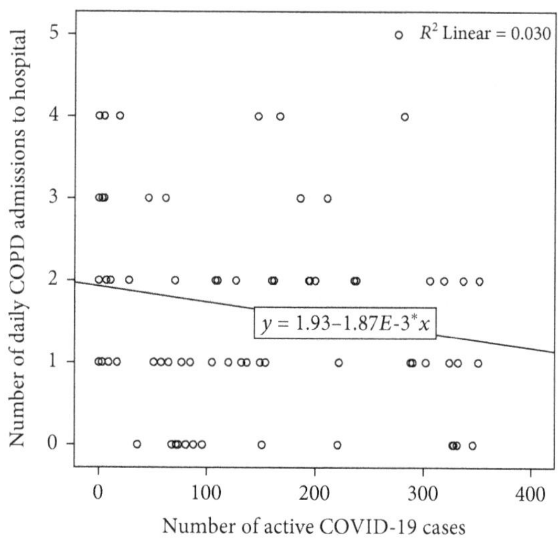

Figure 2: Number of active COVID-19 cases (total and per day) vs. number of AECOPD admissions/day.

respectively, demonstrating a 54.2% drop in admissions. There was no significant difference in the mean age of patients (70.9 years in 2020, 71.7 years in 2019; $p = 0.347$).

The mean hospital length of stay for patients with AECOPD was 6.76 days (5.89-7.6 days, 95% CI) and 6.74 days (5.48-8.04 days, 95% CI) in 2020 and 2019, respectively ($p = 0.704$). The mean number of previous hospital admissions due to AECOPD per patient was 4.79 (3.48-6.11) and

TABLE 2: Oxygen treatment received in AECOPD inpatients during the study period.

	2019, n (%)	2020, n (%)	Chi-square	p value
Venturi mask used (n)	120 (84.5%)	58 (69.0%)	7.541	0.006
Normal face mask/non-rebreather mask (n)	7 (4.9%)	16 (19.0%)	11.508	0.001
No oxygen mask (n)	15 (10.6%)	10 (11.9%)	0.097	0.756

4.05 (3.32-4.78) in 2020 and 2019, respectively ($p = 0.148$). There were no significant differences between the two study groups with respect to demographics, comorbidities, or COPD pre-admission treatment (Table 1).

The mean time from onset of symptoms to hospital admission was longer among patients admitted in 2020, when compared to those admitted in 2019 (232.8 hours (95% CI, 148.08-251.41) vs. 199.7 hours (95% CI, 83.53-382.19)), although this difference did not reach statistical significance ($p = 0.076$) (Figure 1).

A negative correlation was not noted between the number of active COVID-19 cases and AECOPD admissions to hospital (correlation coefficient of -0.208, $R = 0.03$, with a p value approaching statistical significance at 0.082) as illustrated in Figure 2.

None of the patients included in the study tested positive for the SARS-CoV-2 virus on RT-PCR testing; however, not all the patients were swabbed. Among the 2020 cohort, 83% ($n = 99$) of patients were screened for the virus, 62% ($n = 74$) were swabbed once, 17% ($n = 20$) were swabbed twice, and 4% ($n = 5$) were swabbed three times. The number of swabs were related to hospital protocols in place at the time which were largely based on the clinical suspicion of COVID-19, the persistence of fever or symptoms despite conventional treatment, or suspicious findings on computed tomography. Patients were kept in isolation until a negative swab was confirmed, as per hospital protocol at the time.

There was a significant reduction in patients who were administered nebulised treatment (salbutamol ± ipratropium bromide) as an inpatient in 2020, when compared to 2019 (60.4% [$n = 58$] vs. 84.9% [$n = 191$]; chi − square = 23.162, $p \leq 0.001$). In addition, a higher proportion of AECOPD patients in 2020 received supplemental oxygen therapy *via* a normal face mask or a non-rebreather mask during their hospital stay (19% vs. 4.9%, chi − square = 12.024, $p = 0.002$) (Table 2).

No difference in escalation of care was noted between 2020 and 2019 ($p = 0.457$) (Table 3).

The proportion of inpatient deaths with an AECOPD was significantly higher in 2020 compared to 2019 (19.3% [$n = 23$] vs. 8.5% [$n = 22$], respectively, chi-square 9.125; $p = 0.003$), as demonstrated in Figure 3.

To determine predictors of mortality, 2020 and 2019 cohorts were both included in a logistic regression analysis. When analysed individually using the chi-square test and the independent samples t-test, four continuous variables and nine categorical variables were found to be significantly related to mortality outcome (Tables 4 and 5). Other predictors yielding p values larger than the 0.05 criterion were excluded.

TABLE 3: Escalation of care of patients hospitalised with AECOPD (analysed using Fisher's exact test).

Escalation of care	2019	2020	Fisher exact test	Df	p value
NIV (n)	24	9			
ICU admission (n)	8	6	1.589	2	0.457
Tracheal intubation (n)	4	3			

NIV: non-invasive ventilation; ICU: intensive care unit.

To correct for other predictors of mortality, a logistic regression model was fitted to relate mortality outcome to predictors described above (Table 6).

The logistic regression model identifies four significant predictors. Year is the best predictor of mortality outcome and is followed by the lack of use of SABA rescue treatment, active malignancy, and increased length of stay. The Nagelkerke pseudo R-square value (0.654) indicates that this 4-predictor parsimonious logistic regression model explains 65.4% of the total variation in the mortality outcome.

5. Discussion

In this study, we noted a significant decrease in the number of admissions to Mater Dei Hospital in 2020, compared to 2019. Furthermore, an increased mortality was noted among the 2020 cohort, where the year 2020 was found to be a significant predictor for inpatient mortality. A significant reduction in nebuliser and controlled oxygen use was noted, although this did not significantly impact mortality.

The fall in the AECOPD hospital admission rate between 2019 and 2020 in Malta is likely multifactorial. It is difficult to quantify any single contributing effect and may include potentially improved air quality due to a reduction in air pollution and particulate matter after the closure of businesses and industry and reduced air, sea, and vehicular traffic, increased use of facial masks with a potential resulting decrease in other seasonal respiratory viruses, mandatory shielding of people (including those with respiratory disease, those over 65 years of age, and those on oral corticosteroids and immunosuppressant medication), and fear of presenting to health services due to risk of exposure to the SARS-CoV-2 virus. A similar trend was noted in a study conducted in Hong Kong. Chan (2020) reported that during the first three months of 2020, the admission rate for AECOPD decreased by 44%, compared to the average admission rate in previous years. In this study, the decrease was attributed to masking and increased social distancing [12]. In contrast to Hong Kong, during the period studied, mandatory mask wearing

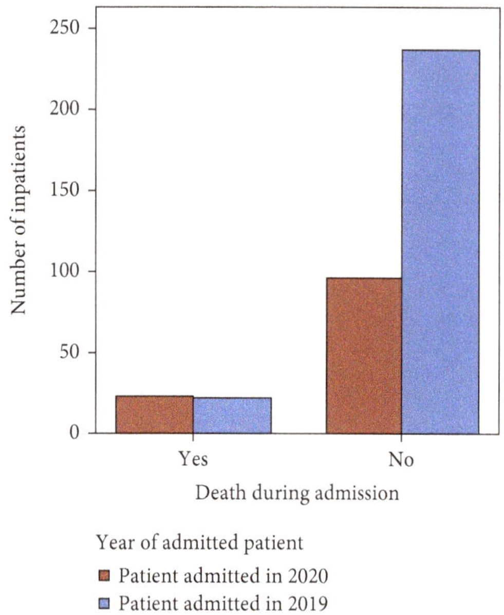

Figure 3: Mortality in 2019 and 2020 during admission.

in public was not yet implemented in Malta. The enforcement of mandatory wearing of masks in enclosed public spaces began on the 3rd May 2020 [13]. During this time, people above the age of 65 years and those immunocompromised were encouraged to isolate and to work from home. As of Saturday 17th October 2020, it became mandatory to wear a face mask in indoor and outdoor spaces [14].

It is a well-known fact that pollution contributes heavily to COPD exacerbations, morbidity, and mortality [15]. A study exploring the air quality of the major capital cities worldwide confirmed that with the lockdown measures imposed during the COVID-19 pandemic, there was a reduction in the concentration of PM2.5 (particulate matter less than 2.5 micrometers in diameter) and an improvement in the overall air quality, providing a potential factor for the reduced COPD admissions rate [16]. A study conducted in Bergamo presented evidence that particulate matter may increase transmission of COVID-19. These results may explain why areas having high levels of air pollution also have a higher COVID-19 case concentration [17]. In contrast to expectations, PM2.5 in Malta did not show any reductions following the implementation of COVID-19 measures, unlike nitrogen dioxide (NO_2), as a major source of PM2.5 is dust from the Sahara Desert [18].

There are various conflicting guidelines regarding whether nebulised treatment is appropriate during the COVID-19 pandemic. NICE and the British Thoracic Society (BTS) recognise that unlike NIV, nebulised medication may not be a viral AGP and does not pose a significant risk for infection with COVID-19 [19, 20]. Contrary, the Global Initiative for Asthma (GINA) advises against nebulised medication use, advocating for the use of pressurised meter dose inhalers (pMDIs) [21].

Between patient groups, a significant decrease in the use of nebulised treatment was noted, as well as a reduction in the administration of controlled oxygen via the venturi mask was noted. This could be explained by fear of hypoxaemia in admitted patients suspected of having the SARS-CoV-2 viral infection. As mentioned above, guidelines concerning the use of nebulised treatment differ widely between academic bodies. NICE advises that as the aerosol from nebulised medication is derived from a non-patient source, it therefore does not carry patient-derived particles and does not carry risk for transmission of COVID-19. There was a shift from controlled oxygen administration to normal face mask and non-rebreather mask supplemental oxygen when comparing 2019 to 2020. This was due to infection control measures implemented at the hospital during the study period limiting the use of venturi masks. Somogyi et al. (2004) demonstrated that venturi oxygen masks can produce a flow of potentially infectious exhaled air during patient expiration [22]. According to Hui et al. (2014), the maximum distances of exhaled air during the application of venturi masks and non-rebreather masks are 0.4 m and <0.1 m, respectively [23]. Following the study period, hospital policies regarding treatment algorithms mentioned above were changed.

This study demonstrated a significant increase in mortality for AECOPD patients admitted during the 2020 COVID-19 pandemic, even though none of these patients tested positive for COVID-19. Based on our results, we hypothesised that lack of controlled oxygen and nebulised treatment would be the predictors towards explaining the difference in mortality. On univariate analysis, thirteen predictors were found to be significant predictors of mortality among all AECOPD inpatient admissions. Among these variables, only differences in oxygen given upon admission and nebulised therapy were significantly different between 2019 and 2020. However, on logistic regression, these two variables did not persist as predictors of mortality. Furthermore, from the predictors found to be significant (active malignancy, length of stay, and SABA pre-admission treatment), none were found to be significantly different between the two cohorts.

Several meta-analyses indicate that COPD patients are at an increased risk of disease severity and mortality if they contract COVID-19 [11, 24–28]. It is therefore recommended that strict adherence to preventer medications is maintained to limit the risk of exacerbations at such a time. The Canadian Thoracic Society highlights this in their updated guidelines [24]. Kaye et al. (2020) found that this recommendation resulted in a general increase in treatment adherence [29]. Of note, during the initial phase of the pandemic, fewer patients attended the outpatient department, resulting in fewer COPD patients being seen by a respiratory specialist. This may have led to poorer control of COPD and contributed to the outcomes.

We cannot therefore explain the difference in mortality found through the results of this study. These results may indicate that the study was relatively underpowered, despite all AECOPD admissions during the study period being included.

6. Limitations

All data were collected from online medical records; therefore, the day-to-day ward round notes and treatment charts

Table 4: Continuous variables significantly related with inpatient mortality (analysed using independent samples t-test).

	Mortality	Sample size	Mean	Standard deviation	p value
Patient age on admission (years)	Yes	45	76.71	8.064	<0.001
	No	333	70.75	9.091	
Total number of previous AECOPD admissions (n)	Yes	45	1.47	1.791	<0.001
	No	328	4.67	6.644	
Length of stay in hospital (days)	Yes	45	11.73	12.027	0.003
	No	333	6.05	5.717	
Days since last admission (days)	Yes	45	2.07	0.863	0.049
	No	325	1.79	0.888	

Table 5: Categorical variables that were significantly related with inpatient mortality (analysed using the chi-square test).

	Death during admission	Alive on discharge	Chi-square	p value
Year of admission (2019/2020, n)	22/23	237/96	9.125	0.003
Active malignancy (yes/no, n)	16/23	29/304	34.289	<0.001
Hypertension (yes/no, n)	35/6	201/132	9.803	0.002
Ischaemic heart disease (yes/no, n)	17/23	91/242	3.996	0.046
Oxygen given on admission (venturi/normal face mask/no oxygen, n)	2/5/1	175/18/24	25.228	<0.001
Nebuliser treatment (yes/no, n)	1/4	247/68	9.631	0.002
Admission to ICU (yes/no, n)	5/40	9/324	7.859	0.005
SABA pre-admission treatment (yes/no, n)	18/16	250/82	7.865	0.005
Diabetes (yes/no, n)	18/23	87/246	5.713	0.017

ICU: intensive care unit; SABA: short-acting beta-agonist.

Table 6: Predictors of inpatient mortality identified by the logistic regression model.

	Model fitting criteria -2 log likelihood of reduced model	Likelihood ratio tests Chi-square	Df	p value
Intercept	14.583	0.000	0	
Year of admission	26.393	11.810	1	0.001
SABA pre-admission treatment	24.360	9.777	1	0.002
Active malignancy	23.580	8.997	1	0.003
Length of stay	18.558	3.975	1	0.046

SABA: short-acting beta-agonist.

were not reviewed as these are not available online. A discharge summary was not available for cases where inpatient death occurred, limiting the data available on severity of the AECOPD and treatment received during the hospital stay. Data collection was also limited by the accuracy and completeness of data documented in the discharge summary and online medical records. This study did not evaluate any difference in outpatient mortality in those suffering with COPD, so no comment can be made on any increase in out-of-hospital deaths due to the lack of presentation suggested by the decrease in hospital admissions.

7. Conclusions

In conclusion, we noted a statistically significant decrease in hospital admissions of patients with AECOPD during the COVID-19 pandemic in 2020, when compared to 2019. The year 2020 was proved to be a significant predictor for inpatient mortality, with a significantly higher inpatient mortality rate in 2020 compared to 2019. The decrease in nebulised medication administered and controlled oxygen treatment noted in the study period did not prove to be a significant predictor of mortality when corrected for other variables, and we cannot therefore explain with certainty the difference in mortality found in this retrospective cohort study.

References

[1] WHO, "coronavirus disease (COVID-19) dashboard," https://covid19.who.int/.

[2] A. Brodeur, D. M. Gray, A. Islam, and S. Bhuiyan, "A literature

review of the economics of Covid-19," *IZA Discussion Paper No. 13411*https://ssrn.com/abstract=3636640.

[3] N. van Doremalen, T. Bushmaker, D. H. Morris et al., "Aerosol and surface stability of SARS-CoV-2 as compared with SARS-CoV-1," *The New England Journal of Medicine*, vol. 382, no. 16, pp. 1564–1567, 2020.

[4] V. G. Press, A. S. Gershon, F. C. Sciurba, and D. P. Blagev, "Concerns about coronavirus disease-related collateral damage for patients with COPD," *Chest*, vol. 158, no. 3, pp. 866–868, 2020, Epub 2020 May 28.

[5] "Times of Malta Website," https://timesofmalta.com/articles/view/first-coronavirus-case-reported-in-malta.776288.

[6] J. T. Lau, S. Griffiths, K. C. Choi, and H. Y. Tsui, "Avoidance behaviors and negative psychological responses in the general population in the initial stage of the H1N1 pandemic in Hong Kong," *BMC Infectious Diseases*, vol. 10, no. 1, p. 139, 2010.

[7] N. Grech, R. Xuereb, K. England, R. G. Xuereb, and M. Caruana, "When the patients stayed home: the impact of the COVID-19 pandemic on acute cardiac admissions and cardiac mortality in Malta," *Journal of Public Health*, 2021.

[8] A. P. Kansagra, M. S. Goyal, S. Hamilton, and G. W. Albers, "Collateral Effect of Covid-19 on Stroke Evaluation in the United States," *New England Journal of Medicine*, vol. 383, no. 4, pp. 400-401, 2020.

[9] A. Truffa Giachet, U. Barbero, F. Ugo et al., "Reduced rate of hospital admissions for ACS during Covid-19 outbreak in Northern Italy," *The New England journal of medicine (United States)*, vol. 383, no. 1, pp. 88-89, 2020.

[10] T. M. Berghaus, P. Karschnia, S. Haberl, and M. Schwaiblmair, "Disproportionate decline in admissions for exacerbated COPD during the COVID-19 pandemic," *Respiratory Medicine*, p. 106120, 2020.

[11] J. M. Leung, M. Niikura, C. W. T. Yang, and D. D. Sin, "COVID-19 and COPD," *European Respiratory Journal*, vol. 56, no. 2, p. 2002108, 2020.

[12] K. Chan, "Significant reduction in hospital admissions for acute exacerbation of chronic obstructive pulmonary disease in Hong Kong during coronavirus disease 2019 pandemic," *Respiratory Medicine*, vol. 171, p. 106085, 2020.

[13] "Masks to be required when shopping or on the bus," 2020, April 2021, https://timesofmalta.com/articles/view/masks-to-be-required-when-shopping-or-on-the-bus.789347.

[14] "COVID-19 frequently asked questions," 2020, April 2021, https://deputyprimeminister.gov.mt/en/health-promotion/covid-19/Pages/frequently-asked-questions.aspx.

[15] N. N. Hansel, M. C. McCormack, and V. Kim, "The effects of air pollution and temperature on COPD," *COPD: Journal of Chronic Obstructive Pulmonary Disease*, vol. 13, no. 3, pp. 372–379, 2016.

[16] D. Rodríguez-Urrego and L. Rodríguez-Urrego, "Air quality during the COVID-19: PM2.5 analysis in the 50 most polluted capital cities in the world," *Environmental Pollution*, vol. 266, Part 1, p. 115042, 2020.

[17] L. Setti, F. Passarini, G. De Gennaro et al., "SARS-Cov-2RNA found on particulate matter of Bergamo in Northern Italy: first evidence," *Environmental Research*, vol. 188, p. 109754, 2020.

[18] Malta, Environment and Resources Authority, "A preliminary assessment related to the impact of Covid-19 measures on air quality in Malta," *Environment and Resources Authority*, pp. 1–10, 2020, https://era.org.mt/wp-content/uploads/2020/12/Covid-19-and-Air-Quality_MT-Report_Final.pdf.

[19] Public Health England, NHS: National Services Scotland, and Department of Health and Social Care, & Public Health Wales (PHW), "COVID-19: guidance for the remobilisation of services within health and care settings," *Infection Prevention and Control Recommendations*, 2020, https://www.gov.uk/government/publications/wuhan-novel-coronavirus-infection-prevention-and-control.

[20] British Thoracic Society BTS, "COVID-19: information for the respiratory community," *British Thoracic Society*, 2020, https://www.brit-thoracic.org.uk/covid-19/covid-19-information-for-the-respiratory-community/.

[21] M. Cazzola, J. Ora, A. Bianco, P. Rogliani, and M. G. Matera, "Guidance on nebulization during the current COVID-19 pandemic," *Respiratory Medicine*, vol. 176, p. 106236, 2021.

[22] R. Somogyi, A. Vesely, T. Azami et al., "Dispersal of respiratory droplets with open vs closed oxygen delivery masks," *Chest*, vol. 125, no. 3, pp. 1155–1157, 2004.

[23] D. S. Hui, M. T. Chan, and B. Chow, "Aerosol dispersion during various respiratory therapies: a risk assessment model of nosocomial infection to health care workers," *Hong Kong Medical Journal*, vol. 20, Suppl 4, pp. 9–13, 2014.

[24] M. Bhutani, P. Hernandez, J. Bourbeau et al., "Key highlights of the Canadian Thoracic Society's position statement on the optimization of COPD management during the coronavirus disease 2019 pandemic," *Chest*, vol. 158, no. 3, pp. 869–872, 2020.

[25] J. S. Alqahtani, T. Oyelade, A. M. Aldhahir et al., "Prevalence, severity and mortality associated with COPD and smoking in patients with COVID-19: a rapid systematic review and meta-analysis," *PLoS One*, vol. 15, no. 5, p. e0233147, 2020.

[26] Q. Zhao, M. Meng, R. Kumar et al., "The impact of COPD and smoking history on the severity of COVID-19: a systemic review and meta-analysis," *Journal of Medical Virology*, vol. 92, no. 10, pp. 1915–1921, 2020.

[27] D. C. Sanchez-Ramirez and D. Mackey, "Underlying respiratory diseases, specifically COPD, and smoking are associated with severe COVID-19 outcomes: a systematic review and meta-analysis," *Respiratory Medicine*, vol. 171, p. 106096, 2020.

[28] J. Olloquequi, "COVID-19 susceptibility in chronic obstructive pulmonary disease," *European Journal of Clinical Investigation*, vol. 50, no. 10, p. e13382, 2020.

[29] L. Kaye, B. Theye, I. Smeenk, R. Gondalia, M. A. Barrett, and D. A. Stempel, "Changes in medication adherence among patients with asthma and COPD during the COVID-19 pandemic," *The Journal of Allergy and Clinical Immunology: In Practice*, vol. 8, no. 7, pp. 2384-2385, 2020.

14

Impact of Clinical Factors on Generic and Disease-Specific Quality of Life in COPD and Asthma-COPD Overlap with Exacerbations

Zsófia Lázár[1] **Alpár Horváth**[1,2] **Gábor Tomisa,**[1,2] **Lilla Tamási**[1] **and Veronika Müller**[1]

[1]*Dept. Pulmonology, Semmelweis University, 25-29 Tömő Str. 1083 Budapest, Hungary*
[2]*Chiesi Hungary Ltd., Dunavirág u. 2, 1138 Budapest, Hungary*

Correspondence should be addressed to Veronika Müller; muller.veronika@med.semmelweis-univ.hu

Academic Editor: Stefano Centanni

Purpose. The health-related quality of life (HRQL) in chronic obstructive pulmonary disease (COPD) is worsened by frequent exacerbations, and it can be affected by the concomitant presence of bronchial asthma (asthma-COPD overlap (ACO)). The impacts of clinical factors associated with HRQL have not been compared in patients with COPD and ACO experiencing exacerbations. *Patients and Methods.* Patients with COPD (N=705) and ACO (N=148) belonging to C and D groups according to GOLD 2017 were recruited in stable condition. Demographic and clinical data were collected, spirometry was performed, and patients rated the intensity of respiratory symptoms during the previous week. The COPD Assessment Test (CAT) and the EQ-5D 3 level version (dimensions and visual analogue scale (VAS)) were used to assess disease-specific and generic HRQL, respectively. Fisher's exact test, χ^2 test, ANOVA, and Pearson correlation were used for analysis (mean ± SD). Multiple linear regression was applied to identify variables related to CAT and EQ-5D VAS scores. *Results.* The CAT and EQ-5D VAS scores showed similarly low HRQL in COPD and ACO (20.7 ± 6.7 vs. 21.1 ± 6.3 ($p = 0.52$) and 56.2 ± 17.8 vs. 53.7 ± 18.2 ($p = 0.11$)). There was a weak correlation between CAT and EQ-5D VAS scores (COPD: $r = -0.345$, $p < 0.001$; ACO: $r = -0.245$, $p = 0.003$). More patients with COPD had problems related to anxiety/depression in EQ-5D (63.7% vs. 55.4%, $p = 0.06$). Pack-years exerted a negative effect on HRQL measures both in ACO and COPD. Low HRQL in COPD was associated with female gender, dyspnea, cough, gastroesophageal reflux disease, and arrhythmia, while in ACO, it was related to arrhythmia, hypertension, and cough, but less to dyspnea. *Conclusions.* Patients with COPD and ACO experiencing exacerbations have low quality of life, which is influenced by smoking history, symptoms, and comorbidities. These findings have important implications for the development of therapeutic strategies to improve the health status of patients with these conditions.

1. Introduction

Chronic obstructive pulmonary disease (COPD) is characterized by irreversible and progressive airflow limitation, the presence of multiple comorbidities, and reduced quality of life [1]. Several factors have been described to be negatively related to the quality of life measures in COPD such as the lower level of education, an unskilled profession, female gender, and disease severity [2–4]. Comorbidities including peripheral arterial disease, osteoporosis, depression, diabetes, stroke, and myocardial infarction also exert an additional unfavorable effect on the health status [2, 5–7]. Exacerbations are important events in the course of COPD, and notably, patients with frequent exacerbations suffer from poorer quality of life [8, 9]. However, the influence of clinical factors on health status in frequent exacerbators has not been explored.

A subgroup of patients with COPD also show clinical features of bronchial asthma and can be termed to have asthma-COPD overlap (ACO) [10]. Patients with ACO are younger; they have a lower level of dyspnea and smoked less than patients with COPD alone [11]. Of note, the rate of exacerbation was shown to be unchanged [11, 12], but also increased [13, 14] in ACO. Compared to COPD, patients with ACO have more severe airway obstruction [15, 16], more severe wheezing [16], and a different set of comorbidities [17]. Reports on quality of life in ACO vs. COPD showed contradictory findings [12, 18], and health measures have not been studied in frequent exacerbators with overlap disease.

Thus, we aimed to investigate the health-related quality of life (HRQL) in patients with COPD and ACO who experience multiple disease relapses. We compared the clinical features and the disease-specific and a generic HRQL in patients with COPD and ACO belonging to groups C and D as classified according to the Global Initiative for Chronic Obstructive Lung Disease (GOLD) recommendation [1]. Furthermore, the influence of demographic and clinical variables, as well as comorbidities on the health status of patients, was also studied.

2. Material and Methods

2.1. Patients and Study Design. Patients were recruited by 71 respiratory specialists during regular control visits at outpatient pulmonology centers in Hungary between 01 November 2017 and 31 March 2018. Inclusion criteria were age > 18 years, COPD diagnosed >1 year ago by a respiratory specialist (as postbronchodilator $FEV_1/FVC < 0.70$) [1], and exacerbation history equivalent to groups C or D according to GOLD document 2017 [1]. ACO was established when patients showed overlapping clinical characteristics of COPD and bronchial asthma [10] together with a concomitant diagnosis of bronchial asthma established at least one month prior to inclusion. Patients with ACO had a positive bronchial hyperreactivity or reversibility testing (>12% or 200 ml after the inhalation of 400 μg salbutamol) in the past. Exclusion criteria were the presence of severe and untreated comorbidity, inability to fill out the HRQL questionnaires, current systemic steroid or antibiotic treatment, restrictive ventilatory failure, severe cardiac failure, current tuberculosis infection, and active cancer.

The study had a noninterventional longitudinal design. During the first visit, detailed clinical characteristics, information on drug side effects, spirometric variables, and data on symptoms and HRQL were collected, inhaler technique was checked and corrected when necessary. At later visits (after 1 month and 3 months), the inhaler technique was rechecked, education on inhaler use was repeated, and spirometric values, symptom scores, and HRQL variables were recorded. Data of patients with three completed visits were collected for statistical analysis ($N = 944$). During data clearance, 91 patients were excluded for not meeting the inclusion criteria for exacerbation number ($N = 853$). In the present work, data only from the first visit were analyzed in a cross-sectional manner.

The study was approved by the Hungarian Medical Research Council (46367-4/2017/EKU) and the National Institute of Pharmacy and Nutrition (46402-5/2017). Each patient signed a written informed consent. All work was conducted in accordance with the Declaration of Helsinki (1964).

2.2. Data Collection. Demographic and basic clinical data were recorded (age, gender, smoking history, number of moderate, and severe past exacerbations according to categories). Former smoking was defined as smoking stopped at least 6 months earlier. Educational level was noted as completed higher education (higher), completed secondary education (middle), and completed or uncompleted primary education (low). Height, weight, and prebronchodilator spirometry (FVC, FEV_1) were measured [19]. Body mass index (BMI) was calculated, and patients were categorized into four groups [20]: underweight (<20 kg/m^2), normal weight (20 to 24.9 kg/m^2), overweight (25 to 29.9 kg/m^2), and obese (≥30 kg/m^2). Current inhaled therapy regimens (classes of drugs) and the use of short-acting bronchodilators in the past week (≤1/week, 2-3/week, >3/week) were recorded.

Self-reported comorbidities were noted according to predefined categories (gastroesophageal reflux disease (GERD), ischemic heart disease, hypertension, myocardial infarction, arrhythmia, heart failure, cerebrovascular event, osteoporosis, diabetes, glaucoma, and chronic bronchitis). Arrhythmia was defined as an existing chronic arrhythmia or a previous intermittent episode. A previous stroke or a past intermittent cerebrovascular episode was considered a cerebrovascular event. Chronic bronchitis was defined as at least 3 months of productive coughing in 2 or more consecutive years, and it was assessed only in patients with COPD.

Patients rated their level of dyspnea using the Modified British Medical Research Council (mMRC) Questionnaire [21], and they were asked to assess the intensity of symptoms (dyspnea at rest, dyspnea during daily activities, and cough) in the past week on a scale from 0 to 10, where 0 meant no symptoms and 10 referred to unbearable symptoms. Sputum production in the past week was also reported: no sputum (0), a small amount (1), a moderate amount (2), and a significant amount (3).

Quality of life was measured with the disease-specific COPD Assessment Test (CAT), which is a validated 8-item tool used for monitoring COPD [22]. Symptoms were self-assessed by patients on a scale from 0 to 5; the maximal overall score is 40 with higher scores referring to higher symptom burden.

The EQ-5D-3L (3 level version) and the EQ-5D-VAS (visual analogue scale) were applied to evaluate the generic health status [23]. The EQ-5D-3L comprises of 5 dimensions: mobility, self-care, usual activities, pain/discomfort, and anxiety/depression. In each dimension, the disability can be rated by the patients on 3 levels: no problems (1), some problems (2), and extreme problems (3). Due to the lack of available value sets representative for the Hungarian population, a utility score could not be calculated; therefore, the dimensions were individually analyzed. Patients graded their today health using the VAS in the form of a 20 cm vertical line ranging from 0 to 100, where 100 represents the best imaginable and 0 the worst imaginable health status.

2.3. Data Analysis. Categorical variables were analyzed with the Fisher exact and χ^2 tests (combined with post hoc analysis). Continuous variables showed Gaussian distribution and were analyzed using a t-test, ANOVA, and Pearson correlation and presented through their means and standard deviations (SD). Multiple linear regression was applied to identify clinical variables related to CAT and EQ-5D VAS. The SPSS 19.0. software (IBM, Armonk, NY, US) was applied for statistical analysis; p values < 0.05 were considered significant.

3. Results

3.1. Demographic Variables in Patients with COPD and ACO. Among the 853 patients included in the study, 18% and 82% had ACO and COPD alone, respectively (Table 1). Most patients belonged to GOLD group D (COPD patients C/D: 5.0/95.0%, ACO patients: group C/D: 3.4%/96.6%; $p = 0.41$). There was a trend for more male patients with COPD. The BMI was higher in patients with ACO with an increased ratio of obese patients, while we observed a tendency for more underweight patients with COPD. As expected, there were more current smokers with COPD, and more patients were nonsmokers in the ACO group; however, the pack-years were similar in the two groups. FEV_1 and FEV_1/FVC were lower in COPD alone. Inhaled therapy regimens with ICS (inhaled corticosteroid) were more frequently used by patients with ACO, while long-acting muscarinic antagonist and long-acting beta$_2$-agonist (LAMA+LABA) products were applied by more patients with COPD alone. We noted a trend for an increased number of hypertension cases and a higher overall burden of comorbidities in COPD. No difference was noted in age, educational level, and the number of COPD-related emergency room visits and hospitalizations between the two groups.

3.2. Quality of Life and Symptoms in Patients with COPD and ACO. There was a significant but weak correlation between CAT and EQ-5D VAS scores in patients with COPD ($r = -0.345$, $p < 0.001$; Figure 1(a)) and ACO ($r = -0.245$, $p = 0.003$; Figure 1(b)). The CAT score showed a similarly low disease-specific quality of life in both groups, which is line with the predominance of the GOLD D group patients in the populations (Table 2). The EQ-5D VAS tool demonstrated a mean decrease of 2.5 points in ACO compared to COPD; however, it did not reach statistical significance. A trend for more severe anxiety and depression was noted in patients with COPD, and the proportion of patients with any problems (some or extreme problems) in the anxiety/depression dimension was increased in COPD vs. ACO (63.7% vs. 55.4%, $p = 0.06$). We found no difference in the health status between the two groups analyzed according to other EQ-5D dimensions (Table 2).

The intensity of respiratory symptoms and the use of short-acting bronchodilator in the past week were similar in the two groups (Table 2). Of note, approximately half of the patients needed to use a reliever medication more than three times in the previous week, highlighting the high symptom burden.

Interestingly, the CAT score was increased in patients with ACO on LAMA+LABA therapy compared to COPD patients on dual long-acting bronchodilators (Table 3). Data on mono-LAMA and mono-LABA use were not analyzed due to the low number of patients in the ACO group ($n = 2$ and $n = 0$, respectively).

3.3. Clinical Variables Associated with Health Status in Patients with COPD. In patients with COPD, a lower disease-specific quality of life, denoted by a higher CAT score, was associated with pack-years and the increased number of severe exacerbations in the past 12 months (Table 4). The intensity of dyspnea either at rest or during daily activities and the intensity of cough were related to higher CAT scores; however, the amount of sputum showed no association. Among the comorbidities, only GERD was associated with higher CAT scores.

As shown by the EQ-5D VAS score, a better generic HRQL was linked to a higher level of education, while it was negatively associated with female gender, pack-years, arrhythmia, and dyspnea at rest. There was a trend for worse health status in patients with the frequent use of reliever medications.

3.4. Clinical Variables Associated with Health Status in Patients with ACO. In patients with ACO, an increased CAT score was associated with the high intensity of cough in the past week (Table 4). In addition, the frequent use of reliever medications was related to higher CAT scores, and arrhythmia showed a trend for an increase in the CAT score. Unexpectedly, we found a tendency between lower CAT scores and a high number of previous severe COPD-related exacerbation and the presence of obesity (trend toward significance).

The EQ-5D VAS score was positively associated with a higher level of education. There was a negative relationship between the general health status and pack-years, arrhythmia, and the frequent use of short-acting bronchodilators. Moreover, we observed a trend for a negative association between the EQ-5D VAS score and hypertension and the intensity of dyspnea at rest.

4. Discussion

Exacerbations in COPD are associated with worse and deteriorating quality of life [8, 24]. A higher number of hospitalizations due to respiratory symptoms [13, 14] and a lower HRQL [18] were recorded in patients with ACO compared to subjects with asthma or COPD alone. The mechanism of ACO is currently incompletely understood, and more research is needed to identify its specific clinical and physiological characteristics [10]. In the present study, we focused on patients with COPD and ACO with a history of past exacerbations and found that both groups have similarly low HRQL, which is associated with partly shared clinical variables including the burden of respiratory symptoms and comorbidities.

The clinical characteristics of patients with ACO and COPD showed differences. We observed a higher number of women, increased BMI, and somewhat better FEV_1/FVC among patients with ACO, which corroborate previous findings [25]. Interestingly, airway obstruction was less severe in patients with ACO, while previous studies reported decreased [15] or similar [25] FEV_1 compared to patients with COPD. These discrepancies can be explained by the different patient population in our study: (i) we also included never smokers, (ii) patients were diagnosed by respiratory specialists, and

Table 1: Demographic and clinical data of patients with COPD and ACO.

	COPD ($n = 705$)	ACO ($n = 148$)	p value
Men	50.9%	42.6%	0.065
Age (years)	63.7 ± 9.5	62.3 ± 11.2	0.109
Body mass index (kg/m^2) (all patients)	27.8 ± 6.6	29.0 ± 6.2	0.043
Body mass index (categories)			0.048
<20	9.9%	5.4%	0.082
20-24.9	28.6%	21.6%	0.087
25.0-29.9	27.9%	30.4%	0.549
>30	33.6%	42.6%	0.038
Smoking status			<0.001
Current	54.5%	39.2%	<0.001
Past	36.0%	35.1%	0.834
Never	9.5%	25.7%	<0.001
Pack-years	32.3 ± 17.5	31.7 ± 19.4	0.717
Educational level			0.104
Low	44.4%	43.9%	
Medium	51.1%	47.3%	
High	4.5%	8.8%	
No. of hospitalizations and ER visits due to respiratory symptoms in the past year			0.932
0	62.4%	60.8%	
1	27.7%	29.1%	
≥2	9.9%	10.1%	
FVC (L)	2.22 ± 0.70	2.30 ± 0.88	0.239
FVC (% reference)	69.4 ± 17.6	71.3 ± 18.3	0.237
FEV_1 (L)	1.25 ± 0.46	1.34 ± 0.58	0.040
FEV_1 (% reference)	48.6 ± 14.9	52.3 ± 16.2	0.007
FEV_1/FVC	0.56 ± 0.10	0.58 ± 0.10	0.037
Inhaled therapy			<0.001
LAMA	3.1%	1.4%	0.238
LABA	0.7%	0%	0.303
LAMA+LABA	49.2%	25.7%	<0.001
LABA+ICS	3.3%	16.9%	<0.001
LABA+LAMA+ICS	43.7%	56.1%	0.006
Comorbidities			
Gastroesophageal reflux	22.4%	21.0%	0.696
Ischemic heart disease	22.4%	18.9%	0.350
Hypertension	60.9%	52.7%	0.066
Myocardial infarction	4.5%	2.7%	0.312
Arrhythmia	10.8%	6.1%	0.083
Heart failure	7.8%	5.4%	0.311
Cerebrovascular event	5.7%	4.7%	0.647
Osteoporosis	7.4%	9.5%	0.646
Diabetes	12.3%	14.2%	0.167
Glaucoma	2.0%	0.7%	0.270
Benign prostate hyperplasia	13.4%	11.1%	0.623
Total number of comorbidities	1.63 ± 1.49	1.40 ± 1.31	0.090

Table 1: Continued.

Data are shown as mean ± SD. Data were analyzed with Fisher's exact test, t-test, and χ^2 tests (with post hoc analysis). ACO: asthma-COPD overlap; ER: emergency; FVC: forced vital capacity; FEV_1: forced expiratory volume in the 1st second; LAMA: long-acting muscarinic antagonist; LABA: long-acting beta$_2$-agonists; ICS: inhaled corticosteroid.

(iii) patients belonged only to GOLD groups C and D. In spite of the higher FEV_1, dyspnea was as severe in ACO as in COPD (either assessed by mMRC or symptom scores), which might be related to the heightened sensation of dyspnea in this group [26]. We observed a higher prevalence of hypertension and arrhythmia in COPD than in ACO as also shown by others [12].

We did not find a difference in CAT scores between patients with COPD and ACO, which supports previous findings in a cohort with similar symptom burden [27]. Nonetheless, Kurashima et al. found higher CAT scores in Japanese patients with ACO who showed higher scores for cough, phlegm, and dyspnea, but the average CAT score and exacerbation frequency were lower than in our cohort [26]. Furthermore, Park et al. did not show a difference in the disease-specific quality of life between ACO and COPD in a Korean cohort using the CAT tool; however, the Saint George's Respiratory Questionnaire (SGRQ) could detect better HRQL in ACO [12]. On the contrary, ACO was associated with a worse health status assessed by the SGRQ in a US population comprised of patients with different ethnic groups [25]. These and our data suggest that besides exacerbation history, disease-specific health status in ACO might also be influenced by the genetic background of patients.

Our study provides novel data on the relationship between inhaled therapies and HRQL in ACO. We found that patients on dual long-acting bronchodilators have worse CAT scores compared to patients with combination therapies including ICS. This supports the use of ICS in ACO as also stated in the consensus-based document available in the Global Strategy for Asthma Management and Prevention report [10].

Our results demonstrate that different clinical factors modulate disease-specific quality of life in COPD and ACO with exacerbations. The negative influence of smoking history [28], the intensity of dyspnea [29], and the exacerbation number [30] in COPD have already been known, but the unfavorable effect of gastroesophageal reflux disease on CAT score has not been described before. It can be speculated that GERD worsens cough, which is also associated with higher CAT in our cohort; however, further research should give better insight into the mechanism of GERD and HRQL. Contrary to COPD, dyspnea is not associated with CAT scores in ACO, which was rather related to cough as also noted by others [26]. In ACO, the number of severe exacerbations is not associated with higher CAT scores, which

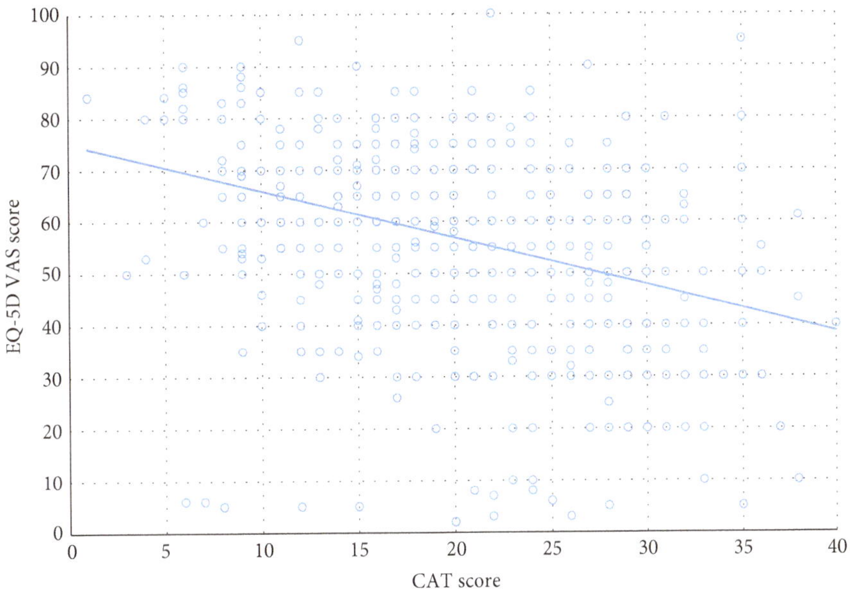

(a)

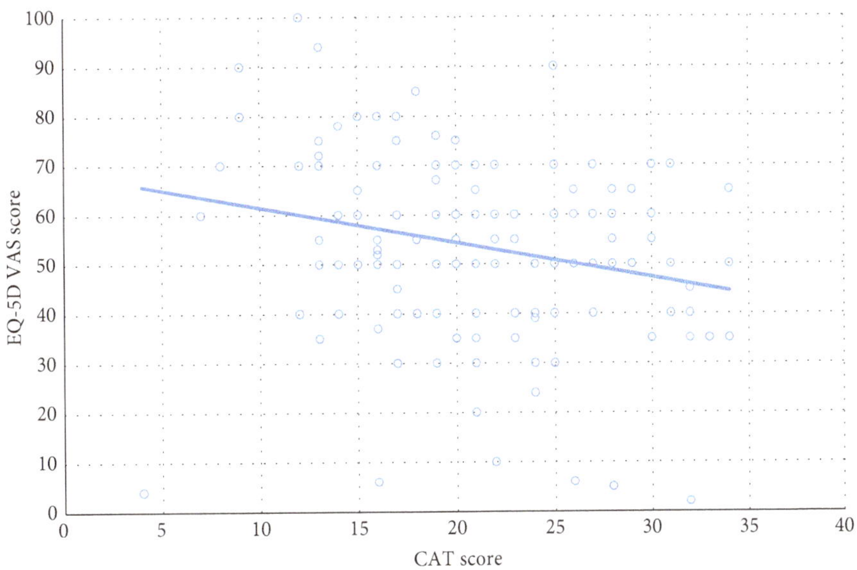

(b)

FIGURE 1: Correlation between the CAT and the EQ-5D VAS scores: (a) COPD, $r = -0.345$, $p < 0.001$; (b) ACO, $r = -0.245$, $p = 0.003$ (Pearson correlation).

could be explained by better recovery induced by the better response to systemic steroids in this population compared to patients with COPD. The association of the frequent use of reliever medications and arrhythmia to CAT scores in ACO might be linked, and it raises attention to the speculative negative effects of reliever abuse on disease-specific HRQL.

The EQ-5D VAS scores were low for both ACO and COPD confirming similarly reduced health status in these groups. This extends previous findings, which showed that patients with ACO have reduced health status, comparable to COPD patients of the exacerbator phenotype [31]. Interestingly, most patients reported some problems in all five dimensions of the EQ-5D, and there was a tendency for a higher proportion of COPD patients with any problems of depression and anxiety. In a Polish COPD cohort, an increased prevalence of both anxiety and depression was noted for frequent exacerbators compared to patients with ACO [32], which is verified in our cohort of exacerbation-matched patients.

The factors influencing generic health, as reflected by EQ-5D VAS scores, in patients with ACO and COPD are partly shared. We show that contrary to smoking status, which does not influence HRQL in this and in other COPD cohorts [7], pack-years do exert a negative influence on EQ-5D VAS score in both groups. Dyspnea at rest is the only

TABLE 2: Symptoms and quality of life in patients with COPD and ACO.

	COPD	ACO	p value
CAT score	20.7 ± 6.7	21.1 ± 6.3	0.522
EQ-5D VAS score	56.2 ± 17.8	53.7 ± 18.2	0.110
EQ-5D scores			
Mobility	1.54 ± 0.52	1.51 ± 0.54	0.511
Self-care	1.48 ± 0.56	1.48 ± 0.58	0.928
Usual activities	1.83 ± 0.55	1.89 ± 0.53	0.304
Pain/discomfort	1.74 ± 0.57	1.69 ± 0.55	0.318
Anxiety/depression	1.76 ± 0.66	1.66 ± 0.66	0.074
mMRC score	2.5 ± 0.8	2.4 ± 0.8	0.692
Severity of symptoms in the past week			
Dyspnea at rest	3.64 ± 3.06	3.67 ± 3.33	0.900
Dyspnea during daily activities	4.27 ± 2.98	4.60 ± 2.92	0.216
Cough	5.09 ± 2.19	4.93 ± 2.41	0.425
Sputum production	1.67 ± 0.64	1.69 ± 0.64	0.738
Use of short-acting bronchodilators in the past week (% all patients)			0.274
≤1	22.5%	20.4%	
2-3	29.5%	23.1%	
>3	48.0%	56.5%	

Data are shown as mean ± SD. Data were analyzed with t-test, Mann-Whitney test, and χ^2 test. CAT: COPD Assessment Test; mMRC: Modified British Medical Research Council Questionnaire.

TABLE 3: Quality of life measures according to maintenance inhaled therapy.

	CAT		p value	EQ-5D VAS score		p value
	COPD	ACO		COPD	ACO	
LAMA+LABA	20.5 ± 6.9	23.0 ± 6.3	0.033	59.4 ± 16.1	59.5 ± 15.3	0.963
LABA+ICS	20.4 ± 6.0	20.4 ± 6.0	0.958	50.9 ± 23.9	47.8 ± 18.4	0.619
LABA+LAMA+ICS	20.9 ± 6.8	20.4 ± 6.3	0.545	52.9 ± 18.3	53.4 ± 18.3	0.853

Data are shown as mean ± SD. Data were analyzed with t-test.

symptom related to health status both in COPD and ACO, which might be partly explained by the altered dimensions of dyspnea in patients with COPD [29]. Prebronchodilator FEV_1 did not show a relation to HRQL; however, other lung function values including specific airway resistance and readouts of hyperinflation could better evaluate the beneficial effect of bronchodilators on dyspnea and quality of life [33], but these parameters were not measured in our study. We corroborated previous findings on the negative effect of cardiovascular comorbidities in COPD [2] by showing that HRQL is associated with cardiovascular comorbidities including arrhythmia (COPD and ACO) and hypertension (ACO). Like others [4], we also found that female patients have lower HRQL if they have COPD, but not ACO. However, higher classes of education are associated with better HRQL in both groups as already shown for COPD [7].

We analyzed the correlation between the disease-specific and generic HRQL measures in ACO for the first time. We found that the CAT and EQ-5D VAS scores were more weakly correlated in ACO than in COPD, which can be explained by the higher influence of nonrespiratory symptoms on the general health status in ACO.

Our study was performed in a large cohort of COPD patients diagnosed by respiratory specialists; however, it has few limitations. First, comorbidities which are known to influence HRQL in COPD and might also affect it in ACO such as psychiatric disorders and peripheral artery disease [7] were not studied. Second, comorbidities were self-reported by patients, which might limit their validity. Third, utility score could not be calculated for EQ-5D-3L. Furthermore, we did not measure bronchial reversibility, although a subgroup of patients with COPD alone show a clinically relevant bronchial reversibility linked with inflammatory processes [34]. Importantly, reversibility was related to dyspnea and quality of life in a recent COPD cohort [35].

5. Conclusions

In conclusion, patients with COPD and ACO experiencing exacerbations have similarly reduced disease-specific and

TABLE 4: Estimates yielded from multiple regression analysis to predict factors associated with quality of life measures.

	COPD		ACO	
	CAT	EQ-5D VAS	CAT	EQ-5D VAS
Age	-0.018	0.021	0.031	0.171
Gender				
Male	Ref.	Ref.	Ref.	Ref.
Female	0.403	-3.617[a]	0.177	-4.327
Body mass index (kg/m^2)				
<20	0.549	1.820	-1.351	-0.773
20-24.9	Ref.	Ref.	Ref.	Ref.
25.0-29.9	0.863	-2.160	-1.891	-2.669
>30	0.769	-0.471	-3.407[d]	-7.136
Smoking status				
Current	0.781	0.653	-0.034	-0.491
Ex-smoker	Ref.	Ref.	Ref.	Ref.
Pack-years	0.029[a]	-0.094[a]	-0.006	-0.238[a]
Educational level				
Low	Ref.	Ref.	Ref.	Ref.
Medium	-0.452	4.208[b]	-0.594	3.009
High	-0.903	1.441	-1.046	10.372[e]
No. of hospitalizations and ER visits due to exacerbation in the past year				
0	Ref.	Ref.	Ref.	Ref.
1	-0.722	0.058	-2.598	-0.262
≥2	2.257[b]	-0.443	-6.772[a]	-6.430
FEV$_1$ (% reference)	-0.024	0.072	-0.049	0.143
Comorbidities				
Absence of comorbidity	Ref.	Ref.	Ref.	Ref.
Gastroesophageal reflux	1.578[b]	1.118	0.477	4.149
Ischemic heart disease	-1.104[d]	0.979	-0.476	-0.198
Hypertension	0.098	2.473	1.249	-6.218[e]
Past myocardial infarction	1.409	5.494	9.143	-9.305
Arrhythmia	0.674	-6.298[a]	5.589[e]	-15.852[a]
Heart failure	0.830	-0.031	0.993	-7.320
Past cerebrovascular event	-0.404	-3.174	-1.922	-6.255
Osteoporosis	-1.508	0.213	-0.183	4.052
Diabetes	-0.431	-0.235	-3.067	-1.123
Glaucoma	2.869	-1.372	-[1]	-[1]
Chronic bronchitis	-1.341[a]	2.583	-[2]	-[2]
Severity of symptoms in the past week				
Dyspnea at rest	0.573[c]	-1.286[c]	0.150	-1.302[d]
Dyspnea during daily activities	0.353[c]	-0.398	0.351	0.808
Cough	0.508[c]	0.405	0.939[a]	-0.143
Sputum production, amount small	Ref.	Ref.	Ref.	Ref.
Medium	0.331	-2.587	0.120	1.664
Significant	0.307	-0.706	-1.806	-8.841
Use of short-acting bronchodilators in the past week (% all patients)				
≤1	Ref.	Ref.	Ref.	Ref.
2-3	0.006	2.258	3.870	-11.269[a]
>3	1.194	-3.831[d]	4.593[a]	-6.393

TABLE 4: Continued.

[a]$p < 0.05$, [b]$p < 0.01$, [c]$p < 0.001$, [d]$p = 0.07$, [e]$p = 0.09$. 1: not analyzed due to missing data; 2: not assessed in the ACO group; Ref.: reference category.

generic qualities of life, but patients with COPD seem to have more severe problems in the dimension of anxiety and depression. Pack-years and the frequent use of short-acting bronchodilators exert a negative effect on HRQL measures both in ACO and COPD. HRQL is influenced by symptoms and comorbidities as well. Low HRQL in COPD is associated with the female gender, dyspnea, cough, GERD, and arrhythmia, while it is related to arrhythmia, hypertension, and cough, but less to dyspnea in ACO. Our results aid the development of complex therapeutic strategies to improve the health status of patients with COPD and ACO.

Disclosure

Chiesi Hungary Ltd. had no role in designing the study and was not involved in the analysis and interpretation of data or manuscript preparation or submission for publication.

Acknowledgments

We would like to thank all the colleagues for patient recruitment: K.É. Alb, C. Babka, A. Bánvölgyi, A. Bartha, M. Bárány, É. Bauknecht, M. Beke, Z. Bitay, C. Böcskei, L. Bognár, Z. Bólya, K. Böszörményi, I. Breining, M. Czompó, M. Décsi, T. Donka, M. Egri, E. Frank, R. Fráter, E. Füzesi, K. Gazsó, K. Hajdu, C. Hangonyi, G. Horváth, H. Huszár, L. Jancsikin, E. Juhász, T. Juhász, I. Kerényi, Z. Kerényi, E. Klembucz, F. Kollár, K. Kontz, A. Kukuly, M. Kukuly, C. Kun, É. Lanczki, K. Lévai, J. Maha, K. Major, L. Makk, G. Mészégető, I. Mészáros, E. Mohácsi, I. Nádudvary, E. Nagy, M. Nyírő, L. Osvai, M. Papp, M. Póczi, M. Poncsák, N. Popa, J. Schlezák, M. Szabó, M. Szabó, É. Szabó, G. Szabó, Z. Szász, I. Szereday, I. Szép, S. Tehenes, T. Tóth, V. Tóth, É. Valyon, B. Várnai, J. Várkonyi, E. Vecsey, Z. Vecsey, Z. Vidák, Á. Vincze, and I. Vinkler. This work was supported by Chiesi Hungary Ltd. and Janos Bolyai Research Scholarship of the Hungarian Academy of Sciences (to Zsófia Lázár) (grant number BO/00559/16).

References

[1] C. F. Vogelmeier, G. J. Criner, F. J. Martinez et al., "Global strategy for the diagnosis, management, and prevention of chronic obstructive lung disease 2017 report: GOLD executive summary," *The European Respiratory Journal*, vol. 49, no. 3, p. 1700214, 2017.

[2] H. Y. Kwon and E. Kim, "Factors contributing to quality of life in COPD patients in South Korea," *International Journal of Chronic Obstructive Pulmonary Disease*, vol. 11, pp. 103–109, 2016.

[3] M. Miravitlles, K. Naberan, J. Cantoni, and A. Azpeitia, "Socio-economic status and health-related quality of life of patients with chronic obstructive pulmonary disease," *Respiration*, vol. 82, no. 5, pp. 402–408, 2011.

[4] K. Naberan, A. Azpeitia, J. Cantoni, and M. Miravitlles, "Impairment of quality of life in women with chronic obstructive pulmonary disease," *Respiratory Medicine*, vol. 106, no. 3, pp. 367–373, 2012.

[5] S. Houben-Wilke, R. A. Jörres, R. Bals et al., "Peripheral artery disease and its clinical relevance in patients with chronic obstructive pulmonary disease in the COPD and systemic consequences-comorbidities network study," *American Journal of Respiratory and Critical Care Medicine*, vol. 195, no. 2, pp. 189–197, 2017.

[6] M. E. Wacker, for the COSYCONET study group, R. A. Jörres et al., "Relative impact of COPD and comorbidities on generic health-related quality of life: a pooled analysis of the COSYCONET patient cohort and control subjects from the KORA and SHIP studies," *Respiratory Research*, vol. 17, no. 1, p. 81, 2016.

[7] M. E. Wacker, for the COSYCONET-Consortium, R. A. Jörres et al., "Assessing health-related quality of life in COPD: comparing generic and disease-specific instruments with focus on comorbidities," *BMC Pulmonary Medicine*, vol. 16, no. 1, p. 70, 2016.

[8] T. A. R Seemungal, G .C. Donaldson, E. A. Paul, J. C. Bestall, D. J. Jeffries, and J. A. Wedzicha, "Effect of exacerbation on quality of life in patients with chronic obstructive pulmonary disease," *American Journal of Respiratory and Critical Care Medicine*, vol. 157, no. 5, pp. 1418–1422, 1998.

[9] M. Miravitlles, M. Ferrer, A. Pont et al., "Effect of exacerbations on quality of life in patients with chronic obstructive pulmonary disease: a 2 year follow up study," *Thorax*, vol. 59, no. 5, pp. 387–395, 2004.

[10] "Global strategy for asthma management and prevention," 2017, February 2019 Available from: http://www.ginaasthma.org.

[11] H. Inoue, T. Nagase, S. Morita, A. Yoshida, T. Jinnai, and M. Ichinose, "Prevalence and characteristics of asthma-COPD overlap syndrome identified by a stepwise approach," *International Journal of Chronic Obstructive Pulmonary Disease*, vol. Volume 12, pp. 1803–1810, 2017.

[12] H. J. Park, M. K. Byun, H. J. Kim et al., "Asthma-COPD overlap shows favorable clinical outcomes compared to pure COPD in a Korean COPD cohort," *Allergy, Asthma & Immunology Research*, vol. 9, no. 5, pp. 431–437, 2017.

[13] H. Andersen, P. Lampela, A. Nevanlinna, O. Saynajakangas, and T. Keistinen, "High hospital burden in overlap syndrome of asthma and COPD," *The Clinical Respiratory Journal*, vol. 7, no. 4, pp. 342–346, 2013.

[14] R. de Marco, G. Pesce, A. Marcon et al., "The coexistence of asthma and chronic obstructive pulmonary disease (COPD): prevalence and risk factors in young, middle-aged and elderly people from the general population," *PLoS One*, vol. 8, no. 5, 2013.

[15] B. W. Morgan, M. R. Grigsby, T. Siddharthan et al., "Epidemiology and risk factors of asthma-chronic obstructive pulmonary disease overlap in low- and middle-income countries," *The Journal of Allergy and Clinical Immunology*, vol. 143, no. 4, pp. 1598–1606, 2019.

[16] A. Senthilselvan and J. Beach, Characteristics of asthma and COPD overlap syndrome (ACOS) in the Canadian population," *The Journal of Asthma*, vol. 56, no. 11, pp. 1129–1137, 2019.

[17] A. Bikov, A. Horváth, G. Tomisa, L. Bártfai, and Z. Bártfai, "Changes in the burden of comorbidities in patients with COPD and asthma-COPD overlap according to the GOLD 2017 recommendations," *Lung*, vol. 196, no. 5, pp. 591–599, 2018.

[18] P. Kauppi, H. Kupiainen, A. Lindqvist et al., "Overlap syndrome of asthma and COPD predicts low quality of life," *The Journal of Asthma*, vol. 48, no. 3, pp. 279–285, 2011.

[19] M. R. Miller, J. Hankinson, V. Brusasco et al., "Standardisation of spirometry," *The European Respiratory Journal*, vol. 26, no. 2, pp. 319–338, 2005.

[20] C. Landbo, E. Prescott, P. Lange, J. Vestbo, and T. P. Almdal, "Prognostic value of nutritional status in chronic obstructive pulmonary disease," *American Journal of Respiratory and Critical Care Medicine*, vol. 160, no. 6, pp. 1856–1861, 1999.

[21] C. M. Fletcher, "Standardised questionnaire on respiratory symptoms: a statement prepared and approved by the MRC Committee on the Aetiology of Chronic Bronchitis (MRC breathlessness score)," *BMJ*, vol. 2, p. 1665, 1960.

[22] P. W. Jones, G. Harding, P. Berry, I. Wiklund, W. H. Chen, and N. Kline Leidy, "Development and first validation of the COPD Assessment Test," *The European Respiratory Journal*, vol. 34, no. 3, pp. 648–654, 2009.

[23] R. Brooks, "EuroQol: the current state of play," *Health Policy*, vol. 37, no. 1, pp. 53–72, 1996.

[24] M. Monteagudo, T. Rodríguez-Blanco, M. Llagostera et al., "Factors associated with changes in quality of life of COPD patients: a prospective study in primary care," *Respiratory Medicine*, vol. 107, no. 10, pp. 1589–1597, 2013.

[25] M. Hardin, M. Cho, M. L. McDonald et al., "The clinical and genetic features of COPD-asthma overlap syndrome," *The European Respiratory Journal*, vol. 44, no. 2, pp. 341–350, 2014.

[26] K. Kurashima, Y. Takaku, C. Ohta, N. Takayanagi, T. Yanagisawa, and Y. Sugita, "COPD assessment test and severity of airflow limitation in patients with asthma, COPD, and asthma–COPD overlap syndrome," *International Journal of Chronic Obstructive Pulmonary Disease*, vol. 11, pp. 479–487, 2016.

[27] L. Tamasi, M. Szilasi, and G. Galffy, "Clinical effectiveness of budesonide/formoterol fumarate Easyhaler® for patients with poorly controlled obstructive airway disease: a real-world study of patient-reported outcomes," *Advances in Therapy*, vol. 35, no. 8, pp. 1140–1152, 2018.

[28] H. B. Bringsvor, K. Skaug, E. Langeland et al., "Symptom burden and self-management in persons with chronic obstructive pulmonary disease," *International Journal of Chronic Obstructive Pulmonary Disease*, vol. Volume 13, pp. 365–373, 2018.

[29] C. Morélot-Panzini, H. Gilet, B. Aguilaniu et al., "Real-life assessment of the multidimensional nature of dyspnoea in COPD outpatients," *The European Respiratory Journal*, vol. 47, no. 6, pp. 1668–1679, 2016.

[30] J. Sundh, G. Johansson, K. Larsson et al., "Comorbidity and health-related quality of life in patients with severe chronic obstructive pulmonary disease attending Swedish secondary care units," *International Journal of Chronic Obstructive Pulmonary Disease*, vol. 10, pp. 173–183, 2015.

[31] M. Miravitlles, M. Barrecheguren, and M. Roman-Rodriguez, "Frequency and characteristics of different clinical phenotypes

of chronic obstructive pulmonary disease," *The International Journal of Tuberculosis and Lung Disease*, vol. 19, no. 8, pp. 992–998, 2015.

[32] A. Kania, R. Krenke, K. Kuziemski et al., "Distribution and characteristics of COPD phenotypes - results from the polish sub-cohort of the POPE study," *International Journal of Chronic Obstructive Pulmonary Disease*, vol. Volume 13, pp. 1613–1621, 2018.

[33] P. Santus, D. Radovanovic, S. Henchi et al., "Assessment of acute bronchodilator effects from specific airway resistance changes in stable COPD patients," *Respiratory Physiology & Neurobiology*, vol. 197, pp. 36–45, 2014.

[34] M. Cazzola, B. Boveri, P. Carlucci et al., "Lung function improvement in smokers suffering from COPD with zafirlukast, a CysLT1-receptor antagonist," *Pulmonary Pharmacology & Therapeutics*, vol. 13, no. 6, pp. 301–305, 2000.

[35] J. E. Hansen, A. G. Dilektasli, J. Porszasz et al., "A new bronchodilator response grading strategy identifies distinct patient populations," *Annals of the American Thoracic Society*, vol. 16, no. 12, pp. 1504–1517, 2019.

15

The S100 Protein Family as Players and Therapeutic Targets in Pulmonary Diseases

Zeeshan Sattar,[1] **Alnardo Lora**,[1] **Bakr Jundi**,[1] **Christopher Railwah**,[1] **and Patrick Geraghty**[1,2]

[1]*Division of Pulmonary and Critical Care Medicine, Department of Medicine, State University of New York Downstate Health Sciences University, 450 Clarkson Avenue, Brooklyn, NY 11203, USA*
[2]*Department of Cell Biology, State University of New York Downstate Health Sciences University, 450 Clarkson Avenue, Brooklyn, NY 11203, USA*

Correspondence should be addressed to Patrick Geraghty; patrick.geraghty@downstate.edu

Academic Editor: Kazuyoshi Kuwano

The S100 protein family consists of over 20 members in humans that are involved in many intracellular and extracellular processes, including proliferation, differentiation, apoptosis, Ca_2^+ homeostasis, energy metabolism, inflammation, tissue repair, and migration/invasion. Although there are structural similarities between each member, they are not functionally interchangeable. The S100 proteins function both as intracellular Ca^{2+} sensors and as extracellular factors. Dysregulated responses of multiple members of the S100 family are observed in several diseases, including the lungs (asthma, chronic obstructive pulmonary disease, idiopathic pulmonary fibrosis, cystic fibrosis, pulmonary hypertension, and lung cancer). To this degree, extensive research was undertaken to identify their roles in pulmonary disease pathogenesis and the identification of inhibitors for several S100 family members that have progressed to clinical trials in patients for nonpulmonary conditions. This review outlines the potential role of each S100 protein in pulmonary diseases, details the possible mechanisms observed in diseases, and outlines potential therapeutic strategies for treatment.

1. Introduction to S100 Proteins

In multiple diseases, numerous exogenous and endogenous factors trigger inflammatory cascades. A family of endogenous proinflammatory mediators named damage-associated molecular patterns (DAMPs; also known as alarmins) have become of special interest in the past few decades. During stress reactions or cell injury, DAMPs are released and activate inflammatory pathways [1]. DAMPs function independently when they are intracellular and act in a cytokine-like manner when they are extracellular. Of note, it is suggested that the term "DAMPs" is too broad of a term to characterize all endogenous molecules linked to an inflammatory pathway; thus, there is an ongoing debate on defining DAMPs and classifying them [2]. One family of DAMPs that have been identified to play a significant role in the host immune response in multiple diseases is the S100 protein family.

S100 proteins are involved in both intracellular and extracellular processes including cell apoptosis, migration, protein phosphorylation, calcium balance, differentiation, proliferation, and inflammation [3–6]. The term S100 was first used by Blake Moore to describe proteins that were soluble in 100% saturated ammonium sulfate in 1965 [7]. There are now 25 such S100 proteins/complexes described, which include 16 S100A proteins (S100A1-S100A16) as well as others (such as S100B, S100G, S100P, and S100Z) [8]. The S100 protein family is exclusively expressed in vertebrates. It consists of small (10-14 kDa), acidic, and calcium-binding proteins (CaBPs) with two distinct EF-hand motifs (helix-loop-helix) [9]. This subfamily of CaBPs exists mainly as homodimers but can also exist as monomers (only S100G is stable in this configuration), heterodimers (S100A1/S100B and S100A8/S100A9), or multimers intra- and extracellularly. Their expression is tissue and cell-type specific [10].

Along with Ca^{2+}, S100 proteins also bind many other transition metal ions (e.g., Fe^{2+}, Cu^{2+}, Mn^{2+}, Zn^{2+}, and Ni^{2+}) that result in a conformational change allowing interaction with target proteins [11, 12]. S100 proteins act as DAMP molecules and can work as stimulatory ligands for both immune and nonimmune cells, such as endothelial cells [13]. They do so by binding pattern recognition receptors (PRRs) such as toll-like receptor 4 (TLR4) as well as non-PRR DAMP receptors such as advanced glycation end products (RAGE) [14]. By binding to these receptors, S100 proteins trigger downstream nuclear factor-κB (NF-κB), which results in upregulation of the proinflammatory gene expression [15, 16]. In this review, we outline the potential role of the S100 protein members in pulmonary diseases and detail potential molecular mechanisms they may play in disease initiation and progression. Equally, we outline potential therapeutic approaches to treat pulmonary diseases by targeting S100 proteins.

2. S100 Proteins: Activation, Expression, Interacting Proteins, and Targets

S100 proteins interact with a variety of target proteins including enzymes, cytoskeletal subunits, receptors, transcription factors, and nucleic acids. Therefore, through structural changes, interactions with Ca^{2+}, posttranslational modifications, receptor-mediated transduction, and direct responses S100 proteins mediate many processes.

2.1. S100 Protein Structure, Calcium Bind, and Posttranslation Modifications. Pending on the cellular and extracellular location of S100 proteins, they can interact with many proteins and form dimers. There are two critical steps for S100 protein activation: Ca^{2+} binding [17] and dimer formation [18]. Typically, the S100 proteins are observed as symmetric dimers, with each S100 subunit containing four α-helices [4]. Several heterodimers are reported among family members *in vitro*, but only the S100A8-S100A9 heterodimer is believed to play a significant role *in vivo* [19]. S100 subunits contain two Ca^{2+}-binding domains, a carboxy-terminal canonical domain composed of 12 amino acids and an amino-terminal domain composed of 14 amino acids [4]. Both are connected by a 10-12 residues region, crucial for target interactions. Ca^{2+}-binding affinity drastically increases when a target engages [20–22]. Upon binding Ca^{2+}, S100 proteins undergo conformational rearrangement exposing a hydrophobic cleft that is required for target binding. Therefore, S100 target binding is mostly Ca^{2+}-dependent. Individual S100 family members exhibit differences in surface geometries, hydrophobic residue distribution, and charge density [23]. Several S100 proteins undergo posttranslational modifications, such as oxidative modification, s-nitrosylation, phosphorylation, covalent modification, transglutaminase 2-mediated crosslinking, sumoylation, S-glutathionylation, cysteinylation, the formation of intra- and intersulfinamide bonds, or intracellular localization [24–29]. The activity of S100 proteins is regulated by metal ions, such as calcium, zinc, and copper, that modulate the folding and oligomerization of the protein [30]. Regarding pulmonary disease, few studies focus on the structure or modification of S100 proteins but merely their presence or the impact of deficiency or inhibition on disease initiation or progression.

2.2. S100 Expression Profile. Each S100 family protein is encoded by a separate gene, mostly but not limited to chromosome 1q21 [9]. When examining the expression of each S100 gene between different cell types or tissues, despite structural similarities and clustered genes, each S100 gene has a very specific expression pattern [31–33]. Therefore, we must not expect similar expression patterns for each S100 gene member. Dysregulated expression of multiple S100 family members occurs in most diseases. Epigenetic events are reported in various medulloblastoma cell lines resulting in dysregulated S100 gene expression [34]. DNA de-methylation and hypomethylation [35] and micro-RNA regulation are reported in the regulation of the S100 gene expression. CpG islands are observed in the 5′ regulatory regions of S100A2, S100A6, S100A10, and S100A11 genes, within the proximal promoter and the first two introns [36]. Methylation of these islands is typically associated with a repressed chromatin state and transcription inhibition. But not all S100 genes contain these CpG islands, such as S100P and S100Z genes. Equally, several S100 genes are reported to be upregulated due to several extracellular factors, such as oxidative stress, certain cytokines, and growth factors in many types of cells [37]. Within pulmonary diseases, the expression of S100 genes is reported to be primarily triggered by extracellular responses. Importantly, different subsets of monocytes can have different expression profiles of S100 proteins [38]. Our group demonstrated that the protein tyrosine phosphatase (PTP1B) could negatively regulate the S100A9 expression and reduced S100A9 stimuli responses via regulation of TLR4 signaling [39]. However, there are several other means to regulate the S100A9 expression as it is sensitive to the Src kinase inhibitor PP2 [40] and the STAT3 expression [41]. Therefore, the S100 gene expression varies depending on the cell type, tissue, external stimuli, age, and possible sex.

2.3. Secretion of S100 Proteins. Little is known about the mechanisms that mediate the secretion of S100 proteins. The S100 proteins lack a leader sequence and are not secreted via the classical Golgi pathway. The secretion of S100 proteins appears to occur either passively upon cell necrosis or actively following cell activation. Several S100 proteins undergo secretion following stimulation by particular cell activators, such as serotonin-receptor agonists [42], antidepressants, glutamate, adenosine, IL-1β [43], lysophosphatidic acid, and changes in extracellular Ca^{2+} and K^{+} levels [44]. Some S100 proteins have affinities to lipid structures that may allow them to translocation across the plasma membrane following cell stress or activation [45]. Equally, S100 proteins can interact with phospholipid-binding proteins, such as S100A10 binding to Annexin A2 [46], to induce exocytosis of intracellular S100 proteins to the extracellular domain. S100 protein members, S100A8/S100A9, may be released from necrotic myeloid cells or actively secreted following translocation to the membrane, utilizing an intact microtubule network and PKC activation [47]. Oxidative stress can induce the release of S100 proteins from several cells. S100A8/S100A9 could be released neutrophil extracellular traps (NETs). Therefore, S100 proteins may be readily secreted within the lungs. Expression levels and plasma or BALF levels of several S100 proteins are observed to be altered in the lungs of several pulmonary diseases, as outlined in Section 3 and Table 1.

2.4. S100 Protein Receptors and Targets. Once released to the extracellular space, S100 proteins trigger immune cell activation through binding to different cell surface receptors. S100 proteins primarily trigger inflammation responses through their interactions with toll-like receptor (TLR) 4 and receptor for advanced glycation end products (RAGE) [48]. S100A8 and A9 are known to bind to TLR4 [48], while S100A7, S100A12, S100A8/A9, and S100B interact with RAGE [16, 49, 50]. By interacting with RAGE and/or TLR4, S100 proteins can activate mitogen-activated protein kinases (MAPK) responses and transcription factors, such as NF-κB, resulting in the production of proinflammatory cytokines [50, 51]. S100A6 activates RAGE to promote apoptosis [52]. However, S100B inactivates RAGE [53]. S100 proteins are also known to interact with extracellular matrix metalloproteinase inducer (EMMPRIN) (also known as CD147), G-protein-coupled receptor (GPCR), CD36 [54], FGFR1 [55], CD166 antigen [56], IL-10 receptor [57], neuroplastin-β [58], CD68 [59], and ErbB4 [60] (see Figure 1). It is important to note that S100 protein heterodimers and the presence of calcium may also influence different receptor responses.

3. Linking S100 Proteins to Pulmonary Disease Outcomes

Multiple sources suggest that S100 protein family members augment the inflammatory response and disease outcomes in a variety of different pulmonary diseases.

3.1. S100A1. S100A1 is a small (~10 kDa) protein that predominantly functions to modulate the Ca^{2+} milieu, energy metabolism, and contraction of the cardiac myocytes [61]. It is also shown to be present in vascular endothelial cells and smooth muscle cells, and its absence is associated with a hypertensive phenotype in animal models partly secondary to endothelial cell dysfunction [62, 63]. Teichert-Kuliszewska et al. demonstrated that S100A1 is also expressed in the lung vascular endothelium, and its deficiency in knockout (KO) mice leads to increased right ventricular (RV) systolic pressure (RVSP) as well as aberrant endothelial-dependent relaxation in response to acetylcholine and decreased availability of nitric oxide (NO) thus predisposing to pulmonary hypertension [61]. Pigs embolized with Sephadex developed RV hypertrophy and, interestingly, showed increased RV S100A1 expression and mild pulmonary hypertension (pH) [64].

3.2. S100A2. S100A2 is linked to both suppressions of tumor progression as well as being a promoter of carcinogenesis [65–69]. Its role in non-small-cell lung cancer (NSCLC) was elucidated by Feng et al. who suggested that hypermethylation of the promoter region of the S100A2 gene led to its downregulation in the early stages of NSCLC carcinogenesis thus contributing to tumor progression [68]. In contrast, some data suggest that overexpression of S100A2 may indicate a poor prognosis in stage 1 NSCLC [70]. EGF-stimulated EGFR phosphorylation induces the S100A2 expression, and S100A2 exhibits antitumor activity by reducing the rate of tumor growth when overexpressed in nude mice with NCI-H2172 cell tumor xenograft model [71].

3.3. S100A3/S100A13. Mutation of the S100A3 gene leads to the replacement of arginine with cysteine at the 77th position of the S100A3 protein along with a mutation of the S100A13 gene leading to decreased expression of both proteins. This is implicated in an atypical genetic variant of early onset interstitial pulmonary fibrosis [72]. The decreased expression of these proteins leads to abnormal calcium homeostasis intracellularly, decreased tolerability of oxidative stress, and altered expression of extracellular matrix proteins. In addition to its role in idiopathic pulmonary fibrosis (IPF), S100A3 is also a potential drug target in lung cancers. Gianni et al. showed that knockdown of S100A3 leads to degradation of RARα, a transcription factor that plays a role in the antiproliferative effects of All-trans retinoic acid (ATRA) [73], by proteasomes thus inducing resistance to the antiproliferative and differentiating effects of ATRA on lung cancer cells [74]. Tumor microvascular density (MVD) is an indicator of tumor neovascularization which advocates recurrence, potential for metastases, and survival of cancerous cells. Overexpression of S100A13 in stage I NSCLC has been associated with enhanced intratumoral MVD. This suggests that S100A13 plays a role in lung cancer progression and metastasis [75]. Similarly, it is associated with a more aggressive invasive phenotype of lung cancer [76].

3.4. S100A4. S100A4 was originally labeled as a specific marker of fibroblasts in different tissues and was termed as FSP-1 (fibroblast-specific-protein-1), but further studies showed that S100A4 is also involved in the fibrogenic of mesenchymal progenitor cells in the lung thus contributing to the pathogenesis of IPF [77]. S100A4 is released by M2 alveolar macrophages, which then activates fibroblasts [77]. Inhibition of the S100A4 expression with niclosamide improved survival in a bleomycin-induced fibrosis model in mice [77]. Bleomycin significantly increases the S100A4 expression in alveolar macrophages [77]. Extracellular S100A4 activates lung fibroblasts by the upregulation of α-SMA, type I collagen, and sphingosine-1-phosphate (S1P) [78]. S100A4 is also involved in the pathogenesis of lung cancer through inhibition of autophagy [79], a process by which defective proteins and organelles are degraded in lysosomes to maintain the cellular milieu [80, 81]. S100A4 inhibits starvation-induced autophagy, thus promoting the proliferation of NSCLC cells through activation of the Wnt/β-catenin pathway in a RAGE-dependent manner [79]. S100A4 regulates oxygen consumption rates, mitochondrial activity, ATP production, and glycolytic activity by regulating mitochondrial complex I subunit NADH dehydrogenase (ubiquinone) Fe-S protein 2 (NDUFS2) [82]. Interestingly, S100A4 has some

Table 1: S100 proteins involved in pulmonary diseases.

Protein	Receptor and interacting proteins	Major cells expressing	Pulmonary disease	Study
S100A1	RAGE	Macrophages, dendritic, epithelial, and endothelial cells	Reduced in pulmonary hypertension	[61]
S100A2	RAGE	Cancer cells, basal, club and ciliated cells	Reported both induced and reduced in non-small-cell lung carcinoma	[71]
S100A3	RAGE, retinoid receptor, RARα, and PML-RARα	Endothelial, epithelial, and lymphatic cells	Reduced in both pulmonary fibrosis and lung cancer models	[72] [74]
S100A4	TLR4, IL-10R, EGFR, ErbB4, HSPG, GPCR, and RAGE	Tumor cells, T cells, neutrophils, and macrophages	Increased in both lung NSCLC and pulmonary fibrosis	[77] [79]
S100A5	RAGE	Macrophages and cancer cells	Increased in nonsmoking NSCLC	[84]
S100A6	RAGE	Most lung cells but predominantly neutrophils, macrophages, and NK cells	Increased in lung cancer cells, idiopathic pulmonary fibrosis, sarcoidosis, and COPD Reduced in CF	[90] [95] [95] [95] [94]
S100A7	RAGE	Epithelial cells and neutrophils	Reduced in rhinosinusitis Increased in lung NSCLC, squamous cell cancer, asthma, bacterial-associated exacerbations, and pulmonary involvement in systemic sclerosis	[100] [98, 105, 219, 220] [99] [102] [101]
S100A8	TLR4, heparan sulfate and N-glycans, S100A9, and RAGE	Many tissues but predominantly monocytes, granulocytes, and epithelial cells	Increased in cystic fibrosis, extracellular levels in COPD, chronic tuberculosis, asthma, acute lung injury, restrictive allograft syndrome, and COVID-19 Reduced intracellular levels in COPD	[93] [107, 109] [116] [118] [112] [121] [136, 137]
S100A9	TLR4, heparan sulfate and N-glycans, RAGE, S100A8, and EMMPRIN	Many cell types but predominantly macrophages, granulocytes, and epithelial cells	Increased in COPD with and without AE, cystic fibrosis, lung cancer, chronic tuberculosis, IPF, acute, exacerbations, asthma, acute lung injury, restrictive allograft syndrome, rhinosinusitis, and COVID-19	[39, 108–110] [93] [122, 221] [116] [123, 124] [118–120] [112, 125] [121] [125] [136, 137]
S100A10	GPCRs, serotonin receptors, CCR10, and AnxA2	Many cell types but predominantly macrophages, granulocytes, and epithelial cells	Increased in lung adenocarcinoma, hypertension, and acute lung injury	[129, 130] [126] [127]
S100A11	RAGE	Ubiquitous expression in various tissues and cell types		[131, 222]

			Increased in lung adenocarcinoma, hypertension, idiopathic pulmonary fibrosis, sarcoidosis, and COPD	[223] [95] [95] [95]
S100A12	TLR4, RAGE, N-glycans, scavenger receptors, and GPCR	Granulocytes and monocytes	Increased in asthma, COPD, ARDS, restrictive allograft syndrome, and COVID-19	[134, 135] [109] [224] [121] [136, 137]
S100A13	RAGE	Ubiquitous expression in various tissues and cell types	Increased in pulmonary fibrosis and lung cancer cells	[72] [75, 225]
S100A14/S100A11P	RAGE	Epithelial cells and cancer cells	Increased in lung adenocarcinoma and NSCLC	[139, 226, 227]
S100A15	GPCR	Cancer cells and neutrophils	Increased in lung adenocarcinoma	[140]
S100A16	Unknown receptor interaction but binds to S100A14	Cancer, epithelial, endothelial cells, and fibroblasts	Increased in lung adenocarcinoma and NSCLC	[141, 142]
S100B	RAGE and FGFR1	Cancer cells, dendritic cells, and lymphocytes	Increased in lung SCL but reduced in NSCLC	[145] [84]
S100G	Annexin A10	Epithelial and cancer cells	Increased in lung NSCLC	[84]
S100P	RAGE and p53	Epithelial and cancer cells	Increased in restrictive allograft syndrome, lung NSCLS, adenocarcinoma, and pulmonary arterial hypertension	[121] [146, 148, 149] [150]
S100Z	S100A1, S100A3, and S100B	Monocytes and dendritic cells	No known pulmonary link	

antitumorigenesis properties as 10% of *S100a4*$^{-/-}$ mice develop spontaneous tumors that are p54 positive, including bronchioalveolar carcinomas [83]. This loss of *S100a4* in mice coincided with elevated *S100a3* and *S100a5* expression in several tissues [83].

3.5. S100A5/S100G. The prognostic value of high levels of expression of S100A5 and S100G mRNA is associated with worse overall survival in the nonsmoking NSCLC patients [84]. Further studies are warranted to further elucidate the role of S100A5 as a prognostic marker in lung cancer. However, differential expression of S100A5 is observed in primary human bronchial epithelial (HBE) isolated from healthy, asthmatic, and COPD donors grown at the air-liquid interface when exposed to fine particulate matter [85].

3.6. S100A6. S100A6 plays a role in the proliferation, apoptosis, cytoskeleton modulation, and stress-induced responses of normal adult cell types as well as several tumorous cells [86]. It is overexpressed in lung cancer cells and serum from cancer patients [87, 88]. S100A6 plays a role in the proliferation, invasion, migration, and angiogenesis of lung cancer cells by degrading p53 acetylation, a process by which p53 gets activated and performs its role as a tumor suppressor [89]. The S100A6 expression is downregulated by overexpression of the microRNA, miRNA-193a, thereby increasing p53 acetylation [90]. Hematopoietic stem cells from *S100a6*$^{-/-}$ mice have impaired self-renewal and regenerative capacity [91]. Chronic exposure to cigarette smoke increases S100A6 lung levels in Wistar rats [92]. Mice deficient for the cystic fibrosis (CF) transmembrane conductance regulator (CFTR) gene develop multiple complications, including severe pulmonary disease. Male *Cftr*$^{-/-}$ mice have elevated lung *S100a8* and *S100a9*, while demonstrating reduced *S100a6* and *S100a13* [93]. A recent study suggests that there is an S100A6 profile in systemic sclerosis and may represent a potential biomarker [94]. Finally, although the levels of S100A6 along with S100A11 are different between IPF, sarcoidosis, and COPD subjects and healthy controls, there was no prognostically significant [95].

3.7. S100A7. The majority of early work looking at S100A7, also called psoriasin, focused on psoriasis [96, 97]. However, several studies suggest that S100A7 may have a role in several respiratory diseases, including lung cancer [98], asthma [99], rhinosinusitis [100], pulmonary complications of systemic sclerosis [101], and bacterial exacerbations [102]. S100A7 is a chemotactic protein for CD4+ T cells and neutrophils present in the skin epidermis [103]. It also functions as a direct bactericidal protein [104]. Kim et al. demonstrated that levels of S100A7 and S100A8/A9 were reduced in chronic rhinosinusitis (CRS) patients with a mixed ball of bacteria and fungi compared to a fungal ball [100]. This implies that the barrier function of the nasal epithelial cells is reduced in mixed

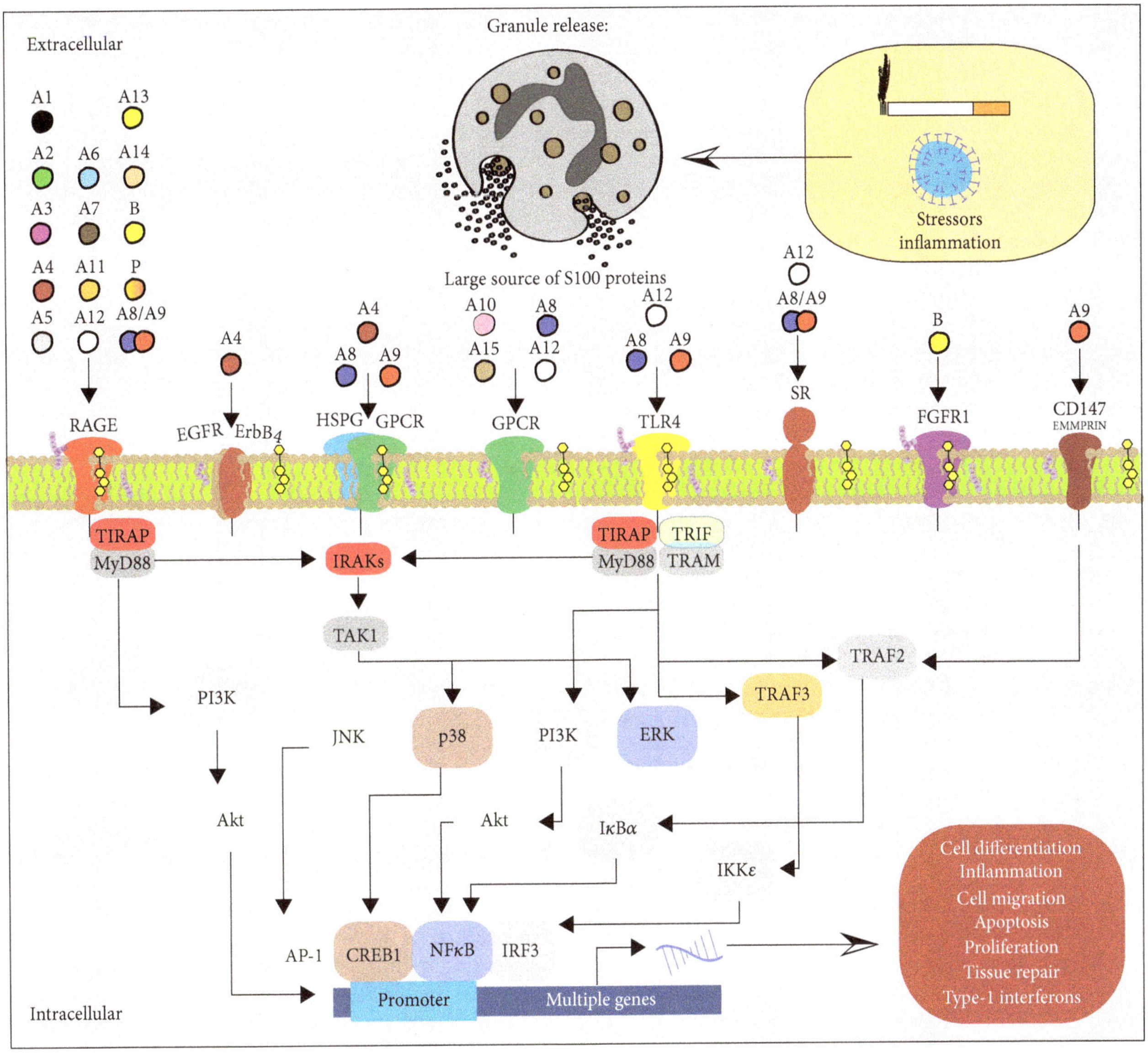

Figure 1: Extracellular functions of S100 proteins. Several factors can trigger S100 proteins to be released or secreted from multiple cell types, including granulocytes. The extracellular S100 proteins interact with several pattern recognition receptors, resulting in proinflammatory signaling pathways that promote cell differentiation, inflammation, migration, apoptosis, proliferation, tissue repair, and a robust type-1 interferon response. Only a portion of the RAGE, HSPG/GPCR, TLR4, and CD147 responses are shown here. RAGE: receptor for advanced glycosylation end products; EGFR: epidermal growth factor receptor; ErbB: v-erb-b2 avian erythroblastic leukemia viral oncogene homolog; HSPG: heparan sulfate proteoglycans; GPCR: Gα9-coupled receptor; TLR4: toll-like receptor 4; SR: scavenger receptor; FGFR1: fibroblast growth factor receptor 1; CD147: cluster of differentiation 147; EMMPRIN: extracellular matrix metalloproteinase inducer; TIRAP: TIR domain containing adaptor protein; MyD88: myeloid differentiation factor 88; IRAK: interleukin 1 receptor-associated kinase; TAK1: transforming growth factor-β- (TGFβ-) activated kinase 1; TRIF: TIR-domain-containing adaptor protein inducing IFNβ; TRAM: translocating chain-associated membrane; TRAF: TNF receptor-associated factor; PI3K: phosphoinositide 3-kinases; Akt: protein kinase B; JNK: JUN N-terminal kinase; ERK: extracellular signal-regulated kinase; AP-1: activator protein 1; CREB1: cAMP-responsive element-binding protein 1; NF-κB: nuclear factor-κB; IRF: interferon regulatory factor; IκBα: nuclear factor of kappa light polypeptide gene enhancer in B cell inhibitor, alpha; IKK: inhibitor of NF-κB kinase.

fungal and bacterial infections thus putting patients at risk of developing an invasive fungal infection.

S100A7 also appears to play a role in the pathogenesis of NSCLC. A study investigating the TGFβ signaling pathway in the progression of NSCLC demonstrated that the TGFβ-induced long noncoding RNA (TBILA) binds to S100A7 thus activating the S100A7/JAB1 pathway leading to NSCLC proliferation and metastasis [98]. The S100A7 expression is induced by activation of the Hippo pathway and acts as a facilitator in the adenosquamous transition of lung cancer cells [105]. S100A7 levels are higher in lung squamous carcinoma and have the potential to be used as a diagnostic marker as its levels are elevated in cancerous cells as compared to nonneoplastic cells [106]. Knockdown of S100A7 leads to decreased phosphorylation of NF-κB thus inhibiting tumor proliferation. This marks S100A7 as a potential therapeutic target for the treatment of lung squamous cell cancers [106].

In asthma, S100A7 plays a role in the interplay between the proinflammatory cytokine IFN-γ and IL-22. The expression of S100A7 is induced by IL-22, and these effects are in turn inhibited by IFN-γ [99]. The expression of S100A7 is enhanced in cases where *S. aureus* is found in the respiratory tract thus stressing the role of this molecule in the epithelial barrier of the lower respiratory tract [102]. S100A7 levels correlate with lung involvement in systemic sclerosis, and the increased expression of psoriasin in the whole saliva has a specificity of 50% and a sensitivity of 85% in detecting lung involvement in this condition [101].

3.8. S100A8 and S100A9. As mentioned above, S100A8 and S100A9 proteins are upregulated in *Cftr*$^{-/-}$ animals, thus suggesting a role of these proteins in the disease process of CF [93]. The anti-inflammatory role of S100A8 in emphysema was investigated by Lin et al., and low intracellular S100A8 levels were observed in emphysema that correlated with disease severity. Furthermore, this protein also has a cytoprotective role, as it is shown that the knockout of this protein leads to oxidative stress-induced cell apoptosis while elevated levels prevent cellular injury [107]. Interestingly, the S100A8/A9 heterodimer may play a role in acute exacerbations of COPD, as it is negatively associated with FEV1% in these patients [108]. Similarly, another study observed elevated S100A8 and S100A9 in COPD samples [109]. Our group has identified S100A9 signaling in smoke and age-related COPD progression [110]. Levels of S100A9 are elevated in older animals as well as animals exposed to cigarette smoke [110]. The unique intracellular and extracellular responses of both of these proteins require further investigation in the lungs. Similar to COPD, it appears that S100A8, S100A9, and the S100A8/A9 heterodimer have opposite effects in acute lung injury (ALI). S100A8 similarly inhibits ALI to dexamethasone [111] while S100A9 and calprotectin (the S100A8/A9 complex) promote neutrophil influx by increasing mast cell degranulation and upregulation of particular chemokines. S100A8 is IL-10 dependent while S100A9 and calprotectin do not induce IL-10 in the airways or tracheal epithelial cells [112].

The S100A8/A9 complex is expressed in tuberculosis (TB) [113–115], as S100A8/A9-expressing neutrophils are observed to assemble in granulomas and S100A8/A9 levels correlated with active disease [113]. This protein also mediates neutrophil accumulation in chronic TB by upregulating the integrin molecule CD11b [116]. The levels of both of these proteins in BALF and sera of asthmatic patients correlate with elevated levels of serum IgE [117]. In addition, they inhibit the apoptosis of neutrophils by increasing the levels of MCP-1, IL-6, and IL-8 through the PI3K/AKT/MAPK/NF-κB pathway [118]. S100A9 enhances the migration of fibrocytes in asthma exacerbations as well as chronic obstructive asthma [119]. S100A9 and/or S100A8/A9 may also have an anti-inflammatory function in asthma by downregulating the function of CD4^{+} Treg cells [120].

Saito et al. elucidated the role of alarmins in chronic lung allograft dysfunction (CLAD), a major contributor to morbidity and mortality in long-term survivors of lung transplantation [121]. The two subtypes of CLAD, restrictive allograft syndrome (RAS) and bronchiolitis obliterans syndrome (BOS), exhibited distinct expression patterns of alarmins including S100A8, S100A9, S100A8/A9, S100A12, S100P, HMGB1 (high mobility group box-1), and soluble RAGE suggesting different biologic profiles of CLAD subtypes. S100A8/A9 overexpression could be involved in the interaction of metastatic lung cancer cells and bone marrow adipocytes leading to bone destruction [122]. S100A8 and S100A9 are upregulated in the acute exacerbations of idiopathic pulmonary fibrosis (IPF) suggesting roles of different signaling pathways like Clathrin-mediated endocytosis signaling, atherosclerosis signaling, and IL2 signaling in the pathogenesis of acute exacerbations of IPF [123]. Serum S100A8/A9 levels are significantly increased in patients with IPF compared with healthy controls and correlate with the diffusing capacity for carbon monoxide (DLCO) and the composite physiologic index [124]. Finally, elevated levels of S100A9 protein are present in the nasal tissues of chronic rhinosinusitis (CRS) subjects. S100A9 mediates the MMP3 expression, resulting in nasal epithelial cell proliferation [125].

3.9. S100A10. S100A10 is believed to be a signature gene involved in blood pressure regulation and maybe a potential target for the detection of risk, prevention, and treatment of hypertension [126]. S100A10 is also one of the cytoskeletal regulatory proteins. It enhances endothelial cell barrier function and is recruited to the caveolin-induced microdomains by high-molecular-weight hyaluronan [127] and potentially could contribute to syndromes of endothelial dysfunction like acute lung injury and sepsis. In primary lung cancers, S100A10 overexpression is associated with higher stage and invasiveness of lung adenocarcinoma [128] as well as lymphatic invasion, cancer stage progression, and poor prognosis in lung squamous cell carcinoma [129]. Increased expression of Kallikrein-related peptidase 6, a serine protease that is normally expressed in mammary tissue, is linked with the enhanced metastatic potential of breast cancer to the lungs and elevated expressions of S100 proteins, like S100A4 and S100A11 [130]. On the contrary, expression at physiological levels leads to suppression of some S100 proteins (S100A4, S100A10, S100A13, S100A16) and thus inhibition of lung metastases.

3.10. S100A11. S100A11 also called S100C or calgizzarin, overexpression is linked with alterations in K-RAS mutated lung adenocarcinomas as well as poorly differentiated lung adenocarcinomas [131]. It is associated with shorter disease-free survival in these tumors. S100A11 levels are increased in the plasma of patients with pulmonary arterial hypertension (PAH) [132]. Hypoxia-induced mitogenic factor, a protein upregulated in animal models of PAH and asthma, is associated with S100A11-mediated smooth muscle cell migration, vesicular exocytosis, and nuclear activation [133].

3.11. S100A12. S100A12 is strongly expressed in the early stages of ALI and early acute respiratory distress syndrome (ARDS) [134]. Possible effects of overexpression include activation of pulmonary endothelium, leukocyte extravasation, and neutrophil accumulation leading to lung injury. Thus, this protein has the potential to be used as a marker of inflammation in ARDS. Contrary to ARDS and ALI, one study demonstrated that this protein blunts inflammatory responses in asthma in murine models [135]. It is also reported to be elevated in COVID-19 patients [136, 137].

3.12. S100A14. The S100A14 expression is associated with a subset of lung adenocarcinoma and has a strong correlation with the invasive and migratory nature of lung adenocarcinoma cells [138]. Its expression is also increased in NSCLC where it has been demonstrated to act as a target of miR-335-3p contributing to NSCLC progression through the pathway involving cancer susceptibility candidate-9, a long noncoding RNA (lncRNA) [139].

3.13. S100A15 and S100A16. Both S100A15 (*S100A7A* gene) and A16 expression are altered in lung cancers. Increased S100A15 expression and decreased DNA methylation of its gene promoter region are associated with poor outcomes in lung adenocarcinoma cases and potentially greater metastasis [140]. The S100A16 expression is increased in NSCLC [141] as well as adenocarcinoma [142] and is a potential marker for prognosis in patients with these varieties of lung cancer.

3.14. S100B. S100B is a nervous system-specific protein and is expressed in glial and Schwann cells [143]. Its levels can rise in response to increased blood-brain barrier permeability [143, 144]. Increased expression of this protein is associated with brain metastases in patients with small cell lung cancer (SCLC) and may indicate poor prognosis as higher levels are linked with shorter survival time [145]. In contrast, increased S100B mRNA expression is associated with better survival in smoking NSCLC patients [84].

3.15. S100P. The S100P expression is associated with the migration, invasiveness, and metastasis of lung cancer [146] as well as the migration of NSCLC [147]. S100P, as an immune-associated gene (IAG) signature, can potentially be used in risk score models to predict the overall survival, stage, lymph node accumulation, tumor metastasis, B cells, and dendritic cell infiltration of lung adenocarcinoma [148]. S100P is sequestered by NORAD, an lncRNA, thereby playing a role in the inhibition of metastatic potential of lung and breast cancers [146]. The transcriptional activation of S100P can be regulated by Porcupine proteins thus contributing to the development of NSCLC [149]. S100P may also play a role in the pathogenesis of pulmonary hypertension in patients with systemic sclerosis as it is overexpressed in these patients [150].

4. Role and Mechanisms of S100 Proteins in Pulmonary Diseases

4.1. S100 Protein-Mediated Signaling in Pulmonary Diseases. In noncancerous pulmonary diseases, several S100 proteins (S100A1, A4, A8, A9, A12, and B) are noted to induce multiple pathways associated with pulmonary disease phenotypes. Here, we will outline the known signaling transduction of these S100 proteins in noncancerous pulmonary diseases. The primary pathways investigated are TLR4 and RAGE-mediated (Figure 1 and Table 1).

Deficiency of *S100a1* results in pulmonary hypertension in mice due to enhanced eNOS activity and nitric oxide levels, via Akt/ERK1/2 pathways, and reduced endothelial cell survival [61]. Alternatively, overexpressing S100A4 in mice results in the development of RAGE-mediated pulmonary arterial hypertension in females [151]. Stimulation with 17β-estradiol increases the S100A4 expression and proliferation in human pulmonary artery smooth muscle cells, and this proliferation is prevented by blocking RAGE signaling [151]. S100A4 also prevents autophagy and induces proliferation in A549 and Lewis lung carcinoma cells, via the RAGE and Wnt pathways [79].

Similarly, S100A9 promotes proliferation of lung fibroblasts and upregulated expression of proinflammatory cytokines (IL-6, IL-8, IL-1β) and collagen type III, via ERK and NF-κB signaling [152]. The S100A8/S100A9 dimer induces the secretion of cytokines, such as MCP-1, IL-6, and IL-8, from bronchial epithelial cells in a TLR4/Akt mediated pathway [118]. This process prevented neutrophil apoptosis in cell coculture experiments [118]. Cigarette smoke is known to modulate the signaling of TLR4 [153], RAGE [154], and EMMPRIN [155]. Our group determined that enhanced S100A9 signaling coincides with lung damage during respiratory syncytial virus (RSV) infection in mice [39]. We determined that S100A9 is enhanced by cigarette smoke exposure and further enhanced during viral exacerbations in mice and human primary lung cells [39]. We also recently demonstrated that cigarette smoke-induced S100A9 contributes to loss of lung function, airspace enlargements, elastin degradation, enhanced phosphorylation of ERK and c-RAF, and altered expression of MMP-3, MMP-9, MCP-1, IL-6, and KC/IL-8 [110]. Equally, elevated S100A9 levels in the lungs correlate with aging [110]. This is also reported in the central nervous system [156] and may occur with other S100 proteins within the lung as S100B blood levels are age-related [157, 158]. Interestingly, p-PKAα interacts with S100A8 in lung tissue obtained from smokers [107]. This interaction alters the phosphorylation of serine within S100A8 and subsequent S100A8 protein destabilization and degradation [107]. Loss of S100A8 increases the percentage of apoptotic A549 cancer cells [107]. S100A8/S100A9 also acts as a chemotactic factor by inducing neutrophil adhesion [159] and can induce ROS-mediated apoptosis, autophagy, mitochondrial damage, and lysosomal activation in various cell types, including lymphocytes, macrophages, endothelial cells, and tumor cells [51]. Expressions of *S100a8* and *S100a9* are both elevated in the lungs of CF transmembrane conductance regulator (*Cftr*) knockout mice, while *S100a6* and *S100a13* are reduced [93]. S100A8/A9 also regulates CD11b expression and neutrophil recruitment during chronic tuberculosis [116]. Interestingly, the downregulation of S100A8 and S100A9 is associated with the differentiation of myeloid cells toward dendritic cells and macrophages

[160]. Alternatively, *S100A9*$^{-/-}$ mice displayed significantly enhanced allergic airway inflammation upon exposure to *Alternaria alternata*, including IL-13, CCL11, CCL24, serum IgE, lung eosinophils, IL-13$^+$IL-5$^+$CD4$^+$ T-helper type 2 cells, airway resistance, and elastance [120]. Recently, we observed that S100A9 expression in chronic rhinosinusitis samples coincides with elevated plasma proteases, and S100A9 protein enhances MMP-7 and MMP-3 production and proliferation in the CCL-30 cell line [125].

Finally, S100A12 and S100B signaling is observed in the lungs. Mice expressing the human S100A12 gene have reduced peribronchial and perivascular inflammation, mucus production, eosinophilia, and airway responsiveness [135]. This was associated with S100A12 induced *Fas* expression and activation of caspase 3 in cultured airway smooth muscle cells, thereby leading to reduced airway smooth muscle [135]. In bronchial epithelial cells, the S100B expression is upregulated due to MyD88-dependent activation of canonical NF-κB in the early stages of fungal infection but later becomes downregulated via TLR-3/9-dependent signaling [161]. CD8+ T cells and NK cells also express and secrete S100B following stimulation [162].

4.2. S100 Proteins in Tissue Repair. Despite S100 proteins being associated with cellular and tissue damage, several members (including S100A7, S100A8/A9, S100A12, and S100A15) are reported to also play a critical role in tissue repair [163]. These S100 proteins are reported to be involved in tissue repair in atherosclerosis, dermatitis, and arthritis [14]. Importantly, S100A4 promotes muscle tissue repair to maintain contractility following heart injury [164]. Within pulmonary diseases, little is reported on the role of S100 proteins in tissue repair. However, intracellular S100A8 was recently shown to protect type II pneumonocytes from smoke-induced cell death [107]. Hiroshima and colleagues demonstrate that S100A9 and S100A8/A9 can reduce neutrophil influx in the LPS model of acute lung injury [112]. Since S100A8/A9 and LPS target TLR4, S100A8/A9 may compete for TLR4 binding with LPS. Interestingly, *S100a9*$^{-/-}$ mice accumulated a lower frequency of CD4+ T regulatory (Treg) cells following exposure to *Alternaria alternata* [120], leading to more lung damage. Equally, despite S100B responses activating intracellular TLRs, during a pulmonary *Aspergillus fumigatus* infection, S100B can itself resolve inflammation via transcriptional inhibition of itself [161]. Therefore, several members of the S100 family could influence cell fate, inflammation, and tissue remodeling within the lungs. There may also be several feedback loops that initially trigger inflammation and subsequently regulates the resolution of these responses to minimize damage and facilitate repair.

5. Targeting S100 Proteins to Treat Pulmonary Diseases

Due to the involvement of S100 proteins in the pathogenesis of numerous diseases as highlighted in this review and mouse models suggest that genetic deletion has minimal effects on normal physiology, there is increasing interest in therapeutic targeting these proteins. Clinical trials to date have primarily focused on nonpulmonary diseases such as systemic lupus erythematosus (SLE), ischemic heart failure, and rheumatoid arthritis. We will discuss S100 inhibitors and clinical trials undertaken with these therapeutics to date (summarized in Table 2).

5.1. Clinical Trials to Date Utilizing the Quinoline-3-Carboxamide Derivatives S100 Protein Inhibitors. In the past decade, several small molecules were identified to block the hydrophobic cleft required for the recognition of S100 targets and thus block their activity, such as paquinimod (ABR-215757), tasquinimod (ABR-215050), and laquinimod (ABR-215062). They are quinoline-3-carboxamide derivatives that primarily block the interaction of S100A8 and S100A9 with RAGE and TLR4 [165, 166]. Laquinimod, a derivative of linomide (Roquinimex), interferes with S100 and its receptor RAGE binding and is proposed as a treatment for multiple sclerosis [167]. Here, we will briefly outline several of the clinical outcomes utilizing these quinoline-3-carboxamide derivatives S100 protein inhibitors primarily in prostate cancer, SLE, and multiple sclerosis. However, few studies in human clinical trials report their findings as of the time of this paper, and pulmonary outcomes are limited.

Phase II randomized, double-blind, placebo-controlled study in men with minimally symptomatic metastatic castrate-resistant prostate cancer (CRPC), tasquinimod improves progression-free survival in patients with metastatic castration-resistant, possibly by reducing the recruitment of MDSCs and inhibiting metastasis [168, 169]. However, when tasquinimod was studied in a global phase III randomized trial in men with bone CRPC and while it significantly improved radiographic progression-free survival, this did not result in an overall survival benefit [170]. A recent phase II study failed to demonstrate the clinical activity of tasquinimod in heavily pretreated patients with advanced hepatocellular, ovarian, renal cell, and gastric cancer, and many experienced adverse events such as fatigue, nausea, decreased appetite, and vomiting [171].

There are multiple published findings from clinical trials with laquinimod, most notably in multiple sclerosis populations. In a large, multicenter phase III clinical trial (ALLEGRO), laquinimod was well tolerated [172]. The most common adverse events were elevated liver enzymes (3.6% on laquinimod, 0.4% on placebo), abdominal pain, back pain, and cough. However, another trial with laquinimod (BRAVO [173]) in patients with relapsing multiple sclerosis showed conflicting results with the efficacy of laquinimod in reducing relapses and MRI measures of inflammation of multiple sclerosis patients. Recently, laquinimod did not reach the primary endpoint of reduction in confirmed disability progression in a phase 3 trial of patients with relapsing multiple sclerosis [167].

Paquinimod is reported to be beneficial in several animal models including systemic sclerosis [174], COPD [110], type 1 diabetes [175], and SLE [176]. Recently, our group observed that treatment of cigarette exposed mice with paquinimod, an S100A9 inhibitor, could preserve lung function [110]. In an SLE-prone mouse study where the animals

TABLE 2: Current drug development targeting S100 proteins.

Therapeutic approach	Agent	Possible S100 protein interaction	Current status	Study
Small molecule inhibition of S100 proteins Quinoline-3-carboxamide derivatives	Tasquinimod (ABR-215050)	Oral administration that blocks S100A8 and S100A9 interacting with RAGE and TLR4	Phase II randomized, double-blind, placebo-controlled studies in men with minimally symptomatic metastatic CRPC	[168–170]
	Paquinimod (ABR-215757)	Oral administration that blocks S100A8/S100A9 interacting with TLR4	Phase I study demonstrated good tolerance in SLE patients, while a phase II study data never published	[176, 177]
	Laquinimod (ABR-215062)	Oral administration that blocks S100A8 and S100A9 interacting with RAGE and TLR4	Conflicting data in several multicenter phase II and III clinical trials in multiple sclerosis populations	[167, 172, 173]
Inhibitors of S100 proteins	Cromolyn (cromoglicic acid)	An antihistaminic drug binds to S100A1, S10012, S100A13, and S100P and disrupts interactions with RAGE	FDA approved 20 years ago as an antihistaminic drug, as a nasal spray (NasalCrom)	[178]
	Amlexanox	Interacts with S100A1, S100A4, and S100A13 to prevent their signaling	Used to treat recurrent aphthous ulcers but discontinued in the USA In Japan, it is used to treat bronchial asthma, allergic rhinitis, and conjunctivitis	[184] [228]
	Phenothiazines, such as trifluoperazine	Disrupt the interaction of S100A4 with myosin-IIA	Used to treat psychotic disorders, anxiety, nausea, and vomiting caused by chemotherapy	[229]
	Pentamidine	Downregulates inflammation mediated S100B	An antimicrobial agent to treat African trypanosomiasis, leishmaniasis, Balamuthia infections, babesiosis, and Pneumocystis pneumonia	[192]
Indirect inhibitors of S100 protein signaling	Arundic acid	Reduces S100B levels	A multicenter, dose-escalating, randomized, double-blind phase I trial was performed in acute ischemic stroke	[194, 230]
	Calcimycin (A23187)	Inhibit S100A4 expression	A calcium ionophore used against gram-positive bacteria and fungi. Also, in *in vitro* fertilization and to make artificial liposomes for cancer drugs	[185]
	Niclosamide (niclocide)	Inhibit S100A4 expression	Oral administered antihelminth drug	[231]
	Sulindac	Inhibit S100A4 expression	A nonsteroidal anti-inflammatory drug	[186]
Gene delivery approaches	Adenoviral-associated vector S100A1 gene delivery	Restored S100A1 levels to restore cardiomyocytes physiologic contractility, cardiac performance, and left ventricular remodeling	Only tested in animal models	[201, 202]
S100 neutralizing antibodies	Anti-S100A4, anti-S100P, anti-S100A9	Prevent extracellular signaling of S100 proteins	Only tested in animal models	[39, 195, 196]
S100 neutralizing peptides	Peptide-Fc fusion proteins (peptibody)	Depletes myeloid-derived suppressor cells getting to tumor and releasing S100 proteins	Only tested in animal models but reduced tumor growth	[197, 199]
Vaccines targeting S100 proteins	Anti-S100A9 vaccine	Prevent S100A9/CD36 signaling in a mouse ischemic stroke model	Only tested in animal models	[200]

developed significant glomerulonephritis resulting in hematuria and proteinuria, treatment with paquinimod was comparable to prednisolone or mycophenolate treatment [176]. A phase 1b study in humans demonstrates good tolerance of paquinimod at 3 mg/kg, but several adverse events, such as arthralgia and myalgia, were reported with the highest dose levels of paquinimod (4.5 mg/day and 6.0 mg/day) [176]. However, although a phase 2 study was initiated, no results have been released as of the time of this paper [177].

5.2. Other Potential Therapeutic Intervention of S100 Proteins. Here, we will briefly outline some alternative approaches to target S100 proteins that could be applied to lung diseases. These include gene delivery approaches, inhibitory antibodies and peptides, vaccines, and chemical inhibitors (see Table 2). Several new compounds were recently identified specifically for S100 proteins that inhibit the interactions of S100P [178], S100A4 [179, 180], S100A9 [179], S100A10 [181], and S100B [182, 183] with their targets.

The antihistaminic drug, cromolyn, binds to S100A1, S10012, S100A13, and S100P and disrupts S100P interacting with RAGE [178]. A cromolyn analog which inhibits S100P was used in pancreatic cell line and mice models to reduce tumor growth and metastasis [178]. Another anti-inflammatory antiallergic immunomodulatory drug, Amlexanox, interacts with S100A1, S100A4, and S100A13 and alters S100 protein signal transduction [184]. Alternatively, phenothiazines interact with multiple S100 family members, such as S100A4 [22], and may influence their signaling.

Equally several compounds are known to inhibit the S100A4 expression, with calcimycin (a calcium ionophore), niclosamide (an antihelminth drug), and sulindac (a nonsteroidal anti-inflammatory drug) are all reported as inhibitors of S100A4 transcription [185, 186]. Interestingly, calcimycin can augment surfactant secretion in cultured type II airway epithelial cells (AEC II) [187, 188]. Equally, niclosamide increases the sensitivity of cancer cells for radiation therapy in lung cancer [189] and alleviates pulmonary fibrosis *in vitro* and *in vivo* by attenuation of epithelial-to-mesenchymal transition, matrix proteins, and Wnt/β-catenin signaling [190]. Sulindac is also linked to lung cancer therapy and pulmonary fibrosis [191]. Whether these responses are due to S100A4 are unknown. Pentamidine is deemed an S100B inhibitor as it reduces several inflammatory markers such as MDA, PGE2, and IL-1, which in turn downregulated S100B [192]. By blocking S100B activity, pentamidine rescues expression of the tumor suppressor factor wtp53 and restores proapoptotic responses in colon cancer [193]. Alternatively, other groups have tried to reduce S100B levels, using arundic acid, and found that treatment with arundic acid at 24-48 hours after the induction of ischemia significantly decreased infarct volumes by approximately 40% [194].

Other approaches to modulate S100 protein activity include neutralizing antibodies [39, 195, 196] and peptide-Fc fusion proteins (peptibodies) directed against S100A8 and S100A9 [197]. Antibody-based therapies are an interesting approach for several of the S100 proteins as they possibly could reduce toxicity and off-target effects but may be limited to only extracellular S100 proteins. Treatment with an anti-S100A4 antibody decreased signs of allergy in a mouse model as well as in allergen-challenged T cells from allergic patients [198]. Inhibiting extracellular S100 protein signaling may be beneficial for COPD, as intracellular S100A8 protects against type II pneumocyte cytotoxicity [107], while extracellular S100A9 contributes to disease progression [110]. Some inhibitory peptides can penetrate cells with S100B inhibitory peptides reported to penetrate tumor cells and reduce growth in a melanoma xenograft model [199]. Immunization with an anti-S100A9 vaccine in a mouse ischemic stroke inhibited long-term thrombus formation, through inhibition of increased S100A9/CD36 signaling, without risk of bleeding or adverse autoimmune responses [200]. In rodent [201] and pig [202] cardiac disease models, adenoviral-associated vector S100A1 gene delivery to cardiac tissue normalized low S100A1 levels and restore cardiomyocytes physiologic contractility, restored cardiac performance, and left ventricular remodeling. Therefore, many approaches exist to modulate S100 protein signaling but most require testing in the setting of pulmonary diseases.

6. The Influence of Neutrophils in the Release of S100 Proteins in Pulmonary Diseases

Finally, we want to briefly discuss the importance of S100 proteins and neutrophils in pulmonary diseases. Neutrophils are the first responders to the site of inflammation and are essential for microbial containment, eradication, and host survival. Dysregulated neutrophil responses are central to the pathophysiology of many inflammatory lung diseases. Approximately 45% of the cytosolic proteins in neutrophils are constituted with S100A8, S100A9, and S100A12 and are released upon injury or infection [203, 204]. Following activation of neutrophils, the S100 proteins are secreted or released and function in an autocrine and paracrine manner. The released S100 proteins induce the production of proinflammatory cytokines, neutrophil degranulation and chemotaxis, leukocyte adhesion and endothelial transmigration, and increased effects of lipopolysaccharide on phagocytes and cells (Figure 1). At the site of inflammation, calprotectin acts as a chemotactic factor by inducing neutrophils adhesion [159] and thereby further exaggerates neutrophil responses.

Rammes et al. have suggested that in monocytes, the non-classical S100A8/A9 secretion constitutes an intact microtubule network and PKC activation [114]. However, in neutrophils, the process by which S100A8/A9 is secreted is not fully elucidated and may be different from the pathway in monocytes since the S100A8/A9 complex is detected in NETs. Secretion of S100A8/A9 is dependent on the production of ROS and required K^+ exchanges through the ATP-sensitive K^+ channel [205]. Schenten et al. indicated that S100A9 is phosphorylated at threonine 113 by the MAPK p38 in activated neutrophils and released to the extracellular space by the process of NETosis [27, 206, 207]. Equally, S100A9 is an activator of the β-2 integrin Mac-1 (CD11b/CD18) on neutrophils [208] and could influence neutrophil trafficking, phagocytosis, ROS production, and T cell activation [209]. However, further research is needed to elucidate the signaling pathway.

With the new human viral disease severe acute respiratory syndrome coronavirus 2 (SARS-CoV-2), there is emerging data identifying the roles of S100 proteins to coronavirus disease 2019 (COVID-19). In preclinical models of SARS-CoV-2 infected animals and patients, there are increased levels of immature neutrophils and dramatically upregulated S100A8 levels [210]. In addition, multivariable analysis of patients' samples demonstrated that elevated S100A9 was independently associated with mortality [211]. Serum S100A8/A9 levels in COVID-19 patients are linked to severity and in-hospital mortality [212] and early indicator of respiratory failure [210]. This suggests that S100 proteins of neutrophil origin could significantly contribute to inflammation and respiratory outcomes in COVID-19 subjects. Higher blood frequency of NETs and neutrophil activation markers including S100A8/A9 are observed in COVID-19 cases associated with thrombosis [213] and in COVID-19 with severe pulmonary outcomes [214]. The presence of S100A8/A9 in fecal is linked to intestinal inflammation in COVID-19 patients [215, 216]. Equally, monocytes with low expression of HLA-DR and high expression of S100A8, A9, and 12 are strongly associated with severe COVID-19 [137]. Serum S100B COVID-19 patients significantly correlate with disease severity and are associated with inflammation markers (ferritin, C-reactive protein, procalcitonin) and organ damage markers (alanine aminotransferase, creatinine) [217]. Recently, paquinimod was shown to resolve SARS-CoV-2 mediated pneumonia by reducing the viral load and a subset of neutrophils in mice [218]. Therefore, neutrophil-associated S100 proteins may represent key players in the pathogenesis of many pulmonary diseases, including COVID-19.

7. Conclusions

In the past two decades, our knowledge of the roles of S100 proteins in pulmonary diseases has grown, and many novel approaches were identified to target members of this protein family as therapeutic options. Despite considerable progress in S100 protein biology, we still know little about posttranslational modifications or heterodimer formation impact on S100 signaling, and the COVID-19 pandemic highlights the potential role of S100 proteins in tissue damage.

Acknowledgments

This work was supported by grants made available to P.G. (the Alpha-1 Foundation (493373 and 614218)).

References

[1] M. E. Bianchi, "DAMPs, PAMPs and alarmins: all we need to know about danger," *Journal of Leukocyte Biology*, vol. 81, no. 1, pp. 1–5, 2007.

[2] T. Gong, L. Liu, W. Jiang, and R. Zhou, "DAMP-sensing receptors in sterile inflammation and inflammatory diseases," *Nature Reviews. Immunology*, vol. 20, no. 2, pp. 95–112, 2020.

[3] E. Leclerc, G. Fritz, S. W. Vetter, and C. W. Heizmann, "Binding of S100 proteins to RAGE: an update," *Biochimica et Biophysica Acta*, vol. 1793, no. 6, pp. 993–1007, 2009.

[4] R. Donato, B. R. Cannon, G. Sorci et al., "Functions of S100 proteins," *Current Molecular Medicine*, vol. 13, no. 1, pp. 24–57, 2013.

[5] S. R. Gross, C. G. Sin, R. Barraclough, and P. S. Rudland, "Joining S100 proteins and migration: for better or for worse, in sickness and in health," *Cellular and Molecular Life Sciences*, vol. 71, no. 9, pp. 1551–1579, 2014.

[6] R. Donato, "Intracellular and extracellular roles of S100 proteins," *Microscopy Research and Technique*, vol. 60, no. 6, pp. 540–551, 2003.

[7] B. W. Moore, "A soluble protein characteristic of the nervous system," *Biochemical and Biophysical Research Communications*, vol. 19, no. 6, pp. 739–744, 1965.

[8] N. Kozlyuk, A. J. Monteith, V. Garcia, S. M. Damo, E. P. Skaar, and W. J. Chazin, "S100 proteins in the innate immune response to pathogens," *Methods in Molecular Biology*, vol. 1929, pp. 275–290, 2019.

[9] I. Marenholz, C. W. Heizmann, and G. Fritz, "S100 proteins in mouse and man: from evolution to function and pathology (including an update of the nomenclature)," *Biochemical and Biophysical Research Communications*, vol. 322, no. 4, pp. 1111–1122, 2004.

[10] L. L. Gonzalez, K. Garrie, and M. D. Turner, "Role of S100 proteins in health and disease," *Biochimica et Biophysica Acta (BBA)-Molecular Cell Research*, vol. 1867, no. 6, p. 118677, 2020.

[11] B. A. Gilston, E. P. Skaar, and W. J. Chazin, "Binding of transition metals to S100 proteins," *Science China. Life Sciences*, vol. 59, no. 8, pp. 792–801, 2016.

[12] T. G. Nakashige, B. Zhang, C. Krebs, and E. M. Nolan, "Human calprotectin is an iron-sequestering host-defense protein," *Nature Chemical Biology*, vol. 11, no. 10, pp. 765–771, 2015.

[13] D. Foell, H. Wittkowski, T. Vogl, and J. Roth, "S100 proteins expressed in phagocytes: a novel group of damage-associated molecular pattern molecules," *Journal of Leukocyte Biology*, vol. 81, no. 1, pp. 28–37, 2007.

[14] C. Xia, Z. Braunstein, A. C. Toomey, J. Zhong, and X. Rao, "S100 proteins as an important regulator of macrophage inflammation," *Frontiers in Immunology*, vol. 8, p. 1908, 2018.

[15] C. R. Silva, B. M. S. Melo, J. R. Silva et al., "S100A9 plays a pivotal role in a mouse model of herpetic neuralgia via TLR4/TNF pathway," *Brain, Behavior, and Immunity*, vol. 88, pp. 353–362, 2020.

[16] M. A. Hofmann, S. Drury, C. Fu et al., "RAGE mediates a novel proinflammatory axis: a central cell surface receptor for S100/calgranulin polypeptides," *Cell*, vol. 97, no. 7, pp. 889–901, 1999.

[17] M. B. Brophy, J. A. Hayden, and E. M. Nolan, "Calcium ion gradients modulate the zinc affinity and antibacterial activity of human calprotectin," *Journal of the American Chemical Society*, vol. 134, no. 43, pp. 18089–18100, 2012.

[18] G. Fritz, H. M. Botelho, L. A. Morozova-Roche, and C. M. Gomes, "Natural and amyloid self-assembly of S100 proteins: structural basis of functional diversity," *The FEBS Journal*, vol. 277, no. 22, pp. 4578–4590, 2010.

[19] M. Ichikawa, R. Williams, L. Wang, T. Vogl, and G. Srikrishna, "S100A8/A9 activate key genes and pathways in colon tumor progression," *Molecular Cancer Research*, vol. 9, no. 2, pp. 133–148, 2011.

[20] N. T. Wright, B. R. Cannon, P. T. Wilder et al., "Solution structure of S100A1 bound to the CapZ peptide (TRTK12)," *Journal of Molecular Biology*, vol. 386, no. 5, pp. 1265–1277, 2009.

[21] J. Markowitz, R. R. Rustandi, K. M. Varney et al., "Calcium-binding properties of wild-type and EF-hand mutants of S100B in the presence and absence of a peptide derived from the C-terminal negative regulatory domain of p53," *Biochemistry*, vol. 44, no. 19, pp. 7305–7314, 2005.

[22] V. N. Malashkevich, K. M. Varney, S. C. Garrett et al., "Structure of Ca2+-bound S100A4 and its interaction with peptides derived from nonmuscle myosin-IIA," *Biochemistry*, vol. 47, no. 18, pp. 5111–5126, 2008.

[23] U. A. Ramagopal, N. G. Dulyaninova, K. M. Varney et al., "Structure of the S100A4/myosin-IIA complex," *BMC Structural Biology*, vol. 13, no. 1, p. 31, 2013.

[24] L. M. Orre, M. Pernemalm, J. Lengqvist, R. Lewensohn, and J. Lehtiö, "Up-regulation, modification, and translocation of S100A6 induced by exposure to ionizing radiation revealed by proteomics profiling," *Molecular & Cellular Proteomics*, vol. 6, no. 12, pp. 2122–2131, 2007.

[25] K. J. Miranda, R. F. Loeser, and R. R. Yammani, "Sumoylation and nuclear translocation of S100A4 regulate IL-1β-mediated production of matrix metalloproteinase-13," *The Journal of Biological Chemistry*, vol. 285, no. 41, pp. 31517–31524, 2010.

[26] S. Y. Lim, M. Raftery, H. Cai et al., "S-nitrosylated S100A8: novel anti-inflammatory properties," *Journal of Immunology*, vol. 181, no. 8, pp. 5627–5636, 2008.

[27] V. Schenten, S. Plançon, N. Jung et al., "Secretion of the phosphorylated form of S100A9 from neutrophils is essential for the proinflammatory functions of extracellular S100A8/A9," *Frontiers in Immunology*, vol. 9, p. 447, 2018.

[28] L. S. Cunden, M. B. Brophy, G. E. Rodriguez, H. A. Flaxman, and E. M. Nolan, "Biochemical and functional evaluation of the intramolecular disulfide bonds in the zinc-chelating antimicrobial protein human S100A7 (psoriasin)," *Biochemistry*, vol. 56, no. 43, pp. 5726–5738, 2017.

[29] D. L. Cecil and R. Terkeltaub, "Transamidation by transglutaminase 2 transforms S100A11 calgranulin into a procatabolic cytokine for chondrocytes," *Journal of Immunology*, vol. 180, no. 12, pp. 8378–8385, 2008.

[30] W. J. Chazin, "Relating form and function of EF-hand calcium binding proteins," *Accounts of Chemical Research*, vol. 44, no. 3, pp. 171–179, 2011.

[31] M. Pedrocchi, B. W. Schäfer, H. Mueller, U. Eppenberger, and C. W. Heizmann, "Expression of ca(2+)-binding proteins of the S100 family in malignant human breast-cancer cell lines and biopsy samples," *International Journal of Cancer*, vol. 57, no. 5, pp. 684–690, 1994.

[32] J. T. Elder and X. Zhao, "Evidence for local control of gene expression in the epidermal differentiation complex," *Experimental Dermatology*, vol. 11, no. 5, pp. 406–412, 2002.

[33] S. S. Cross, F. C. Hamdy, J. C. Deloulme, and I. Rehman, "Expression of S100 proteins in normal human tissues and common cancers using tissue microarrays: S100A6, S100A8, S100A9 and S100A11 are all overexpressed in common cancers," *Histopathology*, vol. 46, no. 3, pp. 256–269, 2005.

[34] J. C. Lindsey, M. E. Lusher, J. A. Anderton, R. J. Gilbertson, D. W. Ellison, and S. C. Clifford, "Epigenetic deregulation of multiple S100 gene family members by differential hypomethylation and hypermethylation events in medulloblastoma," *British Journal of Cancer*, vol. 97, no. 2, pp. 267–274, 2007.

[35] Q. Wang, M. Williamson, S. Bott et al., "Hypomethylation of WNT5A, CRIP1 and S100P in prostate cancer," *Oncogene*, vol. 26, no. 45, pp. 6560–6565, 2007.

[36] W. Lesniak, "Epigenetic regulation of S100 protein expression," *Clinical Epigenetics*, vol. 2, no. 2, pp. 77–83, 2011.

[37] K. Hsu, C. Champaiboon, B. D. Guenther et al., "Anti-infective protective properties of S100 calgranulins," *Anti-Inflammatory & Anti-Allergy Agents in Medicinal Chemistry (Formerly Current Medicinal Chemistry-Anti-Inflammatory and Anti-Allergy Agents)*, vol. 8, no. 4, pp. 290–305, 2009.

[38] M. A. Ingersoll, R. Spanbroek, C. Lottaz et al., "Comparison of gene expression profiles between human and mouse monocyte subsets," *Blood*, vol. 115, no. 3, pp. e10–e19, 2010.

[39] R. F. Foronjy, P. O. Ochieng, M. A. Salathe et al., "Protein tyrosine phosphatase 1B negatively regulates S100A9-mediated lung damage during respiratory syncytial virus exacerbations," *Mucosal Immunology*, vol. 9, no. 5, pp. 1317–1329, 2016.

[40] J. A. Spijkers-Hagelstein, P. Schneider, E. Hulleman et al., "Elevated S100A8/S100A9 expression causes glucocorticoid resistance in MLL-rearranged infant acute lymphoblastic leukemia," *Leukemia*, vol. 26, no. 6, pp. 1255–1265, 2012.

[41] C. Li, F. Zhang, M. Lin, and J. Liu, "Induction of S100A9 gene expression by cytokine oncostatin M in breast cancer cells through the STAT3 signaling cascade," *Breast Cancer Research and Treatment*, vol. 87, no. 2, pp. 123–134, 2004.

[42] A. C. Tramontina, F. Tramontina, L. D. Bobermin et al., "Secretion of S100B, an astrocyte-derived neurotrophic protein, is stimulated by fluoxetine via a mechanism independent of serotonin," *Progress in Neuro-Psychopharmacology & Biological Psychiatry*, vol. 32, no. 6, pp. 1580–1583, 2008.

[43] D. F. de Souza, M. C. Leite, A. Quincozes-Santos et al., "S100B secretion is stimulated by IL-1β in glial cultures and hippocampal slices of rats: likely involvement of MAPK pathway," *Journal of Neuroimmunology*, vol. 206, no. 1-2, pp. 52–57, 2009.

[44] P. Nardin, L. Tortorelli, A. Quincozes-Santos et al., "S100B secretion in acute brain slices: modulation by extracellular levels of Ca(2+) and K (+)," *Neurochemical Research*, vol. 34, no. 9, pp. 1603–1611, 2009.

[45] K. M. Kathir, K. Ibrahim, D. Rajalingam, I. Prudovsky, C. Yu, and T. K. S. Kumar, "S100A13-lipid interactions–role in the non-classical release of the acidic fibroblast growth factor," *Biochimica et Biophysica Acta*, vol. 1768, no. 12, pp. 3080–3089, 2007.

[46] M. Kapoor, Q. Zhou, F. Otero et al., "Evidence for annexin II-S100A10 complex and plasmin in mobilization of cytokine activity of human TrpRS," *The Journal of Biological Chemistry*, vol. 283, no. 4, pp. 2070–2077, 2008.

[47] T. Vogl, S. Ludwig, M. Goebeler et al., "MRP8 and MRP14 control microtubule reorganization during transendothelial migration of phagocytes," *Blood*, vol. 104, no. 13, pp. 4260–4268, 2004.

[48] T. Vogl, K. Tenbrock, S. Ludwig et al., "Mrp8 and Mrp14 are endogenous activators of toll-like receptor 4, promoting lethal, endotoxin-induced shock," *Nature Medicine*, vol. 13, no. 9, pp. 1042–1049, 2007.

[49] O. Turovskaya, D. Foell, P. Sinha et al., "RAGE, carboxylated glycans and S100A8/A9 play essential roles in colitis-associated carcinogenesis," *Carcinogenesis*, vol. 29, no. 10, pp. 2035–2043, 2008.

[50] C. Gebhardt, A. Riehl, M. Durchdewald et al., "RAGE signaling sustains inflammation and promotes tumor development," *The Journal of Experimental Medicine*, vol. 205, no. 2, pp. 275–285, 2008.

[51] S. Ghavami, I. Rashedi, B. M. Dattilo et al., "S100A8/A9 at low concentration promotes tumor cell growth via RAGE ligation and MAP kinase-dependent pathway," *Journal of Leukocyte Biology*, vol. 83, no. 6, pp. 1484–1492, 2008.

[52] E. Leclerc, G. Fritz, M. Weibel, C. W. Heizmann, and A. Galichet, "S100B and S100A6 differentially modulate cell

survival by interacting with distinct RAGE (receptor for advanced glycation end products) immunoglobulin domains," *The Journal of Biological Chemistry*, vol. 282, no. 43, pp. 31317–31331, 2007.

[53] G. Sorci, F. Riuzzi, C. Arcuri, I. Giambanco, and R. Donato, "Amphoterin stimulates myogenesis and counteracts the antimyogenic factors basic fibroblast growth factor and S100B via RAGE binding," *Molecular and Cellular Biology*, vol. 24, no. 11, pp. 4880–4894, 2004.

[54] C. Tondera, M. Laube, and J. Pietzsch, "Insights into binding of S100 proteins to scavenger receptors: class B scavenger receptor CD36 binds S100A12 with high affinity," *Amino Acids*, vol. 49, no. 1, pp. 183–191, 2017.

[55] F. Riuzzi, G. Sorci, and R. Donato, "S100B protein regulates myoblast proliferation and differentiation by activating FGFR1 in a bFGF-dependent manner," *Journal of Cell Science*, vol. 124, no. 14, pp. 2389–2400, 2011.

[56] R. von Bauer, D. Oikonomou, A. Sulaj et al., "CD166/ALCAM mediates proinflammatory effects of S100B in delayed type hypersensitivity," *Journal of Immunology*, vol. 191, no. 1, pp. 369–377, 2013.

[57] O. Dmytriyeva, S. Pankratova, S. Owczarek et al., "The metastasis-promoting S100A4 protein confers neuroprotection in brain injury," *Nature Communications*, vol. 3, no. 1, p. 1197, 2012.

[58] M. Sakaguchi, M. Yamamoto, M. Miyai et al., "Identification of an S100A8 receptor neuroplastin-β and its heterodimer formation with EMMPRIN," *The Journal of Investigative Dermatology*, vol. 136, no. 11, pp. 2240–2250, 2016.

[59] K. Okada, S. Arai, H. Itoh et al., "CD68 on rat macrophages binds tightly to S100A8 and S100A9 and helps to regulate the cells' immune functions," *Journal of Leukocyte Biology*, vol. 100, no. 5, pp. 1093–1104, 2016.

[60] S. Pankratova, J. Klingelhofer, O. Dmytriyeva et al., "The S100A4 protein signals through the ErbB4 receptor to promote neuronal survival," *Theranostics*, vol. 8, no. 14, pp. 3977–3990, 2018.

[61] K. Teichert-Kuliszewska, J. N. Tsoporis, J. F. Desjardins et al., "Absence of the calcium-binding protein, S100A1, confers pulmonary hypertension in mice associated with endothelial dysfunction and apoptosis," *Cardiovascular Research*, vol. 105, no. 1, pp. 8–19, 2015.

[62] J.-F. Desjardins, A. Pourdjabbar, A. Quan et al., "Lack of S100A1 in mice confers a gender-dependent hypertensive phenotype and increased mortality after myocardial infarction," *American Journal of Physiology-Heart and Circulatory Physiology*, vol. 296, no. 5, pp. H1457–H1465, 2009.

[63] S. T. Pleger, D. M. Harris, C. Shan et al., "Endothelial S100A1 modulates vascular function via nitric oxide," *Circulation Research*, vol. 102, no. 7, pp. 786–794, 2008.

[64] P. Ehlermann, A. Remppis, O. Guddat et al., "Right ventricular upregulation of the Ca^{2+} binding protein S100A1 in chronic pulmonary hypertension," *Biochimica et Biophysica Acta*, vol. 1500, no. 2, pp. 249–255, 2000.

[65] S. Wolf, C. Haase-Kohn, and J. Pietzsch, "S100A2 in cancerogenesis: a friend or a foe?," *Amino Acids*, vol. 41, no. 4, pp. 849–861, 2011.

[66] A. V. Biankin, J. G. Kench, E. K. Colvin et al., "Expression of S100A2 calcium-binding protein predicts response to pancreatectomy for pancreatic cancer," *Gastroenterology*, vol. 137, no. 2, pp. 558–568.e11, 2009.

[67] K. Ohuchida, K. Mizumoto, Y. Miyasaka et al., "Over-expression of S100A2 in pancreatic cancer correlates with progression and poor prognosis," *The Journal of Pathology: A Journal of the Pathological Society of Great Britain and Ireland*, vol. 213, no. 3, pp. 275–282, 2007.

[68] G. Feng, X.-c. Xu, E. M. Youssef, and R. Lotan, "Diminished expression of S100A2, a putative tumor suppressor, at early stage of human lung carcinogenesis," *Cancer Research*, vol. 61, no. 21, pp. 7999–8004, 2001.

[69] C. A. Moskaluk, M. K. Abdrabbo, J. Harper et al., "Gastric cancers overexpress S100A calcium-binding proteins," *Cancer Research*, vol. 62, no. 23, pp. 6823–6826, 2002.

[70] H. Wang, Z. Zhang, R. Li et al., "Overexpression of S100A2 protein as a prognostic marker for patients with stage I non small cell lung cancer," *International Journal of Cancer*, vol. 116, no. 2, pp. 285–290, 2005.

[71] K. Lee, S. T. Yun, C. O. Yun, B. Y. Ahn, and E. C. Jo, "S100A2 promoter-driven conditionally replicative adenovirus targets non- small-cell lung carcinoma," *Gene Therapy*, vol. 19, no. 10, pp. 967–977, 2012.

[72] E. A. al-Mutairy, F. A. Imtiaz, M. Khalid et al., "An atypical pulmonary fibrosis is associated with co-inheritance of mutations in the calcium binding protein genes-S100A3andS100A13," *European Respiratory Journal*, vol. 54, no. 1, article 1802041, 2019.

[73] M. Gianni, M. Li Calzi, M. Terao et al., "AM580, a stable benzoic derivative of retinoic acid, has powerful and selective cyto-differentiating effects on acute promyelocytic leukemia cells," 1996.

[74] M. Gianni, M. Terao, M. Kurosaki et al., "S100A3 a partner protein regulating the stability/activity of RARα and PML-RARα in cellular models of breast/lung cancer and acute myeloid leukemia," *Oncogene*, vol. 38, no. 14, pp. 2482–2500, 2019.

[75] S. Miao, T. Qiu, Y. Zhao et al., "Overexpression of S100A13 protein is associated with tumor angiogenesis and poor survival in patients with early-stage non-small cell lung cancer," *Thoracic cancer*, vol. 9, no. 9, pp. 1136–1144, 2018.

[76] A. Pierce, N. Barron, R. Linehan et al., "Identification of a novel, functional role for S100A13 in invasive lung cancer cell lines," *European Journal of Cancer*, vol. 44, no. 1, pp. 151–159, 2008.

[77] W. Zhang, S. Ohno, B. Steer et al., "S100a4 is secreted by alternatively activated alveolar macrophages and promotes activation of lung fibroblasts in pulmonary fibrosis," *Frontiers in Immunology*, vol. 9, p. 1216, 2018.

[78] Y. Li, J. Bao, Y. Bian et al., "S100A4(+) macrophages are necessary for pulmonary fibrosis by activating lung fibroblasts," *Frontiers in Immunology*, vol. 9, p. 1776, 2018.

[79] S. Hou, T. Tian, D. Qi et al., "S100A4 promotes lung tumor development through β-catenin pathway-mediated autophagy inhibition," *Cell Death & Disease*, vol. 9, no. 3, p. 277, 2018.

[80] D. C. Rubinsztein, G. Mariño, and G. Kroemer, "Autophagy and aging," *Cell*, vol. 146, no. 5, pp. 682–695, 2011.

[81] N. Mizushima and M. Komatsu, "Autophagy: renovation of cells and tissues," *Cell*, vol. 147, no. 4, pp. 728–741, 2011.

[82] L. Liu, L. Qi, T. Knifley et al., "S100A4 alters metabolism and promotes invasion of lung cancer cells by up- regulating mitochondrial complex I protein NDUFS2," *The Journal of Biological Chemistry*, vol. 294, no. 18, pp. 7516–7527, 2019.

[83] C. el Naaman, B. Grum-Schwensen, A. Mansouri et al., "Cancer predisposition in mice deficient for the metastasis-associated Mts1(S100A4) gene," *Oncogene*, vol. 23, no. 20, pp. 3670–3680, 2004.

[84] Y. Liu, J. Cui, Y.-L. Tang, L. Huang, C. Y. Zhou, and J. X. Xu, "Prognostic roles of mRNA expression of S100 in non-small-cell lung cancer," *BioMed Research International*, vol. 2018, Article ID 9815806, 11 pages, 2018.

[85] J. Sotty, G. Garçon, F. O. Denayer et al., "Toxicological effects of ambient fine ($PM_{2.5-0.18}$) and ultrafine ($PM_{0.18}$) particles in healthy and diseased 3D organo-typic mucocilary-phenotype models," *Environmental Research*, vol. 176, p. 108538, 2019.

[86] R. Donato, G. Sorci, and I. Giambanco, "S100A6 protein: functional roles," *Cellular and Molecular Life Sciences*, vol. 74, no. 15, pp. 2749–2760, 2017.

[87] T. Wang, Y. Liang, A. Thakur et al., "Diagnostic significance of S100A2 and S100A6 levels in sera of patients with non-small cell lung cancer," *Tumor Biology*, vol. 37, no. 2, pp. 2299–2304, 2016.

[88] X. He, X. Xu, A. Q. Khan, and W. Ling, "High expression of S100A6 predicts unfavorable prognosis of lung squamous cell cancer," *Medical Science Monitor: International Medical Journal of Experimental and Clinical Research*, vol. 23, pp. 5011–5017, 2017.

[89] A. Graczyk, Ł. P. Słomnicki, and W. Leśniak, "S100A6 competes with the TAZ2 domain of p300 for binding to p53 and attenuates p53 acetylation," *Journal of Molecular Biology*, vol. 425, no. 18, pp. 3488–3494, 2013.

[90] P. Li, X. Lv, Z. Zhang, and S. Xie, "S100A6/miR193a regulates the proliferation, invasion, migration and angiogenesis of lung cancer cells through the P53 acetylation," *American Journal of Translational Research*, vol. 11, no. 8, pp. 4634–4649, 2019.

[91] T. H. M. Grahn, A. Niroula, Á. Végvári et al., "S100A6 is a critical regulator of hematopoietic stem cells," *Leukemia*, vol. 34, no. 12, pp. 3323–3337, 2020.

[92] S. P. Zhang, Y. W. Wu, Z. Z. Wu, H. Y. Liu, J. H. Nie, and J. Tong, "Up-regulation of RAGE and S100A6 in rats exposed to cigarette smoke," *Environmental Toxicology and Pharmacology*, vol. 28, no. 2, pp. 259–264, 2009.

[93] C. Guilbault, J. P. Novak, P. Martin et al., "Distinct pattern of lung gene expression in the Cftr-KO mice developing spontaneous lung disease compared with their littermate controls," *Physiological Genomics*, vol. 25, no. 2, pp. 179–193, 2006.

[94] C. Landi, E. Bargagli, A. Carleo et al., "Bronchoalveolar lavage proteomic analysis in pulmonary fibrosis associated with systemic sclerosis: S100A6 and 14-3-3ε as potential biomarkers," *Rheumatology (Oxford)*, vol. 58, no. 1, pp. 165–178, 2019.

[95] M. Doubková, M. Karpisek, J. Mazoch, J. Skrickova, and M. Doubek, "Prognostic significance of surfactant protein A, surfactant protein D, Clara cell protein 16, S100 protein, trefoil factor 3, and prostatic secretory protein 94 in idiopathic pulmonary fibrosis, sarcoidosis, and chronic pulmonary obstructive disease," *Sarcoidosis, Vasculitis, and Diffuse Lung Diseases*, vol. 33, no. 3, pp. 224–234, 2016.

[96] B. D. Hardas, X. Zhao, J. Zhang, X. Longqing, S. Stoll, and J. T. Elder, "Assignment of psoriasin to human chromosomal band 1q21: coordinate overexpression of clustered genes is psoriasis," *The Journal of Investigative Dermatology*, vol. 106, no. 4, pp. 753–758, 1996.

[97] S. Semprini, F. Capon, S. Bovolenta et al., "Genomic structure, promoter characterisation and mutational analysis of the S100A7 gene: exclusion of a candidate for familial psoriasis susceptibility," *Human Genetics*, vol. 104, no. 2, pp. 130–134, 1999.

[98] Z. Lu, Y. Li, Y. Che et al., "The TGFβ-induced lncRNA TBILA promotes non-small cell lung cancer progression in vitro and in vivo via cis-regulating HGAL and activating S100A7/JAB1 signaling," *Cancer Letters*, vol. 432, pp. 156–168, 2018.

[99] D. Pennino, P. K. Bhavsar, R. Effner et al., "IL-22 suppresses IFN-γ-mediated lung inflammation in asthmatic patients," *Journal of Allergy and Clinical Immunology*, vol. 131, no. 2, pp. 562–570, 2013.

[100] D. K. Kim, Y. C. Wi, S. J. Shin, K. R. Kim, D. W. Kim, and S. H. Cho, "Diverse phenotypes and endotypes of fungus balls caused by mixed bacterial colonization in chronic rhinosinusitis," *International forum of allergy & rhinology*, vol. 9, no. 11, pp. 1360–1366, 2019.

[101] C. Baldini, L. Giusti, L. Bazzichi et al., "Association of psoriasin (S100A7) with clinical manifestations of systemic sclerosis: is its presence in whole saliva a potential predictor of pulmonary involvement?," *The Journal of Rheumatology*, vol. 35, no. 9, pp. 1820–1824, 2008.

[102] E. Andresen, C. Lange, D. Strodthoff et al., "S100A7/psoriasin expression in the human lung: unchanged in patients with COPD, but upregulated upon positive S. aureusdetection," *BMC Pulmonary Medicine*, vol. 11, no. 1, pp. 10–10, 2011.

[103] T. Jinquan, H. Vorum, C. G. Larsen et al., "Psoriasin: a novel chemotactic protein," *Journal of Investigative Dermatology*, vol. 107, no. 1, pp. 5–10, 1996.

[104] R. Gläser, J. Harder, H. Lange, J. Bartels, E. Christophers, and J. M. Schröder, "Antimicrobial psoriasin (S100A7) protects human skin from Escherichia coli infection," *Nature Immunology*, vol. 6, no. 1, pp. 57–64, 2005.

[105] R. Wang, Y. Li, E. Hu et al., "S100A7 promotes lung adenocarcinoma to squamous carcinoma transdifferentiation, and its expression is differentially regulated by the Hippo-YAP pathway in lung cancer cells," *Oncotarget*, vol. 8, no. 15, pp. 24804–24814, 2017.

[106] G. Liu, Q. Wu, G. Liu, X. Song, and J. Zhang, "RETRACTED ARTICLE: Psoriasin (S100A7) is a novel biomarker for lung squamous cell carcinoma in humans," *Cancer Cell International*, vol. 15, no. 1, p. 18, 2015.

[107] C. R. Lin, K. Bahmed, G. J. Criner et al., "S100A8 protects human primary alveolar type II cells against injury and emphysema," *American Journal of Respiratory Cell and Molecular Biology*, vol. 60, no. 3, pp. 299–307, 2019.

[108] S. J. Huang, Z. N. Ding, H. X. Xiang, L. Fu, and J. Fei, "Association between serum S100A8/S100A9 heterodimer and pulmonary function in patients with acute exacerbation of chronic obstructive pulmonary disease," *Lung*, vol. 198, no. 4, pp. 645–652, 2020.

[109] X. Huang, Y. Li, X. Guo et al., "Identification of differentially expressed genes and signaling pathways in chronic obstructive pulmonary disease via bioinformatic analysis," *FEBS Open Bio*, vol. 9, no. 11, pp. 1880–1899, 2019.

[110] C. Railwah, A. Lora, K. Zahid et al., "Cigarette smoke induction of S100A9 contributes to chronic obstructive pulmonary disease," *American Journal of Physiology. Lung Cellular and Molecular Physiology*, vol. 319, no. 6, pp. L1021–L1035, 2020.

[111] Y. Hiroshima, K. Hsu, N. Tedla et al., "S100A8 induces IL-10 and protects against acute lung injury," *The Journal of Immunology*, vol. 192, no. 6, pp. 2800–2811, 2014.

[112] Y. Hiroshima, K. Hsu, N. Tedla et al., "S100A8/A9 and S100A9 reduce acute lung injury," *Immunology and Cell Biology*, vol. 95, no. 5, pp. 461–472, 2017.

[113] R. Gopal, L. Monin, D. Torres et al., "S100A8/A9 proteins mediate neutrophilic inflammation and lung pathology during tuberculosis," *American Journal of Respiratory and Critical Care Medicine*, vol. 188, no. 9, pp. 1137–1146, 2013.

[114] A. Rammes, J. Roth, M. Goebeler, M. Klempt, M. Hartmann, and C. Sorg, "Myeloid-related protein (MRP) 8 and MRP14, calcium-binding proteins of the S100 family, are secreted by activated monocytes via a novel, tubulin- dependent pathway," *Journal of Biological Chemistry*, vol. 272, no. 14, pp. 9496–9502, 1997.

[115] A. Voganatsi, A. Panyutich, K. T. Miyasaki, and R. K. Murthy, "Mechanism of extracellular release of human neutrophil calprotectin complex," *Journal of Leukocyte Biology*, vol. 70, no. 1, pp. 130–134, 2001.

[116] N. R. Scott, R. V. Swanson, N. al-Hammadi et al., "S100A8/A9 regulates CD11b expression and neutrophil recruitment during chronic tuberculosis," *The Journal of Clinical Investigation*, vol. 130, no. 6, pp. 3098–3112, 2020.

[117] D. H. Kim, E. Choi, J. S. Lee et al., "House dust mite allergen regulates constitutive apoptosis of normal and asthmatic neutrophils via toll-like receptor 4," *PLoS One*, vol. 10, no. 5, article e0125983, 2015.

[118] D. H. Kim, A. Gu, J. S. Lee et al., "Suppressive effects of S100A8 and S100A9 on neutrophil apoptosis by cytokine release of human bronchial epithelial cells in asthma," *International Journal of Medical Sciences*, vol. 17, no. 4, pp. 498–509, 2020.

[119] C. H. Wang, T. H. Punde, C. D. Huang et al., "Fibrocyte trafficking in patients with chronic obstructive asthma and during an acute asthma exacerbation," *The Journal of Allergy and Clinical Immunology*, vol. 135, no. 5, pp. 1154–1162.e5, 2015.

[120] L. D. Palmer, K. N. Maloney, K. L. Boyd et al., "The innate immune protein S100A9 protects from T-helper cell type 2-mediated allergic airway inflammation," *American Journal of Respiratory Cell and Molecular Biology*, vol. 61, no. 4, pp. 459–468, 2019.

[121] T. Saito, M. Liu, M. Binnie et al., "Distinct expression patterns of alveolar "alarmins" in subtypes of chronic lung allograft dysfunction," *American Journal of Transplantation*, vol. 14, no. 6, pp. 1425–1432, 2014.

[122] G. Luo, M. Tang, Q. Zhao et al., "Bone marrow adipocytes enhance osteolytic bone destruction by activating 1q21.3(S100A7/8/9-IL6R)-TLR4 pathway in lung cancer," *Journal of Cancer Research and Clinical Oncology*, vol. 146, no. 9, pp. 2241–2253, 2020.

[123] A. Carleo, C. Landi, A. Prasse et al., "Proteomic characterization of idiopathic pulmonary fibrosis patients: stable versus acute exacerbation," *Monaldi Archives for Chest Disease*, vol. 90, no. 2, 2020.

[124] C. Machahua, S. A. Guler, M. P. Horn et al., "Serum calprotectin as new biomarker for disease severity in idiopathic pulmonary fibrosis: a cross-sectional study in two independent cohorts," *BMJ Open Respiratory Research*, vol. 8, no. 1, p. e000827, 2021.

[125] M. Boruk, C. Railwah, A. Lora et al., "Elevated S100A9 expression in chronic rhinosinusitis coincides with elevated MMP production and proliferation in vitro," *Scientific Reports*, vol. 10, no. 1, p. 16350, 2020.

[126] T. Huan, T. Esko, M. J. Peters et al., "A meta-analysis of gene expression signatures of blood pressure and hypertension," *PLoS Genetics*, vol. 11, no. 3, pp. e1005035–e1005035, 2015.

[127] P. A. Singleton, T. Mirzapoiazova, Y. Guo et al., "High-molecular-weight hyaluronan is a novel inhibitor of pulmonary vascular leakiness," *American Journal of Physiology. Lung Cellular and Molecular Physiology*, vol. 299, no. 5, pp. L639–L651, 2010.

[128] K. Katono, Y. Sato, S.-X. Jiang et al., "Clinicopathological significance of S100A10 expression in lung adenocarcinomas," *Asian Pacific Journal of Cancer Prevention*, vol. 17, no. 1, pp. 289–294, 2016.

[129] K. Sato, Y. Saiki, K. Arai et al., "S100A10 upregulation associates with poor prognosis in lung squamous cell carcinoma," *Biochemical and Biophysical Research Communications*, vol. 505, no. 2, pp. 466–470, 2018.

[130] G. Pampalakis, E. Zingkou, K. G. Sidiropoulos et al., "Biochemical pathways mediated by KLK6 protease in breast cancer," *Molecular Oncology*, vol. 13, no. 11, pp. 2329–2343, 2019.

[131] T. Woo, K. Okudela, H. Mitsui et al., "Up-regulation of S100A11 in lung adenocarcinoma - its potential relationship with cancer progression," *PLoS One*, vol. 10, no. 11, article e0142642, 2015.

[132] H. Bouzina, R. Hesselstrand, and G. Rådegran, "Plasma insulin-like growth factor binding protein 1 in pulmonary arterial hypertension," *Scandinavian Cardiovascular Journal*, vol. 55, pp. 35–42, 2021.

[133] C. Fan, Z. Fu, Q. Su, D. J. Angelini, J. van Eyk, and R. A. Johns, "S100A11 mediates hypoxia-induced mitogenic factor (HIMF)-induced smooth muscle cell migration, vesicular exocytosis, and nuclear activation," *Molecular & Cellular Proteomics*, vol. 10, no. 3, p. M110.000901, 2011.

[134] H. Wittkowski, A. Sturrock, M. A. van Zoelen et al., "Neutrophil-derived S100A12 in acute lung injury and respiratory distress syndrome," *Critical Care Medicine*, vol. 35, no. 5, pp. 1369–1375, 2007.

[135] M. A. Hofmann Bowman, A. Heydemann, J. Gawdzik, R. A. Shilling, and B. Camoretti-Mercado, "Transgenic expression of human S100A12 induces structural airway abnormalities and limited lung inflammation in a mouse model of allergic inflammation," *Clinical and Experimental Allergy*, vol. 41, no. 6, pp. 878–889, 2011.

[136] W. Wen, W. Su, H. Tang et al., "Immune cell profiling of COVID-19 patients in the recovery stage by single- cell sequencing," *Cell discovery*, vol. 6, no. 1, p. 31, 2020.

[137] J. Schulte-Schrepping, N. Reusch, D. Paclik et al., "Severe COVID-19 is marked by a dysregulated myeloid cell compartment," *Cell*, vol. 182, no. 6, pp. 1419–1440.e23, 2020.

[138] K. Katono, Y. Sato, M. Kobayashi et al., "Clinicopathological significance of S100A14 expression in lung adenocarcinoma," *Oncology research and treatment*, vol. 40, no. 10, pp. 594–602, 2017.

[139] W. Zhao, T. Chen, and Y. Zhao, "Upregulated lncRNA CASC9 contributes to progression of non-small cell lung cancer through inhibition of miR-335-3p and activation S100A14 expression," *Oncotargets and Therapy*, vol. 13, pp. 6027–6036, 2020.

[140] Y. C. Chen, M. C. Lin, C. C. Hsiao et al., "Increased S100A15 expression and decreased DNA methylation of its gene promoter are involved in high metastasis potential and poor outcome of lung adenocarcinoma," *Oncotarget*, vol. 8, no. 28, pp. 45710–45724, 2017.

[141] L. Sun, Z. Zhang, Y. Yao, W. Y. Li, and J. Gu, "Analysis of expression differences of immune genes in non-small cell lung cancer based on TCGA and ImmPort data sets and the application of a prognostic model," *Annals of translational medicine*, vol. 8, no. 8, pp. 550–550, 2020.

[142] K. Saito, M. Kobayashi, R. Nagashio et al., "S100A16 is a prognostic marker for lung adenocarcinomas," *Asian Pacific Journal of Cancer Prevention*, vol. 16, no. 16, pp. 7039–7044, 2015.

[143] L. Peng, L. Xu, and W. Ouyang, "Role of peripheral inflammatory markers in postoperative cognitive dysfunction (POCD): a meta-analysis," *PLoS One*, vol. 8, no. 11, article e79624, 2013.

[144] E. Higgins, G. Edwards, J. Tanguay, and M. Button, "93P: chemoradiotherapy with radical intent for small cell lung cancer (SCLC): a 5 year retrospective review," *Journal of Thoracic Oncology*, vol. 11, no. 4, p. S97, 2016.

[145] S. Mu, H. Ma, J. Shi, and D. Zhen, "The expression of S100B protein in serum of patients with brain metastases from small-cell lung cancer and its clinical significance," *Oncology Letters*, vol. 14, no. 6, pp. 7107–7110, 2017.

[146] B. S. Tan, M. C. Yang, S. Singh et al., "lncRNA NORAD is repressed by the YAP pathway and suppresses lung and breast cancer metastasis by sequestering S100P," *Oncogene*, vol. 38, no. 28, pp. 5612–5626, 2019.

[147] R. Hu, K. E. Huffman, M. Chu, Y. Zhang, J. D. Minna, and Y. Yu, "Quantitative secretomic analysis identifies extracellular protein factors that modulate the metastatic phenotype of non-small cell lung cancer," *Journal of Proteome Research*, vol. 15, no. 2, pp. 477–486, 2016.

[148] Z. Wang and X. Chen, "Establishment and validation of an immune-associated signature in lung adenocarcinoma," *International Immunopharmacology*, vol. 88, p. 106867, 2020.

[149] B. Bartling, G. Rehbein, A. Simm, R. E. Silber, and H. S. Hofmann, "Porcupine expression is associated with the expression of S100P and other cancer-related molecules in non-small cell lung carcinoma," *International Journal of Oncology*, vol. 36, no. 4, pp. 1015–1021, 2010.

[150] M. Moll, R. B. Christmann, Y. Zhang et al., "Patients with systemic sclerosis-associated pulmonary arterial hypertension express a genomic signature distinct from patients with interstitial lung disease," *Journal of scleroderma and related disorders*, vol. 3, no. 3, pp. 242–248, 2018.

[151] Y. Dempsie, M. Nilsen, K. White et al., "Development of pulmonary arterial hypertension in mice over-expressing S100A4/Mts1 is specific to females," *Respiratory Research*, vol. 12, no. 1, p. 159, 2011.

[152] X. Xu, H. Chen, X. Zhu et al., "S100A9 promotes human lung fibroblast cells activation through receptor for advanced glycation end-product-mediated extracellular-regulated kinase 1/2, mitogen-activated protein-kinase and nuclear factor-κB-dependent pathways," *Clinical and Experimental Immunology*, vol. 173, no. 3, pp. 523–535, 2013.

[153] P. Geraghty, A. J. Dabo, and J. D'Armiento, "TLR4 protein contributes to cigarette smoke-induced matrix metalloproteinase-1 (MMP-1) expression in chronic obstructive pulmonary disease," *The Journal of Biological Chemistry*, vol. 286, no. 34, pp. 30211–30218, 2011.

[154] A. B. Robinson, J. A. Stogsdill, J. B. Lewis, T. T. Wood, and P. R. Reynolds, "RAGE and tobacco smoke: insights into modeling chronic obstructive pulmonary disease," *Frontiers in Physiology*, vol. 3, p. 301, 2012.

[155] T. Betsuyaku, M. Tanino, K. Nagai, Y. Nasuhara, M. Nishimura, and R. M. Senior, "Extracellular matrix metalloproteinase inducer is increased in smokers' bronchoalveolar lavage fluid," *American Journal of Respiratory and Critical Care Medicine*, vol. 168, no. 2, pp. 222–227, 2003.

[156] W. R. Swindell, A. Johnston, X. Xing et al., "Robust shifts in S100a9 expression with aging: a novel mechanism for chronic inflammation," *Scientific Reports*, vol. 3, no. 1, p. 1215, 2013.

[157] L. V. Portela, A. B. Tort, D. V. Schaf et al., "The serum S100B concentration is age dependent," *Clinical Chemistry*, vol. 48, no. 6, pp. 950–952, 2002.

[158] M. Wiesmann, U. Missler, D. Gottmann, and S. Gehring, "Plasma S-100b protein concentration in healthy adults is age- and sex-independent," *Clinical Chemistry*, vol. 44, no. 5, pp. 1056–1058, 1998.

[159] C. Ryckman, K. Vandal, P. Rouleau, M. Talbot, and P. A. Tessier, "Proinflammatory activities of S100: proteins S100A8, S100A9, and S100A8/A9 induce neutrophil chemotaxis and adhesion," *Journal of Immunology*, vol. 170, no. 6, pp. 3233–3242, 2003.

[160] P. Cheng, C. A. Corzo, N. Luetteke et al., "Inhibition of dendritic cell differentiation and accumulation of myeloid-derived suppressor cells in cancer is regulated by S100A9 protein," *The Journal of Experimental Medicine*, vol. 205, no. 10, pp. 2235–2249, 2008.

[161] G. Sorci, G. Giovannini, F. Riuzzi et al., "The danger signal S100B integrates pathogen- and danger-sensing pathways to restrain inflammation," *PLoS Pathogens*, vol. 7, no. 3, article e1001315, 2011.

[162] J. Steiner, N. Marquardt, I. Pauls et al., "Human $CD8^+$ T cells and NK cells express and secrete S100B upon stimulation," *Brain, Behavior, and Immunity*, vol. 25, no. 6, pp. 1233–1241, 2011.

[163] J. Goyette, W. X. Yan, E. Yamen et al., "Pleiotropic roles of S100A12 in coronary atherosclerotic plaque formation and rupture," *Journal of Immunology*, vol. 183, no. 1, pp. 593–603, 2009.

[164] M. Schneider, S. Kostin, C. C. Strøm et al., "S100A4 is upregulated in injured myocardium and promotes growth and survival of cardiac myocytes," *Cardiovascular Research*, vol. 75, no. 1, pp. 40–50, 2007.

[165] E. Källberg, T. Vogl, D. Liberg et al., "S100A9 interaction with TLR4 promotes tumor growth," *PLoS One*, vol. 7, no. 3, article e34207, 2012.

[166] P. Björk, A. Björk, T. Vogl et al., "Identification of human S100A9 as a novel target for treatment of autoimmune disease via binding to quinoline-3-carboxamides," *PLoS Biology*, vol. 7, no. 4, p. e97, 2009.

[167] G. Giovannoni, V. Knappertz, J. R. Steinerman et al., "A randomized, placebo-controlled, phase 2 trial of laquinimod in primary progressive multiple sclerosis," *Neurology*, vol. 95, no. 8, pp. e1027–e1040, 2020.

[168] R. Pili, M. Häggman, W. M. Stadler et al., "Phase II randomized, double-blind, placebo-controlled study of tasquinimod in men with minimally symptomatic metastatic castrate-

resistant prostate cancer," *Journal of Clinical Oncology*, vol. 29, no. 30, pp. 4022–4028, 2011.

[169] K. Jennbacken, K. Welén, A. Olsson et al., "Inhibition of metastasis in a castration resistant prostate cancer model by the quinoline-3-carboxamide tasquinimod (ABR-215050)," *Prostate*, vol. 72, no. 8, pp. 913–924, 2012.

[170] C. Sternberg, A. Armstrong, R. Pili et al., "Randomized, double-blind, placebo-controlled phase III study of tasquinimod in men with metastatic castration-resistant prostate cancer," *Journal of Clinical Oncology*, vol. 34, no. 22, pp. 2636–2643, 2016.

[171] B. Escudier, S. Faivre, E. van Cutsem et al., "A phase II multicentre, open-label, proof-of-concept study of tasquinimod in hepatocellular, ovarian, renal cell, and gastric cancers," *Targeted Oncology*, vol. 12, no. 5, pp. 655–661, 2017.

[172] G. Comi, D. Jeffery, L. Kappos et al., "Placebo-controlled trial of oral laquinimod for multiple sclerosis," *The New England Journal of Medicine*, vol. 366, no. 11, pp. 1000–1009, 2012.

[173] On behalf of the BRAVO Study Group, T. L. Vollmer, P. S. Sorensen et al., "A randomized placebo-controlled phase III trial of oral laquinimod for multiple sclerosis," *Journal of Neurology*, vol. 261, no. 4, pp. 773–783, 2014.

[174] M. Stenström, H. C. Nyhlén, M. Törngren et al., "Paquinimod reduces skin fibrosis in tight skin 1 mice, an experimental model of systemic sclerosis," *Journal of Dermatological Science*, vol. 83, no. 1, pp. 52–59, 2016.

[175] S. Tahvili, M. Törngren, D. Holmberg, T. Leanderson, and F. Ivars, "Paquinimod prevents development of diabetes in the non-obese diabetic (NOD) mouse," *PLoS One*, vol. 13, no. 5, article e0196598, 2018.

[176] A. A. Bengtsson, G. Sturfelt, C. Lood et al., "Pharmacokinetics, tolerability, and preliminary efficacy of paquinimod (ABR-215757), a new quinoline-3-carboxamide derivative: studies in lupus-prone mice and a multicenter, randomized, double-blind, placebo-controlled, repeat-dose, dose-ranging study in patients with systemic lupus erythematosus," *Arthritis and Rheumatism*, vol. 64, no. 5, pp. 1579–1588, 2012.

[177] "Exploratory study of changes in disease activity and biomarkers with ABR-215757 in patients with mild active systemic lupus erythematosus (SLE)," ClinicalTrials.Gov identifier: NCT00997100.

[178] T. Arumugam, V. Ramachandran, D. Sun et al., "Designing and developing S100P inhibitor 5-methyl cromolyn for pancreatic cancer therapy," *Molecular Cancer Therapeutics*, vol. 12, no. 5, pp. 654–662, 2013.

[179] P. Björk, E. Källberg, U. Wellmar et al., "Common interactions between S100A4 and S100A9 defined by a novel chemical probe," *PLoS One*, vol. 8, no. 5, article e63012, 2013.

[180] N. G. Dulyaninova, K. M. Hite, W. D. Zencheck et al., "Cysteine 81 is critical for the interaction of S100A4 and myosin-IIA," *Biochemistry*, vol. 50, no. 33, pp. 7218–7227, 2011.

[181] T. R. Reddy, C. Li, P. M. Fischer, and L. V. Dekker, "Three-dimensional pharmacophore design and biochemical screening identifies substituted 1,2,4-triazoles as inhibitors of the annexin A2-S100A10 protein interaction," *ChemMedChem*, vol. 7, no. 8, pp. 1435–1446, 2012.

[182] C. Yoshimura, T. Miyafusa, and K. Tsumoto, "Identification of small-molecule inhibitors of the human S100B-p53 interaction and evaluation of their activity in human melanoma cells," *Bioorganic & Medicinal Chemistry*, vol. 21, no. 5, pp. 1109–1115, 2013.

[183] D. B. Zimmer, R. G. Lapidus, and D. J. Weber, "In vivo screening of S100B inhibitors for melanoma therapy," *Methods in Molecular Biology*, vol. 963, pp. 303–317, 2013.

[184] M. Okada, H. Tokumitsu, Y. Kubota, and R. Kobayashi, "Interaction of S100 proteins with the antiallergic drugs, olopatadine, amlexanox, and cromolyn: identification of putative drug binding sites on S100A1 protein," *Biochemical and Biophysical Research Communications*, vol. 292, no. 4, pp. 1023–1030, 2002.

[185] U. Sack, W. Walther, D. Scudiero et al., "S100A4-induced cell motility and metastasis is restricted by the Wnt/β-catenin pathway inhibitor calcimycin in colon cancer cells," *Molecular Biology of the Cell*, vol. 22, no. 18, pp. 3344–3354, 2011.

[186] U. Stein, F. Arlt, J. Smith et al., "Intervening in β-catenin signaling by sulindac inhibits S100A4-dependent colon cancer metastasis," *Neoplasia*, vol. 13, no. 2, pp. 131–IN8, 2011.

[187] L. Liu, "Inhibition of lung surfactant secretion by KN-62, a specific inhibitor of the calcium- and calmodulin-dependent protein kinase II," *Biochemistry and Molecular Biology International*, vol. 45, no. 4, pp. 823–830, 1998.

[188] E. Vara, J. Arias-Díaz, C. Garcia, J. L. Balibrea, and E. Blázquez, "Glucagon-like peptide-1(7-36) amide stimulates surfactant secretion in human type II pneumocytes," *American Journal of Respiratory and Critical Care Medicine*, vol. 163, no. 4, pp. 840–846, 2001.

[189] M. Xiang, Z. Chen, D. Yang et al., "Niclosamide enhances the antitumor effects of radiation by inhibiting the hypoxia-inducible factor-1α/vascular endothelial growth factor signaling pathway in human lung cancer cells," *Oncology Letters*, vol. 14, no. 2, pp. 1933–1938, 2017.

[190] R. Boyapally, G. Pulivendala, S. Bale, and C. Godugu, "Niclosamide alleviates pulmonary fibrosis in vitro and in vivo by attenuation of epithelial-to-mesenchymal transition, matrix proteins & Wnt/β-catenin signaling: a drug repurposing study," *Life Sciences*, vol. 220, pp. 8–20, 2019.

[191] R. Verma, M. Brahmankar, L. Kushwah, and B. Suresh, "Evaluating the inhibitory potential of sulindac against the bleomycin-induced pulmonary fibrosis in Wistar rats," *Environmental Toxicology and Pharmacology*, vol. 36, no. 3, pp. 769–778, 2013.

[192] C. Cirillo, E. Capoccia, T. Iuvone et al., "S100B inhibitor pentamidine attenuates reactive gliosis and reduces neuronal loss in a mouse model of Alzheimer's disease," *BioMed Research International*, vol. 2015, Article ID 508342, 11 pages, 2015.

[193] L. Seguella, F. Rinaldi, C. Marianecci et al., "Pentamidine niosomes thwart S100B effects in human colon carcinoma biopsies favouring wtp53 rescue," *Journal of Cellular and Molecular Medicine*, vol. 24, no. 5, pp. 3053–3063, 2020.

[194] T. Mori, T. Town, J. Tan, N. Tateishi, and T. Asano, "Modulation of astrocytic activation by arundic acid (ONO-2506) mitigates detrimental effects of the apolipoprotein E4 isoform after permanent focal ischemia in apolipoprotein E knock-in mice," *Journal of Cerebral Blood Flow and Metabolism*, vol. 25, no. 6, pp. 748–762, 2005.

[195] J. Klingelhöfer, B. Grum-Schwensen, M. K. Beck et al., "Anti-S100A4 antibody suppresses metastasis formation by blocking stroma cell invasion," *Neoplasia*, vol. 14, no. 12, pp. 1260–IN47, 2012.

[196] S. Dakhel, L. Padilla, J. Adan et al., "S100P antibody-mediated therapy as a new promising strategy for the treatment of pancreatic cancer," *Oncogene*, vol. 3, no. 3, article e92, 2014.

[197] H. Qin, B. Lerman, I. Sakamaki et al., "Generation of a new therapeutic peptide that depletes myeloid-derived suppressor cells in tumor-bearing mice," *Nature Medicine*, vol. 20, no. 6, pp. 676–681, 2014.

[198] S. Bruhn, Y. Fang, F. Barrenas et al., "A generally applicable translational strategy identifies S100A4 as a candidate gene in allergy," *Science Translational Medicine*, vol. 6, no. 218, p. 218ra4, 2014.

[199] A. Dhar, S. Mallick, P. Ghosh et al., "Simultaneous inhibition of key growth pathways in melanoma cells and tumor regression by a designed bidentate constrained helical peptide," *Biopolymers*, vol. 102, no. 4, pp. 344–358, 2014.

[200] T. Kawano, M. Shimamura, H. Nakagami et al., "Therapeutic vaccine against S100A9 (S100 calcium-binding protein A9) inhibits thrombosis without increasing the risk of bleeding in ischemic stroke in mice," *Hypertension*, vol. 72, no. 6, pp. 1355–1364, 2018.

[201] P. Most, S. T. Pleger, M. Völkers et al., "Cardiac adenoviral S100A1 gene delivery rescues failing myocardium," *The Journal of Clinical Investigation*, vol. 114, no. 11, pp. 1550–1563, 2004.

[202] S. T. Pleger, C. Shan, J. Ksienzyk et al., "Cardiac AAV9-S100A1 gene therapy rescues post-ischemic heart failure in a preclinical large animal model," *Science Translational Medicine*, vol. 3, no. 92, p. 92ra64, 2011.

[203] T. Ravasi, K. Hsu, J. Goyette et al., "Probing the S100 protein family through genomic and functional analysis," *Genomics*, vol. 84, no. 1, pp. 10–22, 2004.

[204] J. Edgeworth, M. Gorman, R. Bennett, P. Freemont, and N. Hogg, "Identification of p8,14 as a highly abundant heterodimeric calcium binding protein complex of myeloid cells," *The Journal of Biological Chemistry*, vol. 266, no. 12, pp. 7706–7713, 1991.

[205] M. R. Tardif, J. A. Chapeton-Montes, A. Posvandzic, N. Pagé, C. Gilbert, and P. A. Tessier, "Secretion of S100A8, S100A9, and S100A12 by neutrophils involves reactive oxygen species and potassium efflux," *Journal of Immunology Research*, vol. 2015, Article ID 296149, 16 pages, 2015.

[206] V. Schenten, S. Bréchard, S. Plançon, C. Melchior, J. P. Frippiat, and E. J. Tschirhart, "$IPLA_2$, a novel determinant in Ca^{2+}- and phosphorylation-dependent S100A8/A9 regulated NOX2 activity," *Biochimica et Biophysica Acta*, vol. 1803, no. 7, pp. 840–847, 2010.

[207] V. Schenten, C. Melchior, N. Steinckwich, E. J. Tschirhart, and S. Brechard, "Sphingosine kinases regulate NOX2 activity via p38 MAPK-dependent translocation of S100A8/A9," *Journal of Leukocyte Biology*, vol. 89, no. 4, pp. 587–596, 2011.

[208] R. A. Newton and N. Hogg, "The human S100 protein MRP-14 is a novel activator of the beta 2 integrin Mac-1 on neutrophils," *Journal of Immunology*, vol. 160, no. 3, pp. 1427–1435, 1998.

[209] S. C. Fagerholm, C. Guenther, M. Llort Asens, T. Savinko, and L. M. Uotila, "Beta2-Integrins and interacting proteins in leukocyte trafficking, immune suppression, and immunodeficiency disease," *Frontiers in Immunology*, vol. 10, p. 254, 2019.

[210] A. Silvin, N. Chapuis, G. Dunsmore et al., "Elevated calprotectin and abnormal myeloid cell subsets discriminate severe from mild COVID-19," *Cell*, vol. 182, no. 6, pp. 1401–1418.e18, 2020.

[211] M. S. Abers, O. M. Delmonte, E. E. Ricotta et al., "An immune-based biomarker signature is associated with mortality in COVID-19 patients," *JCI Insight*, vol. 6, no. 1, 2021.

[212] L. G. de Guadiana Romualdo, M. D. R. Mulero, M. H. Olivo et al., "Circulating levels of GDF-15 and calprotectin for prediction of in-hospital mortality in COVID-19 patients: a case series," *The Journal of Infection*, vol. 82, no. 2, pp. e40–e42, 2021.

[213] E. Petito, E. Falcinelli, U. Paliani et al., "Association of neutrophil activation, more than platelet activation, with thrombotic complications in coronavirus disease 2019," *The Journal of Infectious Diseases*, vol. 223, no. 6, pp. 933–944, 2021.

[214] H. Shi, Y. Zuo, S. Yalavarthi et al., "Neutrophil calprotectin identifies severe pulmonary disease in COVID-19," *Journal of Leukocyte Biology*, vol. 109, no. 1, pp. 67–72, 2021.

[215] M. Effenberger, F. Grabherr, L. Mayr et al., "Faecal calprotectin indicates intestinal inflammation in COVID-19," *Gut*, vol. 69, no. 8, pp. 1543-1544, 2020.

[216] V. Ojetti, A. Saviano, M. Covino et al., "COVID-19 and intestinal inflammation: role of fecal calprotectin," *Digestive and Liver Disease*, vol. 52, no. 11, pp. 1231–1233, 2020.

[217] A. Aceti, L. M. Margarucci, E. Scaramucci et al., "Serum S100B protein as a marker of severity in COVID-19 patients," *Scientific Reports*, vol. 10, no. 1, p. 18665, 2020.

[218] Q. Guo, Y. Zhao, J. Li et al., "Induction of alarmin S100A8/A9 mediates activation of aberrant neutrophils in the pathogenesis of COVID-19," *Cell Host & Microbe*, vol. 29, no. 2, pp. 222–235.e4, 2021.

[219] Y. Liu, J. Cui, Y. L. Tang, L. Huang, C. Y. Zhou, and J. X. Xu, "Prognostic roles of mRNA expression of S100 in non-small-cell lung cancer," *BioMed Research International*, vol. 2018, Article ID 9815806, 11 pages, 2018.

[220] Z. Qi, T. Li, F. Kong et al., "The characteristics and function of S100A7 induction in squamous cell carcinoma: heterogeneity, promotion of cell proliferation and suppression of differentiation," *PLoS One*, vol. 10, no. 6, article e0128887, 2015.

[221] M. W. Nasser, N. A. Wani, D. K. Ahirwar et al., "RAGE mediates S100A7-induced breast cancer growth and metastasis by modulating the tumor microenvironment," *Cancer Research*, vol. 75, no. 6, pp. 974–985, 2015.

[222] L. Núñez-Naveira, L. A. Mariñas-Pardo, and C. Montero-Martínez, "Mass spectrometry analysis of the exhaled breath condensate and proposal of dermcidin and S100A9 as possible markers for lung cancer prognosis," *Lung*, vol. 197, no. 4, pp. 523–531, 2019.

[223] K. Okudela, A. Katayama, T. Woo et al., "Proteome analysis for downstream targets of oncogenic KRAS–the potential participation of CLIC4 in carcinogenesis in the lung," *PLoS One*, vol. 9, no. 2, article e87193, 2014.

[224] H. Bouzina, R. Hesselstrand, and G. Rådegran, "Plasma insulin-like growth factor binding protein 1 in pulmonary arterial hypertension," *Scandinavian Cardiovascular Journal*, vol. 55, no. 1, pp. 35–42, 2021.

[225] M. A. Kovach, K. A. Stringer, R. Bunting et al., "Microarray analysis identifies IL-1 receptor type 2 as a novel candidate biomarker in patients with acute respiratory distress syndrome," *Respiratory Research*, vol. 16, no. 1, p. 29, 2015.

[226] D. Massi, M. Landriscina, A. Piscazzi et al., "S100A13 is a new angiogenic marker in human melanoma," *Modern Pathology*, vol. 23, no. 6, pp. 804–813, 2010.

[227] T. Sugino, N. Ichikawa-Tomikawa, M. Tanaka et al., "Identification of S100A14 as a metastasis-promoting molecule in a murine organotropic metastasis model," *Clinical & Experimental Metastasis*, vol. 36, no. 4, pp. 411–422, 2019.

[228] F. Ding, D. Wang, X. K. Li et al., "Overexpression of S100A14 contributes to malignant progression and predicts poor prognosis of lung adenocarcinoma," *Thorac Cancer*, vol. 9, no. 7, pp. 827–835, 2018.

[229] M. Ichinose, H. Sugiura, H. Nagase et al., "Japanese guidelines for adult asthma 2017," *Allergology International*, vol. 66, no. 2, pp. 163–189, 2017.

[230] V. N. Malashkevich, N. G. Dulyaninova, U. A. Ramagopal et al., "Phenothiazines inhibit S100A4 function by inducing protein oligomerization," *Proceedings of the National Academy of Sciences of the United States of America*, vol. 107, no. 19, pp. 8605–8610, 2010.

[231] L. C. Pettigrew, S. E. Kasner, G. W. Albers et al., "Safety and tolerability of arundic acid in acute ischemic stroke," *Journal of the Neurological Sciences*, vol. 251, no. 1-2, pp. 50–56, 2006.

[232] U. Sack, W. Walther, D. Scudiero et al., "Novel effect of antihelminthic Niclosamide on S100A4-mediated metastatic progression in colon cancer," *Journal of the National Cancer Institute*, vol. 103, no. 13, pp. 1018–1036, 2011.

16

Comparison of Diaphragmatic Stretch Technique and Manual Diaphragm Release Technique on Diaphragmatic Excursion in Chronic Obstructive Pulmonary Disease

Aishwarya Nair,[1] Gopala Krishna Alaparthi,[1] Shyam Krishnan,[1] Santhosh Rai,[2] R. Anand,[3] Vishak Acharya,[3] and Preetam Acharya[3]

[1]*Department of Physiotherapy, Kasturba Medical College, Manipal Academy of Higher Education, Bejai, Mangalore-575004, India*
[2]*Department of Radiodiagnosis, Kasturba Medical College Mangalore, Manipal Academy of Higher Education, Mangalore-575004, India*
[3]*Department of Pulmonary Medicine, Kasturba Medical College, Manipal Academy of Higher Education, Mangalore-575004, India*

Correspondence should be addressed to Gopala Krishna Alaparthi; gopalalaparthi@gmail.com

Academic Editor: Roberto Walter Dal Negro

Background. Chronic Obstructive Pulmonary Disease (COPD) impairs the function of the diaphragm by placing it at a mechanical disadvantage, shortening its operating length and changing the mechanical linkage between its various parts. This makes the diaphragm's contraction less effective in raising and expanding the lower rib cage, thereby increasing the work of breathing and reducing the functional capacity. *Aim of the Study.* To compare the effects of diaphragmatic stretch and manual diaphragm release technique on diaphragmatic excursion in patients with COPD. *Materials and Methods.* This randomised crossover trial included 20 clinically stable patients with mild and moderate COPD classified according to the GOLD criteria. The patients were allocated to group A or group B by block randomization done by primary investigator. The information about the technique was concealed in a sealed opaque envelope and revealed to the patients only after allocation of groups. After taking the demographic data and baseline values of the outcome measures (diaphragm mobility by ultrasonography performed by an experienced radiologist and chest expansion by inch tape performed by the therapist), group A subjects underwent the diaphragmatic stretch technique and the group B subjects underwent the manual diaphragm release technique. Both the interventions were performed in 2 sets of 10 deep breaths with 1-minute interval between the sets. The two outcome variables were recorded immediately after the intervention. A wash-out period of 3 hours was maintained to neutralize the effect of given intervention. Later the patients of group A and group B were crossed over to the other group. *Results.* In the diaphragmatic stretch technique, there was a statistically significant improvement in the diaphragmatic excursion before and after the treatment. On the right side, p=0.00 and p=0.003 in the midclavicular line and midaxillary line. On the left side, p=0.004 and p=0.312 in the midclavicular and midaxillary line. In manual diaphragm release technique, there was a statistically significant improvement before and after the treatment. On the right side, p=0.000 and p=0.000 in the midclavicular line and midaxillary line. On the left side, p=0.002 and p=0.000 in the midclavicular line and midaxillary line. There was no statistically significant difference in diaphragmatic excursion in the comparison of the postintervention values of both techniques. *Conclusion.* The diaphragmatic stretch technique and manual diaphragm release technique can be safely recommended for patients with clinically stable COPD to improve diaphragmatic excursion.

1. Introduction

Chronic Obstructive Pulmonary Disease (COPD) is a common preventable and treatable disease that is usually progressive, characterized by persistent airflow limitation and associated with an enhanced chronic inflammatory response in the airways and the lung to noxious particles or gases [1]. In India, chronic respiratory diseases account for 3% of Disability Adjusted Life Years (DALYs); together COPD, asthma, and other respiratory diseases are the second leading cause of death in the Indian population and fourth in the world according to WHO [2, 3].

The diaphragm, which is the main inspiratory muscle, generates a craniocaudal movement of its dome during contraction [4]. The two striking features in COPD, air trapping and lung hyperinflation, impair the function of the diaphragm, shortening its operating length and changing the mechanical linkage between its various parts thereby placing it at mechanical disadvantage [5]. These pathological changes affect the diaphragm's ability of raising and expanding the lower rib cage which may lead to a decrease in the transverse diameter of the lower ribcage during inspiration. These changes cause an increase in the work of breathing and reduce the functional capacity [6, 7]. Skeletal muscle dysfunction, which is an observed extrapulmonary effect in COPD, affects the severity of the disease, providing a potential target for therapeutic intervention [1]. This dysfunction occurs at a level which affects exercise capacity and dyspnoea levels [8].

Although the main treatment approaches for COPD are pharmacological therapy and pulmonary rehabilitation, there are a number of published studies in the osteopathic and chiropractic literature describing the use of manual therapy techniques [9–12].

Some evidence suggests that manual therapy has the potential to affect and change respiratory mechanics in certain chronic pulmonary diseases, such as chronic asthma and COPD, which includes an increase in flexibility of the chest wall and thoracic excursion. This can indirectly lead to an improvement in exercise capacity and lung function [13, 14]. There is also evidence that respiratory muscle stretching may bring about an improvement in ventilation in patients with COPD by increasing the capacity for chest wall (CW) expansion [15, 16].

According to some studies, stretching of the respiratory muscles improves vital capacity, improves chest wall mobility, and reduces dyspnoea thereby counteracting the effects of COPD [17]. Studies also suggest that a vast variety of manual techniques targets the various components of pulmonary system like musculoskeletal, lymphatic, etc. Studies support that manual therapy of the diaphragm improves its excursion thereby improving respiratory mechanics, facilitating bronchial tree lymphatic flow and reducing airways congestion [18–21].

The diaphragmatic stretch technique or doming of diaphragm technique is designed to relax the resting state of the diaphragm, enhancing its contraction and relaxation functions, thereby creating a greater pressure gradient between the thorax and abdomen [22].

González-Álvarez FJ et al. applied the diaphragm stretch technique to check ribcage and abdominal excursion in healthy subjects and found a significant increase in the same level at xiphoid level [23]. Yelvar YDG studied the immediate effects of manual therapy on inspiratory muscle strength and respiratory functions in patients who were a known case of COPD with no current or ongoing exacerbation, by applying the Redoming of diaphragm technique which showed an improvement in pulmonary function and inspiratory muscle strength [24].

The Manual Diaphragm Release Technique (MDRT) is an intervention intended to directly stretch the diaphragmatic muscle fibres thereby increasing the chest wall mobility [25, 26]. Evidence supports the beneficial effect on diaphragmatic mobility and it can be hypothesised that there is traction of the lower rib cage in a cranial direction and manual compression of the tissues in the area of insertion of the anterior costal diaphragm fibres brought about by the manual action on the underside of the last four costal cartilages which allows lengthening the diaphragm in its insertional zone [27].

In a study conducted by Rocha et al., manual diaphragm release technique improved diaphragmatic mobility, 6-minute walking distance, and inspiratory capacity in patients with clinically stable COPD with no history of exacerbations in the past 6 weeks [27].

Abdelaal Ashraf AM et al. studied the effect of diaphragm as well as costal manipulation on functional capacity and pulmonary function in patients with moderate COPD, not involved in previous rehabilitation program at least 4 months prior to the study and had no recent infectious exacerbations for the 2 months preceding the study wherein both techniques (Doming of Diaphragm and Diaphragm Release) were given and it was found that both techniques were effective tools in improving pulmonary function and functional capacity [28].

There was a lack of retrievable data available regarding comparison of Diaphragmatic stretching technique and Manual Diaphragm Release technique on diaphragmatic excursion in patients with COPD. The aim of the study is to compare the effects of Diaphragmatic stretch and Manual Diaphragm Release technique on diaphragmatic excursion in patients with COPD.

2. Methodology

2.1. Inclusion Criteria

(i) Patients with stable COPD of both genders who are referred for Physiotherapy by a pulmonologist/physician in KMC Hospitals.

(ii) Patients with mild or moderate COPD according to the GOLD criteria, 2016.GOLD 1: Mild FEV1 $\geq$ 80% predicted, GOLD 2: Moderate 50% $\leq$ FEV1 < 80% predicted.

2.2. Exclusion Criteria

(i) Patients with acute exacerbation of COPD.

(ii) Patients with unstable hemodynamic parameters (arterial pressure <100mmHg systolic and <60mmHg for diastolic and mean arterial pressure (MAP) <80mmHg).

(iii) Patients who have undergone recent cardiothoracic or abdominal surgery.

(iv) Patients who have a recent history of chest wall or abdominal trauma; substantial chest wall deformity

(v) History of psychiatric illness.

3. Study Procedure

The study was approved by the Institutional Ethics Committee of Kasturba Medical College Mangalore. Eligible patients

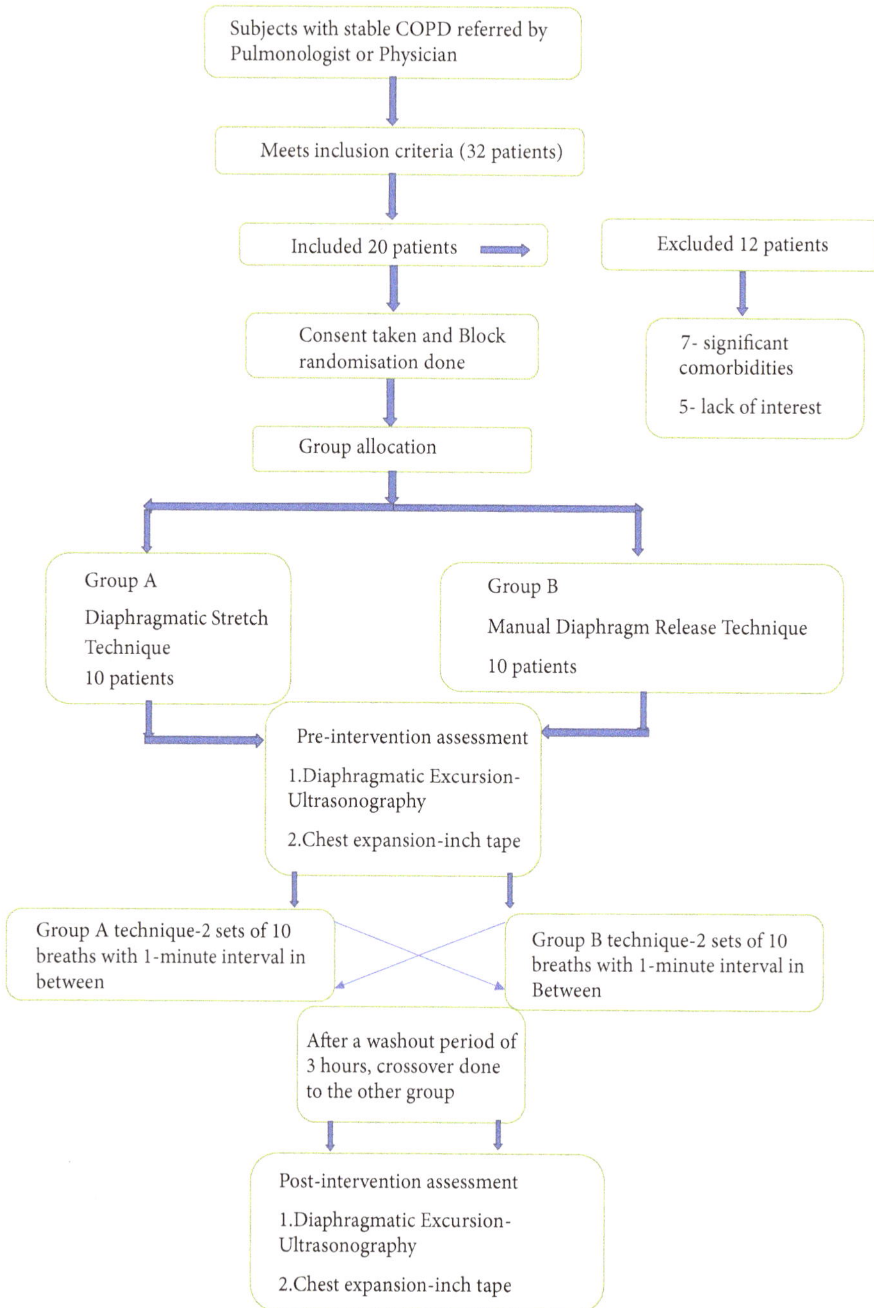

FIGURE 1: Flow diagram of the study.

were selected based on the inclusion and exclusion criteria. The purpose of study was made clear to each patient and a written informed consent was obtained prior to involving them in the study.

The patients were allocated to Group A or Group B by block randomization done by primary investigator. A total of 20 samples were divided into 2 blocks with 10 patients in each. The information about the technique was concealed in a sealed opaque envelope and revealed to the patients only after allocation of groups. After taking the demographic data and baseline values of the outcome measures (diaphragm mobility by ultrasonography performed by an experienced radiologist and chest expansion by inch tape performed by the therapist), Group A subjects underwent the Diaphragmatic Stretch Technique and the Group B subjects underwent the Manual Diaphragm Release Technique. Both the interventions were performed in 2 sets of 10 deep breaths with 1-minute interval between the sets. The two outcome variables were recorded immediately after the intervention. A wash-out period of 3 hours was maintained to neutralize the effect of given intervention. Later the patients of Group A and Group B were crossed over to the other group (Figure 1).

4. Methods to Perform the Techniques

4.1. Diaphragmatic Stretch Technique. The subjects were asked to sit erect for the intervention. The therapist standing behind the subject pass their hands around the thoracic cage, introducing fingers in the subcostal margins. The subject's trunk was rounded slightly to relax the rectus abdominis. As the subject exhaled, the therapist easing their hands caudally grasped the lower ribs at the subcostal margin. This firm, but gentle, traction was maintained as the patient inhales [22].

4.2. Manual Diaphragm Release Technique. The participant was asked to lie supine with relaxed limbs. Positioned at the head of the patient, the therapist made manual contact with the hypothenar region and last three fingers bilaterally to the underside of the seventh to tenth rib costal cartilages. The therapist's forearms were aligned towards the participant's shoulders. In the inspiratory phase, the therapist was gently pulling the points of contact with both hands in the direction of the head and slightly laterally, accompanied the elevation of the ribs.

During exhalation, the therapist's contact was deepened towards the inner costal margin, maintaining resistance. In the subsequent respiratory cycles, the therapist deepened the contact inside the costal margin [27].

5. Description of Outcome Measures

5.1. Diaphragm Excursion. The patient was asked to sit and diaphragm movements were recorded in the B-Mode. The probe was positioned both in the midclavicular and in the midaxillary lines consecutively, in the subcostal area, so that the ultrasound beam will enter to visualize the bilateral diaphragm perpendicularly.

The procedure began at the end of normal expiration with the subjects instructed to inhale as deeply as possible. A fixed point at the edge of the image on the screen and the diaphragm margin at maximal inspiration and again at maximal expiration served as reference points between which measurements were made, where the averages of three values were taken for both maximal inspiration and maximal expiration [29].

5.2. Chest Expansion. The chest expansion was assessed with the patients standing with their hands placed on their head. They were given instructions to "breathe in maximally" and "breathe out maximally." Chest expansion was measured at two levels. Upper chest expansion at the level of the 4th intercostal space and lower chest expansion at the level of the xiphoid process [30].

6. Sample Size Estimation

A pilot study was conducted which involved 5 patients with clinically stable COPD who were crossed over to both groups. Based on the findings of the pilot study, the mean deviation across the crossed over group with respect to midclavicular findings, 90% power, 95% ci, population SD of 0.02, mean value of difference of diaphragmatic stretch technique (0.14), and manual diaphragm release technique (0.08) at midclavicular line and adding 20% nonresponsive error, the total sample was calculated to be 20 subjects using the following formula:

$$\frac{(Z\alpha + Z\beta)^2 \sigma_P{}^2}{2(\mu - \mu_0 - \sigma)^2} \quad (1)$$

where

$Z\alpha$ - 1.96 for 95% CI.

$Z\beta$ - 1.34 for 90% power.

6.1. Data Analysis. The data were fed into the computer having Statistical Package for Social Science (SPSS) version 11.5. The variables are summarised as mean and standard deviation. The pre and post values for the two techniques were measured using ANOVA. The comparison between the post-intervention values of the two techniques was done using ANOVA and Bonferroni test. A p-value less than 0.05 was considered as statistically significant.

TABLE 1: Demographic data of participants.

Variable		Frequency
Age (66.85 ± 8.37)		20
Gender	male	12
	Female	8
Smoking history	yes	9
	No	11
COPD category	mild	11
	Moderate	9

7. Results

We selected 32 patients who were diagnosed with clinically stable COPD within the mild or moderate category of GOLD classification. Out of this, 7 patients had to be excluded due to the presence of significant comorbidities (Coronary Artery Disease, Pleural Effusion, Bronchiectasis); 5 patients dropped out of the study due to lack of interest. A total of 20 patients as per the sample size were included on whom both the techniques were performed. Baseline characteristics of the patients such as Age, Gender, COPD category, history of smoking is presented in Table 1. Diaphragmatic Excursion following Diaphragmatic stretch technique, on the Right side there was a difference of 0.29 ±0.21 (p=0.001) in the mid-clavicular line and 0.25 ±0.20 (p=0.003) in the midaxillary line. On the Left side, there was a difference of 0.24 ±0.24 (p=0.004) in the midclavicular line and 0.35 ±0.25 (p=0.312) in the midaxillary line showed in Table 2.

Diaphragmatic excursion following Manual Diaphragm Release Technique is summarised in Table 3. In Manual Diaphragm Release Technique, on the Right side there was a difference of 0.24 ±0.20(p=0.001) in the midclavicular line and 0.22 ±0.20 (p=0.001) in the midaxillary line. On the Left side, there was a difference of 0.26 ±0.28 (p=0.002) in the midclavicular line and 0.29 ±0.18(p=0.001) in the midaxillary

TABLE 2: Comparison of Diaphragmatic Excursion before and after Diaphragmatic Stretch Technique.

	Right Side (in cms)				Left Side (in cms)			
Midclavicular Line	**Pre**	**Post**	**Difference**	**P <0.05**	**Pre**	**Post**	**Difference**	**P<0.05**
	2.56 ± 0.56	2.86 ± 0.59	0.29 ± 0.21	0.001**	2.57 ± 0.54	2.79 ± 0.52	0.24 ± 0.24	0.004**
Midaxillary Line	**Pre**	**Post**	**Difference**	**P <0.05**	**Pre**	**Post**	**Difference**	**P<0.05**
	2.74 ± 0.63	2.95 ± 0.70	0.25 ± 0.20	0.003**	2.69 ± 0.63	2.85 ± 0.6	0.35 ± 0.25	0.312

Note: ** is highly significant.

TABLE 3: Comparison of Diaphragmatic Excursion before and after the Manual Diaphragm Release Technique.

	Right (in cms)				Left (in cms)			
Midclavicular Line	**Pre**	**Post**	**Difference**	**p<0.05**	**Pre**	**Post**	**Difference**	**p<0.05**
	2.56 ± 0.56	2.78 ± 0.52	0.24 ± 0.20	0.001**	2.57 ± 0.54	2.84 ± 0.59	0.26 ± 0.28	0.002**
Midaxillary Line	**Pre**	**Post**	**Difference**	**p<0.05**	**Pre**	**Post**	**Difference**	**p<0.05**
	2.74 ± 0.63	2.98 ± 0.62	0.22 ± 0.20	0.001**	2.69 ± 0.63	2.95 ± 0.55	0.29 ± 0.18	0.001**

Note: ** is highly significant.

TABLE 4: Comparison of Chest Expansion before and after Diaphragmatic Stretch Technique and Manual Diaphragm Release Technique.

	4th intercostal space (in inches)				Xiphoid process (in inches)			
Diaphragmatic Stretch	**Pre**	**Post**	**Difference**	**p<0.05**	**Pre**	**Post**	**Difference**	**p<0.05**
	34.98 ± 2.95	35.69 ± 2.85	0.76 ± 0.71	0.001	36.10 ± 3.22	36.73 ± 3.26	0.62 ± 0.64	0.001
Manual Diaphragm Release Technique	**Pre**	**Post**	**Difference**	**p<0.05**	**Pre**	**Post**	**Difference**	**p<0.05**
	34.98 ± 2.95	35.80 ± 3.01	0.82 ± 0.06	0.002	36.10 ± 3.22	36.82 ± 3.34	0.72 ± 0.88	0.002

TABLE 5: Comparison of post intervention values of Diaphragmatic Excursion and Chest Expansion between groups.

Diaphragmatic Excursion (in cms)					
Technique		Midclavicular line		Midaxillary line	
		Right side	Left side	Right side	Left side
Diaphragmatic stretch technique		2.86 ± 0.59	2.79 ± 0.52	2.95 ± 0.70	2.85 ± 0.6
Manual diaphragm release technique		2.78 ± 0.52	2.84 ± 0.59	2.95 ± 0.70	2.95 ± 0.55
Difference	Mean ± SD	0.07 ± 0.21	-0.04 ± 0.23	-0.02 ± 0.26	-0.10 ± 0.32
	sig. (p< 0.05)	0.393	1.00	1.00	0.483
Chest expansion (in inches)					
Technique		4th intercostal space		Xiphoid process	
Diaphragmatic stretch technique		35.69 ± 2.85		36.73 ± 3.26	
Manual diaphragm release technique		35.80 ±3.01		36.82 ± 3.34	
Difference	Mean ± SD	-0.11 ± 0.16		-0.09 ± 0.08	
	sig. (p< 0.05)	0.713		0.737	

line. Chest expansion values before and after both techniques are summarised in Table 4. After Diaphragmatic Stretch Technique there was a difference of 0.76 ±0.71 (p=0.001) at the level of 4th intercostal space and 0.62 ±0.64 (p=0.001) at the level of xiphoid process. After Manual Diaphragm Release Technique there was a difference of 0.82 ± 0.06 (p=0.002) at the level of 4th intercostal space and 0.72 ±0.88 (p=0.002) at the level of xiphoid process.

Comparison of post values of both techniques in Diaphragmatic Excursion and Chest Expansion is summarised in Table 5. In Diaphragmatic Excursion, difference in postintervention values at the Midclavicular line on the right side was found to be 0.07 ± 0.21 (p= 0.393) and on the left side was found to be -0.04 ± 0.23 (p= 1.00); Difference in post-intervention values at the Midaxillary line on the right side was found to be -0.02 ± 0.26 (p= 1.00) and on the left side was found to be -0.10 ± 0.32 (p= 0.483). In Chest Expansion, difference in the postintervention values at the level of 4th intercostal space was found to be -0.11 ± 0.16 and at the level of xiphoid process was found to be -0.09 ± 0.08

8. Discussion

The main purpose of the study was to compare the effects of Diaphragmatic Stretch Technique and Manual Diaphragm Release Technique on Diaphragmatic excursion in COPD.

In our study we found that there was a statistically significant difference in the diaphragmatic excursion and chest expansion following both interventions within the groups but there was no significant difference between groups of the two techniques on the two outcome measures.

The Diaphragmatic Stretch Technique was found to have statistically significant within group difference. This can be hypothesised to be due to the acute activation of the muscle spindle caused by muscle stretching, that increases the sensory afferent stimulus, increasing neuromotor response, eventually increasing muscle tension, improving muscle viscoelasticity and consequently decreasing muscle stiffness and increasing thoracic mobility [31–34]. Muscle stretching may stimulate the receptors in the muscle–tendon region i.e. the Golgi tendon organs, thereby causing an inhibitory effect [35, 36].

Noll DR et al reported that one session of manual therapy which included the Redoming of Diaphragm technique, improved the pulmonary function in patients with COPD [11]. Yelvar GDY found that a single session of Manual Therapy which included the Diaphragmatic Release improved the inspiratory muscle strength and pulmonary function in patients with severe COPD [24]. Gonzalez-Alvarez FJ applied the diaphragm stretch technique on healthy subjects and found that there was a significant improvement in ribcage excursion at xiphoid level along with improvement in the posterior chain kinematics [23].

The Manual Diaphragm Release Technique was found to have statistically significant within group difference after may be hypothesised that the technique provided an improvement in the flexibility of the respiratory muscles and the thoracic cavity, as well as an improvement in the length-tension relationship, which allowed a beneficial effect on the performance of respiratory mechanics. This technique may stimulate proprioception and increase the elasticity of adhered fibres, and it acts by eliminating tension in the soft tissues, through low speed movements, which when applied over the area, act on the sensory system through the Golgi tendon organs [37].

However, there is little research that gives scientific support to the effects of such techniques. In the literature there is a deficiency of studies on the action of stretching of the respiratory muscles, affirming to us that this probably occurs because it is a muscular group of complex functioning and, perhaps for this reason, does not present specific techniques [37].

Rocha et al, performed the Manual Diaphragm Release Technique in stable COPD patients and found an improvement in diaphragm mobility [27]. Abdaleel Ashraf AM et al. found that application Diaphragmatic Release technique and Redoming of the Diaphragm technique significantly increased FVC, FEV1 and 6MWT [28]. Braga DKAP et al found that the "diaphragm lift" and double diaphragm brought about an improvement in the maximum expiratory pressure, all the coefficients of the cirtometry and mobility of the thoracic cavity [37].

In our study, we found the between groups values to be statistically nonsignificant. This may be due to a small sample size, which must have hindered with the comparison of both the techniques. It can also be attributed to the fact that the number of repetitions done for both the techniques was not sufficient enough to compare between them.

The limitations of the study are that larger sections of the COPD population should be included. We have measured the immediate effects of the techniques on the diaphragmatic excursion. The skill and expertise of the therapist in performing the techniques are a subjective limitation of the study. Further studies may be done for a longer duration using both the techniques in patients belonging to different COPD subgroups.

9. Conclusion

The Diaphragmatic Stretch Technique and Manual Diaphragm Release Technique can be safely recommended for patients with clinically stable COPD to improve Diaphragmatic Excursion and Chest Expansion.

Disclosure

Aishwarya Nair is the first author.

References

[1] C. F. Vogelmeier, G. J. Criner, F. J. Martinez et al., "Global Strategy for the Diagnosis, Management and Prevention of Chronic Obstructive Lung Disease 2017 Report: GOLD Executive Summary," *Respirology*, vol. 22, no. 3, pp. 575–601, 2017.

[2] P. Rajkumar, K. Pattabi, S. Vadivoo et al., "A cross-sectional study on prevalence of chronic obstructive pulmonary disease (COPD) in India: Rationale and methods," *BMJ Open*, vol. 7, no. 5, Article ID e015211, 2017.

[3] K. Srinath Reddy, B. Shah, C. Varghese, and A. Ramadoss, "Responding to the threat of chronic diseases in India," *The Lancet*, vol. 366, no. 9498, pp. 1744–1749, 2005.

[4] W. D. Reid and G. Dechman, "Considerations when testing and training the respiratory muscles," *Physical Therapy in Sport*, vol. 75, no. 11, pp. 971–982, 1995.

[5] T. Similowski, S. Yan, A. P. Gauthier, P. T. Macklem, and F. Bellemare, "Contractile properties of the human diaphragm during chronic hyperinflation," *The New England Journal of Medicine*, vol. 325, no. 13, pp. 917–923, 1991.

[6] W. P. Dos Santos Yamaguti, E. Paulin, S. Shibao et al., "Air trapping: The major factor limiting diaphragm mobility in chronic obstructive pulmonary disease patients," *Respirology*, vol. 13, no. 1, pp. 138–144, 2008.

[7] A. Aliverti, M. Quaranta, B. Chakrabarti, A. L. P. Albuquerque, and P. M. Calverley, "Paradoxical movement of the lower ribcage at rest and during exercise in COPD patients," *European Respiratory Journal*, vol. 33, no. 1, pp. 49–60, 2009.

[8] G. Choudhury, R. Rabinovich, and W. MacNee, "Comorbidities and systemic effects of chronic obstructive pulmonary disease," *Clinics in Chest Medicine*, vol. 35, no. 1, pp. 101–130, 2014.

[9] R. K. Howell, T. W. Allen, and R. E. Kappler, "The influence of osteopathic manipulative therapy in the management of patients with chronic obstructive lung disease.," *The Journal of the American Osteopathic Association*, vol. 74, no. 8, pp. 757–760, 1975.

[10] W. D. Miller, *The research status of spinal manipulative therapy*, M. Goldstein, Ed., Dept. HEW, Bethesda, Md, USA, 1975.

[11] D. R. Noll, B. F. Degenhardt, J. C. Johnson, and S. A. Burt, "Immediate effects of osteopathic manipulative treatment in elderly patients with chronic obstructive pulmonary disease," *The Journal of the American Osteopathic Association*, vol. 108, no. 5, article 251e9, 2008.

[12] D. R. Noll, J. C. Johnson, R. W. Baer, and E. J. Snider, "The immediate effect of individual manipulation techniques on pulmonary function measures in persons with chronic obstructive pulmonary disease," *Osteopathic Medicine and Primary Care*, vol. 3, no. 9, pp. 1–12, 2009.

[13] S. E. Bockenhauer, K. N. Julliard, K. S. Lo, E. Huang, and A. M. Sheth, "Quantifiable effects of osteopathic manipulative techniques on patients with chronic asthma," *The Journal of the American Osteopathic Association*, vol. 102, no. 7, pp. 371–375, 2002.

[14] R. Engel and S. Vemulpad, "The role of spinal manipulation, soft-tissue therapy, and exercise in chronic obstructive pulmonary disease: A review of the literature and proposal of an anatomical explanation," *The Journal of Alternative and Complementary Medicine*, vol. 17, no. 9, pp. 797–801, 2011.

[15] E. Paulin, A. F. Brunetto, and C. R. Carvalho, "Effects of a physical exercises program designed to increase thoracic mobility in patients with chronic obstructive pulmonary disease," *Jornal de Pneumologia*, vol. 29, no. 5, pp. 287–294, 2003.

[16] M. T. Putt, M. Watson, H. Seale, and J. D. Paratz, "Muscle Stretching Technique Increases Vital Capacity and Range of Motion in Patients With Chronic Obstructive Pulmonary Disease," *Archives of Physical Medicine and Rehabilitation*, vol. 89, no. 6, pp. 1103–1107, 2008.

[17] F. Kakizaki, M. Shibuya, T. Yamazaki, M. Yamada, H. Suzuki, and I. Homma, "Preliminary Report of the Effects of Respiratory Muscle Stretch Gymnastics on Chest Wall Mobility in Patients With Chronic Obstructive Pulmonary Disease," *Journal of Cardiopulmonary Rehabilitation and Prevention*, vol. 19, no. 6, pp. 390-391, 1999.

[18] M. L. Kuchera, F. Do, and W. A. Kuchera, *Osteopathic considerations in systemic dysfunction*, Greyden Press LLC, 1994.

[19] V. M. Frymann, "The osteopathic approach to cardiac and pulmonary problems.," *The Journal of the American Osteopathic Association*, vol. 77, no. 9, pp. 668–673, 1978.

[20] E. G. Stiles, "Manipulative management of chronic lung disease," *Osteopath Ann*, vol. 9, pp. 300–304, 1981.

[21] A. G. Chila, "Osteopathic principles in family medicine: pediatric respiratory care," *Osteopath Ann*, vol. 11, pp. 352–355, 1983.

[22] L. Chaitow, "Osteopathic assessment and treatment of thoracic and respiratory dysfunction," in *Multidisciplinary approaches to breathing pattern disorders*, L. Chaitow, D. Bradley, and C. Gilbert, Eds., pp. 131–169, Churchill Livingstone, London, UK, 2002.

[23] F. J. González-Álvarez, M. C. Valenza, I. Torres-Sánchez, I. Cabrera-Martos, J. Rodríguez-Torres, and Y. Castellote-Caballero, "Effects of diaphragm stretching on posterior chain muscle kinematics and rib cage and abdominal excursion: A randomized controlled trial," *Brazilian Journal of Physical Therapy*, vol. 20, no. 5, pp. 405–411, 2016.

[24] G. D. Yilmaz Yelvar, Y. Cirak, Y. Parlak Demir, M. Dalkilinc, and B. Bozkurt, "Immediate effect of manual therapy on respiratory functions and inspiratory muscle strength in patients with COPD," *International Journal of Chronic Obstructive Pulmonary Disease*, vol. 11, no. 1, pp. 1353–1357, 2016.

[25] F. Ricard and J.-L. Sallé, *Tratado de Osteopatia*, vol. 135, Panamericana, Madrid, Spain, 3rd edition, 2009.

[26] M. De Coster and A. Pollaris, *Osteopatía Visceal*, vol. 38, Paidotribo, Madrid, Spain, 2nd edition, 2005.

[27] T. Rocha, H. Souza, D. C. Brandão et al., "The Manual Diaphragm Release Technique improves diaphragmatic mobility, inspiratory capacity and exercise capacity in people with chronic obstructive pulmonary disease: A randomised trial," *Journal of Physiotherapy*, vol. 61, no. 4, pp. 182–189, 2015.

[28] A. A. Abdelaal, M. M. Ali, and I. M. Hegazy, "Effect of diaphragmatic and costal manipulation on pulmonary function and functional capacity in chronic obstructive pulmonary disease patients: Randomized controlled study," *International Journal of Medical Research & Health Sciences*, vol. 4, no. 4, p. 841, 2015.

[29] K. Okura, A. Kawagoshi, M. Iwakura et al., "Contractile capability of the diaphragm assessed by ultrasonography predicts nocturnal oxygen saturation in COPD," *Respirology*, vol. 22, no. 2, pp. 301–306, 2017.

[30] M. F. Olsén, H. Lindstrand, J. L. Broberg, and E. Westerdahl, "Measuring chest expansion; A study comparing two different instructions," *Advances in Physiotherapy*, vol. 13, no. 3, pp. 128–132, 2011.

[31] H. Minoguchi, M. Shibuya, T. Miyagawa et al., "Cross-over comparison between respiratory muscle stretch gymnastics and inspiratory muscle training," *Internal Medicine*, vol. 41, no. 10, pp. 805–812, 2002.

[32] M. P. McHugh and C. H. Cosgrave, "To stretch or not to stretch: The role of stretching in injury prevention and performance," *Scandinavian Journal of Medicine & Science in Sports*, vol. 20, no. 2, pp. 169–181, 2010.

[33] M. Ito, F. Kakizaki, Y. Tsuzura, M. Yamada, and M. Shibuya, "Immediate effect of respiratory muscle stretch gymnastics and diaphragmatic breathing on respiratory pattern," *Internal Medicine*, vol. 38, no. 2, pp. 126–132, 1999.

[34] A. Mukherjee and A. Chakravarty, "Spasticity mechanisms - for the clinician," *Frontiers in Neurology*, vol. 1, 2010.

[35] T. A. Siatras, V. P. Mittas, D. N. Mameletzi, and E. A. Vamvakoudis, "The duration of the inhibitory effects with static stretching on quadriceps peak torque production," *The Journal of Strength and Conditioning Research*, vol. 22, no. 1, pp. 40–46, 2008.

[36] J. Kokkonen, A. G. Nelson, C. Eldredge, and J. B. Winchester, "Chronic static stretching improves exercise performance," *Medicine & Science in Sports & Exercise*, vol. 39, no. 10, pp. 1825–1831, 2007.

[37] D. K. Braga, D. F. Marizeiro, A. C. Florêncio et al., "Manual therapy in diaphragm muscle: effect on respiratory muscle strength and chest mobility," *Manual Therapy, Posturology & Rehabilitation Journal = Revista Manual Therapy*, vol. 1, no. 14, 2016.

17

Patient Delay in Initiating Tuberculosis Treatment and Associated Factors in Oromia Special Zone, Amhara Region

Muhammed Abdu,[1] **Awraris Balchut**,[2] **Eshetu Girma**,[1] **and Wondwosen Mebratu**[1]

[1]*Wollo University, Ethiopia*
[2]*Debre Birhan University, Ethiopia*

Correspondence should be addressed to Muhammed Abdu; mabdu220@gmail.com

Academic Editor: Stefano Centanni

Background. Tuberculosis (TB) is a major global public health problem. The disease is a leading cause of morbidity and mortality in Ethiopia. Early identification of cases and commencement of effective chemotherapy is an effective method to control the spread of tuberculosis. Delay in diagnosis and starting tuberculosis treatment increases severity, risk of mortality, and transmission of the disease in the community. *Objective.* The purpose of this study is to assess the magnitude of patient delay in initiating tuberculosis treatment and its associated factors among tuberculosis patients in health facilities of Oromia Special Zone, Ethiopia. *Methods.* A facility-based cross-sectional study was conducted in Oromia Special Zone. Data were collected using pretested questionnaires from patients with tuberculosis who are on treatment during the study period. The simple random sampling method was used to select health facilities and study participants. Data were entered using Epi Info version 7.2 and analyzed by SPSS version 23. Bivariate and multivariate logistic regression analyses were used to see the significance of association between the outcome and independent variables. A P value < 0.05 was considered statistically significant. *Results.* Three hundred and eighty-seven tuberculosis patients aged 18 years and above enrolled in the study. Among these, 223 (57.6%) were males, 194 (50.1%) were married, and 206 (53.2%) lived in rural areas. The mean age of respondents was 35 years. The median patient delay was 35 (IQR = 30) days, and 54.4% of patients seek their first consultation after 21 days. Patients who have a basic schooling level (AOR = 0.45, 95% CI: 0.23, 0.89) compared with the college/university level, long distance greater than 10 km (AOR = 3.23, 95% CI: 1.97, 5.42), seeking treatment from informal source and private drug stores (AOR = 3.01, 95% CI: 1.52, 5.95), extrapulmonary tuberculosis (AOR = 2.30, 95% CI: 1.26, 4.23), and poor knowledge about tuberculosis (AOR = 1.58, 95% CI: 1.01, 2.49) were associated factors that predict patient delay. *Conclusion and Recommendation.* A significant proportion of tuberculosis patients delayed to seek treatment. Health promotion and education involving different stake holders will make the community create awareness about tuberculosis that could help reduce delays in initiating tuberculosis treatment.

1. Introduction

1.1. Background. Tuberculosis (TB) is an infectious disease caused by Mycobacterium tuberculosis, a rod-shaped bacillus called "acid fast"; occasionally, the disease can also be caused by Mycobacterium bovis and Mycobacterium africanum [1]. TB is a major public health problem throughout the world, and also, a third of the world's population is estimated to be infected with tubercle bacilli, hence at risk of developing active disease [2].

According to the 2016 WHO report, in 2015, there were an estimated 10.4 million new TB cases of which 5.9 million were children [3]. The advances in TB prevention and control program lead to a decrease in mortality according to the Millennium Development Goals (MDG). In all, effective diagnosis and treatment of TB saved an estimated 43 million infectiousness, drug resistance, relapse, and even death due to TB [4, 5].

The related literature has revealed that patients' first presentation to health facilities is associated with geographical condition, health service, being unemployed, distance, age, sex, poverty, educational status, rural resident, awareness of TB, self-treatment, and stigma [4–6]. Delay in the diagnosis and start of effective treatment of TB patients result in a prolonged period of infectivity in the community and health care workers. On average, an untreated smear-positive TB patient can infect 10 contacts annually and over 20 during the natural history of the disease until death [6–8].

1.2. Statement of the Problem. The End TB Strategy targets to ensure that no family is burdened with catastrophic expenses due to TB [2]. The Sustainable Development Goals (SDGs) for 2030 adopted by the United Nations in 2015 targets to end the global TB epidemic. The WHO End TB Strategy, approved by the World Health Assembly in 2014, calls for a 90% reduction in TB deaths and an 80% reduction in the TB incidence rate by 2030, compared with 2015 [3].

Ethiopia is among the 30 High TB, HIV, and MDR-TB Burden Countries that accounted for 80% of all estimated TB cases worldwide, with an annual estimated TB incidence of 207/100,000 populations and death rate of 33 per 100,000 populations for 2014 [2]. The DR-TB sentinel report of Ethiopia in 2013 showed that the prevalence of MDR-TB is 2.3% among new TB cases and 17.8% among previously treated TB cases [2].

Studies on different parts of the world showed that the magnitude or duration of patient delay was 53.2% in Nepal [4], 72% with greater than 30 days in Colombia [5], 34.8% with a median delay of 32 days in Turkey [7], 65.5% in Iran [9], and 61 and 30 days in Peruvian Amazon and Thailand [10, 11], respectively. In the African region, patient delay, the time from onset of symptom to first consultation to modern health care, is alarmingly prolonged with studies reporting from 71% in Tanzania [12], 61% in Nigeria [13], and 48% in Zimbabwe [14], and also, some studies in Ethiopia showed that there was a patient delay of 62.3% in the North Wollo zone [15], 62% and 52.4% in Bahir Dar town, respectively [16, 17], and 42% in Addis Ababa [18].

Early diagnosis and prompt effective therapy form the key elements of the tuberculosis control program. Delay in diagnosis results in increased infectivity in the community, and it is estimated that an untreated smear-positive patient can infect, on average, 10 contacts annually and over 20 during the natural history of the disease until death [6]. Delay in tuberculosis diagnosis may also lead to a more advanced disease state at presentation, which contributes to late sequelae and overall mortality. Smear-positive cases are more likely to infect other individuals [6].

According to the MOH of Ethiopia hospital statistics data, tuberculosis is the leading cause of morbidity, the third cause of hospital admission (after deliveries and malaria), and the second cause of death in Ethiopia, after malaria [19]. The key elements of TB control and prevention programs are early diagnosis and prompt initiation of effective chemotherapy. Therefore, any delay in diagnosis and consequently treatment of TB patients not only increases infectivity in the community but also may lead to a more advance disease state which may result in more complication and expose them to a higher risk of death [6].

Thus, there are many factors that need to be addressed in order to achieve the goal of reducing the TB burden. As far as the researcher knowledge, these types of studies have not been conducted in the study area. Therefore, this study is aimed at assessing the magnitude of delay for the first consultation and associated factors among tuberculosis patients in Oromia Special Zone.

2. Literature Review

Early tuberculosis treatment is aimed at curing the TB patient and restoring quality of life and productivity, preventing death from active TB or its late effects, preventing relapse of TB, preventing the development and transmission of drug resistance, and decreasing TB transmission to others [1].

The End TB Strategy has three high-level indicators; these are the TB incidence rate, the absolute number of TB deaths, and the percentage of TB patients and their households that experience catastrophic costs as a result of TB disease. Targets for these indicators have been set for 2030 and 2035, with accompanying milestones for 2020 and 2025 [3].

In 1993, the World Health Organization (WHO) declared a state of global emergency for tuberculosis (TB), due to the steady increase of the disease worldwide. In 1995, the DOTs (directly observed treatment, short course) strategy was established as the key intervention to achieve tuberculosis control worldwide [6]. Delay diagnosis or incomplete treatment results in prolonged infectiousness, drug resistance, relapse, and even death. Patients with undiagnosed pulmonary TB primarily act as reservoirs for transmission. The contagion parameter suggests that, where TB is endemic, each infectious case will result in 20–28 secondary infections [4].

In order to remove the threat of TB, communities need to be empowered through awareness of primary issues and healthy behaviors. The TB epidemic cannot be addressed without involving those most affected by the disease, and the resulting consequences of their sickness. The communities can help provide practical solutions to the problems many people face when they fall ill and need diagnosis and proper care as well as lead to more interventions by health care professionals [20].

2.1. Magnitude of Patient Delay. An analytical cross-sectional study conducted in Nepal showed that the magnitude of patient delay was 53.2% with a median delay of 32 days [4]. The study conducted in Colombia, in 1456 new smear-positive pulmonary tuberculosis patients, shows that 72% of the patient had a delay > 30 days between symptom onset and treatment start and 28% had a 3+ bacillary load at diagnosis [5].

A study done in Iran revealed that 65.5% of cases had received delayed treatment with the mean time between onset of symptom, diagnosis, and treatment of 73 days [9]. A cross-sectional quantitative survey done in Peruvian Amazon showed that the median delay from symptom onset to seeking diagnostic testing was 61 days [10]. Only 31.2% of the study subjects took longer than 30 days to seek a medical consultation in Nonthaburi, Thailand [11]. Another study done in China revealed that 95.5% of patients self-presented for evaluation of the illness after a median 58 days of delay after symptom began [21]. Similar studies done in Pradesh India and Hong Kong show that the median patient delays were 15 and 20 days [22, 23].

A community-based study conducted in India indicates that the mean patient delay was 29 days [22]. Another study conducted in Ibadan, Nigeria, showed that 61.8% of patients delay for more than a median of 30 days [13]. The study conducted in Zimbabwe showed that 48% of patients had a delay with a median of 28 days [14]. Similar studies done in Sudan and Ghana revealed that the median patient delay was 27.2 and 59 days, respectively [8, 24].

The studies conducted in Jimma zone, southwest Ethiopia, and East Wollega, western Ethiopia, showed that the median durations of patient delay for treatment were 32 and 28 days [25, 26]. Another study done in Bahir Dar town and pastoralist communities in Bale zone, Southeast Ethiopia, revealed that the median patient delay was 30 and 63 days [17, 27]. An institution-based cross-sectional study done in North Wollo zone of Amhara region revealed that the median patient delay was 36 days and 62.3% when the patient seek their first consultation after 30 days of cut-off point [15].

2.2. Factors That Affect Patient Delay. Residence in the rural areas, DOTs center located more than 5 km away from their residence, and unemployed patients were associated factors with unacceptable patient delay in Nepal [4]. The study conducted in Colombia showed that being uninsured, having unknown HIV status, and coming from a neighborhood with NTP-employed community health workers were significantly associated with patient delay [5], while a similar study conducted in Iran indicates that female gender, smoking, and receiving immunosuppressive drugs were associated with a longer delay time [9].

Similar studies in Thailand and India showed that living in urban area and low family income were associated with patient delay, respectively [11, 22]. A qualitative study done in Peru revealed that the reasons for treatment seeking delay were lack of knowledge and confusion of TB symptoms, fear and embarrassment of receiving TB diagnosis, and patient tendency to self-medicate prior to seeking formal medical attention [28]. Another study done in India revealed that male sex, large family size, completed secondary school, and good knowledge were associated with patient delay [29].

A similar study done in Ibadan, Nigeria, indicates that female sex, place of residence, age group > 45 as compared to ≤45 years, and reported stigma were significantly associated with longer patient delay [13]. Delay in Cameroon is significantly associated with being the main income earner, the belief that TB is stigmatizing, and the use of traditional medicine [30]. The study conducted in Nigeria revealed that patient medicine dealer, private hospital, prayer house, and traditional healer were associated with patient delay [13].

The study conducted in North Wollo zone of Amhara region showed that long distance, rural residence, seeking treatment from traditional healers, and poor knowledge about TB were associated factors that predict patient delay [15]. Another study done in Bahir Dar town showed that illiteracy, having extrapulmonary TB, living greater than a distance of 10 km from TB service in health facilities, and prior visit to holy water, with traditional healer, and with private drug store/pharmacy were determinants of patient delay for the first consultation in health facilities [17]. Another study done in Addis Ababa revealed that patient delay was associated with distance and presence of TB-associated stigma [18]. Tuberculosis (TB) patient delay in Jimma zone is associated with being divorced and uneducated [25]. A similar study done in Wollega showed that patients from urban areas were 46% more likely to present to health care providers and female patients were more delayed to present to health providers than their male counterparts [26]. The study conducted in Mekelle revealed that smear-positive pulmonary TB disease, rural residence, illiteracy, lack of awareness/misperception of cause of pulmonary TB, prior treatment with holy water, treatment by private practitioner, and treatment by drug vendors were associated with patient delay [31].

2.3. Significance of the Study. A good understanding of the predictors of patient delay is important in the TB control program. There are so many strategies performed in Ethiopia like TB screening activities by health extension workers, contact screening, and screening at health facilities [2]. Despite efforts made through different methods to sensitize the community with warning symptoms of TB, still, there is a significant delay in health care seeking among TB patients. Information from this study will be useful for policy makers and health departments at different levels in developing interventions aimed at improving early identification of TB cases so as to initiate effective chemotherapy and check disease transmission in the population. It is also useful to others who do studies in this area.

3. Objectives of the Study

The objectives of this study were to determine the magnitude of patient delay in initiating TB treatment and identify factors associated with patient delay in initiating TB treatment in Oromia Special Zone.

4. Methods

4.1. Study Design. A facility based cross-sectional study was conducted.

4.2. Study Area and Study Period. The study was conducted in Oromia Special Zone, which is one of the eleven zones of the Amhara region. The zone has a population of 558060 in 2018 and five woredas and two town administrations. In the zone, 27 health centers provide TB treatment service, and one hospital provides smear microscopy, radiographic, and GeneXpert service.

4.3. Source Population

4.3.1. Source Population. All TB patients were enrolled one year prior to the study period and on treatment under DOTs program, that is, bacteriologically confirmed (with culture, GeneXpert, and smear), clinically diagnosed, and extrapulmonary patients.

4.3.2. Inclusion and Exclusion Criteria

(1) Inclusion Criteria. All tuberculosis patients enrolled and on treatment during the period of data collection were included.

(2) Exclusion Criteria. Patients who are critically ill, have treatment failure and relapse, lost to follow-up, unable to respond, and aged <18 years were excluded.

4.4. Sample Size and Sampling Procedure

4.4.1. Ssample Size Determination. The sample size was determined using the formula for estimation of single population proportion where $Z_{\alpha/2}$ at 95% CI (1.96), d marginal error 0.05, and P proportional obtained from the previous study done in Bahir Dar (0.52) [17]:

$$n = \frac{(Z_{\alpha/2})^2 * P(1-p)}{d^2},$$
$$n = \frac{(1.96)^2(0.52)(0.48)}{(0.05)^2} = 384. \quad (1)$$

With 5% nonresponse rate, the total sample size of the study was 403, by using the second objective, calculated by Epi Info statistical software (Table 1).

Therefore, the final sample size of the study was 403 which was computed based on the assumption of the single population proportion formula since this provided the larger sample size.

4.4.2. Sampling Technique. Among a total of 28 health facilities in the zone that provides diagnostic and treatment services for DOTs, 22 health facilities were selected randomly. Proportional allocation of patients was made according to the number of TB patients in the selected health facility. Then, all TB patients in the selected health facilities during the study period were included in the study consecutively until the intended sample size was achieved.

4.5. Study Variable

4.5.1. Dependent Variable. The dependent variable is delay in seeking care for tuberculosis patients.

4.5.2. Independent Variables. The independent variables were sociodemographic (age, sex, residence, occupation, religion, etc.) variables, health-seeking behavior (treatment sought before the first visit at public HFs, distance to access HFs), health status (type of TB disease (BC/PTB, CD/PTB, and EP) and HIV status (positive, negative)), knowledge of TB disease (the type of disease, its causes, curability, and type of antituberculosis drugs and duration of treatment), and stigma related to TB disease (feeling ashamed of having tuberculosis, having to hide tuberculosis diagnosis from others, delay to seek treatment due to fear of being diagnosed with TB, isolation due to tuberculosis, tuberculosis affecting the relationship with others, and fear of TB/HIV coinfection).

4.6. Operational Definitions

(1) *Patient Delay.* It is the time interval from the first onset of at least one or more symptom to the first visit to health facility, and a time longer than 21 days was considered indicative of patient delay [16, 18, 27].

(2) *The Onset of Symptom.* It is the day when the patient first becomes aware of the symptom or symptoms.

(3) *Knowledge.* Variables measuring knowledge were asked from the patient. These included knowledge about the type of disease, its causes, curability, and type of antituberculosis drugs and duration of treatment. Those individuals who score above the mean level were considered having good knowledge.

(4) *Stigma.* Variables measuring stigma were assessed using the Likert scale of 10 questions (1 strongly disagree, 2 disagree, 3 agree, and 4 strongly agree).

4.7. Data Collection Techniques

4.7.1. Data Collection Instruments and Procedure. An interview schedule was used to capture data from tuberculosis patients attending TB clinics. Some of the statements used were adapted from the "Diagnostic and treatment delay in tuberculosis, in seven countries of the Eastern Mediterranean Region" used by WHO [6]. Consecutive patients were enrolled after leaving the consultation room. They were asked for consent to be interviewed. Before conducting the data collection process, data collectors, 17 diploma nurse and 5 BSc health workers from the health facility currently working in DOTs clinic (TB clinics) and three supervisors who are TB officers, were recruited.

4.8. Data Quality Management. The questionnaire was first prepared in English and translated to the local language, Afan Oromo and Amharic, and again back translated back to English to ensure the consistency of the questions. The data collectors and supervisors were trained for one day on how to collect data by using structured questionnaires and general information about the contents of the questionnaires and consent forms. Data were collected with close supervision by a principal investigator and supervisors. The questionnaire was pretested on 5% of the sample size in Oromia Special Zone in similar health facilities, which were not included in the sample, and necessary modifications were made whenever needed.

4.9. Data Processing Analysis Procedure. Completed quantitative data were entered into Epi Info version 7.2 software. Then, data were exported to SPSS version 23 and checked for inconsistencies and missing values by running frequencies and other data explorations. Inconsistencies and missing values were cleaned by checking the original questionnaire. Description statistics such as mean, median, standard deviation, and percent were used to describe descriptive variables. Binary logistic regression was employed to investigate the association between independent variables and the outcome variable. Variables that show significant association with

TABLE 1: Sample size calculation by TB patient delay-associated factors.

Associated factors	Prevalence	Power	Confidence interval	AOR	Sample size	Including 5%	Reference
TB-associated stigma	42.1	80	95	2.1	262	275	[18]
Informal treatment source (holy water)	62.3	80	95	2.58	228	239	[15]
Educational level (illiterate)	62	80	95	3.73	144	151	[16]
Distance to HFs	52.4	80	95	3.15	114	120	[17]

the delay in the binary logistic regression at P value ≤ 0.25 were included in the multivariable logistic regression models to identify independent predictors to patient delay. In the multiple logistic regression models, the model association was considered at P value ≤ 0.05.

4.10. Ethical Consideration. Ethical approval was obtained from Wollo University College of Medicine and Health Sciences. A support letter was first requested from the Oromia special zonal health department to woreda health offices and support letter from woreda health offices to health facilities. Verbal consent from respondents was obtained before conducting the face-to-face interview. In order to maintain privacy and avoid the fear of stigmatization, health professionals working in TB units who already knew the serostatus of the clients were assigned to be data collectors. Patients were assured that the interview is private and confidential, their participation is voluntary, and their names were not included in the questionnaire. Data collectors were provided proper advice for the respondents regarding any malpractice they have come across after the interview is completed.

5. Results

5.1. Sociodemographic Characteristics. Three hundred and eighty-seven TB patients with a response rate of 96% were enrolled from 22 treatment and diagnostic centers, whereas the remaining was excluded due to data incompleteness during data analysis. The mean age was 35, years and 226 (58.4%) participants were 18-34 years old and 161 (41.6%) were 35 years and above. In the majority of participants, 57.6% were males, 53.2% lived in rural areas, 81.9% were Muslims, and 50.1% were married and 52.5% did not have any schooling level. Two-thirds of the study participants lived within the 10 km radius to health facilities. The main occupation of the participants was farmer (33.1%), and 13.2% were government or private employees (Table 2).

5.2. Clinical Characteristics of TB Patients. Among the respondents, 136 (35.1%) were bacteriologically confirmed PTB, 145 (37.5%) were clinically diagnosed PTB, and 106 (27.4%) were extrapulmonary TB. The majority of the participants (74.7%) had cough/cough with blood as a symptom of tuberculosis, 63% had night sweating, and 58.1% had loss of appetite. Most of them reported multiple symptoms of tuberculosis in this study (Table 3).

5.3. Health-Seeking Behaviors of TB Patients. A total of 275 patients (71.1%) had not sought informal care for their symptoms between the onset of their illness and their first consultation at a health facility, while 102 (26.4%) had sought care from at least one informal provider. Twenty-one (5.4%) had been treated with holy/hot water, 28 (7.2%) by traditional healers, and 63 (16.3%) by private drug stores/pharmacies.

The majority of patients (192 or 46.9%) made their first consultation at a health center, 119 (30.7%) attended the nearby clinics, and 78 (19.6%) at a hospital. Most patients (57.6%) decided to visit health facilities by themselves; forty-two percent of the patients visited a health facility because they were advised by members of their family or health workers. In this study, 43.4% of patients had chat chewing habit, 10.1% had smoking habit, and 2.3% reported alcohol consumption before tuberculosis diagnosis (Table 4).

5.4. Patient Delay. Overall, 211 (54.5%) with 95% CI (49%, 62%) of patients did seek medical advice after 21 days of the onset of their illness. The median delay from onset of symptoms to first visit of a health provider was 35 (IQR = 30) days, range (23-360 days). A total of 353 patients (91.2%) came within two months, and 34 patients (8.8%) came after 90 days. Of all delays, 28.9% were BCPTB, 33.6% were CDPTB, and 36% were EPTB patients. Patient delay among women was 43.1% and men 56.9%. Based on the place of residence, 113 (58.3%) of urban and 71.5% of rural residents were delayed. Among the respondents, 54.9% with poor knowledge was delayed.

On the bivariate analysis, educational status, basic schooling level, and distance to health facility had significantly increased the risk of delay in seeking health care of TB treatment. Respondents with poor knowledge about tuberculosis and those with prior attendance at holy/hot water and nearby drug stores were associated with patient delay.

Having extrapulmonary TB was 2 times more likely to cause delay in seeking health care of TB treatment. No significant association was found between prolonged patient delay with sex, age, marital status, HIV status, and occupation.

On multivariant analysis, respondents with basic schooling level (AOR = 0.45, 95% CI: 0.23, 0.89) and patients who lived beyond a 10-kilometer radius from health facilities (AOR = 3.23, 95% CI: 1.97, 5.42) were three times more delayed than those within the 10 km radius. The use of prior treatment with holy/hot water (AOR = 3.62, 95% CI: 1.11, 11.84) and from private drug store/pharmacy (AOR = 3.01, 95% CI: 1.52, 5.95) was also significantly associated with patient delay.

Extrapulmonary TB patients were two times more likely to be delayed than those study participants with bacteriologically confirmed pulmonary TB (AOR = 2.30, 95% CI: 1.26, 4.23). Having poor knowledge about tuberculosis was

TABLE 2: Characteristics of tuberculosis patients in DOTs clinics of Oromia zone, Northeast Ethiopia, 2018.

Variables	Frequency ($n = 387$)	Percent
Sex		
Male	223	57.6
Female	164	42.4
Age		
18-34	226	58.4
35-50	98	25.3
≥51	63	16.3
Place of residence		
Rural	206	53.2
Urban	181	46.8
Marital status		
Married	194	50.1
Single	150	38.8
Divorced	23	5.9
Widowed	20	5.2
Educational status		
Did not have any schooling level	203	52.2
Did have basic schooling level	69	17.8
Primary	57	14.8
Secondary	36	9.3
College/university	22	5.7
Religion		
Muslim	317	81.9
Orthodox	47	12.1
Protestant	23	5.9
Ethnic group		
Oromia	249	64.3
Amhara	136	34.9
Tigre	3	0.8

TABLE 3: Clinical characteristics of TB patients in Oromia zone, Northeast Ethiopia, 2018.

Variables	N (%)
Types of symptom	
Cough/cough with blood	289 (74.4%)
Night sweating	244 (63.0%)
Loss of appetite	225 (58.1%)
Fever	216 (55.8%)
Chest pain	192 (49.6%)
Weight loss	163 (42.1%)
TB type	
CDPTB	145 (37.5%)
BCPTB	136 (35.1%)
EPTB	106 (27.4%)
HIV status	
Negative	355 (91.7%)
Positive	28 (7.2%)
Unknown	4
Other comorbid conditions	
No	376 (97.2)
Diabetes	6
Hypertension	5
Smoking habit	
No	348 (89.9%)
Yes	39 (10.1)
Chat chewing habit	
No	219 (56.6%)
Yes	168 (43.4%)

another important factor found to cause patient delay in seeking health care for TB treatment (AOR = 1.58, 95% CI: 1.01, 2.49) (Table 5).

6. Discussions

Early detection of cases and treating TB patients are one of the strategies of WHO to reduce the disease morbidity and mortality throughout the world [3]. In this study, it was observed that a significant proportion of patients delayed more than the acceptable level for patient delay. The magnitude of patient delay in seeking health care was 54.5%, and this is almost similar with studies conducted in Nepal 53.2% [4], Bahir Dar 52.4% [17], and Tigray 53% [31], and it is greater than the previous studies in Thailand 31.2% [11] and Addis Ababa 42.1% [18]. But the result of this study is lower than that of the study done in pastoralist communities in Bale zone 96% [27]. The possible reason for this difference may be due to the study setting and topographic conditions.

The overall median patient delay in this study was 35 days with a range of 23-360 days, which was consistent with a study done in North Wollo zone 36 days [15]. But it was somewhat longer than a study done in northwest Ethiopia, Amhara region, with a median of 30 days Bahir Dar town [16, 17] and east Wollega, eastern Ethiopia [25]. It was much longer than previous studies in Pradesh, India, [32] with a median delay of 15 days and Hong Kong [23] with a median delay of 20 days. But it was much shorter than the previous study in Bale zone a median delay of 63 days [27]. The possible suggestion for differences in delay could be probably by cultural, low socioeconomic status, and lack of information about the availability of free tuberculosis treatment.

Long walking distance between health facility and patient home was a risk factor for seeking health care of tuberculosis treatment. Respondents, who live beyond 10 kilometers from health facilities, have 23% times higher delay in seeking health care as compared to those who live within 10 kilometers. This result was in line with studies done in Nepal [4], North Wollo [15], Bahir Dar [17], and Addis Ababa [18]. This might be low inaccessibly in health service and scattered settlement of population.

Regarding the respondent educational level, having basic schooling level was 45% less likely to delay compared to those

Table 4: Health-seeking behaviors of TB patients in Oromia zone, Northeast Ethiopia, 2018.

Variables	N (%)
Treatment sought prior to first visit in health facilities	
No prior treatment	275 (71.1%)
Private drug store/pharmacy	63 (16.3%)
Traditional healers	28 (7.2%)
Holy/hot water	21 (5.4)
Decision to visit the first health facility was made by	
Patients themselves	223 (57.6%)
Family members	135 (34.9%)
Health workers	29 (7.5%)
Health facility visited at first consultation	
Health centers	192 (49.6%)
Clinics	119 (30.7%)
Hospitals	76 (19.6%)
Knowledge about TB	
Good knowledge	196 (50.6%)
Poor knowledge	191 (49.4%)
TB-associated stigma	
Low stigma	223 (57.6%)
High stigma	164 (42.4%)

who have college or university level. This result is different with studies done in Peruvian Amazon [10], Tanzania [33], Bahir Dar [17], and Bale zone [27]. This difference might be the availability of community health insurance made respondents, who have basic schooling level, seek health care in health facilities at the soonest possible time.

The use of an informal treatment provider was also another strong predictor of patient delay in this study. This is in line with previous studies in Peru [28], Nigeria [34], Bahir Dar town [17], and Tigray [31]. Patients who used holy/hot water as a first consultation were four times more likely to delay in seeking health care for tuberculosis treatment compared to those who did not use. This is consistent with previous studies in North Wollo [15] and Bahir Dar [17]. This might be low reliance of treatment in health facilities and high cultural beliefs of respondents on treatment of TB.

Respondents, whose first consultation in private drug stores or pharmacies, were three times more likely to delay in seeking health care of treatment compared to those who did not. This is in line with the study conducted in Nigeria [34], North Wollo zone [15], and Bahir Dar town [17]. The probable reason for this could be that private drug stores or pharmacies have an advantage of availability in most areas and also, they do not charge for cards and other consultation services.

Extrapulmonary TB constituted 27.4% of all cases in this study. Respondents, with extrapulmonary TB, were two times more likely to delay as compared to bacteriologically confirmed pulmonary TB patients. This study was consistent with the studies in Bahir Dar town [17]. However, findings from studies in European countries reveal that extrapulmonary TB is a more rare form of TB and it is more frequent in African patients [35, 36]. This might be due to a variety of symptoms, could easily be over looked, gradual progress, and less sever clinical manifestation at the beginning. Another probable reason might be that patients with extrapulmonary TB feel reassured about their health conditions and do not proceed with necessary investigation to diagnose in peripheral health facilities.

Having good knowledge about tuberculosis is a very important issue for early seeking of medical consultation. In this study, 49.4% of respondents have poor knowledge about tuberculosis. Respondents, with poor knowledge about TB, were 58% more likely to delay in seeking health care of tuberculosis treatment as compared to those who had good knowledge. This is in line with previous studies conducted in North Wollo zone [15], Amhara region, and WHO in east Mediterranean study in Syria Arab republic [6]. This difference might be dependent upon the respondent's knowledge regarding the TB disease for early seeking of medical care.

Patient delay was not found to be significantly associated with age and sex in this study. Similar findings were reported in North Wollo [15] and Addis Ababa [18]. However, studies conducted in Iran [35]; Ibadan, Nigeria [13]; and Wollega [26] reported that females tend to seek health care lately compared to males. This might be due to work overload at home and the limited role of women's decision making power. Similarly, older age was found to be significantly associated with patient delay in India [32] and Ibadan, Nigeria [13]. This difference might be due to older age people are physically and economically dependent with others in their life.

In this study, stigma was not associated with patient delay in seeking care for TB treatment. This is similar with studies conducted in Bahir Dar [17] and Wollega, eastern Ethiopia [26]. Other several studies showed stigma attached to the TB patient is a contextual factor associated to delay seeking of the health services in Cameroon [30], Ghana [24], which is not the case in this study.

In Ethiopia, all patients with a diagnosis of TB are recommended to be tested for HIV [2]. In this study, 98.9% of respondents were checked for HIV. In this study, those with HIV coinfection had a slightly longer delay in seeking treatment but this was not significant; this is similar to studies in Thailand [5], Tanzania [33], and Nigeria [34]. This may be due to shortage of financial resources in the course of seeking treatment for their HIV care.

The strength of this study is it includes 70% of the health facilities that provide DOTs services in the study area and also participate both public and private health facilities. However, there was some degree of recall bias while patients were trying to remember the symptoms to approximate days of the beginning of the symptoms and starting TB treatment. To minimize this limitation, local religious calendar methods and public holidays, national celebrations, and agricultural events were used to facilitate patient recall to collect information.

Table 5: Factors associated with patient delay in DOTs clinics of Oromia Zone, Northeast Ethiopia, 2018.

Variables	Patient delay		Unadjusted and adjusted OR		*P* values
	No delay	Delay	COR (95% CI)	AOR (95% CI)	
Educational status					
College/university	14	8	1	1	
Did not have any schooling level	73	130	3.12 [1.25, 7.77]	0.74 [0.39, 1.39]	
Have basic schooling level	35	34	1.7 [0.63, 4.57]	0.45 [0.23, 0.89]	0.02*
Primary	37	20	0.95 [0.34, 2.64]	0.67 [0.29, 1.56]	
Secondary	17	19	1.96 [0.65, 5.80]	0.49 [0.17, 1.41]	
Place of residence					
Urban	93	88	1	1	
Rural	83	123	1.57 [1.05, 2.34]	0.99 [0.57, 1.56]	
Distance to the nearest health facilities					
<10 km	142	113	1	1	
≥ 10 km	34	98	3.62 [2.28, 5.75]	3.23 [1.97, 5.42]	0.001***
Treatment sought prior to first visit in health facilities					
No prior treatment	149	126	1	1	
Holy/hot water	4	7	5.03 [1.65, 15.32]	3.62 [1.11, 11.84]	0.034*
Private drug store/pharmacy	15	48	3.78 [2.02, 7.08]	3.01 [1.52, 5.95]	0.001***
Traditional healers	8	20	2.96 [1.26, 6.94]	2.14 [0.81, 5.60]	
TB type					
BCPTB	75	61	1	1	
CDPTB	74	71	1.18 [0.74, 1.89]	1.19 [0.71, 1.99]	
EPTB	27	79	3.59 [2.07, 6.25]	2.30 [1.26, 4.23]	0.001***
Knowledge about TB					
Good knowledge	105	95	1	1	
Poor knowledge	71	116	1.81 [1.20, 2.71]	1.58 [1.01, 2.49]	0.04*

AOR = adjusted odds ratio; COR = crude odds ratio; CI = confidence interval. N.B. **P* value ≤ 0.05, ****P* value ≤ 0.001. Coding of dependent variable: delay = 1 and no delayed = 0.

The result of this study revealed that majority of TB patients in this study area did not present within 21 days from onset of illness to a health facility. Educational status having basic schooling level, distance greater than 10 kilometers, first point of contact at holy/hot water, private drug stores or pharmacies, extrapulmonary TB, and poor knowledge about tuberculosis were found to be predictors for prolonged patient delay for first consultation in health facilities. Patient delays were found to be longer, suggesting the need for increased advocacy, communication, and social mobilization efforts targeted at informing the general population to seek health services early when they experience symptoms suggestive of TB. Health education sessions that emphasized the cause, the availability of treatment, and the curability of tuberculosis should be designed and provided to raise awareness.

Based on results found in this study, the authors recommended that the community should be sensitized continuously on seeking appropriate health care and sensitization programs by using socially and culturally convenient media of communication to ensure that the whole community is reached. The health department of the local government should orient religious leaders, private drug stores or pharmacies, and traditional healers to refer symptomatic people for tuberculosis screening and treatment. A community-based study can be done to capture symptomatic individuals who are not attending health facilities.

Consent

We have informed written consent from participants for possible publication.

Authors' Contributions

M.A., A.B., E.G., and W.M. designed the research study, performed the research, and critically reviewed the paper. M.A. analyzed the data. M.A. wrote the draft paper. All authors approved the final manuscript and agree to be accountable for all aspects of the work.

Acknowledgments

The authors would like to acknowledge data collectors and study participants.

References

[1] FMOH, "Guidelines for clinical and programmatic management of TB," in *TB/HIV and leprosy in Ethiopia*, pp. 2–11, Federal Ministry of Health of Ethiopia, Addis Ababa, 2013.

[2] FMOH, "National Comprehensive Tuberculosis," in *Leprosy and TB/ HIV Training Manual for Health Care Workers. Participants ' Manual*, Federal Ministry of Health of Ethiopia, 2017.

[3] World Health Organization, *Global tuberculosis report*, World Health Organization, 2016.

[4] W. Laohasiriwong, R. K. Mahato, R. Koju, and K. Vaeteewootacharn, "Delay for first consultation and its associated factors among new pulmonary tuberculosis patients of Central Nepal," *Tuberculosis Research and Treatment*, vol. 2016, 8 pages, 2016.

[5] D. A. Rodríguez, K. Verdonck, K. Bissell et al., "Monitoring delays in diagnosis of pulmonary tuberculosis in eight cities in Colombia," *Rev Panam Salud Publica*, vol. 39, no. 1, pp. 12–18, 2016.

[6] World Health Organization, *Diagnostic and treatment delay in tuberculosis [Internet]*, WHO, 2006, WHO-EM/TDR/009/E/10.06/1000.

[7] D. Güneylioglu, A. Yilmaz, S. Bilgin, U. Bayram, and E. Akkaya, "Factors affecting delays in diagnosis and treatment of pulmonary tuberculosis in a tertiary care hospital in Istanbul, Turkey," *Medical Science Monitor*, vol. 10, no. 2, pp. - CR62–CR67, 2004.

[8] E. Y. Mohamed, S. M. Abdalla, A. A. Khamis, A. Abdelbadea, and M. A. Abdelgadir, "Factors associated with patient delay in accessing pulmonary tuberculosis care, Gezira state, Sudan, 2009," *Eastern Mediterranean Health Journal*, vol. 19, no. 2, pp. 114–118, 2013.

[9] A. Farazi and M. Jabbariasl, "Time delay and associated factors in diagnosis and treatment of pulmonary tuberculosis in Markazi Province," *Journal of Community Health Research*, vol. 1, no. 1, pp. 46–53, 2012.

[10] C. M. Ford, C. A. Evans, R. H. Gilman et al., "Factors Associated with Delayed Tuberculosis Test-seeking Behavior in the Peruvian Amazon," *The American Journal of Tropical Medicine and Hygiene*, vol. 81, no. 6, pp. 1097–1102, 2009.

[11] T. Rattananupong, N. Hiransuthikul, V. Lohsoonthorn, C. Chuchottaworn, and S. Medicine, "Factors associated with delay in tuberculosis treatment at 10 tertiary level care hospitals," *The Southeast Asian journal of tropical medicine and public health*, vol. 46, no. 4, pp. 689–696, 2013.

[12] G. B. Tarimo, "1," in *Delay in seeking care among tuberculosis patients attending tuberculosis clinics in Rungwe district, Tanzania*, 71 pages, Doctoral dissertation, Muhimbili University of Health and Allied Sciences, 2012.

[13] A. A. Fatiregun and C. C. Ejeckam, "Determinants of patient delay in seeking treatment among pulmonary tuberculosis cases in a government specialist hospital in Ibadan, Nigeria," *Tanzania Journal of Health Research*, vol. 12, no. 2, 20101–9.

[14] K. C. Takarinda, A. D. Harries, B. Nyathi, M. Ngwenya, T. Mutasa-apollo, and C. Sandy, "Tuberculosis treatment delays and associated factors within the Zimbabwe national tuberculosis programme," *BMC Public Health*, vol. 15, no. 1, 20151–12.

[15] D. Tsegaye, E. Abiy, T. Mesele, and T. Tadesse, "Delay in seeking health care and associated factors among pulmonary tuberculosis patients in North Wollo zone , Northeast Ethiopia : institution based cross-sectional study," *iMedPub Journals*, vol. 7, no. 3, pp. 1–7, 2016.

[16] E. Gebeyehu, M. Azage, and G. Abeje, "Factors Associated with Patient's Delay in Tuberculosis Treatment in Bahir Dar City Administration, Northwest Ethiopia," *BioMed Research International*, vol. 2014, Article ID 701429, 6 pages, 2014.

[17] Y. A. Mekonnen, L. Abebe, N. Fentahun, S. A. Belay, and A. W. Kassa, "Delay for first consultation and associated factors among tuberculosis patients in Bahir Dar town administration , North West Ethiopia," *American Journal of Health Research*, vol. 2, no. 4, pp. 140–145, 2014.

[18] G. S. Adenager, F. Alemseged, H. Asefa, and A. T. Gebremedhin, "Factors Associated with Treatment Delay among Pulmonary Tuberculosis Patients in Public and Private Health Facilities in Addis Ababa, Ethiopia," *Tuberculosis Research and Treatment*, vol. 2017, Article ID 5120841, 9 pages, 2017.

[19] FMOH, *Tuberculosis, leprosy and TB/HIV prevention and control program*, FMOH Addis Ababa, 2008.

[20] K. Mutinda, E. Kabiru, and P. Mwaniki, "Health seeking behavior, practices of TB and access to health care among TB patients in Machakos County, Kenya. A cross-sectional study," *Journal of Biology, Agriculture and Healthcare*, vol. 4, no. 14, pp. 96–107, 2014.

[21] S. Cheng, W. Chen, Y. Yang et al., "Effect of Diagnostic and Treatment Delay on the Risk of Tuberculosis Transmission in Shenzhen, China: An Observational Cohort Study, 1993–2010," *PLoS One*, vol. 8, no. 6, pp. e67516–e67516, 2013.

[22] S. G. Konda, C. A. Melo, P. A. Giri, and A. B. Behera, "Determinants of delays in diagnosis and treatment of pulmonary tuberculosis in a new urban township in India: a cross-sectional study," *International Journal of Medical Science and Public Health*, vol. 3, no. 2, p. 140, 2014.

[23] E. C. C. Leung, C. C. Leung, and C. M. Tam, "Delayed presentation and treatment of newly diagnosed pulmonary tuberculosis patients in Hong Kong," *Hong Kong Medical Journal*, vol. 13, no. 3, pp. 221–227, 2007.

[24] E. Osei, P. Akweongo, and F. Binka, "Factors associated with delay in diagnosis among tuberculosis patients in Hohoe Municipality , Ghana," *BMC Public Health*, vol. 15, no. 1, 20151–11.

[25] T. Ayalew, "Delays in tuberculosis treatment and associated factors in Jimma Zone,Southwest Ethiopia," *Ethiopian Journal of Health Sciences*, vol. 19, no. 1, pp. 29–37, 2009.

[26] T. Wondimu, K. W/Michael, W. Kassahun, and S. Getachew, "Delay in initiating tuberculosis treatment and factors associated among pulmonary tuberculosis patients in East Wollega, Western Ethiopia," *Ethiopian Journal of Health Development*, vol. 21, no. 2, 2007148–56.

[27] A. Hussen, S. Biadgilign, F. Tessema, S. Mohammed, K. Deribe, and A. Deribew, "Treatment delay among pulmonary tuberculosis patients in pastoralist communities in Bale Zone , Southeast Ethiopia," *BMC Research Notes*, vol. 5, no. 1, 20121–10.

[28] V. A. Paz-Soldan, R. E. Alban, C. Dimos Jones, A. R. Powell, and R. A. Oberhelman, "Patient reported delays in seeking treatment for tuberculosis among adult and pediatric TB patients and TB patients co-infected with HIV in Lima, Peru: a qualitative study," *Frontiers in Public Health*, vol. 2, 20141–9.

[29] K. Goel, N. Kondagunta, S. J. Soans, A. R. Bairy, and P. Goel, "Reasons for patient delays & health system delays for tuberculosis in South India," *Indian Journal of Community Health*, vol. 23, no. 2, pp. 87–89, 2011.

[30] A. Cambanis, A. Ramsay, M. A. Yassin, and L. E. Cuevas, "Duration and associated factors of patient delay during tuberculosis screening in rural Cameroon," *Tropical Medicine & International Health*, vol. 12, no. 11, pp. 1309–1314, 2007.

[31] M. M. Mesfin, J. N. Newell, J. D. Walley, A. Gessessew, and R. J. Madeley, "Delayed consultation among pulmonary tuberculosis patients: a cross sectional study of 10 DOTS districts of Ethiopia," *BMC Public Health*, vol. 9, no. 1, 200953.

[32] U. R. Mandi and H. Pradesh, "Delay in diagnosis and treatment among Tb patients registered," *The Indian Journal of Tuberculosis*, vol. 60, pp. 37–45, 2013.

[33] E. R. Wandwalo and O. Mørkve, "Delay in tuberculosis case-finding and treatment in Mwanza Tanzania," *International Journal of Tuberculosis and Lung Disease*, vol. 4, pp. 133–138, 2000, September 1999.

[34] O. I. Babatunde, E. C. Bismark, N. E. Amaechi, E. I. Gabriel, and A. U. R. Olanike, "Determinants of Treatment Delays among Pulmonary Tuberculosis Patients in Enugu Metropolis, South-East, Nigeria," *Health*, vol. 7, no. 11, pp. 1506–1516, 2015.

[35] M. Mondoni, O. Viganò, M. Ferrarese et al., "Haemoptysis and fever in a young refugee from Somalia," *International Journal of Infectious Diseases*, vol. 77, pp. 57–60, 2018.

[36] G. Sotgiu, D. Falzon, V. Hollo et al., "Determinants of site of tuberculosis disease: An analysis of European surveillance data from 2003 to 2014," *PLoS One*, vol. 12, no. 11, article e0186499, 2017.

18

A Case of Isolated Primary Pleural Neurofibroma in a 39-Year-Old Woman

Kritika Krishnamurthy[1] **John Alexis,**[1,2] **Pukhraz Basra,**[1] **and Ana Maria Medina**[1,2]

[1]*AM Rywlin Department of Pathology and Laboratory Medicine, Mount Sinai Medical Centre, Miami Beach, FL, USA*
[2]*Florida International University Herbert Wertheim College of Medicine, Miami, FL, USA*

Correspondence should be addressed to Kritika Krishnamurthy; kritikakrishnamurthy@yahoo.com

Academic Editor: Vinicius C. Antao

Primary benign neurogenic neoplasms of the pleura are exceedingly rare. Neurofibromas rarely involve the pleura. A review of the literarture reveals only a single reported case of isolated pleural neurofibroma. Herein the authors describe another case of isolated primary pleural neurofibroma. A 39-year-old nonsmoker woman presented to the emergency room with complaints of progressively worsening chest pain of one month duration. A computed tomography of the chest revealed a crescent shaped, pleural based mass suspicious for a neurogenic tumor such as an intercostal schwannoma. A PET-CT skull base to midthigh failed to reveal any other masses or abnormalities. A surgical excision of the mass was performed due to the patient's intractable pain. The resected specimen consisted of an ovoid fragment of soft tissue with pale yellow, smooth and glistening cut surface. Microscopic examination revealed the tumor to be composed of spindle cells with wavy nuclei arranged haphazardly in loose collagenous and pale myxoid stroma with rare interspersed mast cells. The spindle cells were diffusely positive for S100 protein and SOX-10, and focally positive for neurofilament. In the absence of any other masses in the patient and no pertinent history, a diagnosis of primary pleural neurofibroma was made. This case emphasizes the need to consider neurofibroma in any spindle cell neoplasm of the pleura irrespective of age or singularity.

1. Introduction

Pleural neoplasms are more commonly metastatic than primary. Primary neoplasms of the pleura are exceedingly rare [1]. They are more often malignant than benign, with malignant mesothelioma being the most common entity. Benign neoplasms include solitary fibrous tumor, lipomatous tumors, adenomatoid tumor, calcifying fibrous tumor, multicystic mesothelioma, and schwannoma [2]. Other benign tumor-like lesions include nodular pleural plaque and mesothelial cysts. Of these, solitary fibrous tumor is the most frequently encountered [3].

Neurofibromas are benign neurogenic tumors that rarely involve the pleura [2]. A review of the literarture reveals only a single reported case of isolated pleural neurofibroma. Herein the authors describe another case of isolated primary pleural neurofibroma.

2. Case Report

The patient is a 39-year-old woman who presented to the emergency room with complaints of progressively worsening chest pain of one month duration. The pain was of gradual onset, moderate in intensity, constant, and localised to the left upper quadrant. She was nonsmoker with no significant medical history. Physical examination was within normal limits. A computed tomography of the chest revealed a crescent shaped, pleural based mass, measuring $6 \times 4.9 \times 3.8$ cm, with some modelling and cortical irregularity of the superior aspect of the left lateral fourth rib suggestive of a long standing process (Figure 1). These imaging findings were suspicious for a neurogenic tumor such as an intercostal schwannoma, though other more aggressive etiologies could not be ruled out. A PET-CT skull base to midthigh failed to reveal any other masses or abnormalities. A CT guided biopsy of the mass was attempted, but the specimen was not diagnostic consisting only of scant adipose tissue.

A surgical excision of the mass was performed due to the patient's intractable pain. Intraoperatively, the pleural mass was ovoid, smooth, well-circumscribed and could be separated from the lung parenchyma. It was resected and sent to pathology.

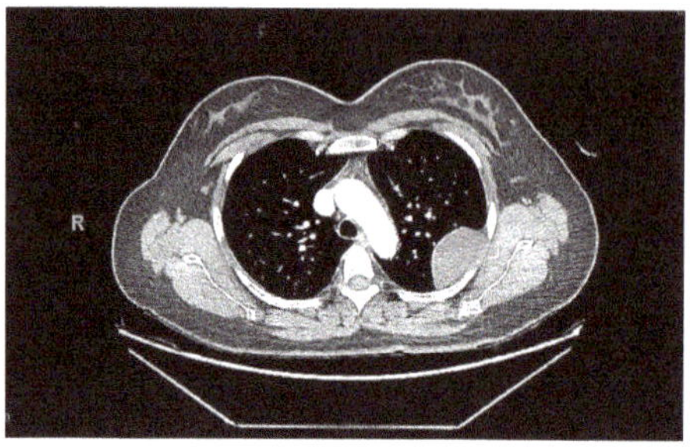

FIGURE 1: A crescent shaped, pleural based mass, measuring 6 × 4.9 × 3.8 cm, with some modelling and cortical irregularity of the superior aspect of the left lateral fourth rib as seen on CT.

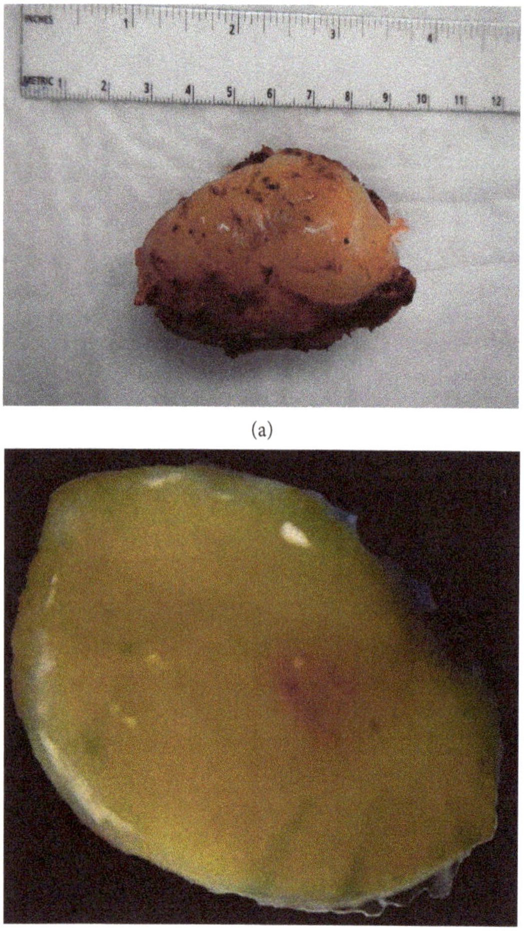

(a)

(b)

FIGURE 2: (a) Well circumscribed, ovoid mass. (b) Yellow, smooth and glistening cut surface.

The resected specimen consisted of an ovoid fragment of soft tissue measuring 7 × 5.3 × 2.4 cm. The cut surface was pale yellow, smooth and glistening (Figures 2(a) and 2(b)). Microscopic examination revealed the tumor to be composed of spindle cells with wavy nuclei arranged haphazardly in loose collagenous and pale myxoid stroma with rare interspersed mast cells (Figures 3(a) and 3(b)). This histopathological picture was suggestive of neurofibroma. On immunohistochemistry, the spindle cells were diffusely positive for S100 protein and SOX-10, and focally positive for neurofilament. CD34 showed some fibrillary positivity while STAT-6 and bcl-2 were negative. CD117 highlighted the mast cells (Figures 4(a)–4(e)). In the absence of any other masses in the patient and no pertinent history, a diagnosis of primary pleural neurofibroma was made.

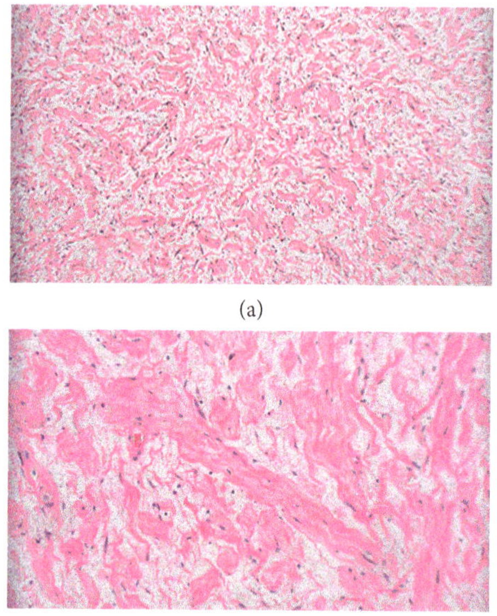

(a)

(b)

FIGURE 3: (a) Spindle cells arranged haphazardly in loose collagenous and pale myxoid stroma (100x). (b) Spindle cells with wavy nuclei (400x).

The patient's post-surgical course was uneventful and continues to be in follow-up with no new complaints at the time of this report.

3. Discussion

Primary benign pleural neoplasms are infrequent [2]. However, it is important to differentiate these uncommon tumors from the more commonly encountered metastatic cancers and malignant mesothelioma as prognosis and management are radically different.

Due to the extensive nerve supply throughout the thorax, neurogenic tumors arise in this location and account for approximately 9% of primary mediastinal tumors in adults [4]. Ribet et al. conducted a retrospective review of 134 cases of neurogenic tumors of the thorax and found them to be benign in 93% of adult cases with nerve sheath tumors comprising 73.5% of adult cases [5].

Benign nerve sheath tumors encountered in the thorax include schwannomas, ganglioneuromas, and neurofibromas [6]. Ratbi et al. studied 17 patients who underwent resection of mediastinal benign neurogenic tumors and found schwannoma in 76.4% cases [7]. The rarity of intrathoracic neurofibromas was further confirmed in a study of 149 intrathoracic neurogenic tumors by Bicakcioglu et al. [8].

Neurofibromas originate from Schwann cells and fibroblasts and may arise in any peripheral nerve. They most often affect patients between 20 and 30 years of age and have no sex

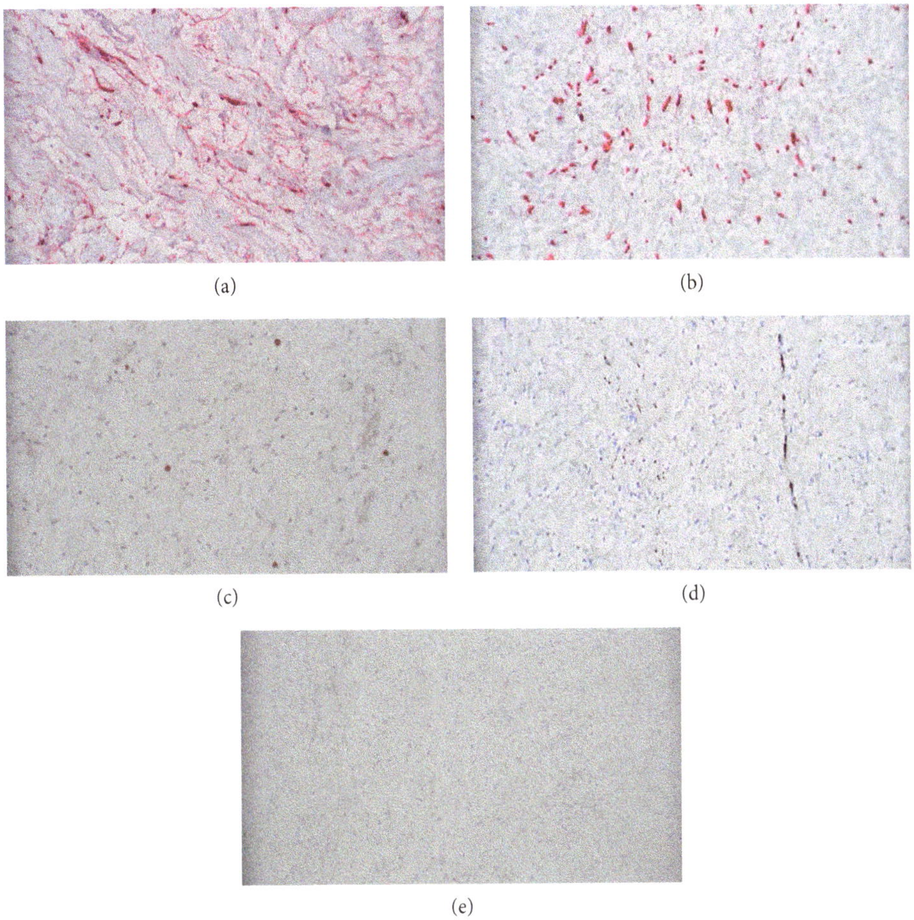

FIGURE 4: (a) Tumor cells diffusely positive for S100 protein (200x). (b) Tumor cells showing SOX-10 positivity (200x). (c) CD117 highlighting mast cells (200x). (d) Neurofilament highlighting the trapped axons (200x). (e) Tumor cells negative for STAT6 (100x).

predilection [9]. Approximately 90% of the neurofibromas are localised and not associated with neurofibromatosis [10]. Localised neurofibromas tend to be slow growing and asymptomatic, although they may expand and cause symptoms due to compression of nerves or other adjacent structures [11]. In our case the patient had a relatively large tumor that may have been compressing adjacent nerves resulting in pain. Gupta et al. described a well-defined homogeneous isodense and non-enhancing mass with rib abnormalities due to bone erosion from the adjacent neurofibroma, similar to the radiologic findings seen in our case [12].

Pleural involvement by neurofibroma is exceedingly rare with only three cases reported so far [12, 13]. Of these, only one case reported by Langman et al., was not associated with neurofibromatosis [13]. Primary pleural neurofibromas arise directly from intercostal nerves and form pleural based masses. The only case of isolated primary pleural neurofibroma is a 71 year old woman who presented with shoulder pain, reported from Europe. Our case is the first reported case of isolated primary pleural neurofibroma in the United States. Though our patient presented with similar complaints of pain as the previous reported case, her younger age of presentation sets her apart.

The differential diagnosis for neurofibromas in the pleura includes but is not limited to neural neoplasms, such as schwannoma and ganglioneuroma, as well as a variety of non-nerve sheath tumors, in particular solitary fibrous tumor, mesothelioma, synovial sarcoma, fibrosarcoma, and undifferentiated pleomorphic sarcoma. The malignant neoplasms such as mesothelioma, synovial sarcoma, fibrosarcoma, and undifferentiated pleomorphic sarcoma can be excluded due to the absence of any features of malignancy in conventional neurofibromas while benign neoplasms such as ganglioneuroma have characteristic histologic features that preclude confusion with neurofibroma.

Differentiating a neurofibroma from a schwannoma and solitary fibrous tumor may sometimes be challenging. The presence of mast cells, which is integral in the development of neurofibromas, is one of the most specific hisopathological features that help clinch the diagnosis of neurofibroma [14, 15]. Immunohistochemistry may also be helpful. Neurofibromas are invariably positive for S-100 protein and negative for STAT6 and bcl-2, in contrast to solitary fibrous tumors which are negative for S-100 protein and positive for STAT6 and bcl-2 [16–18]. In our case, the tumor cells are positive for S-100 protein and negative for bcl-2 and STAT 6, ruling out solitary fibrous tumor. Schwannomas, like neurofibromas, are positive for S-100 protein and SOX-10, and may show focal CD 34 positivity while being bcl-2 negative, thus making them harder to discern from neurofibromas [17, 19]. Localisation of staining for neurofilament protein may be of some value in differentiating the two. Neurofibromas grow within the nerve of origin; accordingly neurofilament protein will stain axons entrapped within the tumor. Whereas, schwannomas grow peripherally and displace the nerve of origin, hence staining for neurofilament protein will fail to reveal any entrapped axons within the tumor though occasionally axons may be entrapped at the very periphery [20]. However, some recent studies suggest that intralesional axons may be more frequently seen in schwannomas than previously reported [21].

Treatment of localized neurofibromas is complete surgical resection. Neurofibromas grow within and cannot be separated from normal nerve, and complete excision of the neoplasm requires sacrifice of the nerve. This is acceptable in cases of pleural neurofibroma as they do not involve major nerves. Local recurrence after complete excision is unusual [22].

4. Conclusion

This case emphasizes the need to consider neurofibroma in any spindle cell neoplasm of the pleura irrespective of age or singularity. The main differential diagnosis includes schwannomas and solitary fibrous tumor which can be excluded in most cases by histopathology supplemented with immunohistochemistry. Complete surgical resection is curative.

References

[1] W. D. Travis, E. Brambilla, H. K. Muller-Hermelink, and C. C. Harris, *WHO Classification of Tumours. Pathology and Genetics of Tumours of the Lung, Pleura, Thymus and Heart*, vol. 10, IARC Press, Lyon, France, 2004.

[2] L. Granville, A. C. Laga, T. Craig Allen et al., "Review and update of uncommon primary pleural tumors: a practical approach to diagnosis," *Archives of Pathology and Laboratory Medicine*, vol. 129, no. 11, pp. 1428–1443, 2005.

[3] A. Churg, "Localized Pleural Tumors," in *Diagnostic Pulmonary Pathology*, P. T. Cagle, Ed., pp. 719–735, Marcel Dekker, New York, NY, 2000.

[4] M. E. Froudarakis, "Diagnostic work-up of pleural effusions," *Respiration*, vol. 75, no. 1, pp. 4–13, 2008.

[5] M. E. Ribet and G. R. Cardot, "Neurogenic tumors of the thorax," *The Annals of Thoracic Surgery*, vol. 58, no. 4, pp. 1091–1095, 1994.

[6] K. G. Davidson, P. R. Walbaum, and R. J. McCormack, "Intrathoracic neural tumours," *Thorax*, vol. 33, no. 3, pp. 359–367, 1978.

[7] M. B. Ratbi, F. El Oueriachi, A. Arsalane, M. M. El Hammoumi, and H. El Kabiri, "Surgery of benign neurogenic tumors in adults: single institution experience," *Pan African Medical Journal*, vol. 19, p. 288, 2014.

[8] P. Bicakcioglu, F. Demirag, A. Yazicioglu, K. Aydogdu, S. Kaya, and N. Karaoglanoglu, "Intrathoracic- neurogenic tumors," *The Thoracic and Cardiovascular Surgeon*, vol. 62, no. 02, pp. 147–152, 2014.

[9] D. Resnick and G. Niwayama, "Soft tissues," in *Diagnosis of Bone and Joint Disorders*, D. Resnick, Ed., pp. 4552–4554, Saunders, Philadelphia, PA, 3rd edition, 1995.

[10] F. M. Enzinger and S. W. Weiss, "Benign Tumors of Peripheral Nerves," in *Soft Tissue Tumors*, pp. 821–888, Mosby, St Louis, MO, 3rd edition, 1995.

[11] E. B. Kesieme, A. E. Dongo, C. Affusim, G. Prisadov, K. Okonta, and C. Imoloamen, "Late presentation of giant intrathoracic neurofibroma with significant mediastinal shift: a case report and review of the literature," *Case Reports in Pulmonology*, vol. 2013, Article ID 619729, 3 pages, 2013.

[12] A. Gupta, P. Mrigpuri, and H. Kumar, "A case of pleural neurofibroma: a rare pleural tumor," *Indian Journal of Case Reports*, vol. 4, no. 2, pp. 133–135, 2018.

[13] G. Langman, S. Rathinam, and L. Papadaki, "Primary localised pleural neurofibroma: expanding the spectrum of spindle cell tumours of the pleura," *Journal of Clinical Pathology*, vol. 63, no. 2, pp. 116–118, 2010.

[14] M. D. Johnson, J. Kamso-Pratt, C. F. Federspiel, and W. O. Whetsell Jr, "Mast cell and lymphoreticular infiltrates in neurofibromas: comparison with nerve sheath tumors," *Archives of Pathology and Laboratory Medicine*, vol. 113, pp. 1263–1270, 1989.

[15] K. Staser, F. C. Yang, and D. W. Clapp, "Mast cells and the neurofibroma microenvironment," *Blood*, vol. 116, no. 2, pp. 157–164, 2010.

[16] E. Kawahara, Y. Oda, A. Ooi, S. Katsuda, I. Nakanishi, and S. Umeda, "Expression of glial fibrillary acidic protein (GFAP) in peripheral nerve sheath tumors. A comparative study of immunoreactivity of GFAP, vimentin, S-100 protein, and neurofilament in 38 schwannomas and 18 neurofibromas," *The American Journal of Surgical Pathology*, vol. 12, no. 2, pp. 115–120, 1988.

[17] M. De Perrot, S. Fischer, M. A. Bründler, Y. Sekine, and S. Keshavjee, "Solitary fibrous tumors of the pleura," *The Annals of Thoracic Surgery*, vol. 74, no. 1, pp. 285–293, 2002.

[18] E. G. Demicco, P. W. Harms, R. M. Patel et al., "Extensive survey of STAT6 expression in a large series of mesenchymal tumors," *American Journal of Clinical Pathology*, vol. 143, no. 5, pp. 672–682, 2015.

[19] D. Nonaka, L. Chiriboga, and B. P. Rubin, "Sox10: a pan-schwannian and melanocytic marker," *The American Journal of Surgical Pathology*, vol. 32, no. 9, pp. 1291–1298, 2008.

[20] F. J. Rodriguez, A. L. Folpe, C. Giannini, and A. Perry, "Pathology of peripheral nerve sheath tumors: diagnostic overview and update on selected diagnostic problems," *Acta Neuropathologica*, vol. 123, no. 3, pp. 295–319, 2012.

[21] A. F. Nascimento and C. D. Fletcher, "The controversial nosology of benign nerve sheath tumors: neurofilament protein staining demonstrates intratumoral axons in many sporadic schwannomas," *The American Journal of Surgical Pathology*, vol. 31, no. 9, pp. 1363–1370, 2007.

[22] M. D. Murphey, W. S. Smith, S. E. Smith, M. J. Kransdorf, and H. T. Temple, "From the archives of the AFIP. Imaging of musculoskeletal neurogenic tumors: radiologic-pathologic correlation," *Radiographics*, vol. 19, no. 5, pp. 1253–1280, 1999.

19

Prevalence of Latent Tuberculosis Infection in the Middle East and North Africa

Mazin Barry

Department of Internal Medicine, Division of Infectious Diseases, College of Medicine, King Saud University, Riyadh, Saudi Arabia

Correspondence should be addressed to Mazin Barry; mbarry@ksu.edu.sa

Academic Editor: Stefano Centanni

Objective. Data on the prevalence of latent tuberculosis infection (LTBI) in Middle Eastern and North African countries are scarce. We aimed to review all relevant published data in countries belonging to this region to determine the overall prevalence of LTBI in the Middle East and North Africa (MENA) region. *Methods.* In this systematic review PubMed and Google Scholar databases were searched for observational, prospective, retrospective, cross-sectional, and cohort studies providing prevalence data of LTBI in any MENA country. Studies fulfilling the search criteria were incorporated in the review. Overall prevalence of LTBI with 95% confidence intervals (CI) was calculated using the random-effects model; heterogeneity was assessed using I^2 statistics. Gender and age group-based subgroup analyses were performed to evaluate the basis of heterogeneity. *Results.* The total number of overall LTBI studies identified was 956, of which 31 studies from ten countries within the MENA region were included that represented 12,439 subjects. The overall prevalence was 41.78% (95% CI 31.18% to 52.78%, $I^2 = 99.31\%$). By gender-based subgroup analysis, the prevalence of LTBI was 33.12% (95% CI 18.97% to 49.04%, $I^2 = 99.25\%$) and 32.65% (95% CI 19.79% to 47%, $I^2 = 98.89\%$) in males and females, respectively, while in the age-based subgroup analysis, the prevalence of LTBI was 0.44% (95% CI -0.05% to 0.9%), 3.37% (95% CI 2.23% to 4.74%, $I^2 = 0\%$), and 43.81% (95% CI 33.09% to 54.82%, $I^2 = 99.18\%$) for children, adolescents, and adults, respectively. *Conclusion.* This systematic review reveals a high prevalence of LTBI in the MENA region; enhanced LTBI surveillance and prompt infection prevention steps are urgently needed to prevent active tuberculosis, this would help achieve the World Health Organization End TB Strategy 2035, and the United Nations Sustainable Development Goals 2030 target in the MENA region.

1. Introduction

Tuberculosis (TB) is a major health problem, with an estimated 10 million people (range 9 to 11.1 million) developing TB disease in 2018, of which 5.8 million, 3.2 million, and 1 million were men, women, and children, respectively. Two-thirds of cases were from eight countries, India (27%), China (9%), Indonesia (8%), Philippines (6%), Pakistan (5%), Nigeria (4%), Bangladesh (4%), and South Africa (3%) [1]. Latent tuberculosis infection (LTBI) does not induce infectious expression of the disease, although it causes continuous immune response generated towards TB antigens. LTBI has a 10% probability of progressing into active TB disease, 5% during the first two years of acquiring the infection, and 5% during the rest of the individual's lifetime. The detection of LTBI and prevention before it becomes infectious is a crucial component of the WHO-End TB strategy. It has been reported from mathematical models that approximately 30% of the population worldwide are LTBI carriers [2]. Previous studies have documented the rates of LTBI to be 31.2% in Ethiopia [3], 49% in Uganda [4], 55.2% in South Africa [5], 11.2% in Spain [6], 50% in India [7], 51% in Korea [8], and 7.6% in England [9];however, very few studies have been undertaken to estimate the prevalence of LTBI in the Middle East and North Africa (MENA) region.

In previous studies, it has been observed that patients belonging to lower socioeconomic groups, refugees, and migrants [10], patients with abnormal immune responses (post-organ transplant, hemodialysis patients, people living with HIV, etc.), and chronic inflammatory conditions have an increased risk of acquiring TB and its progression to active disease [11–13];further, LTBI in people living with HIV has a 10% probability of progressing into active TB, when left untreated, annually; furthermore, it has been shown that a significant geographical variation in TB infection rates persists across the world, implying that health care workers (HCW) in various countries encounter different risks of acquiring TB [14]. In 2018, 87% of new TB cases occurred in the top thirty high TB burden countries, of which eight countries accounted for two-thirds of all new TB cases, they include India, China, Indonesia, Philippines, Pakistan, Nigeria, Bangladesh, and South Africa, while the occurrence was extremely low in the MENA regions [1], it has also been reported that HCW are at particular risk of LTBI, and hence, annual screening is performed in most standardized health care facilities. In addition, the prevalence of LTBI in HCW has been reported to be higher than that of other community groups around the world [15, 16].

Currently, the direct diagnosis of LTBI is not fully possible [17]. The diagnosis of memory T-cell response against LTBI is performed by either the tuberculin skin test (TST) or interferon-gamma release assays (IGRA) [18]. At present, no gold standard test has been developed to measure LTBI; however, there are increasing advancements in this field looking into tumor necrosis factor, chemokines, interleukin growth factors, and other factors that could enhance LTBI diagnosis [19]. With TST, TB-purified protein derivative (PPD) stimulates a type IV hypersensitivity-delayed type reaction [20–22], its advantage is that it is inexpensive and generally accepted especially in low economic countries including Africa [3], but has several disadvantages, as it has demonstrated poor response in individuals with reduced immunity and those with active TB, requires two-step verification, is operative dependent, and exhibits low specificity in determining reactivation of TB in Bacillus Calmette-Guérin (BCG) vaccinated individuals, it can also cause false-positive results in patients sensitized to naturally existing nontuberculous mycobacteria [18, 23].

On the other hand, IGRA has greater specificity compared to TST [17], it involves only one blood test after incubation with *Mycobacteria tuberculosis*-specific antigens, following which T-cell mediated immune response and interferon- (IFN-) gamma release are measured. The QuantiFERON®-TB-Gold-in-Tube (QFT-GIT) and T-SPOT.TB assay tests are the two commercially available IGRA, in which the former is based on ELISA (enzyme-linked immunosorbent assay) and comprises of peptides from the ESAT-6, CFP-10, and TB7.7 antigens of TB. T-SPOT.TB assay is preferred in immunocompromised patients [24–26]. IGRA provides more conclusive results that would help in decision-making, with only a single visit required for the test, it also eliminates false-positive results in people vaccinated with BCG or sensitized with nontuberculous mycobacteria.

Several previous studies have documented the prevalence of LTBI in many countries of the Middle East and North Africa, in a wide range of population, including HCW, household contacts, people living with HIV, prisoners, refugees, and in patients with varied health problems; however, to our knowledge, there are no published studies that have assessed the overall prevalence within the whole MENA region; hence, we performed a systematic review to evaluate the prevalence of LTBI in the MENA region in different population groups belonging to various age groups.

2. Methods

2.1. Criteria for Considering Studies

2.1.1. Inclusion Criteria. Studies based on the incidence or prevalence of LTBI among people of all ages, origin, socioeconomic, and educational backgrounds, in countries located in the Middle East and North Africa, that are cross-sectional, observational, cohort, prospective, and retrospective studies, with LTBI detection performed with either TST or IGRA or both.

2.1.2. Exclusion Criteria. Systematic reviews, case reports, case series, editorials, letters to the editors, and randomized controlled trials.

2.2. Search Strategy. The author searched PubMed and Google Scholar databases for articles published between January 1, 2000 and November 30, 2018, in the English language. The use of medical subject heading (MeSH) terms for LTBI was employed in the database search combined with the following search terms: (latent tuberculosis OR TB OR LTBI OR *Mycobacterium tuberculosis*) AND (Prevalence OR Epidemiology OR "Country name"). The Middle East countries included were Iran, Iraq, Saudi Arabia, Yemen, Syria, Jordan, United Arab Emirates, Israel, Lebanon, Oman, Kuwait, Qatar, Bahrain, Palestine, Cyprus, and Turkey. North African countries included were Egypt, Libya, Algeria, Morocco, Tunisia, Sudan, Western Sahara, and Mauritania. A broad search strategy was used to ensure that all relevant studies were identified, with no filters included in the searches. Following this, the author independently analyzed the title of the study and its abstract and keywords outlining the record, based on which studies were either included or excluded. No minimal sample size was required to be included in the analysis; however, a sample size of ≥200 was considered as adequate, and a sample size of <200 was considered as inadequate.

2.3. Data Extraction

2.3.1. Study Selection and Data Extraction. A detailed search of PubMed and Google Scholar databases by employing various search terms was performed. The duplicate citations were removed, and the studies for inclusion in the review were selected. The initial screening was based on the citation titles and abstracts, following which, the articles were selected and picked up and their complete text obtained, reviewed, and assessed for their eligibility for inclusion. The bibliographic information of the included studies was also screened to identify additional relevant articles for inclusion; furthermore, the data from relevant studies were abstracted using

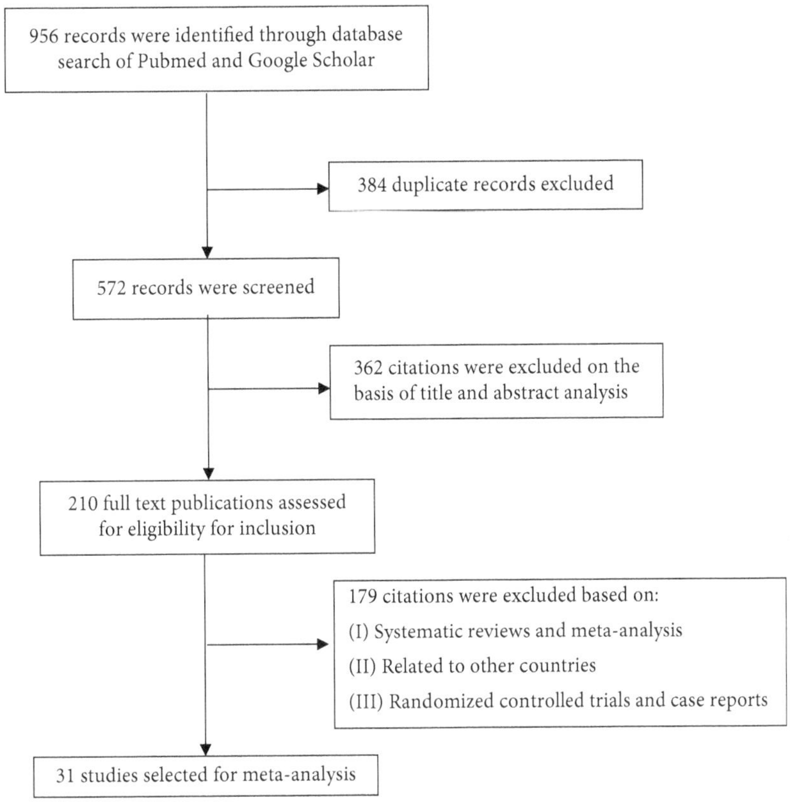

FIGURE 1: Flowchart for study selection.

a data extraction form, and the applicable items for the review were reported in the PRISMA (Preferred Reporting Items for Systematic Reviews and Meta-Analyses) checklist. The following key information has been presented in the data extraction template: first author, period of study and year of publication, country where the research was conducted, study design, number of participants, age at assessment, tools used for assessment, and key findings.

2.3.2. Quality (Risk of Bias) Assessment. The Mirza and Jenkins [27] checklist were referred to for investigating the quality of included studies. The assessment was based on the following nine criteria: clear study aims, adequate sample size, representative sample, inclusion and exclusion criteria, adequate assessment of outcome, response rate reported, adequate description of data, appropriate statistical analysis, and appropriate informed consent obtained. A final total score was calculated for each of the criteria, scored 0 if absent and 1 if present. Thus, the minimum and maximum obtainable scores would be 0 and 9, respectively.

2.4. Statistical Analysis. Analysis was performed using STATA software. The effect sizes were reported as proportions with 95% confidence intervals. The heterogeneity of effects was assessed and quantified by the I^2. The I^2 values greater than 50% were considered to represent substantial heterogeneity. The random-effects model was subjected in cases exhibiting substantial heterogeneity. Subgroup analysis based on sex (male and female), by age strata, and by quality score of the studies (<5 and ≥5) was also performed. A p value less than 0.05 was considered statistically significant for all the analyses undertaken.

3. Results

3.1. Search Results and Study Selection. The database search resulted in a total of 956 citations, of which 384 citations were eliminated due to their duplication, and the rest of the 572 citations were examined. After screening, examination of titles and abstracts resulted in the elimination of 362 citations from the study. Following this, 210 full-text citations were retrieved, and after subjecting them to inclusion and exclusion criteria, a total of 31 studies were identified (Figure 1).

3.2. Study Characteristics. Thirty-one studies representing 12,439 subjects from ten countries within the MENA region were included: thirteen from Turkey, five from both Iran and Saudi Arabia, two from Egypt, and one each from Syria, Israel, Oman, Qatar, Tunisia, and United Arab Emirates. These studies were conducted between 2005 till 2018. The sample size ranged from 34 to 2,650 (Table 1).

3.3. Publication Bias. From the 31 studies, the minimal checklist score was 5 in two studies, while the highest was 9. Details of all included studies clarity, adequacy of sample size, and other details are outlined in Table 2.

3.4. Prevalence of LTBI. The prevalence of LTBI was assessed in 31 studies using random-effects model. A total of 3,981 events were observed among the 12,439 subjects. The proportion of LTBI ranged from 0.44% to 88.15%. The overall

Table 1: Study characteristics.

Study/reference number	Duration of study	Year	Country	Study population	TST and/or QFT	Study design	Sample size	Age (mean ± SD)	Tools	LTBI	Prevalence (95% CI)	Outcome
Nasehi et al. [31]	October to December 2013	2016	Iran	TB laboratory staff and low-risk healthcare workers	TST	Cross-sectional	1006	38.06 ± 7.76 and 37.31 ± 7.32	ANOVA, logistic regression	791	78.62% (75.96, 81.12)	TB laboratory staff the OR of developing LTBI
Mamani et al. [32]	March 2013, 6 months	2016	Iran	Prisoners	TST	Cross-sectional	1208	18-60 years	Wilson procedure with continuity correction	756	62.58% (59.78, 65.32)	High prevalence of LTBI
Bukhary et al. [33]	December 2015	2018	Saudi Arabia	Healthcare workers working in hajj pilgrimage	TST QFT-GIT	Cross-sectional	520	22-62 years	Standardized questionnaire, chi-square test, Fisher exact test	56	10.76% (8.23, 13.75)	Low prevalence of LTBI
Balkhy et al. [34]	July 2010 to March 2013	2017	Saudi Arabia	Primary healthcare workers	TST QFT-GIT	Cross-sectional	1369	<15 to ≥65 years	Chi-square test, McNemar test	146	10.66% (9.07, 12.42)	Low prevalence of LTBI
El-Helaly et al. [35]	August 2009 to May 2011	2014	Saudi Arabia	Preemployment screening of tertiary healthcare workers	TST QFT-GIT	Cross-sectional	1372	18-60 years	Kappa coefficient, chi-square test	421	30.68% (28.25, 33.20)	Fair agreement between TST and QFT-G tests
Hassan and Diab et al. [36]	January to June 2012	2014	Saudi Arabia	Laboratory personnel at a university hospital	QFT-GIT	Cross-sectional	134	21-60 years (33 ± 9.2)	Standardized questionnaire, chi-square test, Fisher's exact test	26	19.4% (13.08, 27.12)	Assessed risk factors involved with LTBI
Abbas et al. [37]	January 2008 to December 2009	2010	Saudi Arabia	Healthcare workers in tertiary care hospital	TST	Cross-sectional	2650	10 to >50 years	ANOVA	291	10.98% (9.81,12.23)	Highest LTBI rates in physicians and nurses
Warrington et al. [38]	January 2016	2018	Syria	Syrian refugees entering Canada	QFT-GIT	Cross-sectional	99	5 to <50 years	Two-tailed independent t-tests	9	9.09% (4.24, 16.55)	Low prevalence of LTBI. No active TB
Mekaini et al. [39]	April to October 2013	2014	UAE	Pediatric population	QFT-GIT	Cross-sectional	669	1-19 years	Kruskal-Wallis one-way ANOVA, chi-square test, Fisher's exact test	3	0.44% (0.09, 1.30)	Low prevalence of LTBI
Shitrit et al. [28]	September and December 2002	2005	Israel	High school students and adults	TST	Cross-sectional	84	18.2 ± 11 years	Pearson correlation coefficient, Student's t -test	57	67.85% (56.77, 77.63)	High prevalence of LTBI
Khamis et al. [40]	January to June 2012	2016	Oman	Healthcare workers exposed		Cross-sectional	291	20 to 65 years	Descriptive statistics	123		High prevalence of

Table 1: Continued.

Study/reference number	Duration of study	Year	Country	Study population	TST and/or QFT	Study design	Sample size	Age (mean ± SD)	Tools	LTBI	Prevalence (95% CI)	Outcome
				to active TB in tertiary care hospital	TST QFT-GIT						42.26% (36.52, 48.17)	LTBI among healthcare workers
Garcell et al. [41]	August 2012 to May 2013	2014	Qatar	Healthcare workers in community hospital	TST QFT-GIT	Cross-sectional	202	39 ± 6.5 years	Test of independence, Student's *t*-test, and Wilcoxon Mann–Whitney	14	6.93% (3.84, 11.35)	Low prevalence of LTBI
Gunluoglu et al. [42]	September to November 2011	2015	Turkey	Chronic renal failure patients undergoing regular hemodialysis	TST QFT-GIT	Cross-sectional	44 (TST); 50 (QFT-GIT)	62.2 years (mean age)	Kappa statistic, Mann–Whitney *U*-test, chi-square, Fisher's exact test, Wilks' lambda test	16 (TST+); 27 (QFT-GIT+)	50% (37.23, 62.76)	High prevalence of LTBI
Duman et al. [43]	Not available	2014	Turkey	Psoriasis patients	TST QFT-GIT	Cross-sectional	61 (psoriasis); 40 (psoriatic arthritis)	44.6 ± 13.1 years	Kolmogorov–Smirnov test, *t*-test, Mann–Whitney *U*-test, chi-square test, multivariable logistic regression, multiple linear regression	52 (psoriasis); 29 (psoriatic arthritis)	80.19% (71.08, 87.46)	High prevalence of LTBI
Babayigit et al. [44]	Not available	2014	Turkey	BCG vaccinated healthcare workers	TST QFT-GIT	Cross-sectional	64	21 to 51 years (32.01 ± 6.28)	Kolmogorov-Smirnov test, Shapiro Wilk test, Mann–Whitney *U*-test, Fisher exact test, Pearson chi-square test, logistic regression analysis	32	50% (37.23, 62.76)	High prevalence of LTBI
Yilmaz et al. [29]	Not available	2012	Turkey	Patients with systemic lupus erythematosus	TST QFT-GIT	Cross-sectional	78	13 to 67 years	Cohen's kappa analysis, chi-square test, Mann–Whitney *U*-test	41	52.56% (40.93, 63.99)	High prevalence of LTBI
Hanta et al. [45]	Not available	2012	Turkey	Patients with rheumatologic diseases	TST QFT-GIT	Cross-sectional	90	41.9 ± 11.9 years	Chi-square test or Fisher's exact test	66	73.33% (62.96, 82.10)	High prevalence of LTBI
Soysal et al. [46]	May 2006 to May 2007	2012	Turkey	Hemodialysis patients	TST T-SPOT.TB	Cross-sectional	411	19 to 84 years	Student's *t*-test, chi-square test or Fisher's exact test, logistic regression analysis	61	14.84% (11.54, 18.65)	Use of T-SPOT.TB in patients with negative TST for diagnosis of LTBI
Caglayan et al. [47]	August 2005	2011	Turkey	Healthcare workers of		Cross-sectional	78	30.51 ± 8.57 years	ANOVA	59		

Table 1: Continued.

Study/reference number	Duration of study	Year	Country	Study population	TST and/or QFT	Study design	Sample size	Age (mean ± SD)	Tools	LTBI	Prevalence (95% CI)	Outcome
				tertiary care hospital	TST QFT-GIT						75.64% (64.60, 84.65)	High prevalence of LTBI
Karadag et al. [48]	Not available	2010	Turkey	Patients with Takayasu arteritis	TST QFT-GIT	Cross-sectional	94	40.2 ± 12.1 years	Student's *t*-test, Wilcoxon rank-sum test, chi-square test, Fisher's exact test	55	58.51% (47.88, 68.58)	High prevalence of LTBI
Inanc et al. [49]	March 2007 to June 2008	2009	Turkey	Patients with rheumatoid arthritis and Ankylosing spondylitis	TST QFT-GIT	Cross-sectional	140	55.4 ± 11.2 years	Chen's kappa analysis, Mann–Whitney *U*-test, chi-square test	85	60.71% (52.11, 68.85)	High prevalence of LTBI
Seyhan et al. [50]	Not available	2010	Turkey	Hemodialysis patients	TST QFT-GIT	Cross-sectional	100	56.2 ± 15.3 years	Student *t*-test, Mann–Whitney *U*-test, chi-square test	56	56% (45.71, 65.91)	High prevalence of LTBI
Hanta et al. [51]	April 2005 to January 2008	2008	Turkey	Patient with rheumatoid arthritis, ankylosing arthritis, and psoriatic arthritis	TST	Cross-sectional	192	43.1 ± 12.7 years	Fisher's exact test	129	67.18% (60.05, 73.77)	TST can be used for diagnosis of LTBI in rheumatologic disease before anti-TNF therapy.
Ozdemir et al. [52]	June to August 2005	2007	Turkey	Healthcare workers in Duzce University hospital	TST QFT-GIT	Cross-sectional	76	18 to 50 years (30.4 ± 5.4)	Cohen's kappa, chi-square test, Student's *t* -test	67	88.15% (78.70, 94.44)	High prevalence of LTBI
Bozkanat et al. [53]	March 2008	2016	Turkey	Healthcare workers in specialist tuberculosis hospital	TST QFT-GIT	Cross-sectional	34	33.0 ± 5.8 years	Kappa test	23	67.64% (49.47, 82.61)	High prevalence of LTBI
Hasanain et al. [54]	December 2015 to January 2017	2018	Egypt	Patients with erectile dysfunction	TST QFT-GIT	Cross-sectional	97	47.9 ± 13.6 years	Chi-square test, Fisher's exact test	29	29.89% (21.02, 40.04)	Prevalence of LTBI was high in patients with high-grade ED
El-Sokkary et al. [55]	August 2012 to	2015	Egypt	Healthcare providers	TST QFT-GIT	Cross-sectional	132	35.2 ± 8.99 years	Chi-square test, Fisher's exact test	78	59.09% (50.19, 67.56)	High prevalence of LTBI

Table 1: Continued.

Study/reference number	Duration of study	Year	Country	Study population	TST and/or QFT	Study design	Sample size	Age (mean ± SD)	Tools	LTBI	Prevalence (95% CI)	Outcome
	January 2013											
Slouma et al. [56]	2007 to 2014	2017	Tunisia	Patients with chronic inflammatory diseases receiving biologic agents since at least 6 months	TST QFT-GIT	Cohort	113	47.67 ± 13.5 years	Student's *t*-test, ANOVA	23	20.35% (13.36, 28.95)	Low prevalence of LTBI
Khazraiyan et al. [57]	January to May 2013	2016	Iran	HIV positive patients	TST QFT-GIT	Cross-sectional	130	19 to 71 years (37.1 ± 8.6)	Chi-square test, Fisher's exact test	38	29.23% (21.58, 37.84)	Low prevalence of LTBI
Jam et al. [30]	January 2006 to February 2007	2010	Iran	Patients with HIV/AIDS	TST	Cross-sectional	262	1 month to >60 years	Chi-square test	63	24.04% (19, 29.68)	Medium prevalence of LTBI
Amiri et al. [58]	June to August 2012	2014	Iran	Homeless people of Tehran	QFT-GIT	Cross-sectional	593	Not available	Logistic regression and chi-square test	277	46.71% (42.63,50.81)	High prevalence of LTBI
											[Overall prevalence 41.78% (31.18, 52.78)]	

QFT-GIT: QuantiFERON-TB Gold In-Tube; TST: tuberculin skin test; LTBI: latent tuberculosis infection; OR: odds ratio; ANOVA: analysis of variance; HIV: human immunodeficiency virus; AIDS: acquired immunodeficiency syndrome; TNF: tumor necrosis factor.

Table 2: Quality assessment of the studies included in the review.

Study	Clear study aims	Adequate sample size	Representative sample	Inclusion and exclusion criteria	Adequate assessment of outcome	Response rate reported	Adequate description of data	Appropriate statistical analysis	Appropriate informed consent obtained	Total score
Nasehi et al., 2016 [31]	1	1	1	1	1	1	1	1	1	9
Mamani et al., 2016 [32]	1	1	1	1	1	1	1	1	1	9
Bukhary et al., 2018 [33]	1	1	1	1	1	0	1	1	1	8
Balkhy et al., 2017 [34]	1	1	1	1	1	0	1	1	1	8
El-Helaly et al., 2014 [35]	1	1	1	1	1	0	1	1	0	7
Hassan and Diab, 2014 [36]	1	0	1	1	0	0	1	1	1	6
Abbas et al., 2010 [37]	1	1	1	1	1	0	1	1	0	7
Warrington et al., 2018 [38]	1	0	1	1	0	0	1	1	0	5
Mekaini et al., 2014 [39]	1	1	1	1	1	0	1	1	1	8
Shitrit et al., 2005 [28]	1	0	1	1	0	1	1	1	1	7
Khamis et al., 2016 [40]	1	1	1	1	1	0	1	1	0	7
Garcell et al., 2014 [41]	1	1	1	1	1	0	1	1	0	7
Gunluoglu et al., 2015 [42]	1	0	1	1	0	1	1	1	1	7
Duman et al., 2014 [43]	1	0	1	1	0	1	1	1	1	7
Babayigit et al., 2014 [44]	1	0	1	1	0	1	1	1	1	7
Yilmaz et al., 2012 [29]	1	0	1	1	0	1	1	1	1	7
Hanta et al., 2012 [45]	1	0	1	1	0	1	1	1	0	6
Soysal et al., 2012 [46]	1	0	1	1	0	0	1	1	0	5
Caglayan et al., 2011 [47]	1	0	1	1	0	1	1	1	0	6
	1	0	1	1	0	1	1	1	0	6

Table 2: Continued.

Study	Clear study aims	Adequate sample size	Representative sample	Inclusion and exclusion criteria	Adequate assessment of outcome	Response rate reported	Adequate description of data	Appropriate statistical analysis	Appropriate informed consent obtained	Total score
Karadag et al., 2010 [48]										
Inanc et al., 2009 [49]	1	1	1	1	1	1	1	1	1	9
Seyhan et al., 2010 [50]	1	0	1	1	0	1	1	1	1	7
Hanta et al., 2008 [51]	1	0	1	1	0	1	1	1	0	6
Ozdemir et al., 2007 [52]	1	0	1	1	0	1	1	1	1	7
Bozkanat et al., 2016 [53]	1	0	1	1	0	1	1	1	0	6
Hasanain et al., 2018 [54]	1	0	1	1	0	0	1	1	1	6
El-Sokkary et al., 2015 [55]	1	0	1	1	0	1	1	1	1	7
Slouma et al., 2017 [56]	1	0	1	1	0	0	1	1	0	5
Khazraiyan et al., 2016 [57]	1	0	1	1	0	0	1	1	1	6
Jam et al., 2010 [30]	1	1	1	1	1	0	1	1	1	8
Amiri et al., 2014 [58]	1	1	1	1	1	0	1	1	0	7

*A sample size of ≥200 was considered as adequate and a sample size of <200 was considered as inadequate. †A response rate of <50% was considered as low = 0, and>50% was considered as high = 1.

prevalence was observed to be 41.78% (95% CI 31.18% to 52.78%, $I^2 = 99.31\%$).

The subgroup analyses revealed the existence of heterogeneity. In the gender-based subgroup analysis, some of the studies failed to mention the gender-based prevalence of LTBI, and hence 14 and 15 studies were excluded from the subgroup analysis of males and females, respectively; hence, the subgroup analysis of males was performed with 17 studies, and that of females with 16 studies. The analysis revealed that the proportion of LTBI ranged from 0.32% to 86.04% and from 0.54% to 90.90% in males and females, respectively. The overall prevalence was estimated to be 33.12% (95% CI 18.97% to 49.04%, $I^2 = 99.25\%$) and 32.65% (95% CI 19.79% to 47%, $I^2 = 98.89\%$) in males and females, respectively.

For the evaluation of age-based prevalence, the WHO classification for age groups was utilized, and the age range for children, adolescents, and adults was taken as <10 years, between 10 and 19 years, and >19 years, respectively; further, three studies, Shitrit et al. [28], Yilmaz et al. [29], and Jam et al. [30], were excluded from this subgroup analysis as the age of subjects in those studies overlapped the age range for children, adolescents, and adults, i.e., 12 years and above, 13 to 67 years, and 1 month to above 60 years, respectively. Moreover, there was no differentiation in the age range for the prevalence of LTBI in these studies; hence, the subgroup analysis of children, adolescents, and adults was performed with 1, 2, and 27 studies, respectively. The prevalence of LTBI in children was observed to be 0.44% (95% CI -0.05% to 0.9%); the prevalence of LTBI in adolescents and adults ranged from 2.46% to 3.55% and 6.93% to 88.15%, respectively. The overall prevalence was observed to be 3.37% (95% CI 2.23% to 4.74%, $I^2 = 0\%$) and 43.81% (95% CI 33.09% to 54.82%, $I^2 = 99.18\%$) for adolescents and adults, respectively.

4. Discussion

After screening 956 studies, a total of 31 scientific papers from ten countries within the MENA region were included in this systematic review [28–58]. The subjects included in these studies were healthcare workers, laboratory staff, medical school students, people living with HIV, and patients with chronic inflammatory diseases. The detection of LTBI in these studies was performed by TST or IGRA or both; furthermore, the studies covered the incidence of LTBI among populations belonging to varying age groups, including children, adolescents, and adults.

In the present study, LTBI prevalence was evaluated by employing the random effects model since high heterogeneity was encountered among studies. The existence of high heterogeneity may have possibly been due to variations in study settings, subjects or participants, methodologies involved, exposure to TB patients, and the control measures taken across the studies.

The overall prevalence of LTBI in the MENA region was found to be 41.78%. In the gender-based subgroup analyses, the prevalence of LTBI was found to be 33.12% and 32.65% in males and females, respectively. As for the age-based prevalence, it was assessed to be 0.44%, 3.37%, and 43.81% in children, adolescents, and adults, respectively; therefore, this systematic review implies a high prevalence of LTBI in the MENA region irrespective of gender, and in order to achieve the WHO End TB 2035 objective, there is an immediate need to scale up measures to stop TB disease and enhance LTBI detection within the MENA region.

There are some strengths and limitations within this study that needs to be highlighted; first, as per our findings, this is the first systematic review on the epidemiology and prevalence of LTBI in the MENA region. As for limitations, studies published in English alone have been included, therefore, other reports from countries with high TB incidence that are published in native or other languages other than English, in national or local journals, have not been included; additionally, studies published in journals indexed in PubMed and Google Scholar were included, while other studies may exist that were published in other indexing databases.

To conclude, this review indicates a high prevalence of LTBI in the MENA region despite the high heterogeneity observed. Future studies should aim towards more rigorous assessment of LTBI prevalence within the MENA region to reach exact estimates as the first important step to hamper TB disease diffusion in these countries.

References

[1] Global tuberculosis report 2018, *World Health Organization*, Licence: CC BY-NC-SA 3.0 IGO, Geneva, 2018, Jan 2019 (https://www.who.int/tb/publications/global_report/en/).

[2] E. L. Corbett, C. J. Watt, N. Walker et al., "The growing burden of tuberculosis: global trends and interactions with the HIV epidemic," *Archives of Internal Medicine*, vol. 163, no. 9, pp. 1009–1021, 2003.

[3] M. Legesse, G. Ameni, G. Mamo, G. Medhin, G. Bjune, and F. Abebe, "Community-based cross-sectional survey of latent tuberculosis infection in Afar pastoralists, Ethiopia, using QuantiFERON-TB Gold In-Tube and tuberculin skin test," *BMC Infectious Diseases*, vol. 11, no. 1, pp. 89–97, 2011.

[4] F. N. Kizza, J. List, A. K. Nkwata et al., "Prevalence of latent tuberculosis infection and associated risk factors in an urban African setting," *BMC Infectious Diseases*, vol. 15, no. 1, pp. 165–173, 2015.

[5] H. Mahomed, T. Hawkridge, S. Verver et al., "Predictive factors for latent tuberculosis infection among adolescents in a high-burden area in South Africa," *The International Journal of Tuberculosis and Lung Disease*, vol. 15, no. 3, pp. 331–336, 2011.

[6] E. E. Àlvarez-León, E. Espinosa-Vega, E. Santana-Rodríguez et al., "Screening for tuberculosis infection in Spanish healthcare workers comparison of the QuantiFERON-TB Gold In-Tube test with the tuberculin skin test," *Infection Control and Hospital Epidemiology*, vol. 30, no. 9, pp. 876–883, 2009.

[7] M. Pai, S. Kalantri, A. N. Aggarwal, D. Menzies, and H. M. Blumberg, "Nosocomial tuberculosis in India," *Emerging Infectious Diseases*, vol. 12, no. 7, pp. 1311–1318, 2006.

[8] K. Lee, M. K. Han, H. R. Choi et al., "Annual incidence of latent tuberculosis infection among newly employed nurses at a tertiary care university hospital," *Infection Control and Hospital Epidemiology*, vol. 30, no. 12, pp. 1218–1222, 2009.

[9] P. Khanna, V. Nikolayevsky, F. Warburton, E. Dobson, and F. Drob-niewski, "Rate of latent tuberculosis infection detected by occupational health screening of nurses new to a London teaching hospital," *Infection Control and Hospital Epidemiology*, vol. 30, no. 6, pp. 581–584, 2009.

[10] M. Mondoni, O. Viganò, M. Ferrarese et al., "Haemoptysis and fever in a young refugee from Somalia," *International Journal of Infectious Diseases*, vol. 77, pp. 57–60, 2018.

[11] M. Sester, U. Sester, P. Clauer et al., "Tuberculin skin testing underestimates a high prevalence of latent tuberculosis infection in hemodialysis patients," *Kidney International*, vol. 65, no. 5, pp. 1826–1834, 2004.

[12] C. D. Hamilton, "Infectious complications of treatment with biologic agents," *Current Opinion in Rheumatology*, vol. 16, no. 4, pp. 393–398, 2004.

[13] American Thoracic Society, "Targeted tuberculin testing and treatment of latent tuberculosis infection," *American Journal of Respiratory and Critical Care Medicine*, vol. 161, pp. 221–247, 2000.

[14] M. J. Field, *Tuberculosis in the Workplace*, National Academy Press, Washington, DC, 2001.

[15] D. Menzies, M. Pai, and G. Comstock, "Meta-analysis: new tests for the diagnosis of latent tuberculosis infection: areas of uncertainty and recommendations for research," *Annals of Internal Medicine*, vol. 146, no. 5, pp. 340–354, 2007.

[16] A. Mathew, T. David, K. Thomas et al., "Risk factors for tuberculosis among health care workers in South India: a nested

case-control study," *Journal of Clinical Epidemiology*, vol. 66, no. 1, pp. 67–74, 2013.

[17] H. Getahun, A. Matteelli, R. E. Chaisson, and M. Raviglione, "Latent mycobacterium tuberculosis infection," *The New England Journal of Medicine*, vol. 372, no. 22, pp. 2127–2135, 2015.

[18] J. Keane and B. Bresnihan, "Tuberculosis reactivation during immunosuppressive therapy in rheumatic diseases: diagnostic and therapeutic strategies," *Current Opinion in Rheumatology*, vol. 20, no. 4, pp. 443–449, 2008.

[19] A. O'Garra, P. S. Redford, F. W. McNab, C. I. Bloom, R. J. Wilkinson, and M. P. R. Berry, "The immune response in tuberculosis," *Annual Review of Immunology*, vol. 31, no. 1, pp. 475–527, 2013.

[20] M. Pai, K. Gokhale, R. Joshi et al., "Mycobacterium tuberculosis infection in health care workers in rural India," *JAMA*, vol. 293, no. 22, pp. 2746–2755, 2005.

[21] Y. A. Kang, H. W. Lee, H. I. Yoon et al., "Discrepancy between the tuberculin skin test and the whole-blood interferon γ assay for the diagnosis of latent tuberculosis infection in an intermediate tuberculosis-burden country," *JAMA*, vol. 293, no. 22, pp. 2756–2761, 2005.

[22] N. Harada, Y. Nakajima, K. Higuchi, Y. Sekiya, J. Rothel, and T. Mori, "Screening for tuberculosis infection using whole-blood interferon-γ and Mantoux testing among Japanese healthcare workers," *Infection Control and Hospital Epidemiology*, vol. 27, no. 5, pp. 442–448, 2006.

[23] N. N. Chegou, J. Heyckendorf, G. Walzl, C. Lange, and M. Ruhwald, "Beyond the IFN-γ horizon: biomarkers for immunodiagnosis of infection with mycobacterium tuberculosis," *The European Respiratory Journal*, vol. 43, no. 5, pp. 1472–1486, 2014.

[24] D. M. Lewinsohn, M. K. Leonard, P. A. LoBue et al., "Official American thoracic society/infectious diseases society of America/centers for disease control and prevention clinical practice guidelines: diagnosis of tuberculosis in adults and children," *Clinical Infectious Diseases*, vol. 64, no. 2, pp. 111–115, 2017.

[25] P. Andersen, M. E. Munk, J. M. Pollock, and T. M. Doherty, "Specific immune-based diagnosis of tuberculosis," *Lancet*, vol. 356, no. 9235, pp. 1099–1104, 2000.

[26] S. M. Arend, K. E. van Meijgaarden, K. de Boer et al., "Tuberculin skin testing and in vitro T cell responses to ESAT-6 and culture filtrate protein 10 after infection with Mycobacterium marinum or M. kansasii," *The Journal of Infectious Diseases*, vol. 186, no. 12, pp. 1797–1807, 2002.

[27] I. Mirza and R. Jenkins, "Risk factors, prevalence, and treatment of anxiety and depressive disorders in Pakistan: systematic review," *BMJ*, vol. 328, no. 7443, p. 794, 2004.

[28] D. Shitrit, G. Izbicki, A. B. Shitrit, M. Raz, J. Sulkes, and M. R. Kramer, "Normal D-dimer levels in patients with latent tuberculosis infection," *Blood Coagulation & Fibrinolysis*, vol. 16, no. 1, pp. 85–87, 2005.

[29] N. Yilmaz, S. Zehra Aydin, N. Inanc, S. Karakurt, H. Direskeneli, and S. Yavuz, "Comparison of QuantiFERON-TB Gold test and tuberculin skin test for the identification of latent mycobacterium tuberculosis infection in lupus patients," *Lupus*, vol. 21, no. 5, pp. 491–495, 2012.

[30] S. Jam, D. Sabzvari, S. SeyedAlinaghi, F. Fattahi, H. Jabbari, and M. Mohraz, "Frequency of mycobacterium tuberculosis infection among Iranian patients with HIV/AIDS by PPD test," *Acta Medica Iranica*, vol. 48, no. 1, pp. 67–71, 2010.

[31] M. Nasehi, A. Hashemi-Shahraki, A. Doosti-Irani, S. Sharafi, and E. Mostafavi, "Prevalence of latent tuberculosis infection among tuberculosis laboratory workers in Iran," *Epidemiology and Health*, vol. 39, p. e2017002, 2017.

[32] M. Mamani, H. Mahmudian, M. M. Majzoobi, and J. Poorolajal, "Prevalence and incidence rates of latent tuberculous infection in a large prison in Iran," *The International Journal of Tuberculosis and Lung Disease*, vol. 20, no. 8, pp. 1072–1077, 2016.

[33] Z. A. Bukhary, S. M. Amer, M. M. Emara, M. E. Abdalla, and S. A. Ali, "Screening of latent tuberculosis infection among health care workers working in Hajj pilgrimage area in Saudi Arabia, using interferon gamma release assay and tuberculin skin test," *Annals of Saudi Medicine*, vol. 38, no. 2, pp. 90–96, 2018.

[34] H. H. Balkhy, K. El Beltagy, A. El-Saed et al., "Prevalence of latent mycobacterium tuberculosis infection (LTBI) in Saudi Arabia; population based survey," *International Journal of Infectious Diseases*, vol. 60, pp. 11–16, 2017.

[35] M. El-Helaly, W. Khan, A. El-Saed, and H. H. Balkhy, "Pre-employment screening of latent tuberculosis infection among healthcare workers using tuberculin skin test and QuantiFERON-TB Gold test at a tertiary care hospital in Saudi Arabia," *Journal of Infection and Public Health*, vol. 7, no. 6, pp. 481–488, 2014.

[36] M. I. Hassan and A. E. Diab, "Detection of latent tuberculosis infection among laboratory personnel at a University Hospital in Eastern Saudi Arabia using an interferon gamma release assay," *Journal of Infection and Public Health*, vol. 7, no. 4, pp. 289–295, 2014.

[37] M. A. Abbas, N. A. AlHamdan, L. A. Fiala, A. K. AlEnezy, and M. S. AlQahtani, "Prevalence of latent TB among health care workers in four major tertiary care hospitals in Riyadh, Saudi Arabia," *The Journal of the Egyptian Public Health Association*, vol. 85, no. 1-2, pp. 61–71, 2010.

[38] P. Warrington, G. Tyrrell, K. Choy, L. Eisenbeis, R. Long, and R. Cooper, "Prevalence of latent tuberculosis infection in Syrian refugees to Canada," *Canadian Journal of Public Health*, vol. 109, no. 1, pp. 8–14, 2018.

[39] L. A. Al Mekaini, O. N. Al Jabri, H. Narchi et al., "The use of an interferon-gamma release assay to screen for pediatric latent tuberculosis infection in the eastern region of the Emirate of Abu Dhabi," *International Journal of Infectious Diseases*, vol. 23, pp. 4–7, 2014.

[40] F. Khamis, A. Al-Lawati, I. Al-Zakwani et al., "Latent tuberculosis in health care workers exposed to active tuberculosis in a tertiary care hospital in Oman," *Oman Medical Journal*, vol. 31, no. 4, pp. 298–303, 2016.

[41] H. Guanche Garcell, E. Crespo Ramirez, A. Kindelan Contreras, and G. F. Gutierrez, "Latent tuberculosis infection in healthcare workers at a community hospital in Qatar," *Journal of Infection and Public Health*, vol. 7, no. 4, pp. 356–359, 2014.

[42] G. Gunluoglu, E. C. Seyhan, R. Kazancioglu et al., "Diagnosing latent tuberculosis in immunocompromised patients measuring blood IP-10 production capacity: an analysis of chronic renal failure patients," *Internal Medicine*, vol. 54, no. 5, pp. 465–472, 2015.

[43] N. Duman, S. Ersoy-Evans, O. Karadağ et al., "Screening for latent tuberculosis infection in psoriasis and psoriatic arthritis patients in a tuberculosis-endemic country: a comparison of the QuantiFERON®-TB Gold In-Tube test and tuberculin skin test," *International Journal of Dermatology*, vol. 53, no. 10, pp. 1286–1292, 2014.

[44] C. Babayigit, B. Ozer, C. Ozer, T. Inandi, N. Duran, and O. Gocmen, "Performance of QuantiFERON-TB Gold In-Tube test and tuberculin skin test for diagnosis of latent tuberculosis infection in BCG vaccinated health care workers," *Medical Science Monitor*, vol. 20, pp. 521–529, 2014.

[45] I. Hanta, S. Ozbek, S. Kuleci, G. Seydaoglu, and E. Ozyilmaz, "Detection of latent tuberculosis infection in rheumatologic diseases before anti-TNFα therapy: tuberculin skin test versus IFN-γ assay," *Rheumatology International*, vol. 32, no. 11, pp. 3599–3603, 2012.

[46] A. Soysal, D. Toprak, M. Koc, H. Arikan, E. Akoglu, and M. Bakir, "Diagnosing latent tuberculosis infection in haemodialysis patients: T-cell based assay (T-SPOT.TB) or tuberculin skin test?," *Nephrol dial transplant*, vol. 27, no. 4, pp. 1645–1650, 2012.

[47] V. Cağlayan, O. Ak, G. Dabak et al., "Comparison of tuberculin skin testing and QuantiFERON-TB Gold-In Tube test in health care workers," *Tüberküloz ve Toraks*, vol. 59, no. 1, pp. 43–47, 2011.

[48] O. Karadag, K. Aksu, A. Sahin et al., "Assessment of latent tuberculosis infection in Takayasu arteritis with tuberculin skin test and Quantiferon-TB Gold test," *Rheumatology International*, vol. 30, no. 11, pp. 1483–1487, 2010.

[49] N. Inanc, S. Z. Aydin, S. Karakurt, P. Atagunduz, S. Yavuz, and H. Direskeneli, "Agreement between Quantiferon-TB gold test and tuberculin skin test in the identification of latent tuberculosis infection in patients with rheumatoid arthritis and ankylosing spondylitis," *The Journal of Rheumatology*, vol. 36, no. 12, pp. 2675–2681, 2009.

[50] E. C. Seyhan, S. Sökücü, S. Altin et al., "Comparison of the QuantiFERON-TB Gold In-Tube test with the tuberculin skin test for detecting latent tuberculosis infection in hemodialysis patients," *Transplant Infectious Disease*, vol. 12, no. 2, pp. 98–105, 2010.

[51] I. Hanta, S. Ozbek, S. Kuleci, and A. Kocabas, "The evaluation of latent tuberculosis in rheumatologic diseases for anti-TNF therapy: experience with 192 patients," *Clinical Rheumatology*, vol. 27, no. 9, pp. 1083–1086, 2008.

[52] D. Ozdemir, A. N. Annakkaya, G. Tarhan et al., "Comparison of the tuberculin skin test and the QuantiFERON test for latent mycobacterium tuberculosis infections in health care workers in Turkey," *Japanese Journal of Infectious Diseases*, vol. 60, no. 2-3, pp. 102–105, 2007.

[53] E. Bozkanat, H. Kaya, O. Sezer et al., "Comparison of tuberculin skin test and QuantiFERON-TB gold in tube test for diagnosis of latent tuberculosis infection in health care workers: a cross sectional study," *The Journal of the Pakistan Medical Association*, vol. 66, no. 3, pp. 270–274, 2016.

[54] A. F. A. Hasanain, A. M. A. Mahran, A. S. Safwat et al., "Latent tuberculosis infection among patients with erectile dysfunction," *International Journal of Impotence Research*, vol. 30, no. 1, pp. 36–42, 2018.

[55] R. H. El-Sokkary, A. M. Abu-Taleb, O. S. El-Seifi et al., "Assessing the prevalence of latent tuberculosis among health care providers in Zagazig City, Egypt using tuberculin skin test and QuantiFERON-TB Gold In-Tube Test," *Central European Journal of Public Health*, vol. 23, no. 4, pp. 324–330, 2015.

[56] M. Slouma, I. Mahmoud, O. Saidane, S. Bouden, and L. Abdelmoula, "Depistage de la tuberculose latente chez les patients candidats a un traitement biologique en Tunisie," *Thérapie*, vol. 72, no. 5, pp. 573–578, 2017.

[57] H. Khazraiyan, Z. A. Liaei, H. E. Koochak, F. A. Ardalan, Z. Ahmadinejad, and A. Soltani, "Utility of QuantiFERON-TB Gold In-Tube test in the diagnosis of latent TB in HIV-positive patients in a medium-TB burden country," *Journal of the International Association of Providers of AIDS Care (JIAPAC)*, vol. 15, no. 2, pp. 101–106, 2015.

[58] F. B. Amiri, M. M. Gouya, M. Saifi et al., "Vulnerability of homeless people in Tehran, Iran, to HIV, tuberculosis and viral hepatitis," *PLoS One*, vol. 9, no. 6, article e98742, 2014.

Diffuse Idiopathic Pulmonary Neuroendocrine Cell Hyperplasia (DIPNECH): A Case of Indolent Pulmonary Nodules Diagnosed with Robotic-Assisted Navigational Bronchoscopy

Adam Purdy, Firas Ido, and Deborah Stahlnecker

Division of Pulmonary and Critical Care, St. Luke's University Health Network, Bethlehem, PA, USA

Correspondence should be addressed to Adam Purdy; adam.purdy@sluhn.org

Academic Editor: Tomonobu Koizumi

Diffuse idiopathic pulmonary neuroendocrine cell hyperplasia (DIPNECH) is an atypical pulmonary disorder with limited understanding. Given the rare nature of this disease, it is essential to obtain adequate tissue pathology to confirm the diagnosis. This disease is mainly diagnosed in middle-aged, nonsmoking females, and it is now accepted as a precursor lesion to pulmonary carcinoid tumors. DIPNECH presents with characteristic radiographic and histologic findings, but its diagnosis, management, and prognosis are often underrecognized and poorly understood. Those with symptoms may present with shortness of breath, wheezing, and persistent cough and are often misdiagnosed with reactive airway disease. Pulmonary function testing may reveal airflow obstruction and air trapping. Imaging is characterized by multiple lung nodules, typically less than 5 mm in size, with a background mosaic attenuation on computed tomography imaging. Histologically, DIPNECH can be suspected based on the presence of hyperplastic neuroendocrine cells. DIPNECH is considered a precursor to invasive neuroendocrine tumor, and up to 50% of patients may have a well-differentiated neuroendocrine tumor at the time of presentation. Here, we present the case of a 46-year-old female with a history of ulcerative colitis on mesalamine who presented with a 6-month history of ongoing shortness of breath, chest tightness, wheezing, and cough. She was initially diagnosed with asthma before imaging later revealed as multiple pulmonary nodules with a diffuse mosaic pattern. Using robotic-assisted navigational bronchoscopy, she underwent sampling of a dominant 1.8 cm right middle lobe pulmonary nodule and pathology was consistent with low-grade neuroendocrine tumor.

1. Introduction

Diffuse idiopathic pulmonary neuroendocrine cell hyperplasia (DIPNECH) is a rare pulmonary disorder that is being reported with increasing frequency. It was not fully recognized and reported until 1992, when it was described in 6 nonsmoking, mainly female patients, who presented with cough and shortness of breath (1). DIPNECH is now recognized by the World Health Organization (WHO) classification of lung tumors as a preneoplastic lesion (2). Surgical lung biopsy is accepted as the "gold standard" for diagnosis. However, navigational bronchoscopy has emerged as a less-invasive and important modality to aid in the diagnosis of this rare disease.

2. Case

We present the case of a 46 year-old-female, never smoker, with a history of ulcerative colitis who initially presented as an outpatient for the evaluation of persistent cough, wheezing, and chest tightness for 6 months. Her review of systems was otherwise negative and her only medication included mesalamine for ulcerative colitis. She had no history of environmental or occupational exposures and denied any allergies. She denied any personal or family history of lung disease. Her vital signs were within normal limits. This patient was evaluated by pulmonology and was diagnosed with cough variant asthma and was started on montelukast

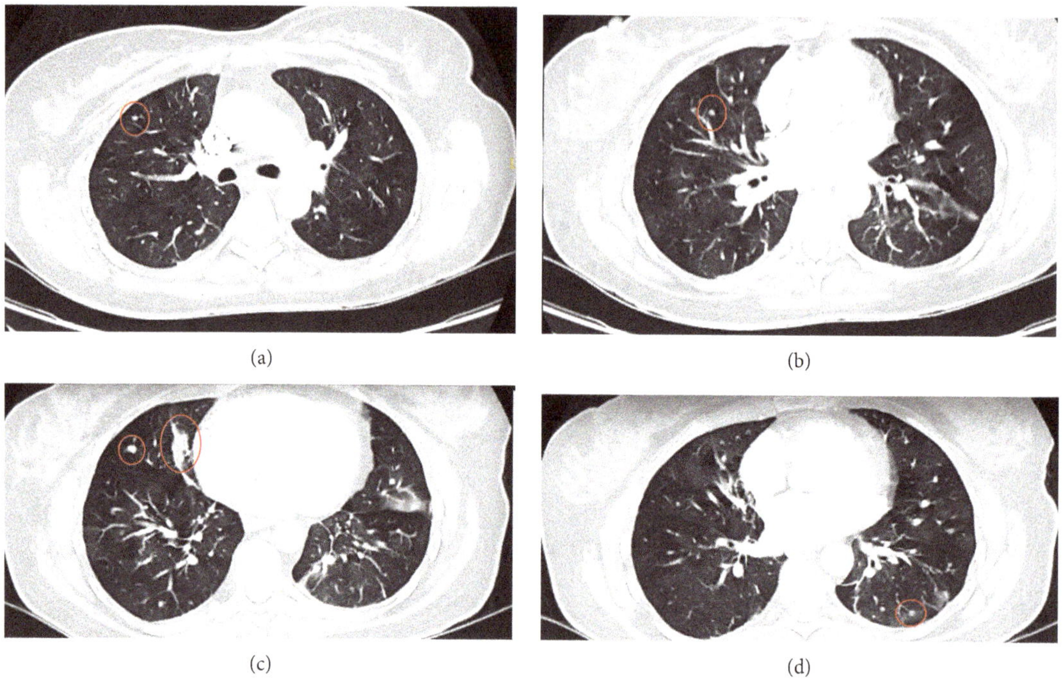

Figure 1: CT chest with diffuse mosaic attenuation and multiple pulmonary nodules: (a) 4 mm right upper lobe nodule; (b) 4 mm right middle lobe nodule; (c) 7 mm lateral right middle lobe nodule with confluent 1.8 cm medial right middle lobe nodule; (d) 4 mm left lower lobe nodule.

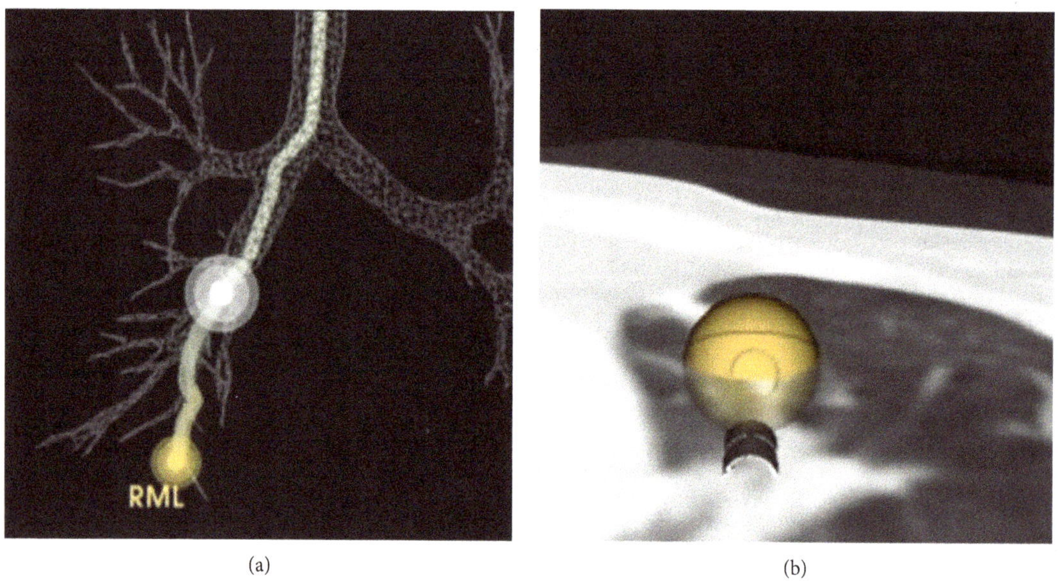

Figure 2: (a) Monarch robotic-assisted navigational bronchoscopy path to the right middle lobe lung nodule. (b) Axial computed tomography imaging superimposed on the robotic-assisted pathway to the right middle lobe lung nodule.

and albuterol as needed. A northeast allergy panel was unremarkable. She subsequently presented to the emergency room with an episode of wheezing and chest tightness and Computed Tomography Angiogram (CTA) revealed multiple lung nodules with mosaic attenuation. The nodules were seen bilaterally in clusters, with the largest measuring up to 1.8 cm in the right middle lobe. Multiple serologic markers were ordered to screen for autoimmune disease including ANA, ANCA, anti-dsDNA, hypersensitivity pneumonitis panel, Sjogren's antibodies, angiotensin converting enzyme, and rheumatoid factor. These were unremarkable other than a positive ANA with titer 1 : 640 homogenous pattern. Due to uncontrolled symptoms, her inhaler regime was escalated to Flovent twice daily with as needed albuterol. A repeat CT chest 3 months later indicated no change in diffuse mosaicism and multiple pulmonary nodules, similar in size, with the

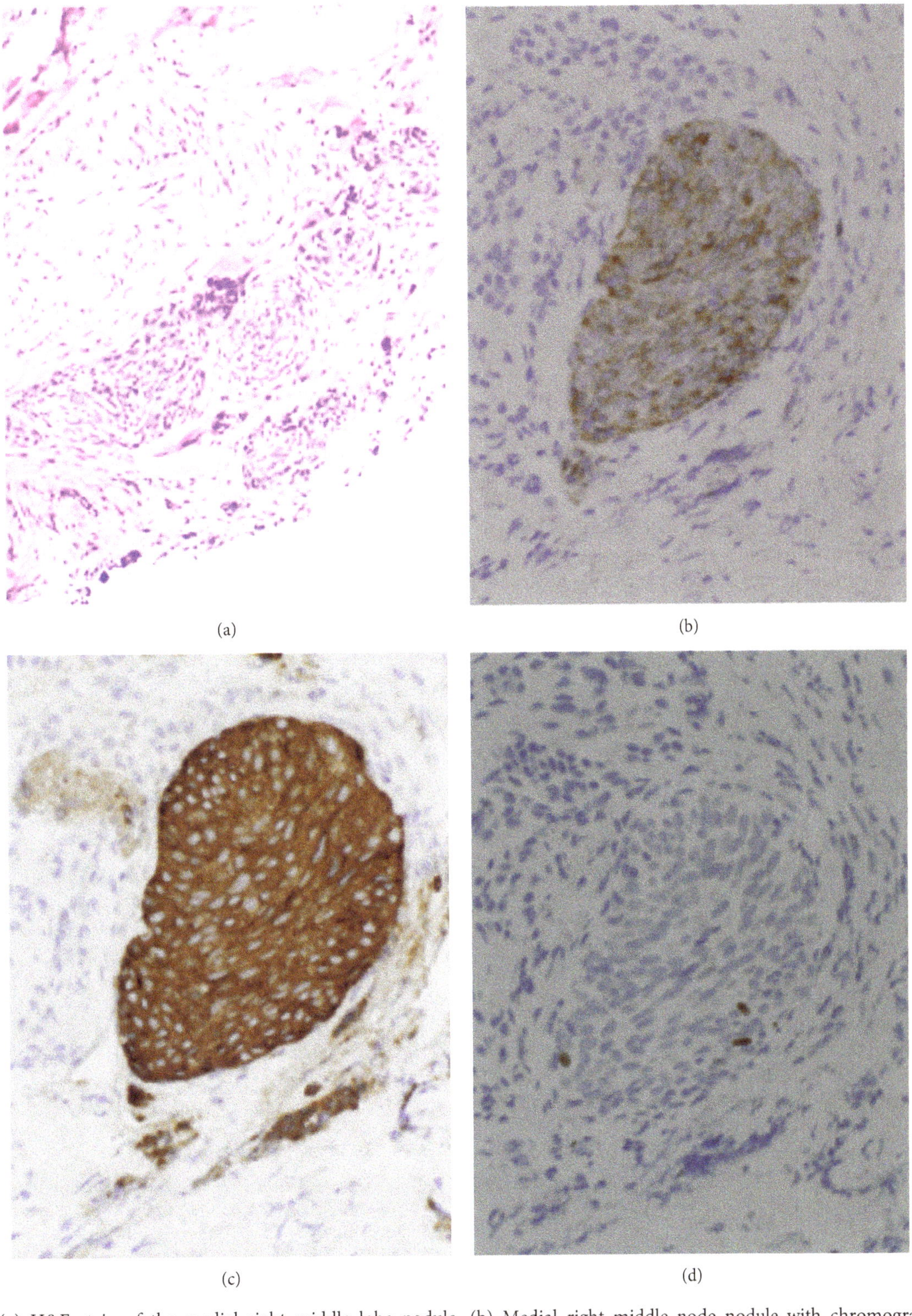

FIGURE 3: (a) H&E stain of the medial right middle lobe nodule. (b) Medial right middle node nodule with chromogranin-positive pathology, a neuroendocrine marker. (c) Medial right middle lobe nodule with synaptophysin-positive pathology, another marker for neuroendocrine cells. (d) Medial right middle lobe nodule with a Ki-67 proliferation marker with only 3 nuclei staining positive.

largest 1.8 cm in the right middle lobe (Figures 1(a)–1(d)). She then underwent robotic-assisted navigational bronchoscopy with fine needle aspiration, brushing, and transbronchial biopsy of the right middle lobe nodule (Figures 2(a) and2(b)). Pathology from the nodule was positive for groups of bland appearing small blue cells, consistent with low-grade neuroendocrine tumor (carcinoid). Pathology was positive for chromogranin and synaptophysin, neuroendocrine markers, and low Ki-67 positivity, indicating low rate of proliferation (Figures 3(a)–3(d)). Endobronchial ultrasound was also performed and Level 7 lymph node was negative for malignancy. The patient was presented at multidisciplinary chest tumor conference and it was recommended that she undergo PET CT scan and surgical resection of the biopsy-proven typical carcinoid tumor in the right middle lobe.

3. Discussion

Diffuse idiopathic pulmonary neuroendocrine cell hyperplasia (DIPNECH) is a rare pulmonary condition. This condition leads to a proliferation of neuroendocrine cells that can be confined to the lung mucosa, cause local invasion, or progress into invasive carcinoid tumors. It is primarily diagnosed in middle-aged, nonsmokers, with a female predominance (3).

Most symptomatic patients present with a long history of cough, shortness of breath, and wheezing. These patients are often misdiagnosed with asthma and there is a significant time lag before the correct diagnosis is made. The average length of time between symptom onset and diagnosis is between 9 and 16 years (4). Most patients have airflow obstruction and air trapping on pulmonary function testing. Radiographic imaging may reveal nodular bronchial wall thickening caused by intraluminal protrusion of proliferating cells, bilateral pulmonary nodules (typically 5 mm or less), ground glass mosaicism consistent with air trapping, and bronchiectasis (3). Pulmonary nodules are assumed to be well-differentiated lung neuroendocrine tumors and most express somatostatin receptors (5). Histologically, the cells are round or spindle-shaped and have a moderate amount of eosinophilic cytoplasm with round to oval nuclei. Constrictive obliterative bronchiolitis, which represents the histological hallmark of DIPNECH, is indicated by mild, chronic inflammatory cell infiltrate and wall thickening and fibrosis of involved airways, leading to narrowing and possible obliteration of the bronchial lumen (2). Due to the presence of neuroendocrine tumorlets and hyperplasia, DIPNECH is considered a precursor to invasive neuroendocrine tumor and, at diagnosis, approximately 50% of patients have a synchronous well-differentiated neuroendocrine tumor (6). Given this, tumors greater than 5 mm in size can be considered carcinoid tumors and should be biopsied (7). It is essential to obtain adequate pathology and bronchoscopy with navigation may be needed for peripheral nodules. Expression of somatostatin receptors in tumorlets and carcinoid cells can be demonstrated by scintigraphy with octreotide or histology (8).

Due to the rare nature of this disease, data on treatment and outcomes are limited. The majority of patients are treated with steroid-based therapy (inhaled and systemic), in an effort to reduce the inflammatory response induced by neuroendocrine cell-secreted neuropeptides (9). Bronchodilator therapy can be beneficial in treating symptoms. Octreotide, a somatostatin analogue, has been used with some success in the presence of somatostatin receptors. This is similarly used to reduce the hormonal hypersecretion of neuroendocrine cells in gastrointestinal and bronchial carcinoids (10). The course of this disease is extremely variable. Many patients will have a slowly progressive or stable clinical course, while fewer may have marked constrictive bronchiolitis, which may progress to severe airflow obstruction.

4. Conclusion

There are no well-established guidelines for the diagnosis, treatment, and management of diffuse idiopathic pulmonary neuroendocrine cell hyperplasia (DIPNECH), given the rarity of this disease. It should not be overlooked given its classification as a preneoplastic process and ability to transform into invasive carcinoid tumor. Our patient was found to have a low-grade carcinoid tumor, and it was recommended that she undergo resection. Given the rarity of DIPNECH, long-term prognosis is variable and this patient must be monitored closely.

References

[1] G. Rossi, A. Cavazza, P. Spagnolo et al., "Diffuse idiopathic pulmonary neuroendocrine cell hyperplasia syndrome," *European Respiratory Journal*, vol. 47, no. 6, pp. 1829–1841, 2016.

[2] J. R. Gosney, J. H. M. Austin, and J. Jett, "Diffuse pulmonary neuroendocrine cell hyperplasia," in *WHO classification of tumours of the lung, pleura, thymus and heart*, pp. 78-79, IARC Press, Lyon, 2015.

[3] A. A. Nassar, D. E. Jaroszewski, R. A. Helmers, T. V. Colby, B. M. Patel, and F. Mookadam, "Diffuse idiopathic pulmonary neuroendocrine cell Hyperplasia," *American Journal of Respiratory and Critical Care Medicine*, vol. 184, no. 1, pp. 8–16, 2011.

[4] S. J. Davies, J. R. Gosney, D. M. Hansell et al., "Diffuse idiopathic pulmonary neuroendocrine cell hyperplasia: an underrecognised spectrum of disease," *Thorax*, vol. 62, no. 3, pp. 248–252, 2007.

[5] A. Gorshtein, D. J. Gross, D. Barak et al., "Diffuse idiopathic pulmonary neuroendocrine cell hyperplasia and the associated lung neuroendocrine tumors: clinical experience with a rare entity," *Cancer*, vol. 118, no. 3, pp. 612–619, 2012.

[6] M.-C. Aubry, C. F. Thomas, J. R. Jett, S. J. Swensen, and J. L. Myers, "Significance of multiple carcinoid tumors and tumorlets in surgical lung specimens: analysis of 28 patients," *Chest*, vol. 131, no. 6, pp. 1635–1643, 2007.

[7] G. Ofikwu, V. R. Mani, A. Rajabalan, A. Adu, L. Ahmed, and D. Vega, "A rare case of diffuse idiopathic pulmonary neuroendocrine cell hyperplasia," *Case Reports in Surgery*, vol. 2015, Article ID 318175, 2015.

[8] L. Righi, M. Volante, V. Tavaglione et al., "Somatostatin receptor tissue distribution in lung neuroendocrine tumours: a clinicopathologic and immunohistochemical study of 218 'clinically aggressive' cases," *Annals of Oncology*, vol. 21, no. 3, pp. 548–555, 2010.

[9] S. Degan, G. Y. Lopez, K. Kevill, and M. E. Sunday, "Gastrin-releasing peptide, immune responses, and lung disease," *Annals of the New York Academy of Sciences*, vol. 1144, no. 1, pp. 136–147, 2008.

[10] S. W. J. Lamberts, A.-J. van der Lely, W. W. de Herder, and L. J. Hofland, "Octreotide," *The New England Journal of Medicine*, vol. 334, no. 4, pp. 246–254, 1996.

21

Pulmonary Arterial Hypertension Specific Therapy in Patients with Combined Post- and Precapillary Pulmonary Hypertension

Hassan Alfraidi,[1,2] **Sultan Qanash**,[1,3] **and Zoheir Bshouty**[1]

[1]*Section of Pulmonary Medicine, Department of Medicine, University of Manitoba, Winnipeg, MB, Canada*
[2]*Division of Cardiology, Department of Medicine, McGill University, Montreal, QC, Canada*
[3]*King Saud Bin Abdulaziz University for Health Sciences, King Abdulaziz Medical City, Jeddah, Saudi Arabia*

Correspondence should be addressed to Zoheir Bshouty; zbshouty@hsc.mb.ca

Academic Editor: Dimitris Georgopoulos

Background. Specific therapy for patients with PAH is associated with good outcomes. Little is known about the effect of this treatment in patients with Cpc-PH (PAPm ≥ 25 mmHg, PAWP > 15 mmHg, DPG ≥ 7 mmHg, and/or PVR > 3 WU). This study evaluates the outcome of treating patients with Cpc-PH using PAH specific therapy. *Methods.* The primary outcome was survival. Secondary outcomes were WHO functional class and 6-minute walk distance (6-MWD). *Results.* Twenty-six patients with Cpc-PH (half with VHD and half with HF) received PAHST. Six patients did not tolerate treatment due to pulmonary edema. No predictors for treatment intolerance were identified. In twenty patients who tolerated the treatment, the mean WHO functional class improved from 2.70 ± 0.21 at initial assessment to 2.22 ± 0.21 ($p < 0.04$) and 2.06 ± 0.21 ($p < 0.03$) at 6 and 9 months, respectively. Mean 6-MWD improved from 276.0 ± 38.50 meters at initial assessment to 343.9 ± 22.99 meters ($p < 0.04$) and 364.6 ± 34.85 meters ($p = 0.07$) at 6 and 9 months, respectively. Twelve patients died during the follow-up period. Mean survival for all patients was 1279.7 ± 193.60 days. *Conclusion.* PAHST may be beneficial in the treatment of Cpc-PH (both short and long term). Prospective randomized controlled trials of PAHST in this population are needed to assess its potential efficacy.

1. Background

Pulmonary Hypertension (PH) is defined as Mean Pulmonary Artery Pressure (PAPm) ≥ 25 mmHg [1]. Pulmonary Arterial Hypertension (PAH) (also termed precapillary PH) is diagnosed when, in addition, PAWP is ≤15 mmHg [1]. Postcapillary PH is defined as PH due to left ventricular dysfunction (either myocardial and/or valvular) when PAWP is >15 mmHg [2, 3]. Isolated postcapillary PH (Ipc-PH) is said to be present when Diastolic Pressure Gradient (DPG = Diastolic PAP − PAWP) is <7 mmHg and PVR ≤ 3 WU [2].

Combined postcapillary and precapillary pulmonary hypertension (Cpc-PH) is a newly recognized entity in which PAWP > 15 mmHg and DPG ≥ 7 mmHg and/or PVR > 3 WU [2–4]. This group was previously referred to as having an "out-of-proportion" elevation in PAPm [3, 4] and represents almost 30% of the PAH patients. In spite of the above, it is worth noting that criteria for what constitutes "out of proportion" are not universally accepted [3, 4]. Some experts [5] have suggested a transpulmonary pressure gradient (TPG = PAPm − PAWP) of >12 mmHg in the setting of PAWP > 15 mmHg as a diagnostic criteria. However, using a fixed TPG or DPG [6, 7] without consideration of Cardiac Output and PAWP in a quite distensible vascular bed is physiologically unsound. In the normal pulmonary circulation, previous studies have shown that the rise in PAPm as a response to a rise in left atrial pressure (LAP) is nonlinear and is highly affected by mean alveolar pressure [8–10]. Raising LAP between zero and 10 mmHg causes hardly any rise in PAPm. As LAP further increases, the rise in PAPm (in proportion to the rise in LAP) increases gradually and approaches a 1 : 1 relationship only at very high LAP (in excess of 25 mmHg) [8–11]. Furthermore, the relationship between PAPm and

LAP in the setting of PAH (and in various disease severities) is not known.

Data from the REVEAL registry has shown that PAH associated with PAWP > 19 mmHg has an increase mortality compared to PAWP < 15 mmHg [12, 13]. Despite the cardinal component of PAH (precapillary), those patients remain untreated with PAHST due to concerns extrapolated from outcomes in the management of patients with heart failure [14, 15]. PAHST is confined mainly to PAH, which mandates the absence of elevated left atrial pressure reflected by PAWP < 15 mmHg [1]. In this study, we evaluated the outcome of treating Cpc-PH with PAHST.

2. Methods

2.1. Study Design. This is a retrospective descriptive study of data obtained from the pulmonary hypertension registry (PHR) at the University of Manitoba (Health Science Centre, Winnipeg, MB). The data in the PHR is collected prospectively from a patient's initial assessment throughout every clinic visit following treatment initiation (approximately every 3 months). The PHR includes comprehensive data related to demographics, comorbidities, prior and concomitant medications, all required investigations to establish a proper diagnosis including invasive and noninvasive hemodynamic parameters, WHO functional class, and 6-minute walk distance (6-MWD). Data collection into the PHR was approved by the University of Manitoba research ethics board.

2.2. Assessments and Definitions. The definition of PH used in the study was based on the latest consensus [5th World Symposium of Pulmonary Hypertension, WSPH, [1]]. PH was defined as resting PAPm ≥ 25 mmHg [1]. All patients underwent right heart catheterization to confirm the diagnosis. All patients with Cpc-PH (as defined above), in addition to having TPG > 12 mmHg vascular compromise > 55% (see below), were included in the study.

We have previously developed a model of the normal pulmonary circulation, which was later adapted to simulate PAH [16]. A set of pulmonary hemodynamic data is entered into the model and through iterations, the model calculates the degree of vascular compromise (measured as percent of pulmonary arterial luminal loss at the precapillary level) that is associated with the entered data [17]. This model is applied to the hemodynamic data of all patients treated at our center. When applying model predictions to all patients in our database with PAH (PAPm ≥ 25 mmHg and PAWP ≤ 15 mmHg), vascular compromise was higher than 55%. This is why a vascular compromise threshold > 55% was used in addition to the criteria of Cpc-PH described above.

PH severity was assessed using WHO functional class and 6-MWD. WHO functional class and 6-MWD were assessed at baseline and at least every 3 months thereafter for one year. After one year, WHO functional class and 6-MWD were assessed every 3–6 months until being lost to follow-up or death. The 6-MWD was performed by trained and certified pulmonary function laboratory technicians according to the American Thoracic Society (ATS) guidelines [18]. Predicted distance for each individual was calculated using reference equations published by Enright and Sherrill in 1998 [19]. The primary end point was survival. Secondary end points included WHO functional class and 6-MWD 6 and 9 months following treatment initiation.

2.3. Treatment Protocol. All patients were initiated on monotherapy with either an endothelin receptor antagonist (ERA) or a phosphodiesterase-5 (PDE-5) inhibitor. Intolerance to a medication prompted a switch to another medication either within the same group or within another group dependent on the cause of the intolerance. The treatment protocol used in the PH clinic is a stepwise approach based on the goal-oriented treatment of PAH [20] as described by Hoeper et al. (and in conjunction with 5th WSPH). Patients who reported inadequate improvement in symptoms or did not achieve 380 meters within 3 to 6 months of monotherapy were stepped up to combination therapy. A drop in 6-MWD of greater than 50 meters was considered clinically significant when assessing individual patients. NYHA classification for dyspnea was recorded, although patients' lack of subjective improvement in symptoms was considered the more relevant clinical response.

2.4. Statistical Analysis. The statistical package used was Statistica. Analysis of variance for repeated measures (ANOVAR) with Tukey's test for specific comparisons was used to compare 6-MWD at 6 and 9 months after treatment initiation to baseline. Friedman ANOVA followed by Wilcoxon signed-rank tests with Bonferroni correction were used to compare WHO functional class at 6 and 9 months after treatment initiation to baseline. Unpaired t-test was used to compare parametric demographics (chi-square was used for nonparametric data), baseline hemodynamics, and functional capacity between patients who did and those who did not tolerate PAHST. Cox proportional hazards regression was used to identify predictors of survival.

3. Results

3.1. Study Population. Between July 2001 and December 2015, twenty-six patients with Cpc-PH underwent initial assessment. Six patients developed pulmonary edema within the first 3 months of treatment that was deemed due to PAHST and were excluded from the short- and long-term outcome analysis. Of the twenty patients who tolerated PAHST, half had a valvular heart disease (VHD) while the other half suffered from heart failure (HF). At our center, patients with VHD are considered for PAHST only if they have persistent PAH or Cpc-PH following valve repair and/or replacement with no evidence of significant residual stenosis and/or regurgitation (of either aortic or mitral valve). In the other ten patients who were diagnosed with HF, six had diastolic dysfunction (DD) with preserved CO and four had systolic dysfunction (SD). Of the six patients who did not tolerate PAHST, four had VHD and two had HF (one DD and one SD). Of the twenty patients who tolerated treatment, 13 (65%) were females and 7 (35%) were males. The mean age (±SE) for all patients was 64.7 ± 2.93 years (females

TABLE 1: Descriptive statistics of patients enrolled in the study.

Variable	Patients who tolerated PAHST*			Patients who did not tolerate PAHST*		
	Number of patients	Mean	SE	Number of patients	Mean	SE
Age	20	64.6	2.93	6	67.4	4.61
CCI	20	3.80	0.36	6	4.0	0.37
PAPm	20	51.3	2.71	6	48.8	3.45
PAWP	20	23.6	0.84	6	27.0	2.80
TPG	20	27.7	2.53	6	21.8	2.27
PVR	19	6.5	0.78	6	7.14	2.47
DPG	20	8.3	1.65	6	4.2	2.06
CO	19	4.46	0.21	6	3.68	0.25
Vascular compromise	19	71.2	1.20	6	71.4	2.47
WHO-baseline	20	2.70	0.21	6	3.00	0.37
WHO-3 months	18	2.33	0.23			
WHO-6 months	18	2.22	0.21			
WHO-9 months	16	2.06	0.21			
6-MWD-baseline	23	276.0	38.50	6	268.0	50.52
6-MWD-3 months	17	360.5	29.01			
6-MWD-6 months	17	343.9	22.99			
6-MWD-9 months	15	364.6	34.85			
6-MWD (% pre)-baseline	23	56.4	6.83	6	58.3	8.99
6-MWD (% pre)-3 months	17	72.6	3.82			
6-MWD (% pre)-6 months	17	72.8	3.58			
6-MWD (% pre)-9 months	15	74.1	4.26			
Survival (in days)	20	1350.8	173.44			

*PAHST = Pulmonary Arterial Hypertension Specific Therapy, CCI = Charlson Comorbidities Index, PAPm = Mean Pulmonary Artery Pressure (mmHg), PAWP = Pulmonary Arterial Wedge Pressure (mmHg), CO = Cardiac Output (L/min), TPG = Transpulmonary Gradient (mmHg), DPG = Diastolic Pressure Gradient (mmHg), PVR = Pulmonary Venous Resistance (WU), WHO = World Health Organization functional class, 6-MWD = 6-minute walk distance (meters), and SE = standard error.

63.0 ± 2.65 and males 67.8 ± 7.01). Basic demographics, invasive hemodynamic data, baseline, 3-month, 6-month, and 9-month WHO, and 6-MWD are shown in Table 1. Data are shown as mean and standard error (SE).

3.2. Treatment. Out of the twenty patients who tolerated treatment, fifteen patients were treated with Bosentan monotherapy, two patients were on Sildenafil monotherapy, and three patients were treated with a combination of both. None of these patients required a change in treatment during the observation period. The six patients who did not tolerate treatment all received Bosentan. All discontinuations were due to pulmonary edema and none because of liver function abnormalities. All patients who tolerated treatment received treatment for at least 6 months and eighteen patients were treated for at least 9 months.

3.3. Right Heart Catheterization (RHC) Data. All patients underwent RHC. Mean (±SE) pulmonary artery pressure was 51.3 ± 2.71 mmHg, mean PAWP was 23.6 ± 0.84 mmHg, mean TPG was 27.7 ± 2.53 mmHg, mean DPG was 8.3 ± 1.65 mmHg, and mean PVR was 6.5 ± 0.78 WU. Based on model predictions, mean vascular compromise was 71.2 ± 1.20%. The rest of the hemodynamic data is shown in Table 1.

3.4. WHO Functional Class. Mean (±SE) WHO functional class for all patients at initial assessment was 2.70 ± 0.21. Mean WHO functional class at 6 and 9 months after treatment initiation was 2.22 ± 0.21 ($p < 0.04$, compared to baseline) and 2.06 ± 0.21 ($p < 0.03$), respectively (Figure 1).

3.5. 6-MWD. Mean (±SE) 6-MWD for all patients at initial assessment was 276.0±38.50 meters (56.4±6.84% predicted). Mean 6-MWD distances at 6 and 9 months after treatment initiation were 343.9 ± 22.99 meters (72.8 ± 3.58% predicted) ($p < 0.04$, compared to baseline) and 364.6 ± 34.85 meters (74.1 ± 4.26% predicted) ($p = 0.073$, compared to baseline), respectively (Figure 2).

3.6. Survival. Out of twenty patients, 12 patients died during the follow-up period (6 years). Mean (±SE) survival for all patients was 1279.7 ± 193.6 days (1383.2 ± 250.4 days for females and 1087.4 ± 311.0 days for males). Kaplan Meier survival curve showed slightly lower survival for patients

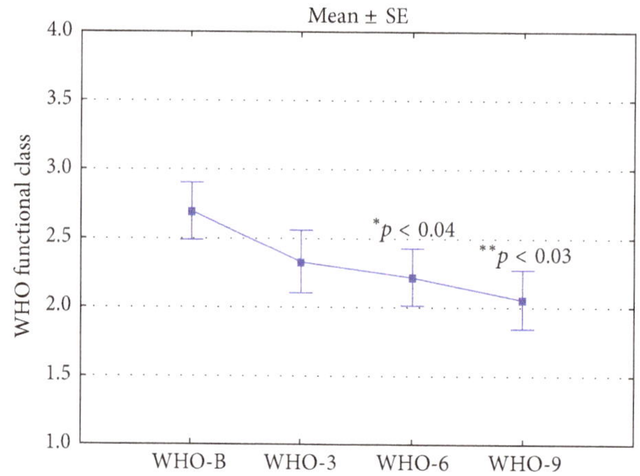

FIGURE 1: WHO functional class at baseline, 3 months, 6 months, and 9 months after initiation of PAHST.

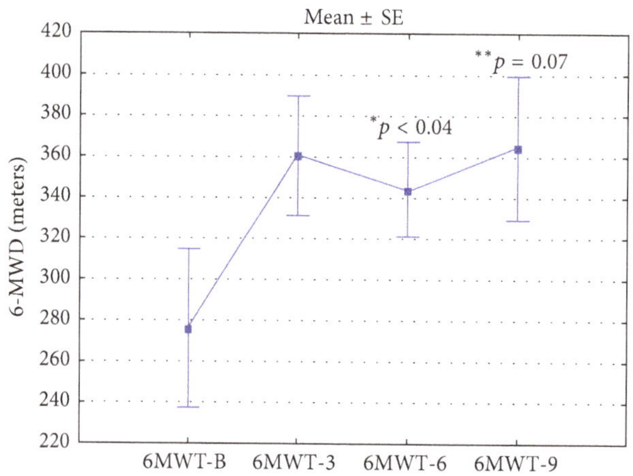

FIGURE 2: 6-minute walk test distance (6-MWT) at baseline, 3 months, 6 months, and 9 months after initiation of PAHST.

with Cpc-PH when compared to patients with pure PAH. A survival rate of 80%, 75%, and 53% at one, two, and three years (Figure 3) was noted, respectively. During the same period of observation, one, two, and three years survival rates in patients with pure PAH in our registry were 89%, 79%, and 67%, respectively. No predictors of survival could be identified among the parameters shown in Table 1.

4. Discussion

In the absence of mitral stenosis, PAWP and LVEDP are both considered accurate surrogates for left atrial pressure [21, 22]. Chronic elevations in left arterial pressure are associated with more than pressure related effects on the pulmonary circulation [23]. Vascular remodeling [24] and endothelial dysfunction [25], resembling PAH, have been described. Combined precapillary and postcapillary PH is a newly recognized entity which has specific hemodynamic parameters that include a PAWP > 15 mmHg, DPG ≥ 7 mmHg, and/or PVR > 3 WU [2–4, 7]. These patients tend to be obese, have more comorbidities, and perform less in 6-MWD [12, 13]. Data from the REVEAL registry has shown that patients with PAH associated with PAWP > 19 mmHg have a higher mortality rate over 2 years when compared to patients with PAWP < 15 mmHg [13].

In the present study, we combined the criteria of Cpc-PH, TPG > 12 mmHg, and we used model predictions of vascular compromise > 55% to ensure that the observed PAPm is out of proportion to the associated rise in PAWP. Calculated mean vascular compromise in both groups (those who tolerated and those who did not tolerate treatment) was higher (71.2 and 71.4%, resp.) than patients with pure PAH (55%) in our database suggesting that these patients had significant precapillary vasculopathy.

Several trials were performed to test the efficacy of PAHST on the treatment of heart failure [13–15]. In these studies, increased mortality and safety concerns have outweighed the beneficial effects on hemodynamics, exercise tolerance, and quality of life [14, 26, 27]. The effect of PAHST on Cpc-PH has been studied with variable outcomes [28–31]. The REVEAL registry has included patients with PAWP 15–18 mmHg. Compared to isolated PAH, PAH with

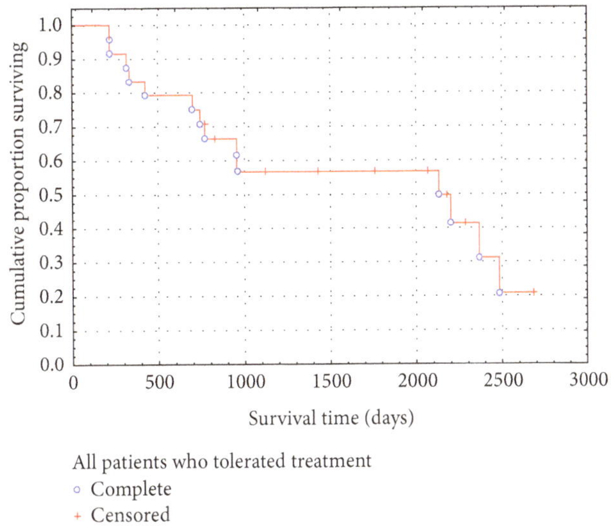

FIGURE 3: Survival rate of the study population receiving PAHST up to 6 years.

PAWP > 19 mmHg is associated with increased mortality [13]. A recent trial in patients with PH and DPG > 20 mmHg who were treated with PAHST had promising results [32].

In the present study, twenty of twenty-six patients with Cpc-PH tolerated PAHST. In those patients, we noted some improvement in WHO functional class and 6-MWD at 6 and 9 months after treatment initiation (Figures 1 and 2).

Pulmonary Arterial Hypertension Specific Therapy has resulted in increased survival at one, two, and three years in patients with PAH (93%, 75% and 66%, resp.) [33]. It is comforting to see that our survival rates in patients with PAH (89%, 79% and 67%, resp.) are comparable to the published survival rates. In our observational study, patients with Cpc-PH who received and tolerated PAHST had slightly lower survival rates of 80%, 75%, and 53%, respectively (Figure 3).

All six patients who did not tolerate PAHST had their treatment discontinued because of developing pulmonary edema and none of these patients sustained end-organ damage or died due to this treatment trial. We could not identify, among the monitored factors, predictors that would identify patients who are more likely to tolerate PAHST.

This study has many limitations including its retrospective design, small sample size, and lack of a control group. The lack of a control group is a legitimate concern as we have no way of predicting whether not treating these patients would have resulted in similar or even better outcomes, although the sustained improvement in WHO functional class and 6-MWD led us to believe that we have not caused harm. It may be considered a pilot study or case series that is alerting us to a group of patients with Cpc-PH, some of whom may benefit from PAHST. Randomized controlled trials, on a much larger scale, are needed to answer the question of benefit and survival in this group of patients. These studies may also help identify predictors of good outcome that would lead to a better selection of patients who are likely to benefit from PAHST.

5. Conclusion

Pulmonary Arterial Hypertension Specific Therapy may be beneficial in the treatment of combined post- and precapillary pulmonary hypertension (both short and long term). Prospective randomized controlled trials of PAHST in this population are needed to assess its potential efficacy.

Disclosure

Dr. Hassan Alfraidi is the principle author. The study includes no identifiable information.

Authors' Contributions

Dr. Hassan Alfraidi contributed in writing the proposal, collecting data, and writing the manuscript. Dr. Sultan Qanash contributed in reviewing the proposal and manuscript. Dr. Zoheir Bshouty contributed in reviewing proposal, data, and manuscript, editing manuscript, revisions, and final review prior to final submission following reviewer's comments.

Acknowledgments

The authors would like to thank the pulmonary hypertension clinic nurse.

References

[1] M. M. Hoeper, H. J. Bogaard, and R. Condliffe, "Definitions and diagnosis of pulmonary hypertension," *Journal of the American College of Cardiology*, vol. 62, no. 25, pp. D42–D50, 2013.

[2] N. Galiè, M. Humbert, JL. Vachiery, S. Gibbs, I. Lang et al., "2015 ECS/ERS Guidelines for the diagnosis and treatment of pulmonary hypertension," *European Heart Journal*, vol. 37, no. 1, pp. 67–119, 2015.

[3] M. Guazzi and B. A. Borlaug, "Pulmonary hypertension due to left heart disease," *Circulation*, vol. 126, no. 8, pp. 975–990, 2012.

[4] J.-L. Vachiéry, Y. Adir, J. A. Barberà et al., "Pulmonary hypertension due to left heart diseases," *Journal of the American College of Cardiology*, vol. 62, no. 25, pp. D100–D108, 2013.

[5] R. Naeije, J.-L. Vachiery, P. Yerly, and R. Vanderpool, "The transpulmonary pressure gradient for the diagnosis of pulmonary vascular disease," *European Respiratory Journal*, vol. 41, no. 1, pp. 217–223, 2013.

[6] C. Gerges, M. Gerges, M. B. Lang et al., "Diastolic pulmonary vascular pressure gradient: A predictor of prognosis in "out-of-proportion" pulmonary hypertension," *CHEST*, vol. 143, no. 3, pp. 758–766, 2013.

[7] E. Tampakakis, P. J. Leary, V. N. Selby et al., "The diastolic pulmonary gradient does not predict survival in patients with pulmonary hypertension due to left heart disease," *JACC: Heart Failure*, vol. 3, no. 1, pp. 9–16, 2015.

[8] H. P. Chaliki, D. G. Hurrell, R. A. Nishimura, R. A. Reinke, and C. P. Appleton, "Pulmonary venous pressure: Relationship to pulmonary artery, pulmonary wedge, and left atrial pressure in normal, lightly sedated dogs," *Catheterization and Cardiovascular Interventions*, vol. 56, no. 3, pp. 432–438, 2002.

[9] R. K. Albert and W. J. E. Lamm, "Left atrial pressure can be accurately transmitted to the pulmonary artery despite Zone 1 conditions," *American Journal of Respiratory and Critical Care Medicine*, vol. 167, no. 7, pp. 1016–1020, 2003.

[10] N. Saouti, N. Westerhof, P. E. Postmus, and A. Vonk-Noordegraaf, "The arterial load in pulmonary hypertension," *European Respiratory Review*, vol. 19, no. 117, pp. 197–203, 2010.

[11] R. Ilsar, B. P. Bailey, T. A. Dobbins, and D. S. Celermajer, "The Relationship Between Pulmonary Artery and Pulmonary Capillary Wedge Pressure for the Diagnosis of Pulmonary Vascular Disease," *Heart, Lung and Circulation*, vol. 19, no. 1, pp. 38–42, 2010.

[12] D. B. Badesch, G. E. Raskob, C. G. Elliott et al., "Pulmonary arterial hypertension: baseline characteristics from the REVEAL registry," *CHEST*, vol. 137, no. 2, pp. 376–387, 2010.

[13] A. E. Frost, H. W. Farber, R. J. Barst, D. P. Miller, C. G. Elliott, and M. D. McGoon, "Demographics and outcomes of patients diagnosed with pulmonary hypertension with pulmonary capillary wedge pressures 16 to 18 mm Hg: Insights from the REVEAL registry," *CHEST*, vol. 143, no. 1, pp. 185–195, 2013.

[14] R. M. Califf, K. F. Adams, W. J. McKenna, and et al, "A randomized controlled trial of epoprostenol therapy for severe congestive heart failure: the Flolan International Randomized Survival Trial (FIRST)," *American Heart Journal*, vol. 134, no. 1, pp. 44–54, 1997.

[15] M. Packer, J. McMurray, B. M. Massie et al., "Clinical effects of endothelin receptor antagonism with bosentan in patients with severe chronic heart failure: Results of a pilot study," *Journal of Cardiac Failure*, vol. 11, no. 1, pp. 12–20, 2005.

[16] Z. Bshouty and M. Younes, "Distensibility and pressure-flow relationship of the pulmonary circulation. II. Multibranched model," *Journal of Applied Physiology*, vol. 68, no. 4, pp. 1514–1527, 1990.

[17] Z. Bshouty, "Vascular compromise and hemodynamics in pulmonary arterial hypertension: Model predictions," *Canadian Respiratory Journal*, vol. 19, no. 3, pp. e15–e17, 2012.

[18] "ATS statement: guidelines for the six-minute walk test," *American Journal of Respiratory and Critical Care Medicine*, vol. 166, no. 1, pp. 111–117, 2002.

[19] P. L. Enright and D. L. Sherrill, "Reference equations for the six-minute walk in healthy adults," *American Journal of Respiratory and Critical Care Medicine*, vol. 158, no. 5, part 1, pp. 1384–1387, 1998.

[20] M. M. Hoeper, I. Markevych, E. Spiekerkoetter, T. Welte, and J. Niedermeyer, "Goal-oriented treatment and combination therapy for pulmonary arterial hypertension," *European Respiratory Journal*, vol. 26, no. 5, pp. 858–863, 2005.

[21] E. D. Flores, R. A. Lange, and L. D. Hillis, "Relation of mean pulmonary arterial wedge pressure and left ventricular end-diastolic pressure," *American Journal of Cardiology*, vol. 66, no. 20, pp. 1532-1533, 1990.

[22] R. K. F. De Oliveira, E. V. M. Ferreira, R. P. Ramos et al., "Usefulness of pulmonary capillary wedge pressure as a correlate of left ventricular filling pressures in pulmonary arterial hypertension," *The Journal of Heart and Lung Transplantation*, vol. 33, no. 2, pp. 157–162, 2014.

[23] N. R. Dayeh, J. Ledoux, and J. Dupuis, "Lung Capillary Stress Failure and Arteriolar Remodelling in Pulmonary Hypertension Associated with Left Heart Disease (Group 2 PH)," *Progress in Cardiovascular Diseases*, vol. 59, no. 1, pp. 11–21, 2016.

[24] J. B. West and O. Mathieu-Costello, "Vulnerability of pulmonary capillaries in heart disease," *Circulation*, vol. 92, no. 3, pp. 622–631, 1995.

[25] M. Farrero, I. Blanco, M. Batlle et al., "Pulmonary hypertension is related to peripheral endothelial dysfunction in heart failure with preserved ejection fraction," *Circulation: Heart Failure*, vol. 7, no. 5, pp. 791–798, 2014.

[26] G. D. Lewis, R. Shah, K. Shahzad et al., "Sildenafil improves exercise capacity and quality of life in patients with systolic heart failure and secondary pulmonary hypertension," *Circulation*, vol. 116, no. 14, pp. 1555–1562, 2007.

[27] P. Botha, G. Parry, J. H. Dark, and G. A. MacGowan, "Acute Hemodynamic Effects of Intravenous Sildenafil Citrate in Congestive Heart Failure: Comparison of Phosphodiesterase Type-3 and -5 Inhibition," *The Journal of Heart and Lung Transplantation*, vol. 28, no. 7, pp. 676–682, 2009.

[28] D. Bonderman, S. Ghio, S. B. Felix et al., "Riociguat for patients with pulmonary hypertension caused by systolic left ventricular dysfunction: A phase IIb double-blind, randomized, placebo-controlled, dose-ranging hemodynamic study," *Circulation*, vol. 128, no. 5, pp. 502–511, 2013.

[29] R. Jiang, L. Wang, C.-T. Zhu et al., "Comparative effectiveness of sildenafil for pulmonary hypertension due to left heart disease with HFrEF," *Hypertension Research*, vol. 38, no. 12, pp. 829–839, 2015.

[30] E. S. Hoendermis, L. C. Y. Liu, Y. M. Hummel et al., "Effects of sildenafil on invasive haemodynamics and exercise capacity in heart failure patients with preserved ejection fraction and pulmonary hypertension: A randomized controlled trial," *European Heart Journal*, vol. 36, no. 38, pp. 2565–2573, 2015.

[31] E. Kaluski, G. Cotter, M. Leitman et al., "Clinical and hemodynamic effects of bosentan dose optimization in symptomatic heart failure patients with severe systolic dysfunction, associated with secondary pulmonary hypertension - A multi-center randomized study," *Cardiology*, vol. 109, no. 4, pp. 273–280, 2008.

[32] C. Gerges, M. Gerges, N. Skoro-Sajer et al., "Hemodynamic thresholds for precapillary pulmonary hypertension," *CHEST*, vol. 149, no. 4, pp. 1061–1073, 2016.

[33] T. Thenappan, S. J. Shah, S. Rich, L. Tian, S. L. Archer, and M. Gomberg-Maitland, "Survival in pulmonary arterial hypertension: A reappraisal of the NIH risk stratification equation," *European Respiratory Journal*, vol. 35, no. 5, pp. 1079–1087, 2010.

22

Rare Primary Pulmonary Marginal Zone Lymphoma Presenting with Incidental Pulmonary Nodules

Saad Ullah,[1] **Mirza Ali,[2] and Mingchen Song[1]**

[1]*Division of Pulmonary and Critical Care Medicine, Southern Illinois University, Springfield, IL, USA*
[2]*Department of Internal Medicine, Southern Illinois University, Springfield, IL, USA*

Correspondence should be addressed to Saad Ullah; saadullah_98@hotmail.com

Academic Editor: Samer Al-Saad

Pulmonary malignancies carry a significant morbidity and mortality and are one of the leading causes of cancer-related deaths worldwide. Primary pulmonary lymphoma is a rare malignancy which should be considered in the differential of solitary pulmonary nodule or lung mass especially in a low-risk patient presenting with constitutional symptoms. Here, we describe a case of an elderly male who presented to our clinic with incidental pulmonary nodules and subsequent workup revealed low grade B cell non-Hodgkin's lymphoma consistent with diagnosis of primary pulmonary marginal zone lymphoma.

1. Introduction

Primary pulmonary lymphoma (PPL) is a rare neoplasm accounting for 0.5-1% of pulmonary malignancies [1]. It can present with nonspecific symptoms or, in some cases, it can be detected as an incidentaloma during surveillance of other thoracic pathologies. Here, we present a case of an elderly male who was seen at his primary care physician's (PCP) office for follow-up of ascending aortic aneurysm. Computed tomography (CT) of the chest without contrast revealed pleural-based right upper lobe, central right lower lobe, and left upper lobe pulmonary nodules. Pathology confirmed the diagnosis of low-grade B-cell non-Hodgkin's lymphoma (NHL) consistent with marginal zone lymphoma.

2. Case Presentation

An 83-year-old male with past medical history of mild Alzheimer's dementia, nonischemic cardiomyopathy, aortic regurgitation, and an ascending aortic aneurysm measured at 4.1 cm presented to the pulmonology clinic with an abnormal CT of the chest. He was seen by his PCP recently for follow-up of ascending aortic aneurysm and had a CT chest without contrast performed which showed 14.8 mm pleural-based nodular density in the posterior medial right upper lobe, irregular 20.5 mm right lower lobe nodule, and a 2 mm left upper lobe partially calcified nodule [Figure 1(a)]. He had no respiratory or constitutional symptoms. He was a lifelong nonsmoker without any significant occupational exposures. [^{18}F]Fluorodeoxyglucose-positron emission tomography with CT (^{18}F –FDG PET/CT) was performed showing multiple ^{18}F –FDG avid nodules in the right upper lobe, right lower lobe, and left upper lobe [Figure 1(b)]. Initially thought to be inflammatory in nature, a 3-month follow-up CT chest was recommended; however, the patient opted for CT-guided transthoracic biopsy. Because the tissue sample was a core needle biopsy of a pleural-based nodule, it did not include any bronchial epithelium; therefore, the presence of lymphoepithelial lesions could not be evaluated. Immunohistochemical staining showed CD20 positive neoplastic B cells with CD3 positive small benign T cells. CD21 stain was also positive within the residual dendritic cell network, such that the marginal zones appeared to be expanded. These findings support a histopathologic diagnosis of low-grade B-cell NHL most consistent with marginal zone lymphoma [Figure 2]. The patient was referred to oncology for further management.

3. Discussion

Primary pulmonary lymphoma (PPL) is a rare clinicopathologic entity, which comprises less than 0.3% of all primary

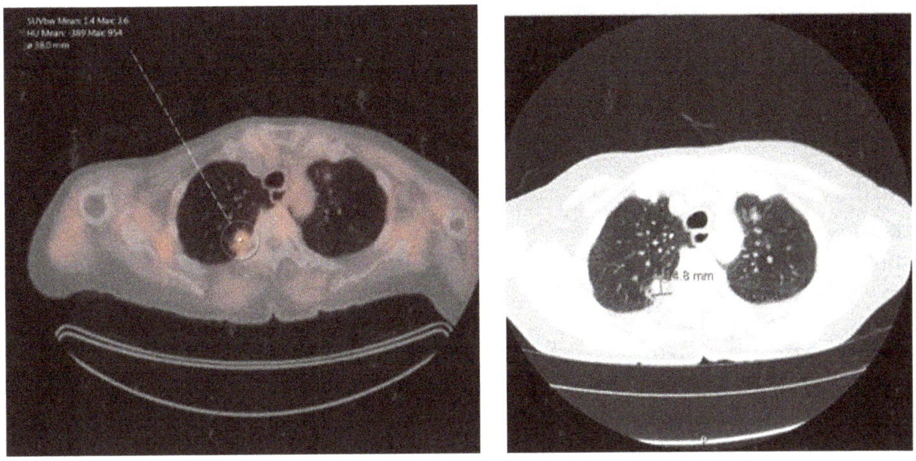

FIGURE 1: (a) On the left of the picture and (b) on the right of the picture. (a) PET CT showing increased uptake in the nodule. (b) CT Chest without contrast: 14.8 mm pleural-based mass-like density in the posterior medial right upper lobe.

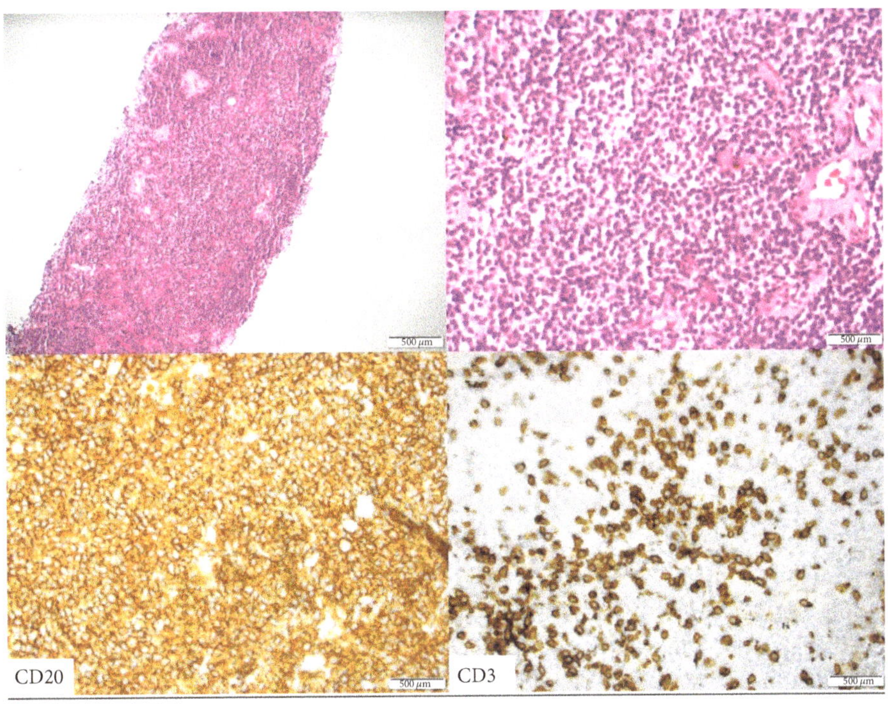

FIGURE 2: The two pathology pictures are low and high power of hematoxylin and eosin-stained slides showing proliferation of small lymphocytes, a few of them exhibiting monocytoid morphology. The bottom left is CD20 immunostaining highlighting the neoplastic B cells. Bottom right is CD3 immunostaining highlighting the background benign small T cells consistent with diagnosis of marginal zone lymphoma.

lung malignancies, less than 1% of all cases of NHL, and 3% to 4% of all extranodal NHL [2–4]. It is defined as a lymphoma localized to the lung in a patient with no prior history of extrapulmonary disease at the time of diagnosis or up to 3 months thereafter [2, 5].

The most common type of PPL is the marginal zone lymphoma (MZL) of mucosa-associated lymphoid tissue (MALT), otherwise known as MALT lymphoma or "MAL-Toma," which comprises 70-80% of all cases of PPL [6]. These MALT lymphomas are thought to arise from clonal proliferation of marginal zone B cells of bronchial-associated lymphoid tissue (BALT) [2]. Approximately 40-50% of pulmonary MALT lymphomas are positive for t(11;18)(q21;q21) [7]. This unique translocation is responsible for the creation of a fusion RNA transcript from the *API2 (apoptosis inhibitor 2)* and the *MALT1* genes which induces activation of the NF-κB pathway resulting in cell proliferation [8, 9]. Unlike gastric MALT lymphoma which is associated with *Helicobacter pylori*, MALT lymphoma of the lung has not been linked to any infectious or specific autoimmune conditions, although there have been case reports associated with tuberculosis [10]. Like gastric MALT lymphoma, it is postulated that pulmonary MALT lymphoma can progress to high-grade diffuse large B-cell lymphoma (DLBCL); however, this has not been well studied [1].

The clinical presentation is highly variable. Most patients are clinically asymptomatic or present with constitutional symptoms, cough, hemoptysis, or dyspnea; B-symptoms are uncommon. Median age at time of diagnosis is 60 years, however, it has also been diagnosed in younger individuals who are usually immunocompromised [2]. One-third of patients have concurrent autoimmune conditions such as rheumatoid arthritis, Sjögren's syndrome, and systemic lupus erythematosus and up to 40% of patients have monoclonal gammopathy as well [11].

Radiographic appearance is variable, ranging from consolidations to inconspicuous nodules or masses. The presence of ground glass opacities, air bronchograms, and bronchiectasis may confound the diagnosis suggesting an infectious or inflammatory process. Presence of air bronchograms is due to relative airway-sparing nature of the disease [2]. Hilar lymphadenopathy is present in approximately 30% of cases [12].

Histologic confirmation is required for definitive diagnosis and is characterized by reactive lymphoid follicles with diffuse infiltration by small lymphocytes and lymphoid proliferation which leads to expansion of the marginal zone; lymphoepithelial lesions (infiltrates of 5 or more neoplastic B-cells into the bronchial epithelium) support the diagnosis but are not required for diagnosis [2]. Lymphoepithelial lesions can be detected with immunohistochemical stains for cytokeratin (which highlights epithelial cells only but not lymphocytes) and CD20 (which highlights lymphocytes but not epithelial cells). As the MALT lymphoma grows, the bronchial wall and adjacent lung parenchyma can be replaced but necrosis or airway obstruction is rare [2].

Primary pulmonary MALT lymphoma is associated with a good prognosis; 5-year and 10-year survival rates are 90% and 70%, respectively [13, 14]. Currently, there are no established guidelines for the management of pulmonary MZL. Considering the indolent course of disease, observation and treatment for symptomatic disease are both reasonable options. Treatment can be considered for symptomatic patients. Therapeutic options include surgical resection, chemotherapy, and radiation therapy. Localized or peripheral lesions can be treated with surgical resection or moderate-dose radiation therapy [15, 16]. Patients with widespread disease not amenable to resection may be treated with single agent chemotherapy, such as rituximab, which has been shown to be effective [17]. Combination chemotherapy with cyclophosphamide, vincristine, and prednisone (CVP) can be considered as well [18]. There is no consensus on whether surgical resection is associated with better outcomes. Further prospective clinical research is greatly needed to determine the optimal treatment modality.

4. Conclusion

Nonspecific presentation and indolent course make the diagnosis of primary pulmonary lymphoma very challenging and often lead to misdiagnosis or delayed diagnosis. This diagnosis should especially be suspected in individuals who present with lung nodules but lack usual risk factors for primary non-small-cell and small-cell lung cancer, similar to our patient.

References

[1] Z. Zhu, W. Liu, O. Mamlouk, J. E. O'Donnell, D. Sen, and B. Avezbakiyev, "Primary pulmonary diffuse large B cell non-hodgkin's lymphoma: a case report and literature review," *American Journal of Case Reports*, vol. 18, pp. 286–290, 2017.

[2] S. Piña-Oviedo, A. Weissferdt, N. Kalhor, and C. A. Moran, "Primary pulmonary lymphomas," *Advances in Anatomic Pathology*, vol. 22, no. 6, pp. 355–375, 2015.

[3] J. Cadranel, M. Wislez, and M. Antoine, "Primary pulmonary lymphoma," *European Respiratory Journal*, vol. 20, no. 3, pp. 750–762, 2002.

[4] W. L. Rush, J. A. W. Andriko, J. K. Taubenberger et al., "Primary anaplastic large cell lymphoma of the lung: A clinicopathologic study of five patients," *Modern Pathology*, vol. 13, no. 12, pp. 1285–1292, 2000.

[5] J. William, D. Variakojis, A. Yeldandi, and K. Raparia, "Lymphoproliferative Neoplasms of the Lung: A Review," *Archives of Pathology & Laboratory Medicine*, vol. 137, no. 3, pp. 382–391, 2013.

[6] A. G. Nicholson and N. L. Harris, "Marginal zone B-cell lymphoma of the mucosa-associated lymphoid tissue (MALT) type," in *WHO Classification of Tumours, Pathology and Genetics, Tumours of the Lung, Pleura, Thymus and Heart*, W. D. Travis, E. Brambilla, H. K. Müller-Hermelink, and C. C. Harris, Eds., pp. 88–90, IARC Press, Lyon, France, 2004.

[7] E. D. Remstein, P. J. Kurtin, R. R. Einerson, S. F. Paternoster, and G. W. Dewald, "Primary pulmonary MALT lymphomas show frequent and heterogeneous cytogenetic abnormalities, including aneuploidy and translocations involving API2 and MALT1 and IGH and MALT1," *Leukemia*, vol. 18, no. 1, pp. 156–160, 2004.

[8] P. Farinha and R. D. Gascoyne, "Molecular pathogenesis of mucosa-associated lymphoid tissue lymphoma," *Journal of Clinical Oncology*, vol. 23, no. 26, pp. 6370–6378, 2005.

[9] P. G. Isaacson, "Update on MALT lymphomas," *Best Practice & Research Clinical Haematology*, vol. 18, no. 1, pp. 57–68, 2005.

[10] F. Tiruneh, A. Awan, R. Amin, S. Afreen, A. Musa, and W. Davis, "A rare case of pulmonary mucosa-associated lymphoid tissue lymphoma transforming into diffuse large B-cell lymphoma," *Cureus*, 2017.

[11] P. J. Kurtin, J. L. Myers, H. Adlakha et al., "Pathologic and clinical features of primary pulmonary extranodal marginal zone B-cell lymphoma of MALT type," *The American Journal of Surgical Pathology*, vol. 25, no. 8, pp. 997–1008, 2001.

[12] S. S. Hare, C. A. Souza, G. Bain et al., "The radiological spectrum of pulmonary lymphoproliferative disease," *British Journal of Radiology*, vol. 85, pp. 848–864, 2012.

[13] M. N. Koss, L. Hochholzer, and P. W. Nichols, "Primary non-Hodgkin's lymphoma and pseudolymphoma of lung: a study of 161 patients," *Human Pathology*, vol. 14, pp. 1024–1038, 1983.

[14] J.-F. Cordier, E. Chailleux, D. Lauque et al., "Primary pulmonary lymphomas; a clinical study of 70 cases in nonimmunocompromised patients," *Chest*, vol. 103, no. 1, pp. 201–208, 1993.

[15] S. Ahmed, S. J. Kussick, A. K. Siddiqui et al., "Bronchial-associated lymphoid tissue lymphoma: a clinical study of a rare disease," *European Journal of Cancer*, vol. 40, no. 9, pp. 1320–1326, 2004.

[16] R. W. Tsang, M. K. Gospodarowicz, M. Pintilie et al., "Stage I and II malt lymphoma: results of treatment with radiotherapy," *International Journal of Radiation Oncology, Biology, Physics*, vol. 50, no. 5, pp. 1258–1264, 2001.

[17] I. Okamura, H. Imai, K. Mori et al., "Rituximab monotherapy as a first-line treatment for pulmonary mucosa-associated lymphoid tissue lymphoma," *International Journal of Hematology*, vol. 101, no. 1, pp. 46–51, 2014.

[18] J. H. Kim, S.-H. Lee, J. Park et al., "Primary pulmonary non-Hodgkin's lymphoma," *Japanese Journal of Clinical Oncology*, vol. 34, no. 9, pp. 510–514, 2004.

23

Azathioprine Hypersensitivity Syndrome during Treatment of Severe Interstitial Lung Disease with Anti-Neutrophil Cytoplasmic Antibody-Associated Vasculitis

Eri Nakano,[1,2] Tomohiko Asakawa,[1] Mea Asou,[1] Eri Nohara,[1] Tomoyuki Seki,[1] and Makoto Araki[1]

[1]*Department of Internal Medicine, Suwa Central Hospital, Chino, Nagano 391-8503, Japan*
[2]*National Hospital Organization, Tokyo National Hospital, Takeoka, Kiyose, Tokyo 204-8585, Japan*

Correspondence should be addressed to Makoto Araki; makoto.araki@gmail.com

Academic Editor: Shih-Yi Lee

Azathioprine is used to treat anti-neutrophil cytoplasmic antibody- (ANCA-) associated vasculitis. Azathioprine hypersensitivity syndrome is often missed. An 81-year-old man undergoing treatment for interstitial pneumonia developed a high fever and was diagnosed with ANCA-associated vasculitis based on an elevated myeloperoxidase- (MPO-) ANCA titer and renal biopsy findings. After induction therapy, his clinical symptoms improved, but his MPO-ANCA remained elevated (>300 $U{\cdot}L^{-1}$) and hematuria persisted. Prednisolone plus azathioprine was administered as maintenance therapy. Three exacerbations of the inflammatory response occurred during the subsequent 3 months. In each instance, we suspected opportunistic infection or a flare-up of vasculitis. The first exacerbation was treated with an increased prednisolone dose and antibiotics. At the onset of the second exacerbation, which was accompanied by systemic erythema, we stopped azathioprine and administered antibiotics. The third exacerbation, which occurred the day after restarting azathioprine, involved a fever with chills and an acute inflammatory reaction; we therefore suspected an azathioprine allergy. A drug provocation test was performed, and a hyperinflammatory response was observed. The patient received prednisolone (15 $mg{\cdot}day^{-1}$) monotherapy; no further fever was observed during the subsequent 2 months. We therefore diagnosed azathioprine hypersensitivity syndrome. Under treatment with prednisolone (5 $mg{\cdot}day^{-1}$) and mycophenolate mofetil (1 $g{\cdot}day^{-1}$) (replacing the azathioprine), no signs of relapse or infection have occurred for more than two years. Renal function and the pulmonary lesions are stable, although the high MPO-ANCA titer and hematuria persist. The diagnosis of azathioprine hypersensitivity is often delayed because of the difficulty in identifying the relationship between immunosuppressive agents and hypersensitivity and in distinguishing this from infection or relapse of the primary disease. The misdiagnosis of azathioprine hypersensitivity leads to unnecessary treatment; thus, clinicians should consider allergic reactions specific to azathioprine when switching from induction to maintenance therapy.

1. Introduction

In the treatment of anti-neutrophil cytoplasmic antibody- (ANCA-) associated vasculitis (AAV), powerful immunosuppressive drugs are usually used, which can lead to treatment-related deaths from infection. Therefore, management of vasculitis flare-ups and opportunistic infections is always important in AAV. Azathioprine (AZA) is the standard AAV maintenance therapy. AZA hypersensitivity syndrome was previously considered to be a rare side effect of AZA, but a recent report found that it occurs in 9% of AZA patients [1]. This syndrome is often misdiagnosed as infection or disease exacerbation and thus is prone to mistreatment; a thorough understanding of its clinical manifestations is therefore required. We report a case of AZA hypersensitivity syndrome that occurred during the treatment of severe interstitial lung disease with AAV.

Table 1: Laboratory findings during the course of the disease.

	At diagnosis	⓪	①	②	③	④	2 years after MMF therapy	Units
WBC	12,570	10,990	10,840	10,100	19,650	16,410	6,030	/μL
Hb	12.2	12.1	12.1	12.3	14	11.8	10.4	mg/dL
Plt	43.7	35.8	32.8	19.4	52.6	26.7	34.0	$10^4/\mu$L
Alb	2.5	3.1	3.1		3.0	2.4	3.8	mg/dL
LDH	209	264	232	300	244	334	206	IU/L
AST	29	18	36	24	35	50	22	IU/L
ALT	37	15	30	26	28	39	10	IU/L
CPK	54	19	17	38	20	38	43	IU/L
BUN	20.9	26.1	28.5	20.8	34.1	70.4	18.2	mg/dL
Cr	0.93	1.40	1.55	1.30	1.66	6.34	1.24	mg/dL
Na	137	140	138	139	137	136	141	mEq/L
K	4.6	4.6	5.5	4.2	4.3	4.9	4.0	mEq/L
Cl	104	104	102	103	101	103	100	mEq/L
CRP	19.92	2.22	9.23	10.87	16.19	31.19	0.43	mg/dL
Urine protein	2+	–	–	2+	±	2+	–	
Urine occult blood	3+	3+	3+	3+	3+	3+	2+	
Urine sediment (RBC)	50-99	50-99	50-99	>100	>100	>100	50-99	/HPF
β-D-Glucan		9.6		11.9	7.7			pg/mL
CMV-antigenemia		neg.		neg.	neg.			
SP-D				<17.2	23.7			mg/dL
KL-6					1,220		469	U/mL
IgG		731		583				mg/dL
Anti-MPO-ANCA	>300	>300		>300		>300	>300	U/mL
Anti-GBM-Ab	<2.0					<2.0		U/mL
Anti-PR3-ANCA	<1.0							U/mL
Anti-nuclear antibody	×40							

ANCA: anti-neutrophil cytoplasmic antibodies; CMV: cytomegalovirus; GBM: glomerular basement membrane; KL-6: Krebs von den Lungen-6; MMF: mycophenolate mofetil; MPO: myeloperoxidase; PR3: proteinase 3; SP-D: surfactant protein d; RBC: red blood cell.

2. Case Presentation

An 81-year-old man with no history of smoking had been undergoing treatment for chronic interstitial pneumonia and paroxysmal atrial fibrillation for 6 years. Incomplete investigations had failed to identify the cause of the interstitial pneumonia. A high fever, worsening of renal function, and myeloperoxidase- (MPO-) ANCA positivity had been noted 6 months earlier (Table 1). A renal biopsy revealed global sclerosis in 2 of 12 glomeruli and 3 glomeruli with glomerular basement membrane necrosis. Crescent formation was not observed. AAV was diagnosed based on the pauci-immune pattern of immunofluorescent staining. As the patient had a resolved hepatitis B virus (HBV) infection (negative for Hbs antigen and positive for Hbc antibody), we decided to perform the standard recommended induction therapy, with prednisolone (PSL) and six courses of intravenous cyclophosphamide (CYC) [2].

After induction therapy, the inflammatory response promptly improved. Renal function remained almost unchanged, but hematuria persisted. We decided to ignore this, considering the impact of direct oral anticoagulants. Lung function did not return, and home oxygen therapy was introduced. The ANCA titer remained over 300 U·mL^{-1}. As there was no change in the Vasculitis Damage Index (VDI) (score of 5; pulmonary fibrosis, chronic breathlessness, impaired lung function, hypertension, and estimated glomerular filtration rate < 50 mL·min^{-1}·1.73 m$^{(2)-1}$), we considered organ failure and decided to shift from induction therapy to maintenance therapy. AZA was selected as an adjunctive immunosuppressive agent to the current PSL (10 mg·day^{-1}) regimen. Owing to the potential for hepatic impairment due to AZA, we titrated AZA (25 mg·day^{-1}) in hospital.

After 10 days of AZA administration (Day 10), blood tests revealed a white blood cell (WBC) count of 10,840 μL^{-1}, a creatine (Cr) level of 1.55 mg·dL^{-1}, and a C reactive protein (CRP) level of 9.23 mg·dL^{-1}; a mild worsening of the inflammatory response and renal function was also observed (Figure 1, ①, Table 1, ①). The patient had no fever and stable breathing. A chest computed tomography (CT) scan was performed, which showed a worsening right lower lobe infiltration shadow, but could not distinguish between an exacerbation of interstitial pneumonia and infection (Figure 2). The high ANCA titers and persistent hematuria remained. Beta-D-glucan and cytomegalovirus- (CMV-) antigenemia tests were

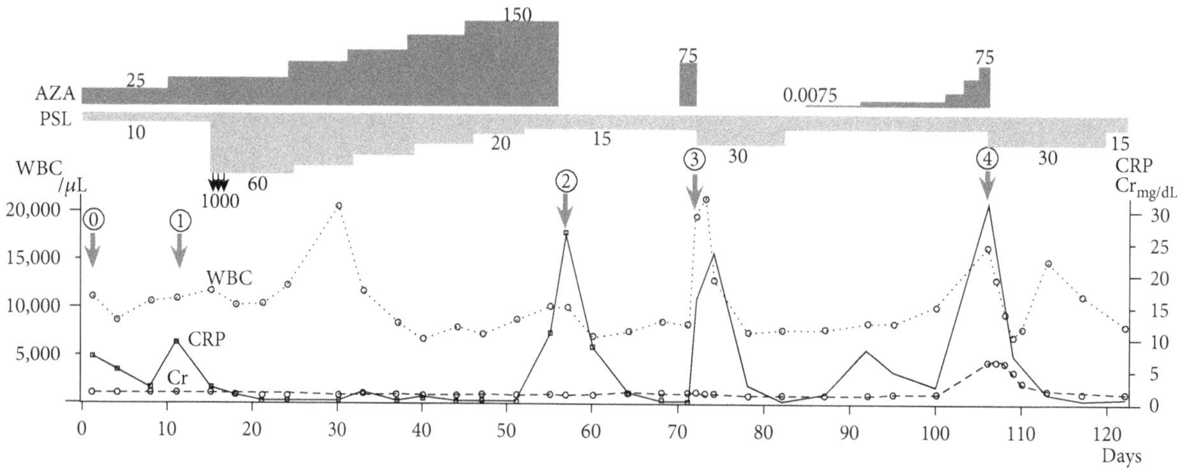

FIGURE 1: WBC, CRP, and Cr levels at about 4 months after the start of AZA and trends in PSL and AZA medication doses. Blood test results for the days indicated by the bold arrow are shown in Table 1. AZA: azathioprine; PSL: prednisolone.

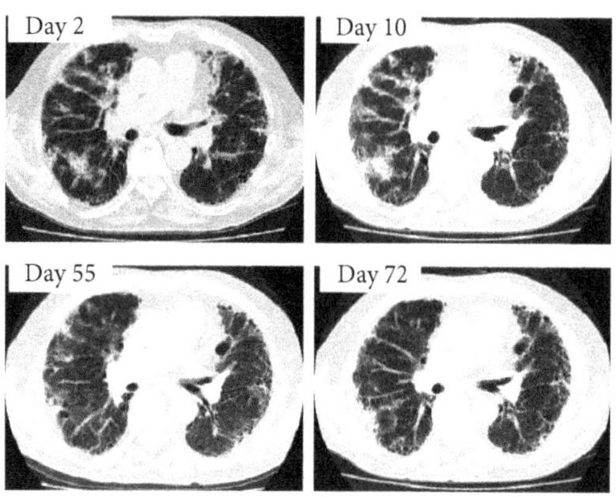

FIGURE 2: Changes in chest CT. Date is the number of days after starting AZA. Day 2: diffuse shading, and a regional infiltrative shadow in the right lower lobe is observed. Day 10: scattered nonregional increases in concentration are the same as before. No apparent exacerbation. Day 55: scattered irregular infiltrative shadows in both peripheral lungs and nondistrictal frosted concentrations are observed. Day 72: distinct infiltrative shadows scattered in the periphery of both lungs, with no significant changes.

negative. There were no abnormal findings in the sputum culture, including mycobacteria. In the absence of clear findings, we decided to treat the infection and vasculitis. For the bacterial pneumonia, ceftriaxone 2 g·day^{-1} was administered for 2 weeks. For the vasculitis, high-dose methylprednisolone therapy (1,000 mg·day^{-1} for 3 days) was performed. Thereafter, the patient was phased down from 60 mg·day^{-1} PSL while AZA treatment was phased up.

On Day 52, the patient was discharged with prescriptions for PSL (15 mg·day^{-1}) and AZA (150 mg·day^{-1}). However, 3 days later, the patient developed a fever of 40.3°C with chills and was urgently admitted to our hospital (Figure 1, ②). Systemic erythema was observed without mucosal damage (Figure 3(a)). A skin biopsy was performed, and the patient was diagnosed with erythema exudativum multiforme based on mild neutrophil infiltration in the shallow dermis (Figure 3(b)). However, we did not know whether this was caused by the drug or the infection. A CT scan was performed, but the invasive shadow of the right lower lobe had improved. Blood tests and imaging studies showed that neither pneumonia nor vasculitis was likely (Figure 2, Table 1, ②). As lymphocytopenia (444 μL^{-1}), probably owing to AZA, was observed, we considered this to be the cause of the infection, discontinued AZA, and commenced levofloxacin (500 mg·day^{-1}) for 14 days. On Day 10 of hospitalization (Day 65), the CRP level was 1.54 mg·dL^{-1} and the inflammatory response had improved.

On Day 71, as his general condition improved, the patient resumed AZA (75 mg·day^{-1}). The next day, at 15:00, the patient developed a fever of 39.3°C with shivering chills (Figure 1, ③). Although blood tests showed a WBC count of 8,330 μL^{-1} and a CRP level of 0.17 mg·dL^{-1} on Day 71, these counts worsened, to a WBC count of 19,650 μL^{-1} and a CRP level of 16.19 mg·dL^{-1} in less than 30 hours (Table 1, ③). We performed a systemic search, which included the respiratory (Figure 2) and urinary tracts, but neither test findings nor urine and blood cultures produced significant evidence of infection. The antibiotic combination of imipenem/cilastatin (0.5 g·12 h^{-1}) was administered, AZA was discontinued, and the dose of PSL was transiently increased to 30 mg as the patient was considered to be under high stress.

As the disease worsened after the administration of AZA, we thought it was likely drug-related, although there was no eosinophilia. However, the high MPO-ANCA titer and microscopic hematuria findings did not rule out a relapse of AAV. In addition, there were few alternative drugs available to treat this patient owing to the severe lung damage and history of HBV infection. Therefore, approximately 2 weeks after the third fever (Day 85), we initiated a drug provocation test with the patient's consent. The dose of AZA was increased to 0.75, 1.5, 3, 6, 12.5, 25, and 50, then 75 mg·day^{-1} at intervals of 2 to 3 days. We monitored the patient's vital signs throughout the course, and the patient did not develop a fever or rash during the 3 weeks of escalation. Up to Day 16 of the drug provocation test (Day 100, AZA 12.5 mg·day^{-1}), the WBC count (10,090 μL^{-1}), CRP

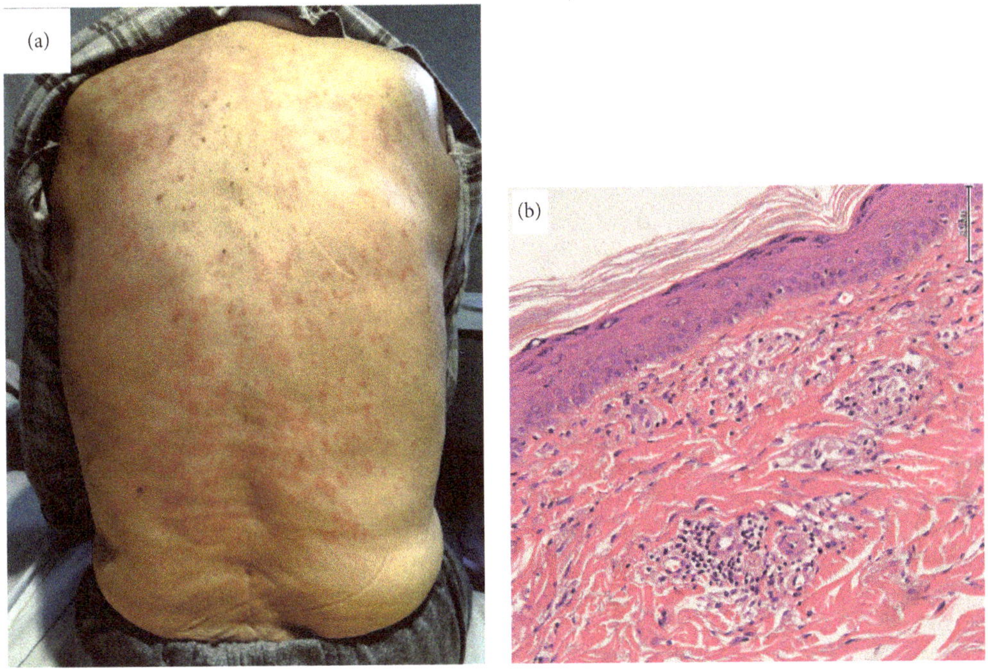

(a) (b)

Figure 3: (a) There is a rash all over the body, mainly on the back. (b) Mild focal neutrophilic infiltration in the superficial dermis and mild to moderate perivascular lymphocytic infiltration. There are no vasculitis findings. Haematoxylin and eosin stain. 200x.

level (2.56 mg·dL^{-1}), and Cr level (1.49 mg·dL^{-1}) were acceptable. On Day 106 (AZA 75 mg·day^{-1}), there was no fever but the inflammatory response increased and renal function worsened, as the WBC count (16,410 μL^{-1}), CRP level (31.19 mg·dL^{-1}), and Cr level (6.4 mg·dL^{-1}) increased (Figure 1, ④, Table 1, ④). AZA was immediately discontinued, and the dose of PSL was doubled to 30 mg·day^{-1}. No antibiotics were used. Renal function returned, indicated by a drop in the Cr level from 6.4 to 1.5 mg·dL^{-1} after 11 days, and the inflammatory response improved. We decided to confirm that the disease would not recur in the absence of AZA. The patient received PSL (15 mg) monotherapy for 2 months without the occurrence of fever or exacerbated inflammatory response; renal function did not worsen. The patient was therefore diagnosed with AZA hypersensitivity syndrome.

Mycophenolate mofetil (MMF) was selected as an additional immunosuppressive agent. The dose of PSL was reduced, and MMF was introduced 2 months after the discontinuation of AZA. Taking into account renal function and old age, the dose of MMF was set at 1 g. For more than 2 years, PSL (5 mg·day^{-1}) and MMF (1 g·day^{-1}) have been administered and there was no fever or acute inflammatory reaction. The patient's breathing and renal function have stabilized. The high MPO-ANCA titer and urine occult blood findings remain unchanged.

3. Discussion

AZA hypersensitivity is a relatively common condition that requires a change in treatment and should not be overlooked. However, in practice, the diagnosis is often difficult because the syndrome mimics infection or the recurrence of AAV. Infection is the main cause of death in AAV, and, in a case of severe pulmonary impairment with a poor reserve capacity, such as this one, the possibility of respiratory infection during a hyperinflammatory response must always be considered. In this case, the MPO-ANCA was persistently >300 U·L^{-1} and urine occult blood was >50 red blood cells per high-power field; thus, the possibility of AAV relapse should be considered. We think that it is meaningful to report how we responded to the allergic reaction to this immunosuppressive drug in such a situation.

AZA hypersensitivity syndrome, a recently proposed concept, is a febrile rash disease that appears, on average, 13.3 days (5–28 days) after the initiation of AZA [3]. This syndrome used to be considered rare, but recently, it has been reported to occur in 9% of patients receiving AZA; thus, it is an important side effect to be aware of [1]. Background diseases, such as AAV, Crohn's disease, ulcerative colitis, autoimmune hepatitis, and chronic rheumatoid arthritis, have been reported with AZA hypersensitivity syndrome, but there is no significant trend. Overall, 49% of AZA hypersensitivity syndromes present with cutaneous symptoms, and the typical rash is Sweet's syndrome-like neutrophilic dermatosis [4]. Symptoms other than fever and rash, such as nausea, vomiting, and meningitis, have also been reported [5]. However, as none are specific to AZA hypersensitivity, it is often overlooked, the symptoms being considered to be dermatosis associated with the underlying disease or infection [6].

In this case, we had difficulty diagnosing AZA hypersensitivity syndrome. In general, most fevers during collagen disease therapy are aggravations of the underlying disease or infections [7], so drug allergies are unlikely to be considered. Moreover, although drug fever has been reported not only with AZA but also with other immunosuppressive agents, such as CYC, mizoribine, and MMF [8–10], allergic reactions to immunosuppressive agents are difficult to recognize in a patient. In the present case, the worsening of the inflammatory response on Day 10 was considered to be either infection or exacerbation of AAV, not an allergic reaction to AZA. The reasons were that the fever was mild, there was no rash, high MPO-ANCA titer and hematuria persisted, and the CT scan showed an infiltrative shadow in the right lower lobe. Furthermore, the acute inflammatory reaction on Day 55 should be diagnosed as AZA hypersensitivity because there was no change in imaging findings and a typical skin rash appeared. However, we did not consider it to be AZA-induced hypersensitivity, as most hypersensitivity cases occur within the first month of treatment. We also did not find that the hypersensitivity was suppressed by high doses of prednisolone.

AZA hypersensitivity syndrome is thought to be mainly caused by the accumulation of toxic metabolites in conjunction with a decrease in thiopurine methyltransferase (TPMT) activity [1]. Unfortunately, TPMT activity could not be measured in this case. Currently, there is no reliable skin test or *in vitro* study for the diagnosis of AZA hypersensitivity. As we did not want to use rituximab (RTX) or methotrexate (MTX) because of the patient's history of the patient's background, such as a history of hepatitis B infection or pulmonary fibrosis, we decided to confirm the diagnosis of AZA using a drug provocation test. We titrated a small dose of AZA, which was the same drug he used at home, and administered increasing doses (Figure 1, PSL dose is fixed at 15 mg·day^{-1}), as performed previously [11]. In this test, the absence of a response at low doses of AZA and the onset of AZA hypersensitivity syndrome at higher doses probably represented dose dependency, as the cause of AZA hypersensitivity is thought to be a decrease in the activity of TPMT. Allergy to AZA was further demonstrated by the absence of inflammatory reactions in the reverse test (2 months of PSL monotherapy).

A similar case of renal impairment owing to AZA hypersensitivity syndrome has been reported in which the Cr level rose on Day 10 from 1.5 to 5.2 mg·dL^{-1} after the administration of 150 mg of AZA. When AZA was resumed after 9 months of CYC treatment, fever and acute renal failure, with a Cr level of 3.0 mg·dL^{-1}, developed within a few hours owing to suspected recurrence of AZA hypersensitivity [12]. Interstitial damage has been suggested as a mechanism for this renal impairment [12, 13].

Remission is defined as the complete absence of clinical disease activity [14]; however, it is difficult to assess when severe respiratory failure occurs, such as in this case. This case switched from induction therapy to maintenance therapy because the VDI score did not worsen. However, it was unclear whether the kidneys were in remission because the urine occult blood (occasionally with dysmorphic erythrocytes) was always positive, partly owing to the antithrombotic therapy. Furthermore, the MPO-ANCA was always high in this case. There is currently a debate about whether MPO-ANCA predicts the future recurrence of AAV, but it is generally not recommended as an indicator, and the risk of recurrence must be judged in relation to the general condition of the patient [2]. However, it has been reported that a positive ANCA at the start of maintenance therapy is associated with a higher risk of AAV recurrence [15], which could not be ignored in this case. It is unclear why ANCA was always high in this case, but the clinical course suggests that there was no morbidity. According to a report, 1 in 56 patients with AAV had a consistently high MPO-ANCA level but did not relapse [16]. There is also a report that MPO-ANCA patients with persistently elevated MPO-ANCA levels do not relapse but do develop chronic renal failure [17]. Additionally, a study has shown that differences in the epitopes of ANCA determine whether they are pathogenic [18].

When switching to maintenance therapy, AAV should be treated with a combination of low-dose PSL and an immunosuppressive agent. The European League Against Rheumatism recommends, in order of priority, AZA, RTX, MTX, and MMF as maintenance therapy and considers leflunomide (LEF) when these are not available. RTX has the serious side effects of opportunistic infection and viral reactivation. When RTX is used to treat lymphoma, HBV reactivation is observed in 8% of patients with HBsAg-negative and anti-HBc-positive HBV [19]. In this case, the HBV-DNA level was below the measurement sensitivity level, and, although it was possible to monitor the HBV-DNA level periodically, we decided not to because of the risk of opportunistic infection. MTX and LEF could not be used in this case of severe lung damage because of interstitial pneumonia. AZA is recommended over MMF for the treatment of AAV because patients treated with MMF had a higher relapse rate than those treated with AZA in the IMPROVE trial [20]. Additionally, the side effects of MMF include the risk of viral infections, gastrointestinal symptoms, myelosuppression, and CMV infection. However, MMF causes fewer adverse events in the lungs than MTX. Therefore, we decided to use MMF in this case, considering the patient's renal function. Although there is no established recommendation for the duration of remission maintenance therapy for AAV, it is desirable to continue for at least 24 months after the induction of maintenance therapy.

4. Conclusion

AZA hypersensitivity syndrome is a Sweet's syndrome-like febrile rash that occurs within 4 weeks of AZA initiation. Infection and flare-ups are a concern in the treatment of AAV, which is heightened if AAV is accompanied by severe lung damage. In such circumstances, immunosuppressive drug allergies can go unnoticed and are prone to misdiagnosis and overtreatment. Clinicians should be aware of this case and consider the possibility of allergic reactions specific to AZA when switching from induction therapy to maintenance therapy.

References

[1] A. C. Hessels, J. S. F. Sanders, A. A. J. M. van de Ven et al., "Azathioprine hypersensitivity syndrome in a cohort of anti-neutrophil cytoplasmic antibody-associated vasculitis patients," *The Journal of Allergy and Clinical Immunology: In Practice*, vol. 7, no. 3, pp. 1004–1009, 2019.

[2] M. Yates, R. A. Watts, I. M. Bajema et al., "EULAR/ERA-EDTA recommendations for the management of ANCA-associated vasculitis," *Annals of the Rheumatic Diseases*, vol. 75, no. 9, pp. 1583–1594, 2016.

[3] C. Choonhakarn and S. Chaowattanapanit, "Azathioprine-induced Sweet's syndrome and published work review," *The Journal of Dermatology*, vol. 40, no. 4, pp. 267–271, 2013.

[4] J. J. Bidinger, K. Sky, D. F. Battafarano, and J. S. Henning, "The cutaneous and systemic manifestations of azathioprine hypersensitivity syndrome," *Journal of the American Academy of Dermatology*, vol. 65, no. 1, pp. 184–191, 2011.

[5] A. James, J. Blagojevic, S. W. Benham, R. Cornall, and J. Frater, "Azathioprine hypersensitivity presenting as septic shock with encephalopathy," *BMJ Case Reports*, vol. 2013, no. mar18 1, article bcr2012008340, 2013.

[6] N. Cyrus, R. Stavert, A. R. Mason, C. J. Ko, and J. N. Choi, "Neutrophilic dermatosis after azathioprine exposure," *JAMA Dermatology*, vol. 149, no. 5, pp. 592–597, 2013.

[7] W. J. Zhou and C. D. Yang, "The causes and clinical significance of fever in systemic lupus erythematosus: a retrospective study of 487 hospitalised patients," *Lupus*, vol. 18, no. 9, pp. 807–812, 2009.

[8] B. Y. Thong, K. P. Leong, J. Thumboo, E. T. Koh, and C. Y. Tang, "Cyclophosphamide type I hypersensitivity in systemic lupus erythematosus," *Lupus*, vol. 11, no. 2, pp. 127–129, 2002.

[9] K. Matsushita, A. Ozaki, H. Inoue et al., "Stevens-Johnson syndrome induced by mizoribine in a patient with systemic lupus erythematosus," *Modern Rheumatology*, vol. 16, no. 2, pp. 113–116, 2014.

[10] M. Szyper-Kravitz, P. Sheinberg, Y. Sidi, Y. Schiffenbauer, E. Trubniykov, and Y. Shoenfeld, "Hypersensitivity to mycophenolate mofetil in systemic lupus erythematosus: diagnostic measures and successful desensitization," *International Archives of Allergy and Immunology*, vol. 138, no. 4, pp. 334–336, 2005.

[11] K. Brockow, B. Przybilla, W. Aberer et al., "Guideline for the diagnosis of drug hypersensitivity Reactions," *Allergo Journal International*, vol. 24, no. 3, pp. 94–105, 2015.

[12] E. Reinhold-Keller, W. H. Schmitt, and W. L. Gross, "Azathioprine toxicity mimicking a relapse of Wegener's granulomatosis," *Rheumatology (Oxford)*, vol. 40, no. 7, pp. 831-832, 2001.

[13] K. Bir, A. M. Herzenberg, and S. Carette, "Azathioprine induced acute interstitial nephritis as the cause of rapidly progressive renal failure in a patient with Wegener's granulomatosis," *The Journal of Rheumatology*, vol. 33, no. 1, pp. 185–187, 2006.

[14] D. Geetha, Q. Jin, J. Scott et al., "Comparisons of guidelines and recommendations on managing antineutrophil cytoplasmic antibody-associated vasculitis," *Kidney International Reports*, vol. 3, no. 5, pp. 1039–1049, 2018.

[15] M. C. Slot, J. W. C. Tervaert, M. M. Boomsma, and C. A. Stegeman, "Positive classic antineutrophil cytoplasmic antibody (C-ANCA) titer at switch to azathioprine therapy associated with relapse in proteinase 3-related vasculitis," *Arthritis and Rheumatism*, vol. 51, no. 2, pp. 269–273, 2004.

[16] J. De'Oliviera, G. Gaskin, A. Dash, A. J. Rees, and C. D. Pusey, "Relationship between disease activity and anti-neutrophil cytoplasmic antibody concentration in long-term management of systemic vasculitis," *American Journal of Kidney Diseases*, vol. 25, no. 3, pp. 380–389, 1995.

[17] C. F. Franssen, C. A. Stegeman, W. W. Oost-Kort et al., "Determinants of renal outcome in anti-myeloperoxidase-associated necrotizing crescentic glomerulonephritis," *Journal of the American Society of Nephrology*, vol. 9, no. 10, pp. 1915–1923, 1998.

[18] A. J. Roth, J. D. Ooi, J. J. Hess et al., "Epitope specificity determines pathogenicity and detectability in ANCA-associated vasculitis," *The Journal of Clinical Investigation*, vol. 123, no. 4, pp. 1773–1783, 2013.

[19] C. Hsu, H. H. Tsou, S. J. Lin et al., "Chemotherapy-induced hepatitis B reactivation in lymphoma patients with resolved HBV infection: a prospective study," *Hepatology*, vol. 59, no. 6, pp. 2092–2100, 2014.

[20] T. F. Hiemstra, M. Walsh, A. Mahr et al., "Mycophenolate mofetil vs azathioprine for remission maintenance in antineutrophil cytoplasmic antibody-associated vasculitis: a randomized controlled trial," *JAMA*, vol. 304, no. 21, pp. 2381–2388, 2010.

24

Efficacy of Omalizumab Therapy in an Asthmatic with Low IgE

Divya R, Rajesh Venkitakrishnan, Jolsana Augustine, and Melcy Cleetus

Department of Pulmonary Medicine, Rajagiri Hospital Chunangamvely, Aluva, 683112, Kochi, Kerala, India

Correspondence should be addressed to Rajesh Venkitakrishnan; rajeshdhanya@rediffmail.com

Academic Editor: Antonio Corrado

Asthma is one of the most common respiratory diseases encountered in clinical practice. Although the vast majority of asthmatics can be adequately controlled with inhaled steroids and other preventer medications, a small proportion remain uncontrolled. Anti-IgE treatment with omalizumab has been proposed in patients as a preferred approach in step 5 asthma therapy according to GINA guidelines. Although therapy with this molecule is approved for patients with atopic asthma and pretreatment serum IgE levels of 30-1500 only, there have been a few reports of its efficacy in subjects outside this reference IgE range. We report the case of a middle-aged lady with severe corticosteroid-dependent asthma and low serum IgE levels who was successfully treated with 9 months of omalizumab therapy. She gained good asthma control and was tapered off steroid use by the fifth month of therapy with omalizumab. The case report stresses the need for further investigation into expanding the spectrum of omalizumab usage in asthma beyond the current IgE suitability range.

1. Introduction

Asthma is an extremely common chronic disease across the globe that affects 7%-13% of the population as per estimates in the first decade of the 21st century [1]. The true burden of asthma in India is not known. Although earlier studies reported a median prevalence of 3%, there is growing evidence to suggest that this may be a gross underestimate [2]. Reviews on the topic state that 10% of patients with asthma are poorly controlled. This subgroup contributes to high utilization of health care resources and has worse quality of life [3].

The 2020 Global Initiative for Asthma (GINA) guidelines recommended that omalizumab be considered a preferred therapy in step 5 care for patients with severe persistent asthma after appropriate phenotype evaluation. The drug is approved for allergic asthmatics with a pretreatment total serum IgE level between 30 and 1500 IU/mL and body weight within a specified range, which is the range over which the drug can reduce enough free IgE to ensure a therapeutic effect. The suitability of the drug in severe asthmatics with IgE values < 30 IU/mL is not well defined although a few case reports suggest clinical benefits. [4, 5] We share the case of a middle-aged lady with severe steroid-dependent asthma and low serum IgE levels in whom successful asthma control was achieved with 9 months of omalizumab therapy. She remains off systemic steroids at 9 months of anti-IgE therapy and continues to be under follow-up.

2. Case Report

A 58-year-old lady, nurse by profession, residing in the United States, presented to us in the second half of 2019. Her history was remarkable for systemic hypertension, dyslipidemia, and chronic persistent asthma. She denied any history of smoking or tobacco product use. She did not have any environmental or professional exposure to agents triggering her asthma. Her asthmatic symptoms dated back to late adolescence and had progressed in severity since then, with significant worsening over the last 3 years. She was steroid dependent for the last 15 months. Despite being on a maintenance dose of 10 mg of prednisolone per day, she used to experience nocturnal symptoms and needed salbutamol inhalations on an average 3-4 times a week. She used to get exacerbations once a month needing hiking up of prednisolone dose to 40 mg per day for 5-7 days. Her detailed evaluation was done in the United States. Her spirometry showed persistent obstructive ventilatory defect. Her compliance to

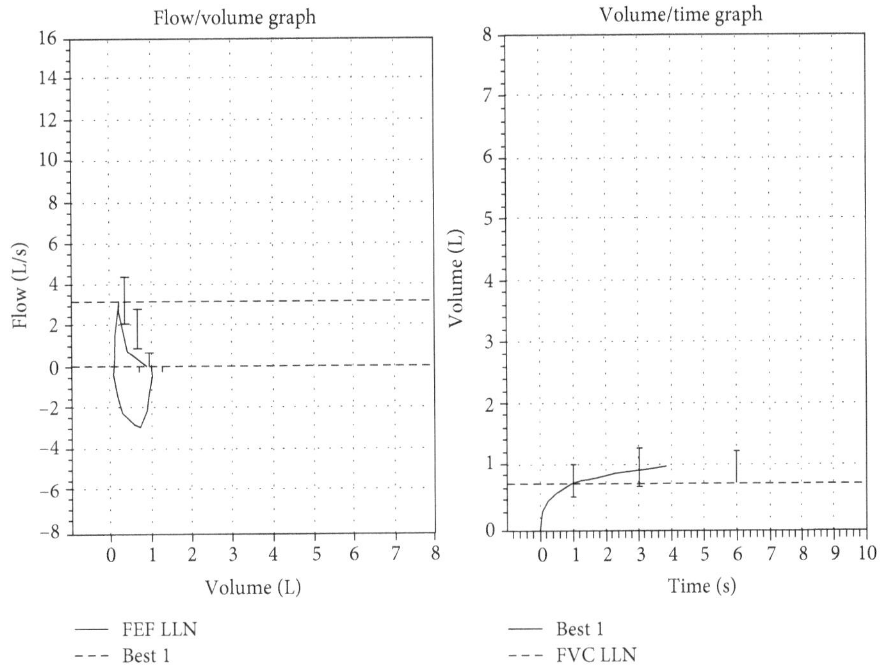

Results			
Parameter	ATS/ERS best	Pred	% pred.
FVC (L)	0.98	1.26	78
FEV1 (L)	0.73	0.98	74
FEV1 ratio	0.74	0.74	100
PEF (L/min)	191	277	69
FEF25-75 (L/s)	0.53*	2.07	26

*Below lower limit of normality (LLN)

FIGURE 1: Spirogram before initiation of omalizumab.

medications was ascertained, inhaler technique was supervised, and medications were optimised. Thyroid abnormalities, gastroesophageal reflux, allergic rhinitis, and vocal cord dysfunction were ruled out by appropriate evaluations. She was obese (BMI 33) with no snoring or excessive daytime sleepiness measured by the Epworth scale. Cardiac function as measured by ECG and 2D ECHO were normal. CT chest showed no parenchymal shadows, bronchiectasis, or mucoid impaction. She had no features of anxiety or depression ascertained during a formal psychology evaluation. Her IgE levels were <10 mg/mL on multiple occasions in the United States as well as during her current evaluation. She was considered for therapy with biological agents (omalizumab) but therapy with this agent was not instituted as her IgE levels were below the range approved for therapy. She was having significant steroid adverse effects including truncal obesity and osteopenia.

With this background, she presented to our outpatient department. Her blood counts revealed a normal total leucocyte count (7700 per cubic mm [3]) with 6 percent eosinophils. Renal functions, hepatic functions, serum electrolytes, fasting lipid profile, and thyroid functions were normal. She was evaluated at the difficult asthma clinic where her compliance to medications was ascertained, inhaler technique was supervised, and medications were optimised (budesonide 1600 mcg per day, tiotropium 18 mcg per day, addition of montelukast-levocetirizine combination, and sustained release theophylline). The reports of evaluations done in the United States were crosschecked. Her spirometry (Figure 1) showed persistent obstructive ventilatory defect (postbronchodilator FEV1 74% predicted). Serum IgE levels repeated at our institution revealed a value of 7.5 IU/mL. She had inadequate response at one month of our therapy with exacerbations needing escalation of systemic steroids. Considering the burden of her disease, adverse drug effects, and its impact on her life, she was given the option of off label omalizumab therapy which she readily accepted after detailed briefing regarding the uncertainty in efficacy. She was initiated on omalizumab 150 mg subcutaneously once monthly, while continuing her baseline drugs. She began to get subjective improvement in her nocturnal symptoms after the second dose and tapering of prednisolone was attempted after the second dose. She was totally off systemic steroids by the sixth month of therapy and her rescue use of beta 2 agonists reduced to one per week on an average. A total of 9 doses of omalizumab were given. The improvement in steroid dose, asthma symptoms, and early morning PEFR are shown in Table 1. She had only 2 exacerbations needing hiking up of steroids during these nine months of therapy as opposed to 7 in the 6 months prior to omalizumab initiation (Figure 2). Her asthma control improved significantly (baseline ACT score of 13 improving to 22 at the end of 9 months). Her postbronchodilator FEV1 improved by 3% over the 9 months of therapy. She remains under reasonable control with 800 mcg per day of

Table 1: Improvement in steroid use, asthma control, and lung function with omalizumab therapy.

	Mean prednisone dose (mg/day)	ACT values	Early morning PEFR (litres/mt)
Baseline	10	22	280
Month 2	7.5	22	290
Month 3	5	18	300
Month 4	2.5	14	300
Month 5	1.25	12	300

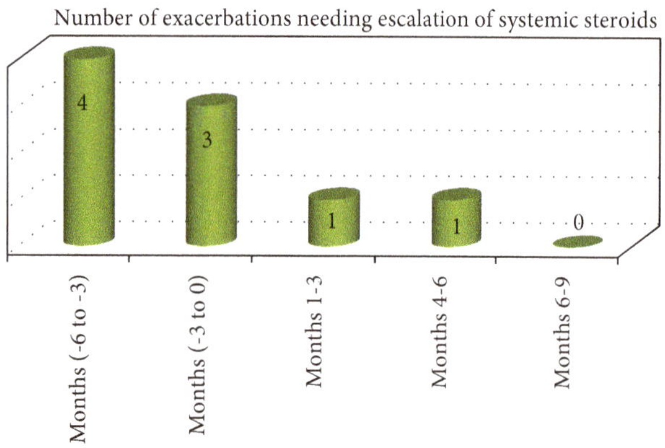

Figure 2: Exacerbations needing escalation of steroid use before and after initiation of anti-IgE treatment.

budesonide, tiotropium, sustained release theophylline, and montelukast. She plans to return to the United States in the next 2 months.

3. Discussion

Omalizumab is a humanized monoclonal antibody with affinity for IgE molecule at its binding site of the high-affinity IgE receptor. Current GINA guidelines recommend omalizumab as a preferred therapy in step 5 care for patients with severe persistent allergic asthma after appropriate phenotype evaluation. Omalizumab is approved as an add-on therapy for moderate to severe allergic asthma in adults and children above 6 years of age. However, the drug is approved only for asthmatics with a pretreatment total serum IgE level between 30 and 1500 IU/mL. Administration in patients with a serum IgE level < 30 IU/L was discouraged, possibly because in the initial report of patients with bronchial hyperreactivity, none had such low IgE concentrations [6]. However, there have been subsequent reports of successful omalizumab therapy in subjects with IgE levels below this reference range, patients with negative skin prick tests and nonallergic asthmatics [4, 5, 7–10].

The success of omalizumab therapy in nonallergic patients with severe asthma has been linked to the "non-anticirculating IgE" effects of omalizumab. Excellent reviews have attempted to elucidate the mechanisms of action of this monoclonal antibody other than the anti-IgE effect [11]. A 2-year study by de Llano and colleagues reported that omalizumab therapy achieved significant improvements in asthma control in nonallergic asthmatic patients [12]. A real-life trial by Grimaldi-Bensouda and colleagues found that omalizumab elicited a marked reduction of hospitalizations and emergency department visits regardless of the atopic status [13]. A randomized study in patients with nonatopic asthma showed that omalizumab, when compared with placebo, was able to lower the frequency of asthma exacerbations and to induce also a significant FEV1 increase; a sharp decrease of FcεRI expression on basophils and plasmacytoid dendritic cells was also noticed in this study [14]. Such experimental findings prompted Lommatzsch and colleagues to hypothesize at least two possible explanations for the unexpected effects of omalizumab in nonallergic asthma [15]. The first hypothesis implies that these apparently nonallergic patients could be sensitized to unrecognized allergens resulting in a local airway-limited sensitization. The immune response is such cases remain confined within the airways, with no systemic spreading. The second is based on the potential ability of omalizumab to restore the antiviral protective action of dendritic cells, which can be defective in both allergic and nonallergic asthmatic patients. These cells lose the ability to produce interferon upon FcεRI activation by antiallergen, as well as by antiviral and antibacterial IgE. Omalizumab can neutralize this negative effect on innate immunity, and it can reduce the exacerbations induced by respiratory viruses as was noted in the PROSE study by Teach et al. [16] In this study, administration of omalizumab (in addition to standard asthma treatment) to asthmatic children aged 6-17 years residing in the inner city before return to school reduced asthma exacerbations in winter, particularly among those with a recent exacerbation.

A study by Johansson et al. [17] suggests that the proportion of disease-relevant allergen-specific IgE antibody fraction (the percentage of allergen-specific IgE antibody to total IgE) is a predictor of the success of anti-IgE therapy rather than total serum IgE levels. Recommended doses of omalizumab efficiently eliminate IgE antibodies if the IgE antibody fraction is <1% of total IgE but have inadequate clinical effect if the fraction is >3-4%. Hence, it may be quite possible that subjects with a low total serum IgE level have higher fractions of a relevant allergen-specific IgE which is blocked by omalizumab. However, a demonstration of a larger proportion of disease-specific IgE antibody fraction may be challenging in real-world clinical practice as opposed to a research setting.

It may be prudent to restrict omalizumab administration criteria to atopic asthmatics within the currently mentioned IgE range till the time the potential mechanisms of non-IgE-mediated action are clearly substantiated. However, off label use in carefully selected patients being managed at experienced centres may be justified with informed consent from patients. It may be reasonable to expect that further basic and clinical research may expand the suitability criteria of omalizumab use in allergic states.

4. Summary and Conclusion

We report the successful off label use of omalizumab in a lady with severe steroid-dependent asthma who had an IgE level of <10 IU/mL. Mechanisms of beneficial effects rendered by omalizumab in nonallergic asthmatics have been incompletely elucidated, and understanding in this arena is evolving. Studies reporting the efficacy of anti-IgE therapy in this subset of asthmatics are few, and the present article may be expected to add further impetus to exploring new horizons of omalizumab use in allergic states.

References

[1] S. S. Braman, "The global burden of asthma," *Chest*, vol. 130, no. 1, pp. 4S–12S, 2006.

[2] A. N. Aggarwal, K. Chaudhry, S. K. Chhabra et al., "Prevalence and risk factors for bronchial asthma in Indian adults: a multicentre study," *Indian Journal of Chest Diseases and Allied Sciences*, vol. 48, no. 1, pp. 13–22, 2006.

[3] P. J. Barnes, B. Jonsson, and J. B. Klim, "The costs of asthma, *European Respiratory Journal*, vol. 9, no. 4, pp. 636–642, 1996.

[4] O. Matsuno, C. Komori, Y. Hang, T. Matsumoto, and S. Minamoto, "Effectiveness of omalizumab in a patient with severe asthma, low serum IgE level, and lack of sensitized allergens induced by oral steroid therapy: the usefulness of impulse oscillation for assessment of omalizumab therapy," *Journal of Asthma*, vol. 49, no. 8, pp. 839–842, 2012.

[5] Y. Sugino, R. Sanda, Y. Takagi et al., "A case of severe asthma responsive to omalizumab treatment despite a low serum IgE level and lack of sensitized allergens," *Arerugī*, vol. 59, no. 11, pp. 1572–1579, 2010.

[6] M. R. Sears, B. Burrows, E. M. Flannery, G. P. Herbison, C. J. Hewitt, and M. D. Holdaway, "Relation between airway responsiveness and serum IgE in children with asthma and in apparently normal children," *The New England Journal of Medicine*, vol. 325, no. 15, pp. 1067–1071, 1991.

[7] N. Asai, Y. Ohkuni, A. Komatsu, R. Matsunuma, K. Nakashima, and N. Kaneko, "Severe persistent asthma responsive to off-label use of omalizumab despite high and low levels of total serum IgE," *Jornal Brasileiro de Pneumologia*, vol. 37, no. 4, pp. 567–570, 2011.

[8] J. Ankerst, A. Nopp, S. G. O. Johansson, J. Adédoyin, and H. Öman, "Xolair Is Effective in Allergics with a Low Serum IgE Level," *International Archives of Allergy and Immunology* vol. 152, no. 1, pp. 71–74, 2010.

[9] F. Menzella, R. Piro, N. Facciolongo, C. Castagnetti, A. Simonazzi, and L. Zucchi, "Long-term benefits of omalizumab in a patient with severe non-allergic asthma," *Allergy, Asthma & Clinical Immunology*, vol. 7, no. 1, 2011.

[10] M. van den Berge, R. G. Pauw, J. G. R. de Monchy, C. A. van Minnen, D. S. Postma, and H. A. M. Kerstjens, "Beneficial Effects of Treatment With Anti-IgE Antibodies (Omalizumab) in a Patient With Severe Asthma and Negative Skin-Prick Test Results," *Chest*, vol. 139, no. 1, pp. 190–193, 2011.

[11] C. Pelaia, C. Calabrese, R. Terracciano, F. de Blasio, A. Vatrella, and G. Pelaia, "Omalizumab, the first available antibody for biological treatment of severe asthma: more than a decade of real-life effectiveness," *Therapeutic Advances in Respiratory Disease*, vol. 12, p. 175346661881019, 2018.

[12] L. P. de Llano, M. d. C. Vennera, F. J. Álvarez et al., "Effects of Omalizumab in Non-Atopic Asthma: Results from a Spanish Multicenter Registry," *Journal of Asthma*, vol. 50, no. 3, pp. 296–301, 2013.

[13] L. Grimaldi-Bensouda, M. Zureik, M. Aubier et al., "Does Omalizumab Make a Difference to the Real-life Treatment of Asthma Exacerbations?," *Chest*, vol. 143, no. 2, pp. 398–405, 2013.

[14] G. Garcia, A. Magnan, R. Chiron et al., "A proof-of-concept, randomized, controlled trial of omalizumab in patients with severe, difficult-to-control, nonatopic asthma," *Chest*, vol. 144, no. 2, pp. 411–419, 2013.

[15] M. Lommatzsch, S. Korn, R. Buhl, and J. C. Virchow, "Against all odds: anti-IgE for intrinsic asthma?," *Thorax*, vol. 69, no. 1, pp. 94–96, 2013.

[16] S. J. Teach, M. A. Gill, A. Togias et al., "Preseasonal treatment with either omalizumab or an inhaled corticosteroid boost to prevent fall asthma exacerbations," *Journal of Allergy and Clinical Immunology*, vol. 136, no. 6, pp. 1476–1485, 2015.

[17] S. G. O. Johansson, A. Nopp, H. Öman et al., "The size of the disease relevant IgE antibody fraction in relation to 'total-IgE' predicts the efficacy of anti-IgE (Xolair) treatment," *Allergy*, vol. 64, no. 10, pp. 1472–1477, 2009.

25

Clinical and Radiological Presentations of Various Pulmonary Infections in Hospitalized Diabetes Mellitus Patients: A Prospective, Hospital-Based, Comparative, Case Series Study

Pravesh Vishwakarma,[1] Kauser Usman,[2] Rajiv Garg,[3] Jyoti Bajpai,[3] Rishi Sethi,[1] and Akshyaya Pradhan[1]

[1]*Department of Cardiology, King George's Medical University, Lucknow, Uttar Pradesh 226003, India*
[2]*Department of Internal Medicine, King George's Medical University, Lucknow, Uttar Pradesh 226003, India*
[3]*Department of Respiratory Medicine, King George's Medical University, Lucknow, Uttar Pradesh 226003, India*

Correspondence should be addressed to Jyoti Bajpai; jyotibajpai33@gmail.com

Academic Editor: Yongchun Shen

Background. Diabetes mellitus is associated with increased rate of respiratory tract infections. The objective was to compare demographic, clinical, serum biochemical, and typical and atypical radiological profiles among hospitalized diabetics and nondiabetics with lower respiratory tract infection. *Material and Methods.* A prospective, hospital-based, consecutive, comparative observational study of 12-month study duration was conducted. Patients aged 13–90 years diagnosed with lower respiratory tract infection with or without diagnosed diabetes mellitus participated in the study. Demographic, clinical, serum biochemistry, and radiological profiles of diabetics ($n = 44$) and nondiabetics ($n = 53$) were compared. *Results.* Diabetics were older than nondiabetics at presentation ($p < 0.0001$). Difference in mean random blood sugar (RBS) ($p < 0.001$), fasting blood sugar (FBS) ($p < 0.001$), and postprandial blood sugar (PPBS) ($p < 0.0001$) was significant between diabetics and nondiabetics. Nondiabetics more frequently presented with fever ($p = 0.0032$), chest pain ($p = 0.0002$), and hemoptysis ($p = 0.01$) as compared to diabetics. Diabetics more frequently presented with extreme temperatures (hypothermia or hyperpyrexia) ($p = 0.022$), lower serum sodium levels ($p = 0.047$), and lower partial arterial pressure ($p < 0.001$) than nondiabetics. The mean pneumonia patient outcomes research team (PORT) risk score was higher in diabetics (124.84 ± 41.31) compared to nondiabetics (77.85 ± 39.77) ($p < 0.001$). Diabetics more commonly displayed bilateral lesions with multilobe or lower lobe involvement, the most common type of lesion being exudative. *Conclusion.* Diabetic patients usually had severe pulmonary infection and poor prognosis as suggested by higher mean PORT risk score. They also more frequently presented with bilateral lesions with multilobe or lower lobe involvement as evidenced by radiography as compared to nondiabetic patients.

1. Introduction

Diabetes mellitus is a vastly prevalent chronic metabolic disorder escalating at an alarming rate around the globe. India has contributed substantially to this global burden. Prevalence of diabetes in India increased from 26 million in 1990 to 65 million in 2016 [1]. This metabolic disorder is identified by hyperglycemia resulting from reduced insulin secretion, reduced glucose usage, and increased glucose production [2, 3]. The hyperglycemic state, lowered immunity, pulmonary microangiopathy, and pulmonary dysfunction are frequently accompanied by sequelae such as severe hospital-acquired pneumonia, severe pulmonary infections with antimicrobial resistance, and chronic complications such as renal failure, coronary disease, diabetic nephropathy, and diabetic retinopathy [4].

The lung is a target organ affected by diabetes mellitus—-pulmonary and vascular functions are closely associated. Acute and chronic respiratory infections such as tuberculosis and pneumonia as well as other rare infectious diseases are frequently observed in diabetic patients [5]. Pulmonary infections are one of the most frequently encountered infections in diabetic patients. Several studies have revealed that pulmonary infections in diabetics predispose this subset of patients to more severe clinical manifestations, longer duration of diabetes, longer duration of treatment, more frequent complications, and increased mortality [2, 5–10]. Moreover, certain types of pulmonary infections are more prevalent among diabetics than nondiabetics. The clinical spectrum and radiological presentation of such infections differ from those of nondiabetics. Further investigations are warranted to determine the pattern of infection in these patients. Against this background, we conducted the present study with the objective to compare demographic, clinical, serum biochemical, and typical and atypical radiological profiles among hospitalized diabetics and nondiabetics with lower respiratory tract infection.

2. Materials and Methods

2.1. Study Design and Patient Population. A prospective, hospital-based, consecutive, comparative, case series study comparing diabetics and nondiabetics with lower respiratory tract infection was conducted at a tertiary care centre King George's Medical University, U.P., Lucknow, in India over a 12-month period from September 2007 to August 2008. All patients aged 13–90 years admitted in inpatient wards of Gandhi Memorial and Associated Hospitals (Department of Internal Medicine and Department of Pulmonary Medicine), King George's Medical University, U.P., Lucknow, with diagnosis of lower respiratory tract infection with or without evidence of diabetes mellitus were included in the study.

Patients who (i) had died within 8 hours of admission, (ii) could not be investigated, (iii) had impaired fasting plasma glucose or impaired glucose tolerance, (iv) had malignancy, or (v) refused to provide written informed consent were excluded from the study. The study was approved by the Institutional Ethics Committee prior to the start of the study. Written informed consent to use the patient's clinical records for scientific purposes was obtained from each patient before study enrolment.

2.2. Data Collection for All Study Patients. After explaining the study and obtaining written informed consent, all patients provided a complete clinical history and underwent a thorough physical examination. Patient demographics such as age and gender and presenting symptoms such as fever, cough, expectoration, hemoptysis, chest pain, and dyspnea were recorded. During the physical examination, hypotension (systolic blood pressure < 90 mmHg or use of vasopressor), tachycardia (pulse rate > 110/min), tachypnea (respiratory rate > 30/min), hyperpyrexia (temperature > 104°F), or hypothermia (temperature < 95°F) was recorded. A battery of basic biochemical and hematological tests was performed for all patients. Similarly, chest radiographs for all patients were obtained.

2.3. Additional Data Collection for Diabetic Patients. Patients with initial blood glucose levels or a prior diagnosis of diabetes provided a detailed history including duration of diagnosed diabetes mellitus and ongoing treatment. Glycemic monitoring (fasting and postprandial blood sugar) along with measurement of hemoglobin A_{1c} (HbA_{1c}) was performed at the time of admission to determine the level of glycemic control. In addition, the presence of diabetes-related complications was investigated by evaluating patient hospital records, current clinical manifestations, blood or urine biochemistry abnormalities, and when necessitated specific tests.

2.4. Lower Respiratory Tract Infection. Lower respiratory tract infection was diagnosed by the presence of ≥2 of the following symptoms: (i) fever, (ii) new or increasing cough or sputum production, (iii) dyspnea, (iv) chest pain, or (v) new focal signs on chest examination in addition to the presence of at least one opacity on chest radiography consistent with infectious pathology and/or isolation of suspected microorganism from sputum, pleural fluid, or blood. The validated pneumonia severity index (PSI)/pneumonia patient outcomes research team (PORT) score [11, 12] was used to categorize risk class of the patient at the time of admission [13].

2.5. Diabetes Mellitus. Diabetes mellitus was diagnosed according to the standard American Diabetic Association guidelines [14]. The criteria for diagnosis are as follows: (i) symptoms of hyperglycemia and random plasma glucose ≥ 200 mg/dL; random was defined as any time of day regardless of time since last meal; the classic symptoms of hyperglycemia include polyuria, polydipsia, and unexplained weight loss; (ii) fasting plasma glucose ≥ 126 mg/dL; fasting was defined as no calorie intake for at least 8 hours; or (iii) 2-hour plasma glucose ≥ 200 mg/dL during an oral glucose tolerance test. The test was performed as described by the World Health Organization using a glucose load containing an equivalent of 75 g anhydrous glucose dissolved in water.

2.6. Impaired Fasting Glucose and Impaired Glucose Tolerance. Patients were diagnosed with impaired fasting glucose or impaired glucose tolerance by fasting glucose ≥ 100 mg/dL but <126 mg/dL or 2-hour values in the oral glucose tolerance test (OGTT) of >140 mg/dL but <200 mg/dL. All cases in the present study were subjected to the oxidase method to avoid interference from lipid, bilirubin, uric acid, and antidiabetic drugs.

2.7. Assessment of Glycemic Control. Assessment of glycemic control, i.e., differentiation of diabetic patients into controlled or uncontrolled, was done by measuring HbA_{1c} as outlined by the American Diabetic Association [14]. Patients with glycated HbA_{1c} levels < 7% were considered to have controlled diabetes mellitus, while patients with levels beyond this were considered to have uncontrolled diabetes mellitus.

2.8. Chest Radiography. Posterior-anterior chest X-ray views were taken in all patients, and if required, lateral views were also taken. Lesions were described according to (i) site, (ii) zone of involvement, or (iii) nature. Sites of the lesion were

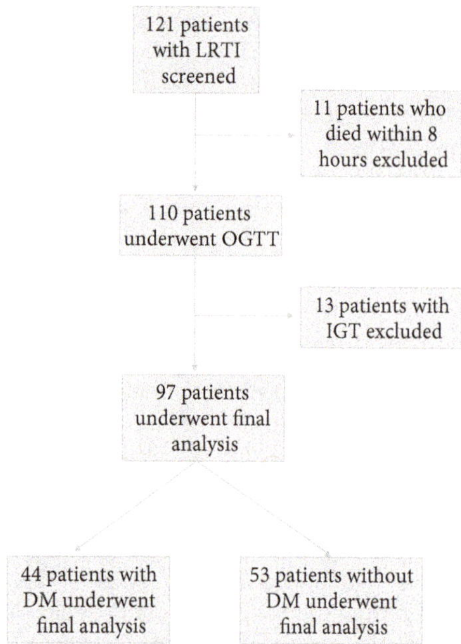

FIGURE 1: Flow diagram of the study.

either unilateral (right or left) or bilateral. Zones of involvement included upper, middle, or lower zones. The upper zone lied above the right anterior border of the second rib. The middle zone lied between the right anterior border of the second and fourth ribs. The lower zone lied between the right anterior border of the fourth rib and diaphragm. The lesions were categorized as exudative, consolidation, pleural effusion, cavitation, pneumothorax, or hydropneumothorax. Exudative lesions were lesions with predominantly small shadows merging with each other to produce shadows resembling cotton wool or clone-like in appearances. Consolidation lesions were patchy, opaque, exudative lesions of segmental or lobar distribution with homogenous density. Pleural effusions were identified as homogenous, dense, and opaque effusions with ill-defined upper limits that were laterally high with filling of costophrenic angle. Cavitations were single or multiple, clear-cut, homogenous, low-density cavities filled with air. Pneumothorax was defined as an area of hyperluscency with absence of bronchovascular markings and presence of collapsed lung margins. The pleural cavity is filled with air. Hydropneumothorax was defined as the presence of both air and fluid in the pleural space.

2.9. Statistical Analysis. Continuous variables are presented as mean ± standard deviation, while categorical variables are presented as frequency and percentages. Continuous variables were compared using the Student t-test. Categorical variables were compared using either the chi-square test or Fisher exact test. A p value < 0.05 was considered statistically significant. The statistical evaluation of data was done using the Statistical Package for the Social Sciences (SPSS; Chicago, IL, USA) program, version 14.

TABLE 1: Demographic profile of diabetics and nondiabetics with pulmonary infections.

Variable	Diabetics ($n = 44$)	Nondiabetics ($n = 53$)	p value
Age (years) (mean ± SD)	54.73 ± 12.18	41.15 ± 18.77	<0.0001
Age, n (%)			
<30 years	0 (0%)	19 (35.8%)	
30–60 years	29 (65.9%)	26 (49.1%)	<0.0001
>60 years	15 (34.1%)	8 (15.1%)	
Males, n (%)	32 (72.7%)	35 (66.0%)	0.4

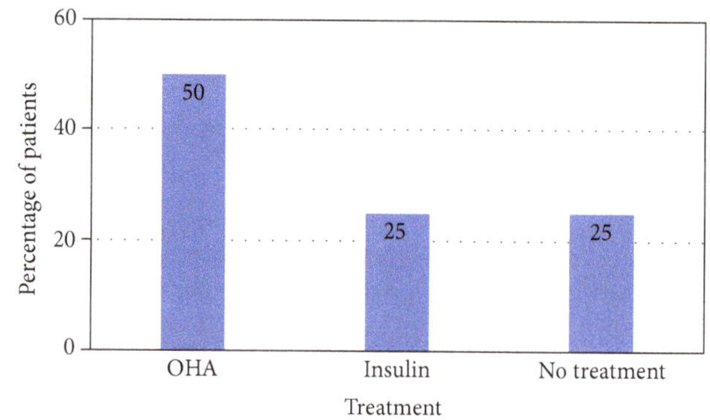

FIGURE 2: Prehospital treatment profile for patients with diabetes mellitus in the study. OHA: oral hypoglycemic agent.

3. Results

A total of 121 patients fulfilled the study inclusion criteria and were enrolled in the study. Out of these 121 patients, 11 patients died within 8 hours of hospitalization and could not be further investigated. These patients were excluded from the study analysis. Of the 110 patients with lower respiratory tract infections, 44 (40.0%) patients had blood sugar levels within diabetic range on OGTT (4 of which were diagnosed during hospital stay), 53 (48.2%) had blood sugar levels within normal range, and 13 (11.8%) had impaired glucose tolerance and were therefore excluded from the study. Thus, 97 patients constituted the study population. 44 (40.0%) patients were diagnosed as diabetic and were designated as cases and the remainder 53 (48.2%) patients were diagnosed as nondiabetic and were designated as controls. The study flow is illustrated in Figure 1.

3.1. Demographic Profile of Diabetics and Nondiabetics with Pulmonary Infections. The mean age of diabetics and nondiabetics with pulmonary infection was 54.73 ± 12.18 and 41.15 ± 18.77 years, respectively. Diabetics were significantly older than nondiabetics ($p < 0.0001$). The study population with pulmonary infection was predominantly middle aged (30-60 years; 66% and 49% in case and control groups, respectively). Males comprised of 32 patients in (72.7%) diabetics and 35 (66.0%) nondiabetics, respectively ($p = 0.48$). The demographic profile of diabetics and nondiabetics with pulmonary infections is demonstrated in Table 1.

TABLE 2: Blood sugar levels of diabetics versus nondiabetics and uncontrolled diabetes mellitus versus controlled diabetes mellitus.

Variable	Diabetics ($n = 44$)	Nondiabetics ($n = 53$)	p value	Uncontrolled diabetes mellitus ($n = 28$)	Controlled diabetes mellitus ($n = 16$)	p value
RBS (mg/dL)	189.84 ± 91.34	101.08 ± 21.05	<0.001	206.36 ± 95.15	167.81 ± 78.00	0.20
FBS (mg/dL)	189.25 ± 85.62	101.02 ± 37.36	<0.001	201.5 ± 88.67	167.81 ± 78.07	0.20
PPBS (mg/dL)	275.76 ± 29.83	133.25 ± 29.83	<0.0001	298.37 ± 113.08	262.88 ± 89.14	0.05

Data are expressed as mean ± standard deviation. RBS: random blood sugar; FBS: fasting blood sugar; PPBS: postprandial blood sugar.

TABLE 3: HbA_{1c} levels, albuminuria levels, and complications of diabetes.

Variable	Diabetics ($n = 44$)
HbA_{1c}, n (%)	
<7% (controlled)	16 (36.4%)
>7% (uncontrolled)	28 (63.6%)
Albuminuria, n (%)	
>300 mg/day	20 (45.5%)
<300 mg/day	10 (22.7%)
Nil	14 (31.8%)
Complications of diabetes	
Nephropathy, n (%)	22 (50.0%)
Retinopathy, n (%)	19 (43.2%)
Neuropathy, n (%)	3 (6.8%)
None, n (%)	16 (36.4%)

3.2. Diabetic Profile of Pulmonary Infection Patients. The mean duration of diabetes in patients with pulmonary infection was found to be 6.23 ± 5.01 years. Orally administered antihyperglycemic agents were the most prescribed treatment used by half of the diabetics. A quarter of the diabetics used insulin, while the other quarter of patients was not adhering to any treatment. Prehospital treatment profile of the diabetic population is displayed in Figure 2. The difference in mean random blood sugar (RBS) ($p < 0.001$), fasting blood sugar (FBS) ($p < 0.001$), and postprandial blood sugar (PPBS) ($p < 0.0001$) between diabetics and nondiabetics was statistically significant. However, the difference in mean RBS ($p = 0.20$), FBS ($p = 0.20$), and PPBS ($p = 0.05$) between uncontrolled and controlled diabetic patients was not statistically significant, although these values were lower in controlled diabetics. The blood sugar levels of these groups are detailed in Table 2. Of the 44 diabetics, 16 (36.4%) patients had controlled diabetes, while 28 (63.6%) had uncontrolled diabetes. Twenty (45.5%) diabetic patients had albuminuria > 300 mg/day, 10 (22.7%) diabetics had albuminuria < 300 mg/day, and 14 (31.8%) diabetics did not have albuminuria. Nephropathy and retinopathy were the most common complications observed in 22 (50.0%) and 19 (43.2%) diabetics, respectively. HbA_{1c} levels, albuminuria levels, and complications of diabetes are described in Table 3.

3.3. Clinical Profile of Pulmonary Infection in Diabetic and Nondiabetic Patients. Nondiabetics more frequently presented with fever ($p = 0.0032$), chest pain ($p = 0.0002$), and hemoptysis ($p = 0.01$) as compared to diabetics. Diabetics had more comorbidities than nondiabetics ($p = 0.021$). Diabetics more frequently presented with extreme temperatures (hypothermia or hyperpyrexia) ($p = 0.022$), lower serum sodium levels ($p = 0.047$), and lower partial arterial pressure ($p < 0.001$) than nondiabetics. The mean PORT risk score was higher in diabetics (124.84 ± 41.31) compared to nondiabetics (77.85 ± 39.77) ($p < 0.001$). Majority of diabetic patients fell into PORT score class IV and V, while the majority nondiabetic patients fell into classes I–III ($p < 0.001$). The clinical profile of pulmonary infections in diabetics and nondiabetics is demonstrated in Table 4, and PORT score class of diabetics and nondiabetics is illustrated in Figure 3.

3.4. Radiological Profile of Pulmonary Infections in Diabetic and Nondiabetic Groups. Unilateral right- and left-sided lesions were more prevalent in nondiabetics (Figure 4), while bilateral lesions were more prevalent in diabetics (Figure 5) ($p = 0.022$). Upper, middle, lower, and multilobe involvement was observed in 10 (22.7%), 2 (4.5%), 16 (36.4%), and 13 (29.5%) diabetics and 12 (22.6%), 7 (13.2%), 18 (34.0%), and 8 (15.1%) nondiabetics, respectively, although this finding was not statistically significant. The radiological profile of pulmonary infections in diabetic and nondiabetics is detailed in Table 5.

4. Discussion

Diabetes mellitus has evidenced to consequence unfavorable outcomes in patients with respiratory tract infections. Several earlier studies have investigated the frequency and pattern of respiratory infections in both diabetic and nondiabetics. Saibal et al. [3] reported a mean age of 56.3 ± 12.2 and 35.7 ± 10.5 years in diabetics and nondiabetics with community-acquired pneumonia, respectively. Wang et al. [15] observed a mean age of 60.8 and 59.1 years in diabetics and nondiabetics with pulmonary tuberculosis, respectively. Fernández et al. [16] found a median age of 76.1 and 60.1 years in diabetics and nondiabetics with community-acquired pneumonia, respectively. Park et al. [17] observed a median age of 66.0 and 42.0 years in uncontrolled diabetics and nondiabetics with pulmonary tuberculosis, respectively. Similarly, Alisjahbana et al. [18] revealed a median age of 45.0 and

TABLE 4: Clinical profile of pulmonary infections in diabetics and nondiabetics.

Variable	Diabetics ($n = 44$)	Nondiabetics ($n = 53$)	p value
Symptoms			
Fever, n (%)	28 (63.6%)	47 (88.7%)	0.0032
Cough, n (%)	32 (72.7%)	44 (83.0%)	0.22
Expectoration, n (%)	21 (47.7%)	26 (49.1%)	0.90
Chest pain, n (%)	5 (11.4%)	24 (45.3%)	0.0002
Hemoptysis, n (%)	9 (20.5%)	24 (45.3%)	0.01
Dyspnea, n (%)	26 (59.1%)	31 (58.5%)	0.88
Conscious	36 (81.8%)	50 (94.4%)	0.053
Unconscious	8 (18.2%)	3 (5.7%)	
Associated comorbidities			
Heart failure, n (%)	3 (6.8%)	0 (0%)	0.021
Renal failure, n (%)	7 (15.9%)	1 (1.9%)	
Chronic liver disease, n (%)	0 (0%)	1 (1.9%)	
None, n (%)	37 (84.1%)	51 (96.2%)	
Systolic blood pressure, n (%)			
≤90 mmHg	6 (13.6%)	2 (3.8%)	0.08
>90 mmHg	38 (686.4%)	51 (96.2%)	
Pulse rate, n (%)			
≥100/min	19 (43.2%)	25 (47.2%)	0.69
<100/min	25 (56.8%)	28 (52.8%)	
Respiratory rate, n (%)			
≥30/min	19 (43.2%)	21 (39.6%)	0.72
<30/min	25 (56.8%)	32 (60.4%)	
Temperature, n (%)			
<95°F	7 (15.9%)	1 (1.9%)	0.022
94–104°F	36 (81.8%)	52 (98.1%)	
>104°F	1 (2.3%)	0 (0%)	
TLC, n (%)			
≥12,000 per cmm	20 (45.5%)	34 (64.2%)	0.064
<12,000 per cmm	24 (54.5%)	19 (35.8%)	
Serum sodium, n (%)			
<130 mEq/dL	13 (29.5%)	7 (13.2%)	0.047
≥130 mEq/dL	31 (70.5%)	46 (86.8%)	
Blood urea, n (%)			
≥60 mg/dL	8 (18.2%)	5 (9.4%)	0.2
<60 mg/dL	36 (81.8%)	48 (90.6%)	
Arterial pH, n (%)			
<7.35	20 (45.5%)	17 (32.1%)	0.18
>7.35	24 (54.5%)	36 (67.9%)	
pO2			
<60 mmHg	25 (56.8%)	51 (96.2%)	<0.001
≤60 mmHg	19 (43.2%)	2 (3.8%)	
PORT risk score (mean ± SD)	124.84 ± 41.31	77.85 ± 39.77	<0.001
Tubercular, n (%)	15 (34.1%)	21 (39.6%)	0.57
Nontubercular, n (%)	29 (65.9%)	32 (60.4%)	
Sputum microscopy, n (%)			
AFB positive	9 (20.5%)	16 (30.2%)	0.50
AFB negative	6 (13.6%)	5 (9.4%)	

Table 4: Continued.

Variable	Diabetics ($n = 44$)	Nondiabetics ($n = 53$)	p value
Mantoux test, n (%)			
Positive	8 (18.2%)	10 (18.9%)	0.99
Negative	7 (15.9%)	10 (18.9%)	

TLC: total leukocyte count; pO2: partial pressure of oxygen; AFB: acid-fast bacteria; PORT: pneumonia patient outcomes research team.

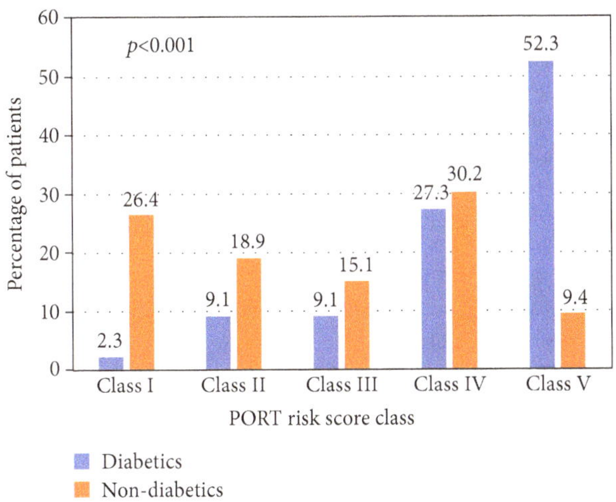

Figure 3: PORT risk score classes of diabetics and nondiabetics with pulmonary infections in the study. PORT: patient outcomes research team.

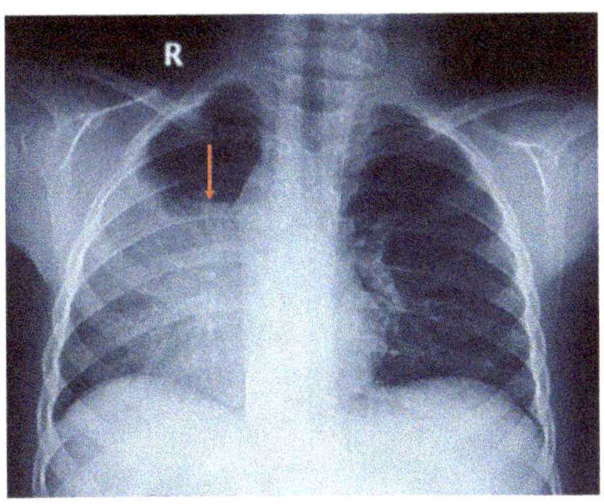

Figure 4: Chest X-ray showed right side mid and lower zone consolidation in nondiabetic patients.

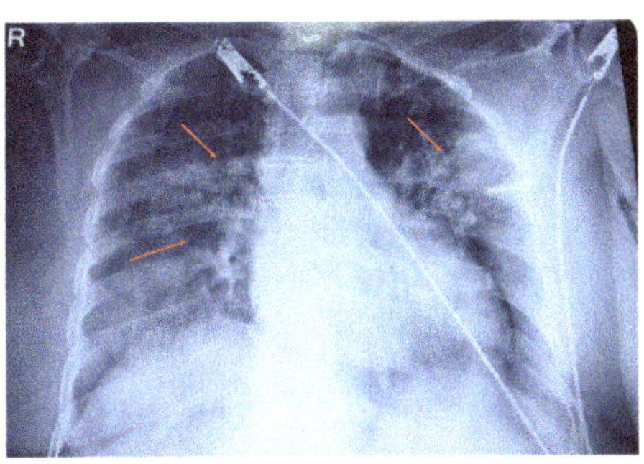

Figure 5: Chest X-ray showed bilateral multifocal mid and lower zone infiltrates/exudates in diabetic patients.

Table 5: Radiological profile of pulmonary infections in diabetics and nondiabetics.

	Diabetics ($n = 44$)	Nondiabetics ($n = 53$)	p value
Site of lesion			
Unilateral (right), n (%)	16 (36.4%)	29 (54.7%)	0.022
Unilateral (left), n (%)	9 (20.5%)	14 (26.4%)	
Bilateral, n (%)	19 (43.2%)	10 (18.9%)	
Zone of lesion			
Upper, n (%)	10 (22.7%)	12 (22.6%)	0.68
Middle, n (%)	2 (4.5%)	7 (13.2%)	
Lower, n (%)	16 (36.4%)	18 (34.0%)	
Multilobed, n (%)	13 (29.5%)	8 (15.1%)	
Nature of lesion			
Exudative, n (%)	20 (45.5%)	14 (26.4%)	0.34
Consolidation, n (%)	16 (36.4%)	24 (45.3%)	
Milliary, n (%)	2 (4.5%)	2 (3.8%)	
Fibrocavitary, n (%)	5 (11.4%)	3 (5.7%)	
Pleural, n (%)	11 (25.0%)	18 (34.0%)	

27.0 years in diabetics and nondiabetics with pulmonary tuberculosis, respectively. In line with these findings, the present study revealed a mean age of 54.73 ± 12.18 and 41.15 ± 18.77 years in diabetics and nondiabetics with lower respiratory infections, respectively. These findings reveal a trend of higher mean age in diabetics than nondiabetics with respiratory infections [2]. This trend may be explained by greater prevalence of comorbidities in diabetic patients above the age of 60 years. Due to these comorbidities and weakening immune system parallel to increase in age, diabetics become more prone to various infections [16].

Symptomatology did not differ between diabetics and nondiabetics with lower respiratory infections. The most common clinical presentations were fever, cough, and expectoration in the present study. Similarly, in the study by Chandra et al. [6], the most common clinical manifestations were fever, cough, and shortness of breath. Moreover, in the study by Alisjahbana et al. [18], cough, weight loss, and fever were the common symptoms. Wang et al. [15] found higher presentation with fever and hemoptysis in diabetic patients with pulmonary tuberculosis. Interestingly, Saibal et al. [3] revealed altered mental status and hypotension as the predominant clinical features in diabetic patients with community-acquired pneumonia.

The PSI/PORT score is a validated tool used as a clinical predictor to stratify patients according to the severity of community-acquired pneumonia. The present study revealed that the majority of patients with diabetes with lower respiratory infections fell into classes IV and V, while contrastingly nondiabetics fell into classes I-III. CURB-65 is another risk stratification tool used to stratify patients with community-acquired pneumonia. The study by Saibal et al. [3] revealed higher CURB-65 score in diabetics than nondiabetics. These findings evidence a higher clinical risk for diabetics than nondiabetics, regardless of the tools used for risk stratification.

Diabetics are more prone to unusual radiographic presentation. Lesions with predominant bilateral [9], lower [6, 15, 19], and multilobe involvement [3, 6, 17] with higher incidences of pleural effusion [3, 6, 15] have been identified in diabetics. In the present study, the radiological presentation of diabetics was characteristic of bilateral, lower, and multilobe involvement with exudative and consolidative lesions. This difference in these clinical manifestations in diabetics and nondiabetics may be explained by altered capillary permeability, less vigorous and more vulnerable immune systems, and altered neutrophil and macrophage function observed in diabetics [3]. Other authors have asserted these disparities may be due to demography and patient selection process [15]. The effect of diabetes mellitus on the radiological presentation of pulmonary tuberculosis is critical because misinterpretations may hinder appropriate diagnosis and treatment.

4.1. Study Limitations. The study has a few limitations. The first is the small sample size and short duration of the study period. Secondly, we did not adjust for possible confounding factors.

5. Conclusion

Diabetic patients usually had severe pulmonary infection and poor prognosis as suggested by higher mean PORT risk score. They also more frequently presented with bilateral lesions with multilobe or lower lobe involvement as evidenced by radiography as compared to nondiabetic patients.

References

[1] N. Tandon, R. M. Anjana, V. Mohan et al., "The increasing burden of diabetes and variations among the states of India: the Global Burden of Disease Study 1990-2016," *The Lancet Global Health*, vol. 6, no. 12, pp. e1352–e1362, 2018.

[2] F. Ahmadi, S. Moogahi, and H. Bahrami, "Determining frequency and pattern of infections associated with diabetes based educational hospitals in Ahvaz city; Iran," *Diabetes & Metabolic Syndrome: Clinical Research & Reviews*, vol. 13, no. 4, pp. 2441–2444, 2019.

[3] M. Saibal, S. Rahman, L. Nishat et al., "Community acquired pneumonia in diabetic and non-diabetic hospitalized patients: presentation, causative pathogens and outcome," *Bangladesh Medical Research Council Bulletin*, vol. 38, no. 3, pp. 98–103, 2012.

[4] A. Cheepsattayakorn and R. Cheepsattayakorn, "Pulmonary infectious diseases in association with diabetes mellitus," *Journal of Lung, Pulmonary & Respiratory Research*, vol. 4, no. 3, pp. 1–4, 2017.

[5] J. M. Pavlovic, A. D. Pavlovic, M. V. Bulajic et al., «Prevalence of diabetes mellitus (DM) in tuberculosis (TB) patients: clinical and radiologic features in the TB-DM association based on a five-year hospital study," *Le Infezioni in Medicina*, vol. 1, pp. 22–27, 2018.

[6] N. Chandra, K. Premkumar, M. Subbalaxmi, P. Umabala, and Y. S. N. Raju, "Incidence of infections in hospitalized subjects with diabetes mellitus," *Journal of Clinical and Scientific Research.*, vol. 6, no. 4, pp. 216–224, 2017.

[7] J. B. Kornum, R. W. Thomsen, A. Riis, H. H. Lervang, H. C. Schonheyder, and H. T. Sorensen, "Type 2 diabetes and pneumonia outcomes: a population-based cohort study," *Diabetes Care*, vol. 30, no. 9, pp. 2251–2257, 2007.

[8] S. R. Masoodi, A. I. Wani, R. A. Misgar, V. K. Gupta, M. I. Bashir, and A. H. Zargar, "Pattern of infections in patients with diabetes mellitus–data from a tertiary care medical centre in Indian sub-continent," *Diabetes and Metabolic Syndrome: Clinical Research and Reviews*, vol. 1, no. 2, pp. 91–95, 2007.

[9] L.-K. Huang, H.-H. Wang, Y.-C. Lai, and S. C. Chang, "The impact of glycemic status on radiological manifestations of pulmonary tuberculosis in diabetic patients," *PLoS One*, vol. 12, no. 6, article e0179750, 2017.

[10] C. Alves, J. Casqueiro, and J. Casqueiro, "Infections in patients with diabetes mellitus: a review of pathogenesis," *Indian Journal of Endocrinology and Metabolism*, vol. 16, no. 7, pp. 27–36, 2012.

[11] D. L. Kasper, E. Braunwald, A. S. Fauci et al., *Harrison's Principles of Internal Medicine 16th Edition*, McGraw-Hill Professional Publishing, 2005.

[12] L. A. Mandell, R. G. Wunderink, A. Anzueto et al., "Infectious Diseases Society of America/American Thoracic Society consensus guidelines on the management of community-acquired pneumonia in adults," *Clinical Infectious Diseases*, vol. 44, Supplement_2, pp. S27–S72, 2007.

[13] M. J. Fine, T. E. Auble, D. M. Yealy et al., "A prediction rule to identify low-risk patients with community-acquired pneumonia," *The New England Journal of Medicine*, vol. 336, no. 4, pp. 243–250, 1997.

[14] American Diabetes Association, "Standards of medical care in diabetes — 2007," *Diabetes Care*, vol. 30, Supplement 1, pp. S4–S41, 2006.

[15] C. S. Wang, C. J. Yang, H. C. Chen et al., "Impact of type 2 diabetes on manifestations and treatment outcome of pulmonary tuberculosis," *Epidemiology and Infection*, vol. 137, no. 2, pp. 203–210, 2009.

[16] J. Pardo Seco, M. Cebey-López, R. Gil Prieto et al., "Differences between diabetic and non-diabetic patients with community-acquired pneumonia in primary care in Spain," *BMC Infectious Diseases*, vol. 19, no. 1, pp. 973–977, 2019.

[17] S. Park, J. Shin, J. Kim et al., "The effect of diabetic control status on the clinical features of pulmonary tuberculosis," *European Journal of Clinical Microbiology & Infectious Diseases*, vol. 31, no. 7, pp. 1305–1310, 2012.

[18] B. Alisjahbana, E. Sahiratmadja, E. J. Nelwan et al., "The effect of type 2 diabetes mellitus on the presentation and treatment

response of pulmonary tuberculosis," *Clinical Infectious Diseases*, vol. 45, no. 4, pp. 428–435, 2007.

[19] F. Bacakoğlu, Ö. K. Başoğlu, G. Çok, A. Sayıner, and M. Ateş, "Pulmonary tuberculosis in patients with diabetes mellitus," *Respiration*, vol. 68, no. 6, pp. 595–600, 2001.

Comparison between the Interferon γ Release Assay—QuantiFERON Gold Plus (QFT-Plus)—and Tuberculin Skin Test (TST) in the Detection of Tuberculosis Infection in Immunocompromised Children

Cory Primaturia, Lelani Reniarti, and Heda M. N. Nataprawira

Department of Child Health, Faculty of Medicine Universitas Padjadjaran/Dr. Hasan Sadikin General Hospital, Jl. Pasteur No. 38 Bandung 40161, Indonesia

Correspondence should be addressed to Heda M. N. Nataprawira; heda_1155@yahoo.com

Academic Editor: Kazuyoshi Kuwano

Background. Immunocompromised patients are at a higher risk of having latent tuberculosis infection (LTBI). QuantiFERON-TB Gold Plus (QFT-Plus) has been proven to perform effectively in LTBI detection among immunocompromised adults and can overcome the limitations of the tuberculin skin test (TST). However, the role of QFT-Plus in detecting LTBI in immunocompromised paediatric patients has not been well established. Therefore, the aim of this study was to assess the test agreement between QFT-Plus and the TST in LTBI detection among immunocompromised children. *Method.* In this cross-sectional study, we enrolled immunocompromised paediatric patients, aged between 5 and 18 years, who were treated with corticosteroids and/or chemotherapy from June to November 2019. We categorized them into three groups based on the following diseases: hematologic malignancies and nephrological and immunological diseases. We recorded the patient characteristics and QFT-Plus and TST results, in which the positive result of the TST was induration ≥ 5 mm. Within the same group, comparisons between the two tests were performed using the McNemar test, and results were statistically significant for p values of <0.05. The kappa index was used to assess the agreement between the two test results. *Results.* Among 71 patients (median age: 11.8 years) who underwent TST and QFT-Plus testing, 52% were females, and 69% had a normal nutritional status. Chemotherapy was the most common treatment modality for hematologic malignancy compared to other immunosuppressive treatments. The total number of patients with positive QFT-Plus and TST results was 11/71 (15.5%) and 4/71 (5.6%), respectively, among whom 3/11 patients had positive results in both tests, and one patient with positive TST results exhibited a discrepancy, as this was not followed by positive QFT-Plus results. QFT-Plus generated more positive results than the TST in immunocompromised children (McNemar, $p = 0.039$ ($p < 0.05$)). The diagnostic agreement between the tests was fair ($K = 0.345$, 95% CI: 0.05–0.745). *Conclusion.* QFT-Plus detected LTBI more effectively than the TST in immunocompromised children.

1. Introduction

Tuberculosis (TB) is still one of the health global problems in the world, including the children population. Based on the Global Tuberculosis Report 2019, Indonesian children with new and relapse TB cases are about 11% of the total TB incidence as estimated in 2018. However, there are many cases of TB that remain unrecognized, incorrectly diagnosed, and unreported. The World Health Organization (WHO) reported that Indonesia is a country with the third highest TB incidence, after India and China [1]. Currently, the TB eradication program is not only focused on treatment but also on prevention by conducting contact investigations and diagnosing latent tuberculosis infection (LTBI) so that the infection does not develop into TB disease by giving isoniazid (INH) prophylaxis treatment [1, 2]. Latent tuberculosis infection (LTBI) is a condition associated with a persistent immune response to the *Mycobacterium tuberculosis* (Mtb) antigen that produces neither any clinical manifestations nor X-ray findings indicating the presence of the disease [3]. LTBI treatment coverage reported low in Indonesia, especially child contacts < 5 years old is about 11% [4]. The studies on LTBI of the immunocompromised population are still limited, while the prevalence of LTBI has been estimated to affect almost one-third (2.3 billion) of the global population [5]. Screening for LTBI is a crucial component of the World Health Organization's (WHO) End TB Strategy [1, 5].

Immunocompromised adult patients with solid organ transplant (SOT), hematopoietic stem cell transplant (HSCT), and hematologic malignancy were reported to have a higher risk of progression to active TB, with a risk between 20 and 74 times greater than the general population [6–10]. Therefore, early detection of LTBI through screening immunocompromised patients is recommended [9, 11, 12]. The latest diagnostic method for LTBI involving the use of interferon-gamma release assays (IGRAs) was developed to replace the tuberculin skin test (TST) [9, 12–16]. The limitations of the TST, including the resulting high percentage of false-negative results in the case of immunocompromised patients, have previously been reported [12, 13, 17, 18]. The use of IGRAs is an alternative diagnostic approach for LTBI detection, and this technique has been observed to be more effective than the TST in the case of immunocompromised adult patients [14, 15, 19].

QuantiFERON-TB Gold Plus (QFT-Plus) is the latest generation of IGRAs. The QFT-Plus kit consists of two tubes of specific TB antigens (TB1 and TB2) and is able to stimulate interferon gamma (IFN-γ) production in the CD4 and CD8 cells on the exposure to the Mtb-specific antigen [13, 15]. The ability of QFT-Plus to detect the CD8 cell response to the Mtb antigen makes QFT-Plus better than the TST in detecting immune-mediated cell responses in an immunocompromised population with a low CD4 count [14, 20]. To the best of our knowledge, there are limited studies that have been conducted on the adult immunocompromised population, and the results of studies on immunocompromised children still remain unclear. Therefore, the aim of this study was to assess the test agreement between QFT-Plus and the TST in LTBI detection among immunocompromised children.

2. Materials and Methods

2.1. Ethical Approval. This study was approved by the ethical committee of RSUP Dr. Hasan Sadikin General Hospital, Bandung, under the identification number LB.02.01/X.6.5/122/2019, on 26 April 2019 and followed the principles outlined in the Declaration of Helsinki.

2.2. Study Setting. The study was conducted at the immunocompromised children's ward of RSUP Dr. Hasan Sadikin Hospital, a zonal referral hospital that caters to the West Java province, in Bandung.

2.3. Study Design and Population. This was an observational analytical study with a cross-sectional design, and it involved immunocompromised children who were hospitalized from June to November 2019. All of the patients were simultaneously tested using QFT-Plus (Qiagen, Hilden, Germany) and the TST after screening them based on the eligibility criteria. The patients with positive and indeterminate results by either QFT-Plus or the TST were treated isoniazid prophylaxis 10 mg/kg/day for 6 months [3]. The inclusion criteria for this study were children aged 5–18 years who were in an immunocompromised condition, including children who were undergoing chemotherapy, immunosuppressive therapy, or steroid therapy with drug doses of 1.5 mg/kg BW/day or 15 mg/day for >1 month, and those who were tested via both QFT-Plus and the TST [12, 15–17]. The exclusion criteria were as follows: patients suspected of having TB and those with a history of receiving TB therapy or of being clinically (cough ≥ 2 weeks, fever ≥ 2 weeks, body weight loss, and malaise) or microbiologically (bacteriologically positive in the rapid molecular test, GeneXpert) diagnosed with TB [2]. The characteristics of each patient were recorded (sex, age, nutritional status, history of chemotherapy, therapy duration, vaccination history, and laboratory findings, including haemoglobin, haematocrit, erythrocyte, leukocyte, thrombocyte, lymphocyte, and albumin levels). For nutritional status, we measured body mass index (BMI) for age, in which defined according to WHO child growth standard deviation (SD) or *Z* scores and were classified using the following cut-offs: for normal status (BMI for age < -2–+2 SD), moderately malnourished (BMI for age < -2 SD), and severely malnourished (BMI for age < -3 SD) [21].

2.4. QuantiFERON Gold Plus (QFT-Plus). A blood sample measuring as much as 5 mL was drawn from each patient's vein and was then transferred into a lithium heparin blood tube. During the delivery process, the blood samples were stored at 2–8°C in order to maintain lymphocyte viabilities. Subsequently, the enzyme-linked immunosorbent assay (ELISA) method was used to calculate the IFN-γ levels in response to the exposure to the specific Mtb antigen (cocktail peptide early secretory antigen target (ESAT-6), culture filtrate protein CFP-10 (TB1) without TB7.7, and six short peptides (TB2)). The results were considered positive if the interferon concentration at ≥0.35 IU/L or ≥25% in the control tube was negative, and they were considered indeterminate if the concentration was <0.35 IU/mL or <25% with a mitogen concentration of <0.5 IU/mL [20].

2.5. Tuberculin Skin Test (TST). The TST was performed using 0.1 mL of purified protein derivative (PPD RT23) that was injected intradermally into the volar surface of the hand. The PPD was stored in a cold environment (2–8°C). An induration assessment was performed 48-72 h following the injection. The results of the TST were interpreted by a paediatrician who determined them to be positive if the induration was found to be ≥5 mm [2].

2.6. Data Management and Statistical Analysis. Data were expressed in numbers (percentages) or median and were

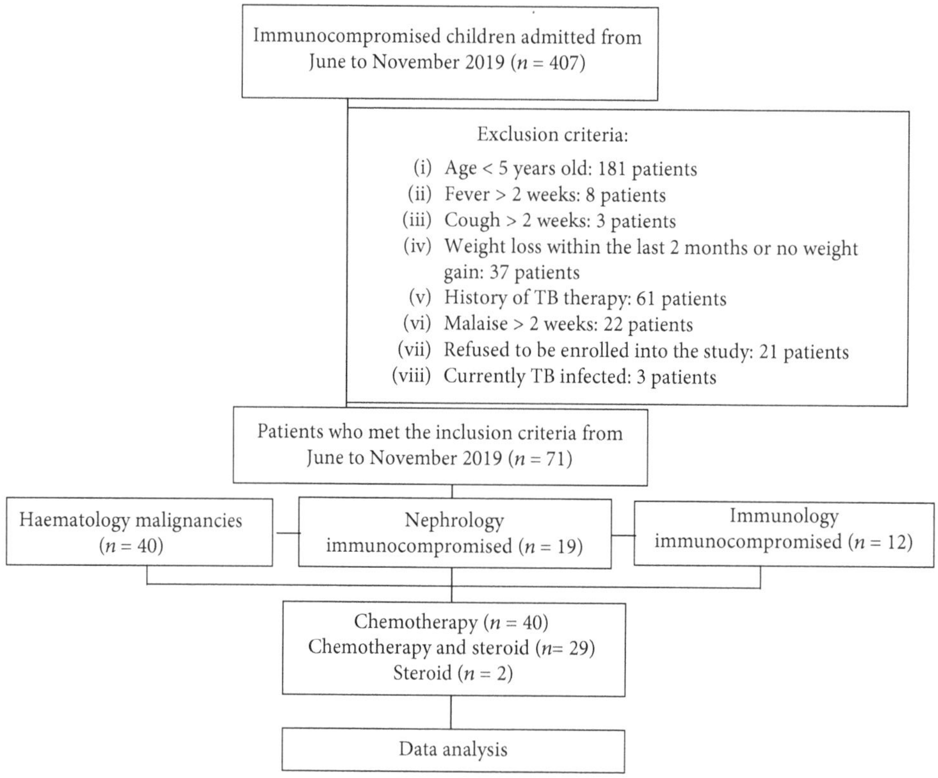

FIGURE 1: Flow diagram. TB: tuberculosis.

analysed using the IBM SPSS Statistics (version 23.0) software. The concordance between the QFT-Plus and TST assay results was assessed using kappa coefficients and was interpreted according to the Landis and Koch classification. Consequently, the Cohen's kappa test results were classified as follows: a score of <0.2 indicated slight reliability; 0.21–0.40, fair reliability; 0.41–0.60, moderate reliability; 0.61–0.80, substantial reliability; and 0.81–1, almost ideal reliability [22]. All the reported p values were calculated with the statistical significance set at a p value of less than 0.05.

3. Results

3.1. Population Characteristics. We prospectively included 407 consecutive immunocompromised patients who were undergoing chemotherapy and steroid treatment from July to November 2019. During this time period, there were only 71 patients who were eligible as per the study criteria. The procedure involved in patient selection is presented in Figure 1.

The types of hematological cancer in this study were acute lymphoblastic leukaemia, acute myeloblastic leukaemia, chronic lymphoblastic leukaemia, lymphoma, and solid malignant tumors (osteosarcoma, ovarian tumors, and retinoblastoma). The nephrological and immunological conditions in this study were nephrotic syndrome, steroid resistance, and systemic lupus erythematosus (SLE). The characteristics of the patients are presented in Table 1.

Among the 71 patients who had undergone QFT-Plus and the TST, the baseline clinical characteristics between the sexes were nearly equal. The median age was 11.8 years old, and most of the patients had a normal nutritional status (69.0%). Regarding the treatment that the patients underwent, 56.3% of them received chemotherapy while 40.8% received a combination of chemotherapy and steroid treatment; the duration of therapy was more than 3 months in most cases (59.2%). There were 57 (80.3%) patients who had undergone GeneXpert evaluation, and all of them generated negative rapid molecular test results. Further, 67 (94.4%) patients had Bacillus Calmette–Guérin (BCG) scars and histories of receiving BCG vaccinations. The nutritional status, history of chemotherapy, and duration of administration of immunosuppressive drugs were compared between the TST and QFT-Plus test groups as shown in Table 2.

The percentage of patients with a normal nutritional status who received positive results on the TST was 6.1% and that of patients who received positive results with QFT-Plus was 14.3%; contrarily, 10% of severely malnourished patients generated positive results on the TST and 30% exhibited positive results with QFT-Plus. Based on the therapy history, three patients (7.5%) who were treated with chemotherapy and one (2.5%) patient who was treated with chemotherapy and steroid treatment together received positive TST results; further, 26% and 15% of patients who underwent chemotherapy and steroid treatment together and chemotherapy alone, respectively, received positive QFT-Plus results, and one patient received indeterminate QFT-Plus results. Based on the duration of therapy, i.e., ≤3 months or >3 months, the percentage of the patients who generated positive results on the TST did not differ to a large extent (3.3% and 7.3%) between the two groups whereas the percentages of those with positive QFT-Plus tests were 13.3% and 17.1% in the

TABLE 1: Characteristics of the patients.

Characteristics	Number ($n = 71$)	%
Sex		
Male	34	47.9
Female	37	52.1
Age (year)		
5–9	18	25.4
10–14	31	43.7
15–18	22	31.0
Median (SD): 11.8 years		
Range: 5-18		
Nutritional status		
Normal	49	69.0
Moderately malnourished	12	16.9
Severely malnourished	10	14.1
History of chemotherapy		
Chemotherapy	40	56.3
Chemotherapy+steroid	29	40.8
Steroid	2	2.8
Duration of therapy		
≤3 months	30	40.8
>3 months	41	59.2
Patient classification		
Hematology	40	56.3
Nephrology	19	26.8
Immunology	12	16.9
Rapid molecular test (GeneXpert)		
Negative	57	80.3
Not done	14	19.7
BCG scar/history of BCG vaccination		
Positive	67	94.4
Negative	4	5.6
History of contact with TB adult patient		
Positive	2	3
Negative	69	97

SD: standard deviation; BCG: Bacillus Calmette–Guérin; TB: tuberculosis.

two groups, respectively. All the immunocompromised conditions did not lead to significant differences in both the TST and QFT-Plus groups ($p > 0.05$). BCG vaccination status in these two groups statically did not show significant differences.

The laboratory examination that was performed included tests to determine the levels of haemoglobin, haematocrit, erythrocytes, leukocytes, thrombocytes, lymphocytes, and albumin (Table 3). There were no significant differences in the laboratory results between the TST and QFT-Plus test ($p > 0.05$).

In this study, the total number of patients with positive results in QFT-Plus and the TST was 11/71 (15.5%) and 4/71 (5.6%), respectively, out of whom 3/11 patients had positive results in both tests, and one patient with positive TST results exhibited a discrepancy as the positive TST results were not followed by positive QFT-Plus results. The comparison between QFT-Plus and the TST for use in LTBI diagnosis yielded statistically significant differences ($p = 0.039$), as shown in Table 4. The agreement value associated with the results of both the diagnostic approaches based on the kappa index was 0.345 ($K < 0.4$) (95% CI: 0.05–0.745), and it was subsequently classified as being fair.

4. Discussion

This study has demonstrated that the number of patients who exhibited positive TST results was smaller (5.6%) than that of those with positive QFT-Plus results (15.5%) associated with LTBI, with a kappa score indicating fair reliability. Compared to the results of previous studies on adult immunocompromised patients [14], our study is quite similar to those studies, with the result for IGRA test (15.1%) and TST (10.9%) with a moderate kappa score [14]. In a previous report, QFT-Plus positive results were compared to TST ones (93.7% and 73.7%, respectively) yielding higher kappa scores in an HIV-affected population [23].

Blood cancer patients have a higher case index of LTBI compared to other immunocompromised groups of patients. Blood cancer has been associated with severe immunocompromised states long before chemotherapy was developed to treat this condition [9, 10, 15, 24]. Further, blood cancer patients are associated with higher risks of developing neutropenia or leukopenia, and therefore, the risk of LTBI also increases in them [25]. This study compared results between patients who were treated with chemotherapy for ≤3 months and those who were treated for >3 months. In the QFT-Plus group, we observed that positive results were exhibited by 13.7% of the patients who were treated for ≤3 months and by 16.6% of the patients who were treated for >3 months, and these results were relatively similar to those of the TST group. We speculated that a longer duration of therapy could aggravate the immunocompromised status of a patient and increase the risk of LTBI. QFT-Plus produced more specific results than the TST because this test contains protein antigens, ESAT-6, CFP-10, and TB 7.7, that cannot be obtained via the BCG vaccination [18, 19]. We observed a discrepancy in the TST results of one of the patients who did not receive a corresponding positive QFT-Plus result. This result can be caused by the lower specificity of the TST, which is influenced by BCG vaccination.

In immunocompromised patients, false-negative results arise due to the lower production levels of cytokines, such as IFN-γ and tumor necrosis factor (TNF-α), that play roles in the immune response against Mtb. This is due to a defective T-cell response corresponding to the production of interleukin-2 (IL-2), which is caused by T-cell receptor phosphorylation that results in disturbances in ZAP-70 (Zeta-chain-associated protein kinase 70) activation, mitogen-activated protein kinase (MAPK) protein activation related to IL-2 gene transcription, and the production of protein after T-cell stimulation against the antigen [26].

Further, IGRAs have their own disadvantages, such as higher costs, the need for advanced laboratory facilities,

Table 2: TST and QFT-Plus results based on nutritional status, chemotherapy history, therapy duration, and patient groups.

Variables assessed	TST ($n = 71$) +	−	Total (n)	p value	QFT-Plus +	Indeterminate	−	Total	p value
Nutritional status									
Normal	3	46	49	0.72	7	1	41	49	0.76
Moderately malnourished	0	12	12		1	0	11	12	
Severely malnourished	1	9	10		3	0	7	10	
Therapy									
Chemotherapy	4	36	40	0.19	6	1	33	40	0.11
Chemotherapy+steroid	0	29	29		5	0	24	29	
Steroid	0	2	2		0	0	2	2	
Duration of therapy									
≤3 months	2	27	29	1.0	5	0	24	29	0.67
>3 months	2	40	42		6	1	35	42	
Patient classification									
Hematological	3	37	40	0.45	6	1	33	40	0.26
Nephrological	0	19	19		1	0	18	19	
Immunological	1	11	12		4	0	8	12	
BCG status									
Positive	4	63	67	1.0	11	1	55	67	0.65
Negative	0	4	4		0	0	4	4	

TST: tuberculin skin test; QFT-Plus: QuantiFERON Gold Plus.

Table 3: Laboratory findings based on the TST and QFT-Plus results.

Laboratory findings	TST (median value and range) Positive	Negative	p value
Haemoglobin (g/dL)	10.6 (9.1-12.1)	11.5 (6.2-17.2)	0.385
Haematocrit (%)	30.5 (27.2-35.0)	33.9 (17.0-52.0)	0.353
Erythrocytes (millions/m^3)	4.1 (3.4-4.4)	4.1 (0.13-21.74)	0.768
Leukocytes (/m^3)	4940 (3880-16040)	9690 (1070-354120)	0.601
Thrombocytes (thousand/m^3)	411 (283-670)	320 (3-580)	0.178
Lymphocytes (%)	18 (13-47)	17.5 (1-70)	0.606
Albumin (g/dL)	3.5 (3.1-3.9)	3.3 (0.8-38)	0.513
	QFT-Plus (median value and range) Positive	Negative	p value
Haemoglobin (g/dL)	11.2 (9.1-16.3)	11.55 (6.2-17.2)	0.952
Haematocrit (%)	32.0 (26-45)	34 (17-52)	0.634
Erythrocytes (millions/m^3)	4.0 (3.3-5.1)	4.1 (0.13-21.74)	0.567
Leukocytes (/m^3)	7370 (3770-19800)	9690 (1070-354120)	0.393
Thrombocytes (thousand/m^3)	372 (199-524)	320 (3-670)	0.279
Lymphocytes (%)	15.5 (5-47)	18.5 (1-70)	0.294
Albumin (g/dL)	3.1 (1.79-3.9)	3.3 (0.8-38)	0.648

*Based on the Mann-Whitney test. TST: tuberculin skin test; QFT-Plus: QuantiFERON Gold Plus.

and the need to maintain lymphocyte viability [19, 27–29]. IGRAs can also generate indeterminate results in cases in which the patient has an immunological disorder that involves low IFN-γ production towards a mitogen or excessive IFN-γ production in the control tube. Patients with immunosuppression are usually at a higher risk of receiving indeterminate results owing to the inadequacy of their body's response toward mitogens in a positive control situation [30]. Indeterminate results are also related to a child's age, and therefore, our study excluded children below 5 years old because of their immature immune response [31, 32]. In our study, we had one (1.4%) patient whose results were considered to be indeterminate and the patient was treated with INH prophylaxis.

Table 4: The comparison between the QFT-Plus and TST results in diagnosing LTBI.

QFT-Plus	TST		Total (%); (95% CI)
	Positive	Negative	
Positive	3	8	11 (15.5%); (8.9–25.71)
Indeterminate	0	1	1 (1.4%); (0.2–7.6)
Negative	1	58	59 (83.1%); (72.7–90.1)
Total	4	67	71
%	(5.6%)	(94.4%)	
95% CI	2.2%–3.6%	86.4%–97.8%	

p (McNemar test) = 0.039; $K = 0.345$ (95% CI: 0.05–0. 745) (SE 0.161). TST: tuberculin skin test; QFT-Plus: QuantiFERON Gold Plus; LTBI: latent tuberculosis infection.

Indeterminate results are suspected to arise due to low levels of albumin and lymphocytes [14, 29, 30, 33]. Along with the results of QFT-Plus and the TST, this study also analysed the median values of the haemoglobin, haematocrit, erythrocyte, leukocyte, thrombocyte, lymphocyte, and albumin levels; however, the results of this analysis did not reveal any significant differences ($p > 0.05$). The median value of the lymphocyte and leukocyte levels in this study was influenced by the hyperleukocytosis states of three hematological malignancy patients with the highest leukocyte count of 300000/mm^3. The number of lymphocytes in patients with indeterminate results was reported to be lower than that of patients with determinate results (1200 cells/mL vs. 1820 cells/mL) [14]. In addition, indeterminate results are generated more frequently in immunocompromised patients owing to anaemia, lymphopenia, hypoproteinaemia, and hypoalbuminemia. Based on our study results, malnutrition did not affect the TST and IGRA results.

The percentage of patients with a normal nutritional status who received positive results on the TST was 6.1% and that of patients with positive QFT-Plus results was 17.1%, while in the severely malnourished patients the percentages of those that received positive results on the TST and QFT-Plus were 10% and 30%, respectively. The nutritional status plays a role in influencing the TST and IGRA test results, as the weight per age (<-2.63) and body mass index per age (<-2.51) lower the odds ratio of the positive TST results and increase the incidence of indeterminate IGRA results. Malnourished patients are at a higher risk of getting infected by Mtb because of their impaired immune responses; however, indeterminate results due to low mitogen response levels are also frequently reported in these patients [32]. In this study, all the malnourished patients exhibited determinate results, and only one (1.4%) patient was found to generate indeterminate results among those with a normal nutritional status.

4.1. Study Limitation. Further follow-ups were not conducted for patients with the possibility of having the TB disease who were administered isoniazid prophylaxis and who received positive QFT-Plus or TST results. Additionally, neither the concentration of viable lymphocytes due to improper specimen handling nor the inability of the patient's lymphocytes to generate IFN-γ was measured in this study.

4.2. Suggestion. The QTF-Plus examination needs to be routinely performed in the case of immunocompromised children in order to facilitate the proper establishment of a diagnosis protocol for LTBI so that an early intervention could accordingly be administered. It is beneficial if a further study is conducted using diagnostic test; therefore, the sensitivity and specificity of the QTF-Plus and TST can be measured in identifying LTBI progressivity to active TB disease, so that TB disease can be prevented and it will have an impact on the reduction of treatment cost.

5. Conclusions

The results of this study confirm that QFT-Plus® detects LTBI more effectively than the TST in immunocompromised children.

Acknowledgments

This project was funded partially by UBC Medical, Indonesia, in the provision of the IGRA QuantiFERON-TB Gold Plus products.

References

[1] World Health Organization, *Global Tuberculosis Report 2019*, World Health Organization, Geneva, 2019.

[2] Kementerian Kesehatan Republik Indonesia, *Petunjuk teknis manjemen dan tatalaksana TB anak*, Kemenkes RI, Jakarta, 2016.

[3] World Health Organization, *Latent Tuberculosis Infection Updated and Consolidated Guidelines for Programmatic Management*, World Health Organization, Geneva, 2018.

[4] N. I. Paton, L. Borand, J. Benedicto et al., "Diagnosis and management of latent tuberculosis infection in Asia: review of current status and challenges," *International Journal of Infectious Diseases*, vol. 87, pp. 21–29, 2019.

[5] R. M. G. J. Houben and P. J. Dodd, "The global burden of latent tuberculosis infection: a re-estimation using mathematical modelling," *PLoS Medicine*, vol. 13, no. 10, article e1002152, 2016.

[6] D. Bumbacea, S. M. Arend, F. Eyuboglu et al., "The risk of tuberculosis in transplant candidates and recipients: a TBNET consensus statement," *The European Respiratory Journal*, vol. 40, no. 4, pp. 990–1013, 2012.

[7] M. Kamboj and K. A. Sepkowitz, "The risk of tuberculosis in patients with cancer," *Clinical Infectious Diseases*, vol. 42, no. 11, pp. 1592–1595, 2006.

[8] C. C. Dobler, K. Cheung, J. Nguyen, and A. Martin, "Risk of tuberculosis in patients with solid cancers and haematological malignancies: a systematic review and meta-analysis," *The European Respiratory Journal*, vol. 50, no. 2, article 1700157, 2017.

[9] L. Anibarro and A. Pena, "Tuberculosis in patients with haematological malignancies," *Mediterranean Journal of Hematology and Infectious Diseases*, vol. 6, pp. 1–9, 2014.

[10] J. Landry and D. Menzies, "Preventive chemotherapy. Where has it got us? Where to go next?," *The International Journal of Tuberculosis and Lung Disease*, vol. 12, no. 12, pp. 1352–1364, 2008.

[11] P. Mishra, R. Kumar, M. Mahapatra et al., "Tuberculosis in acute leukemia: a clinico-hematological profile," *Hematology*, vol. 11, no. 5, pp. 335–340, 2006.

[12] R. Smith, A. Cattamanchi, K. R. Steingart et al., "Interferon-γ release assays for diagnosis of latent tuberculosis infection: evidence in immune-mediated inflammatory disorders," *Current Opinion in Rheumatology*, vol. 23, no. 4, pp. 377–384, 2011.

[13] M. R. Ryu, M. S. Park, E. H. Cho et al., "Comparative evaluation of quantiFERON-TB gold in-tube and quantiFERON-TB gold plus in diagnosis of latent tuberculosis infection in immunocompromised patients," *Journal of Clinical Microbiology*, vol. 56, pp. 1–10, 2018.

[14] L. Richeldi, M. Losi, R. D'Amico et al., "Performance of tests for latent tuberculosis in different groups of immunocompromised patients," *Chest*, vol. 136, no. 1, pp. 198–204, 2009.

[15] E. Y. Kim, J. E. Lim, J. Y. Jung et al., "Performance of the tuberculin skin test and interferon-γ release assay for detection of tuberculosis infection in immunocompromised patients in a BCG-vaccinated population," *BMC Infectious Diseases*, vol. 9, no. 1, pp. 1–8, 2009.

[16] U. Mack, G. B. Migliori, M. Sester et al., "LTBI: latent tuberculosis infection or lasting immune responses to M. tuberculosis? A TBNET consensus statement," *The European Respiratory Journal*, vol. 33, no. 5, pp. 956–973, 2009.

[17] S. Nayak and B. Acharjya, "Mantoux test and its interpretation," *Indian Dermatology Online Journal*, vol. 3, no. 1, pp. 2–6, 2012.

[18] H. Esmail, Barry CE 3rd, and R. J. Wilkinson, "Understanding latent tuberculosis: the key to improved diagnostic and novel treatment strategies," *Drug Discovery Today*, vol. 17, no. 9-10, pp. 514–521, 2012.

[19] A. Trajman, R. E. Steffen, and D. Menzies, "Interferon-gamma release assays versus tuberculin skin testing for the diagnosis of latent tuberculosis infection: an overview of the evidence," *Pulmonary Medicine*, vol. 2013, Article ID 601737, 11 pages, 2013.

[20] European Centre for Disease Prevention and Control Guidance, *Use of interferon-gamma release assays in support of TB diagnosis*, European Centre for Disease Prevention and Control, Stockholm, 2011.

[21] WHO, "WHO child growth standards," *Developmental Medicine and Child Neurology*, vol. 51, no. 12, pp. 1–336, 2006.

[22] M. L. McHugh, "Lessons in biostatistics interrater reliability: the kappa statistic," *Biochem Medica*, vol. 22, pp. 276–282, 2012.

[23] G. B. Klautau, N. V. F. da Mota, M. J. C. Salles, M. N. Burattini, and D. S. Rodrigues, "Interferon-γ release assay as a sensitive diagnostic tool of latent tuberculosis infection in patients with HIV: a cross-sectional study," *BMC Infectious Diseases*, vol. 18, no. 1, pp. 1–8, 2018.

[24] A. J. Minn, "Interferons and the immunogenic effects of cancer therapy," *Trends in Immunology*, vol. 36, no. 11, pp. 725–737, 2015.

[25] K. A. al-Anazi, A. M. al-Jasser, and D. A. P. Evans, "Infections caused by mycobacterium tuberculosis in patients with hematological disorders and in recipients of hematopoietic stem cell transplant, a twelve year retrospective study," *Annals of Clinical Microbiology and Antimicrobials*, vol. 6, no. 1, pp. 1–7, 2007.

[26] L. Encinales, J. Zuñiga, J. Granados-Montiel et al., "Humoral immunity in tuberculin skin test anergy and its role in high-risk persons exposed to active tuberculosis," *Molecular Immunology*, vol. 47, no. 5, pp. 1066–1073, 2010.

[27] M. Pai, C. M. Denkinger, S. V. Kik et al., "Gamma interferon release assays for detection of Mycobacterium tuberculosis infection," *Clinical Microbiology Reviews*, vol. 27, no. 1, pp. 3–20, 2014.

[28] F. R. Sztajnbok, N. L. Boechat, D. C. Sztajnbok, S. B. Ribeiro, S. K. Oliveira, and C. C. Sant'Anna, "The challenge of pediatric tuberculosis in face of new diagnostic techniques," *Jornal de Pediatria*, vol. 85, no. 3, pp. 183–193, 2009.

[29] R. N. Van Zyl-Smit, R. J. Lehloenya, R. Meldau, and K. Dheda, "Impact of correcting the lymphocyte count to improve the sensitivity of TB antigen-specific peripheral blood-based quantitative T cell assays (T-SPOT.®TB and QFT-GIT)," *Journal of Thoracic Disease*, vol. 8, no. 3, pp. 482–489, 2016.

[30] J. C. Sharninghausen, A. E. Shapiro, D. M. Koelle, and K. H. Nina, "Risk factors for indeterminate outcome on interferon gamma release assay in non-US-born persons screened for latent tuberculosis infection," *Open Forum Infectious Diseases*, vol. 5, no. 8, 2018.

[31] E. Critselis, V. Amanatidou, G. Syridou et al., "The effect of age on whole blood interferon-gamma release assay response among children investigated for latent tuberculosis infection," *The Journal of Pediatrics*, vol. 161, no. 4, pp. 632–638, 2012.

[32] S. Jenum, S. Selvam, D. Mahelai et al., "Influence of age and nutritional status on the performance of the tuberculin skin test and QuantiFERON-TB Gold in-Tube in young children evaluated for tuberculosis in Southern India," *The Pediatric Infectious Disease Journal*, vol. 33, no. 10, pp. e260–e269, 2014.

[33] L. E. Baldassari, J. Feng, G. Macaron et al., "Tuberculosis screening in multiple sclerosis: effect of disease-modifying therapies and lymphopenia on the prevalence of indeterminate TB screening results in the clinical setting," *Multiple Sclerosis Journal - Experimental, Translational and Clinical*, vol. 5, no. 3, 2019.

Postpartum Pulmonary Hypertension Masquerading as Submassive Pulmonary Embolism

Mahmood Mubasher,[1] Amir Hanafi,[1] Tausif Syed,[1] Abir Zinal,[1] Ibrahim Y. Abubeker,[1] Mouhand F. H. Mohamed,[2] Mohan Rao,[1] Ryan Hoefen,[1] and Mohammed Danjuma[2]

[1]*Rochester Regional Health-Unity Hospital, Rochester, NY, USA*
[2]*Internal Medicine Department, Hamad General Hospital, Hamad Medical, Corporation, Doha, Qatar*

Correspondence should be addressed to Mouhand F. H. Mohamed; dr.m.oraiby@hotmail.com

Academic Editor: Inger F. Oey

Postpartum pulmonary hypertension (PPPHT) is an extremely rare disorder, with few reported cases. Late diagnosis and treatment are associated with significant morbidity and mortality. We present an 18-year-old female patient who presented four-week postpartum with a typical submissive pulmonary embolism picture subsequently diagnosed as postpartum pulmonary hypertension. The patient had an excellent response to treatment, with a dramatic improvement in her functional status. The authors aim to urge physicians to keep this rare disorder in mind as timely and accurate diagnosis is crucial for management—additionally, the importance of counseling patients about the imminent risks associated with planned future pregnancies.

1. Background

The sixth world symposium on pulmonary hypertension defines pulmonary hypertension (PHT) as the mean pulmonary artery pressure (mPAP) > 20 mmHg or pulmonary vascular resistance (PVR) > 3 Wood units [1]. Patients with PHT typically present with progressive fatigue and shortness of breath; this eventually leads to the development of right heart failure. PHT secondary to left heart disease (Type 2 PHT) continues to be the most common type of pulmonary hypertension [2, 3]. PPPHT is a rare variant of PHT. The period of the most considerable risk is within 30 days after delivery [4]. Clinical manifestations vary; presentation as acute massive pulmonary embolism was reported [4, 5]. Whilst its exact pathogenesis remains uncertain, the interaction of a host of factors may play a role in the evolution and progression of PPPHT. The most notable amongst these factors includes the role of cardiac output during pregnancy and delivery and autotransfusion from the uteroplacental circulation to the systemic circulation, along with the release of uterine pressure on the inferior vena cava after delivery suddenly increasing the preload [6, 7]. The second factor is a possible underlying placental hypoxia that induces the release of biological factors that impact on vascular remodeling and vasoconstriction through their effect on the endothelium and smooth muscles [8]. Thirdly (although not supported by robust evidence), amniotic fluid embolism during labor that inadvertently reached the pulmonary circulation could potentially induce an inflammatory reaction that leads to an increase in pulmonary vascular resistance [9]. Recent advances in clinical therapeutics of PTH have seen a significant reduction in maternal mortality attributable to it from 30-50% to 17-30% [10].

2. Case Presentation

An 18-year-old female patient with a past medical history significant for iron deficiency anemia presented four-week postpartum (first pregnancy) with a one-week history of chest pain and shortness of breath. The patient described a left-sided chest pain as not radiating, constant and stabbing in nature, moderate to severe, pleuritic, and not related to physical activity. The pain was associated with worsening shortness of breath and palpitations. The patient reported associated exertional dyspnea, dizziness, and fatigue that restricted her ability to take care of her baby. She denied fever, orthopnoea, paroxysmal nocturnal dyspnea, or lower limb swelling. The patient had recently returned from a twenty-eight-hour car journey. Apart from anemia, her pregnancy and delivery were both uneventful. The patient has no allergies, no family history of cardiovascular, or clotting disorders.

On examination, the patient was distressed, tachycardic, and tachypneic and had normal blood pressure. She required FiO_2 of 44% to maintain normal saturation. Heartbeat was regular: soft heart sounds without murmurs, gallops, or rubs. There was no parasternal heave and no clinical signs of fluid overload. Moreover, there were no clinical features of endocarditis. She had normal vesicular breath sounds bilateral, with no crackles or wheezes. Lower limb examination was normal without signs of deep vein thrombosis.

Her EKG showed sinus tachycardia with T wave inversion in leads V1-3 (Figure 1).

Biochemical investigations showed a D-dimer of 3331 ng/ml (<500 ng/ml), BNP of 1034 pg/ml (<125 pg/ml), mildly elevated troponin I, and microcytic anemia. Otherwise, renal function, electrolytes, liver function tests, and thyroid hormones were within normal limits. Transthoracic echocardiogram showed a severely dilated right ventricle with globally reduced right ventricular systolic function and a left ventricular ejection fraction of 45-50% (Figure 2). CT pulmonary angiogram showed a dilated pulmonary trunk with no evidence of pulmonary embolism (Figure 3). An extensive venous thromboembolic workup including ultrasound Doppler of both lower limbs, CT venogram of the pelvis and lower limbs, and V/Q scan was negative.

Cardiac MRI showed a severely dilated right ventricle with a strain pattern with significant global reduced right ventricular systolic function, no signs of dysplasia or myocarditis, normal coronary anatomy, and no septal defects. Coronary angiography showed no coronary artery disease or dissection. Right heart catheterization (RHC) revealed the following: right atrial pressure = 12 mmHg (normal range 1-8 mmHg), right systolic ventricular pressure = 45 mmHg (normal range 15-30 mmHg), mean pulmonary artery pressure = 31 mmHg (normal range 10-22), pulmonary capillary wedge pressure = 7 mmHg (normal range 6-15), cardiac output = 2.97 L/min (normal range00204-8 mmHg), and cardiac index of 1.74/min/m^2 (normal range 2.8-4.2), respectively.

Eventually, the patient was diagnosed with postpartum pulmonary hypertension. She was admitted and treated in the intensive care unit under the direct care of a pulmonary hypertension team. Her management was guided by a close follow-up of her hemodynamics. Given the high risk of sudden deterioration at any given point, inotropic support was considered and planned. Luckily, the patient's blood pressure remained normal. Good perfusion pressure was supported by normal lactate measures and absence of end-organ damage. Intravenous furosemide infusion was initiated with close monitoring of volume status, which was well tolerated without the need for inotropic support along with parenteral iron. The patient was discharged on torsemide and spironolactone.

3. Outcome and Follow-Up

On review three weeks postdischarge, her functional status was back to premorbid levels with improved exercise tolerance. Repeated transthoracic echocardiogram revealed no significant interval changes. Repeat right heart catheterization showed mild pulmonary hypertension, normal right and left ventricular filling pressures, and normalization of the cardiac output and index. The patient was counseled about the importance of contraception and the risks of pregnancy, given the associated mortality risk. However, a few months later, the patient became pregnant, and after a multidisciplinary meeting and recounseling, she underwent a therapeutic abortion. She remains to follow in the pulmonology clinic and is doing well.

4. Discussion

Postpartum pulmonary hypertension is an infrequent yet serious entity that can easily be overlooked. Keeping it in mind is very important as early diagnosis and appropriate treatment can have a significant impact on the patient's morbidity and mortality.

The presentation of our patient's submassive pulmonary embolism picture bore a resemblance to other published reports [4, 5]. As was the case with our patient, an extensive workup is usually advised to rule out venous thromboembolism. According to the PIOPED II trial [11], the sensitivity of CT pulmonary angiogram (CTPA) in this regard is about 83%. With high pulmonary embolism probability, the negative predictive value is 95% and increases to 97% if combined by negative CT venogram [11]. Even though amniotic fluid embolism is commonly seen during or immediately after labor, V/Q scan was done to rule it out as the diagnostic yield of CTPA with regard to amniotic fluid embolism is very low. Our patient had sex during the puerperium, which may have made her at risk of having air embolism, in which the penis is thought to act as a piston forcing air into the vagina [12–14]. However, the absence of air in echocardiogram made this unlikely. Coronary artery disease and dissection were ruled out by coronary angiography. Cardiac MRI ruled out myocarditis and arrhythmogenic right ventricular dysplasia as well as the unroofed coronary sinus. Right heart catheterization (RHC) confirmed the PHT as the primary cause of right heart strain, and the normal pulmonary capillary wedge pressure excluded a left ventricular cause of the PHT. The low cardiac output and low cardiac index are likely secondary to the decreased preload secondary to PHT.

It is difficult to know whether the pregnancy and labor-induced stress unmasked a preexisting PHT or if this is a new onset PHT. Owing to the absence of preexisting PHT in our patient, the lack of prior symptoms, the event-free pregnancy, and the start of symptoms three-

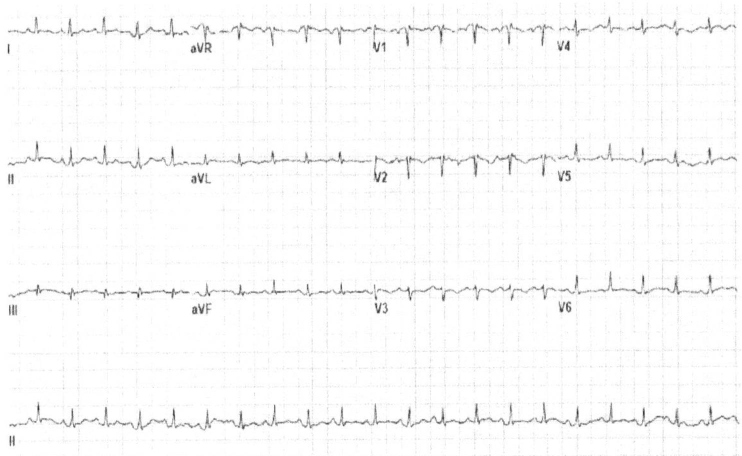

FIGURE 1: Electrocardiogram of the patient showing sinus tachycardia with T wave inversion in leads V1-3.

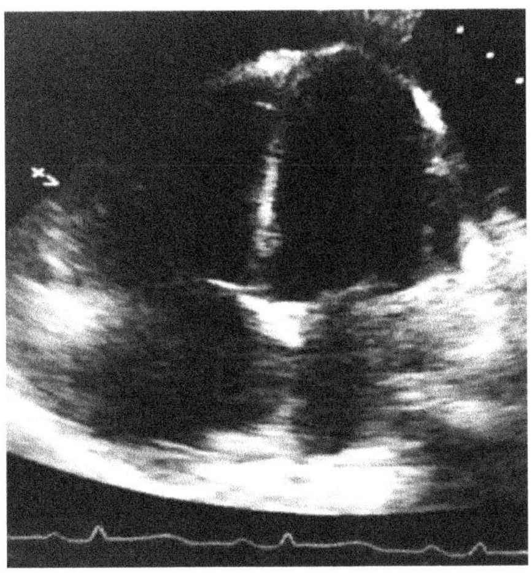

FIGURE 2: Transthoracic echocardiogram showing marked dilatation of right ventricle with globally reduced right ventricular systolic function.

week postpartum, we strongly believe that PPPHT is the correct diagnosis. Patients with PPPHT should be treated in intensive care units under the care of a pulmonary hypertension specialist team. Patients may require supplementary oxygen to maintain adequate oxygenation. Fluid overload should be treated with diuretics; however, the presence of right heart failure (RHF) makes treatment challenging. Patients often require an invasive assessment of hemodynamics to prevent loss of the preload the patient depends on to maintain cardiac output. Our patient had a dramatic improvement of symptoms and normalization of functional status with diuretics alone without the need for pulmonary hypertension-targeted treatments. Treatment of iron deficiency may help in controlling PHT, as previously reported in several studies, which showed that iron deficiency in patients with PHT was considered an important contributing factor [15].

In refractory cases, balloon atrial septostomy is considered a bridge for lung transplantation as it increases preload, cardiac output, and systemic oxygen transport [16]. However, this should be done in a stepwise manner to avoid refractory hypoxemia that may increase mortality [17, 18]. Lung transplant is indicated in the World Health Organization (WHO) functional class III or IV during escalating therapy, rapidly progressive disease, and the continuous need for parenteral targeted pulmonary hypertension therapy. The average five-year survival posttransplantation is around 45-50% [19]. Although the overall progression and prognosis of PPPHT are not well understood, dramatic response to diuretics, lack of need of parenteral targeted pulmonary hypertension therapy, and the normalization of functional status are all favorable prognostic factors.

Even in patients with a good prognosis, future pregnancies are contraindicated. Advice on effective contraceptive methods must be given. Progestogen-only methods and intrauterine devices can be used in women with PHT. Injectable progesterone-only methods and estrogen-containing contraceptives may increase the risk of venous thromboembolism [6, 20, 21]. Dual contraception is indicated in women taking Bosentan due to the interaction between the drug and progesterone-based methods of contraception [6, 16]. Although our understanding of the progression and prognosis of PPPHT is limited, the tough decision of therapeutic abortion was taken after a multidisciplinary meeting and a detailed discussion with the patient and was supported by the current pulmonary artery hypertension guidelines that recommend avoidance of pregnancy and termination of it if it happened [16].

5. Limitation

It is difficult to ascertain or conclude whether the pregnancy and labor-induced stress unmasked a preexisting PHT or if this is a new onset PHT. However, the favorable response to treatment is in keeping with new-onset PPPHT.

6. Conclusions

Postpartum pulmonary hypertension is an extremely rare disorder that has a significant impact on patients' morbidity and mortality. Early diagnosis and appropriate management

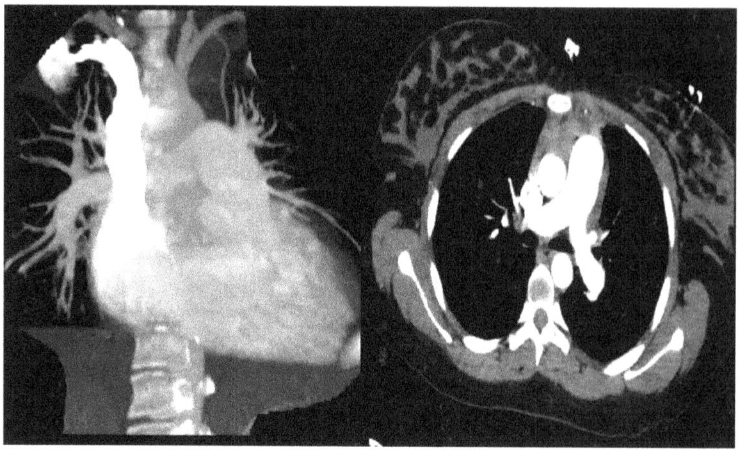

FIGURE 3: CT pulmonary angiogram showing dilated pulmonary trunk, with no evidence of pulmonary embolism.

under the direct supervision of pulmonary hypertension specialists are essential. Postpartum pulmonary hypertension is considered a relative contraindication for further pregnancies. Clinicians should counsel patients on adopting proper contraceptive plans.

Authors' Contributions

MM is responsible for conceptualization, methodology, data curation, visualization, and project administration. MM and AH wrote and prepared the original draft. MM, AH, TS, AZ, IY, MFHM, MR, RH, and MD wrote the review and edited the file. MD performed the supervision. All authors have read and agreed to the published version of the manuscript.

Acknowledgments

We acknowledge the Qatar National Library (QNL) for funding the publication of this article. We acknowledge the patient for allowing us to share the details of her case. We also acknowledge all the medical personnel involved in the care of this patient.

References

[1] G. Simonneau, D. Montani, D. S. Celermajer et al., "Haemodynamic definitions and updated clinical classification of pulmonary hypertension," *European Respiratory Journal*, vol. 53, no. 1, article 1801913, 2019.

[2] G. Simonneau, I. M. Robbins, M. Beghetti et al., "Updated clinical classification of pulmonary hypertension," *Journal of the American College of Cardiology*, vol. 54, no. 1, pp. S43–S54, 2009.

[3] R. J. Oudiz, "Pulmonary hypertension associated with left-sided heart disease," *Clinics in Chest Medicine*, vol. 28, no. 1, pp. 233–241, 2007.

[4] J. P. Escalante, A. Diez, M. Figueroa Casas et al., "Postpartum pulmonary hypertension," *Medicina*, vol. 75, no. 1, pp. 44–47, 2015.

[5] E. Demerouti, A. Manginas, S. Rammos, G. Athanassopoulos, G. Karatasakis, and G. Pavlides, "Postpartum pulmonary arterial hypertension: two cases covering a wide spectrum of presentations," *Hellenic journal of cardiology*, vol. 53, no. 6, pp. 472–475, 2012.

[6] K. M. Olsson and X. Jais, "Birth control and pregnancy management in pulmonary hypertension," *Seminars in Respiratory and Critical Care Medicine*, vol. 34, no. 5, pp. 681–688, 2013.

[7] Endorsed by the European Society of Gynecology (ESG), the Association for European Paediatric Cardiology (AEPC), and the German Society for Gender Medicine (DGesGM), V. Regitz-Zagrosek, C. B. Lundqvist et al., "ESC guidelines on the management of cardiovascular diseases during pregnancy: the Task Force on the Management of Cardiovascular Diseases during pregnancy of the European Society of Cardiology (ESC)," *European Heart Journal*, vol. 32, no. 24, pp. 3147–3197, 2011.

[8] S. J. Sheppard and R. A. Khalil, "Risk factors and mediators of the vascular dysfunction associated with hypertension in pregnancy," *Cardiovascular & Hematological Disorders-Drug Targets*, vol. 10, no. 1, pp. 33–52, 2010.

[9] P. Olley and W. Whitaker, "Postpartum pulmonary hypertension," *Obstetrics and Gynecology*, vol. 29, no. 3, pp. 369–377, 1967.

[10] B. M. Weiss, L. Zemp, B. Seifert, and O. M. Hess, "Outcome of pulmonary vascular disease in pregnancy: a systematic overview from 1978 through 1996," *Journal of the American College of Cardiology*, vol. 31, no. 7, pp. 1650–1657, 1998.

[11] P. Reinartz, B. Nowak, J. Wildberger, W. Schaefer, and U. Buell, "PIOPED II in the diagnosis of pulmonary embolism: evolution or stagnation?," *Journal of Nuclear Medicine*, vol. 47, suppl 1, pp. 20P–20P, 2006.

[12] P. A. Batman, J. Thomlinson, V. C. Moore, and R. Sykes, "Death due to air embolism during sexual intercourse in the puerperium," *Postgraduate Medical Journal*, vol. 74, no. 876, pp. 612-613, 1998.

[13] B. D. Lifschultz and E. R. Donoghue, "Air embolism during intercourse in pregnancy," *Journal of Forensic Sciences*, vol. 28, no. 4, pp. 1021-1022, 1983.

[14] A. Truhlar, V. Cerny, P. Dostal et al., "Out-of-hospital cardiac arrest from air embolism during sexual intercourse: case report and review of the literature," *Resuscitation*, vol. 73, no. 3, pp. 475–484, 2007.

[15] E. Soon, C. M. Treacy, M. R. Toshner et al., "Unexplained iron deficiency in idiopathic and heritable pulmonary arterial hypertension," *Thorax*, vol. 66, no. 4, pp. 326–332, 2011.

[16] N. Galiè, M. M. Hoeper, M. Humbert et al., "Guidelines for the diagnosis and treatment of pulmonary hypertension: the task force for the diagnosis and treatment of pulmonary hypertension of the European Society of Cardiology (ESC) and the European Respiratory Society (ERS), endorsed by the International Society of Heart and Lung Transplantation (ISHLT)," *European Heart Journal*, vol. 30, no. 20, pp. 2493–2537, 2009.

[17] J. Sandoval, J. Gaspar, T. Pulido et al., "Graded balloon dilation atrial septostomy in severe primary pulmonary hypertension. A therapeutic alternative for patients nonresponsive to vasodilator treatment," *Journal of the American College of Cardiology*, vol. 32, no. 2, pp. 297–304, 1998.

[18] A. M. Keogh, E. Mayer, R. L. Benza et al., "Interventional and surgical modalities of treatment in pulmonary hypertension," *Journal of the American College of Cardiology*, vol. 54, no. 1, pp. S67–S77, 2009.

[19] E. P. Trulock, L. B. Edwards, D. O. Taylor et al., "Registry of the International Society for Heart and Lung Transplantation: Twenty-third Official Adult Lung and Heart-Lung Transplantation Report–2006," *The Journal of Heart and Lung Transplantation*, vol. 25, no. 8, pp. 880–892, 2006.

[20] A. R. Hemnes, D. G. Kiely, B. A. Cockrill et al., "Statement on pregnancy in pulmonary hypertension from the Pulmonary Vascular Research Institute," *Pulmonary Circulation*, vol. 5, no. 3, pp. 435–465, 2016.

[21] S. Mantha, R. Karp, V. Raghavan, N. Terrin, K. A. Bauer, and J. I. Zwicker, "Assessing the risk of venous thromboembolic events in women taking progestin-only contraception: a meta-analysis," *BMJ*, vol. 345, no. aug07 2, article e4944, 2012.

Hypersensitivity Pneumonitis Associated with Red-Vented Bulbul: A New Encounter of Bird Related Hypersensitivity Pneumonitis

W. D. N. L. Amarasinghe,[1] **R. Jayasekara**,[1] **B. D. W. Jayamanne**,[2] **T. D. K. Nalaka**,[3] **W. A. D. L. Amarasiri**,[4] **R. Punchihewa**,[5] **and A. Fernando**[1]

[1]*Central Chest Clinic, Colombo, Sri Lanka*
[2]*Department of Public Health, Faculty of Medicine, University of Kelaniya, Sri Lanka*
[3]*Department of Radiology, National Hospital of Sri Lanka, Sri Lanka*
[4]*Department of Physiology, Faculty of Medicine, University of Colombo, Sri Lanka*
[5]*Department of Pathology, National Hospital for Respiratory Diseases, Welisara, Sri Lanka*

Correspondence should be addressed to W. D. N. L. Amarasinghe; amaranadee@gmail.com

Academic Editor: Akif Turna

Bird related hypersensitivity pneumonitis (HP) is becoming more common than other forms of HP around the world. We present two cases of HP, associated with exposure to visiting birds which had nested within their homes in semi urban areas of Colombo, Sri Lanka. A 65-year-old female (case 1) and a 61-year-old male (case 2) presented to the chest clinic complaining of gradually progressive and persistent chronic dry cough and dyspnoea during the year 2018. Both were found to have close contact with red-vented bulbuls (Konda kurulla) in their homes for more than 6 months prior to onset of symptoms and denied any other risk exposures in detail history taking. In both patients, high-resolution computed tomography chest (HRCT) showed centrilobular nodules of ground glass density with significant lobular air trapping. Video-assisted thoracoscopic (VATs) lung biopsy of case 1 showed patchy and focal interstitial thickening with lymphocytic infiltrate, minimal fibrosis, and few noncaseating granulomata within the interstitium. Transbronchial lung biopsy of case 2 showed thickened alveolar septae with lympho-histiocytic infiltrate and occasional neutrophils and eosinopils. Both showed severe reduction in forced vital capacity (FVC) at presentation. Multidisciplinary diagnosis of HP associated with red-vented bulbuls was made. Both achieved good improvement in clinical, lung function, and radiological assessment following removal of offending antigen exposure and treatment with oral corticosteroids.

1. Introduction

Hypersensitivity pneumonitis (HP) is an immunologically-mediated inflammatory lung disease caused by repetitive inhalation of antigens in a susceptible host [1–3]. Potential causative agents are grouped as microbes, animal proteins, and chemicals [1, 4, 5]. Bird related HP is becoming the commonest form caused by high- and low-molecular-weight proteins found in feathers, faeces, and other animal products commonly of pigeons, parrots, parakeets, love birds, cockatoos, budgerigars, and fowl [4, 6–8]. We report two cases that presented to the Central Chest Clinic, Sri Lanka with a multidisciplinary diagnosis of subacute HP associated with red-vented bulbuls. There have been no previously published reports of HP associated with red-vented bulbuls or any other visiting birds. Hence, this is the first paper to study this association.

2. Case Presentations

Both patients were retired professionals from semiurban areas in Colombo who denied exposure to any organic or inorganic particles, which can cause HP, within the last two years. However, repeated questioning revealed that there had been close contact with red-vented bulbuls which frequented their

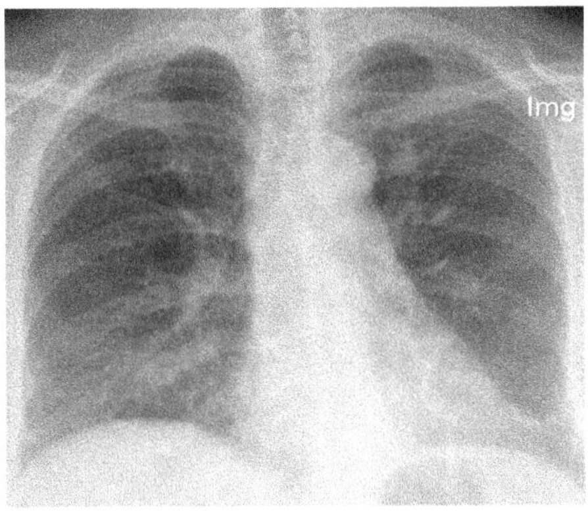

FIGURE 1: Chest X-ray shows patchy opacifications in right mid zone and reticular nodular shadows in mid zones of both lung fields.

houses. The birds nested in chandeliers hung directly above the sofas in their living rooms where these patients spent most of their leisure times. Though there had been debris falling on to the sofa as the birds moved within the nests above, they had not attempted to remove the nests as they enjoyed their presence. The living rooms had been kept closed during the periods when the birds reproduced, to protect the eggs and nestlings. Additionally, both patients had closely handled the nestlings until they fledged. This confirmed that there had been continuous exposure to antigens of red vented bulbuls for around 8–10 hours per day for 10–18 months with a proximity of 2–3 meters in a closed or partially closed environment, in these patients.

2.1. Case 1. A 65-year female presented to the clinic with insidious-onset persistent and progressive dyspnoea, cough, and wheezing for six months. She was a diagnosed diabetic and had a history of allergic rhinitis. She revealed close contact with red-vented bulbul birds for around one-and-half years. Erythrocyte sedimentation rate (ESR) was 41 mm/h. Chest radiography showed patchy opacifications in right mid zone and reticular nodular shadows in mid zones of both lung fields (Figure 1). Saturation at rest was 95% and there was 7% desaturation during the 6-minute walk test where she walked a distance of 480 meters. Spirometry and body plethysmography showed severe restriction and air trapping (FVC 49.5%, total lung capacity-TLC-76%, residual volume-RV-110%, RV/TLC-158%), with reduction in diffusing capacity with patchy parenchymal involvement (carbon monoxide diffusing capacity-DLCO-67%, carbon monoxide transfer coefficient-KCO-99%). HRCT showed centrilobular nodules of ground glass density in upper zones, basal ground glass opacities, and significant lobular air trapping (Figure 2). Video-assisted thoracoscopic lung biopsy showed patchy and focal interstitial thickening with lymphocytic infiltrate, minimal fibrosis, and several noncaseating granulomata within the interstitium (Figure 3).

2.2. Case 2. A 61-year-old male presented with insidious-onset, persistent and progressive dyspnoea and dry cough for four months. At the onset, he had low grade fever and constitutional symptom which subsided over a few weeks. He was a known hypertensive. He revealed close contact with red-vented bulbuls for around ten months. ESR was 78 mm/h. Chest radiography showed reticular nodular shadows in mid and lower zones of both lung fields (Figure 4). Spirometry showed severe restriction (FVC 52.8%, TLC-56%, RV-65%) with a normal diffusing capacity (DLCO-86%, KCO-180%). HRCT showed centrilobular nodules of ground glass density in all three zones and significant lobular air trapping (Figure 5). Bronchial wash cytology revealed inflammatory cells (249/cumm) with predominant lymphocytes (80%). Transbronchial lung biopsy showed thickened alveolar septae with lympho-histiocytic infiltrate and occasional neutrophils and eosinophils. Some of the alveolar spaces contained foamy histiocytes. Fibrosis was not evident.

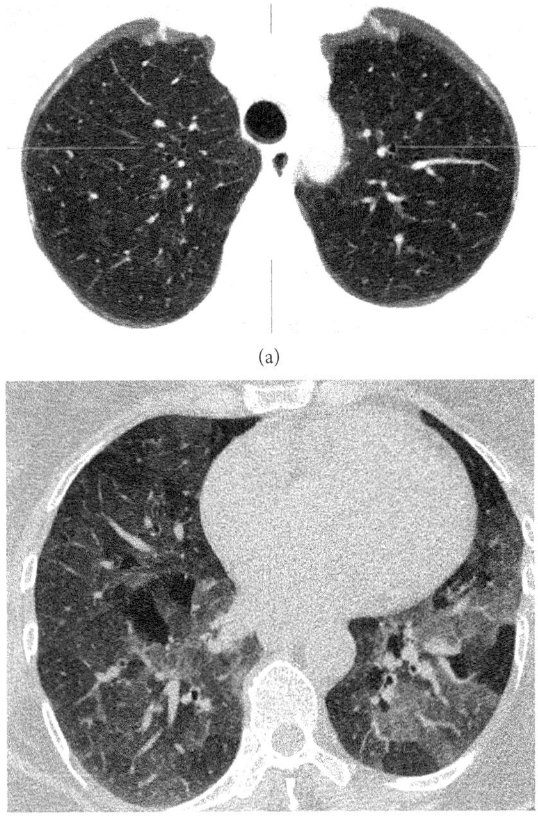

(a)

(b)

FIGURE 2: HRCT chest demonstrating upper lobe predominant centrilobular nodules of ground glass density (a). Expiratory HRCT films shows air trapping in lobules that had decreased attenuation on inspiratory film and centrilobular nodules of ground glass density (b).

A diagnosis of subacute HP associated with exposure to red vented bulbuls was made for both cases at a multidisciplinary meeting for interstitial lung diseases held at the National hospital of Sri Lanka. The patient of case 1 achieved good clinical and lung function improvement (FVC 91.9%) by about two months and that of case 2 showed clinical and lung function improvement (FVC 72%) around the third month of treatment with oral prednisolone (0.5 mg/kg) tail down regimen and the avoidance of the offending exposure. Both patients did not have any recurrences following avoidance of

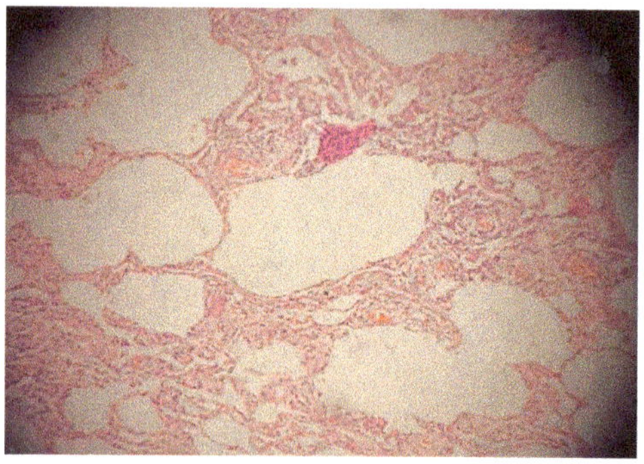

(a)

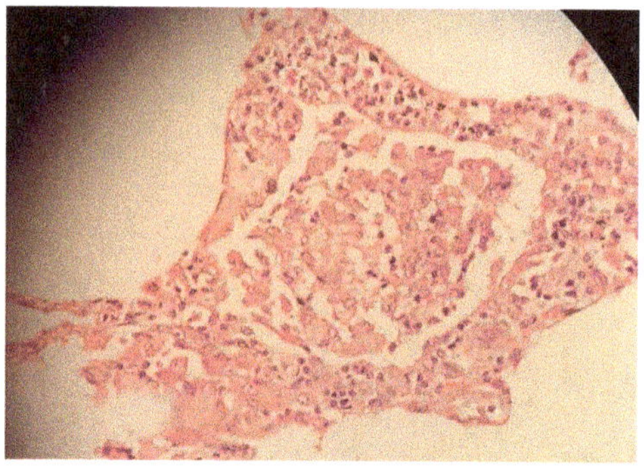

(b)

Figure 3: VATS biopsy shows interstitial thickening with few noncaseating granulomata (a). High power view of a noncaseating granulomata (b).

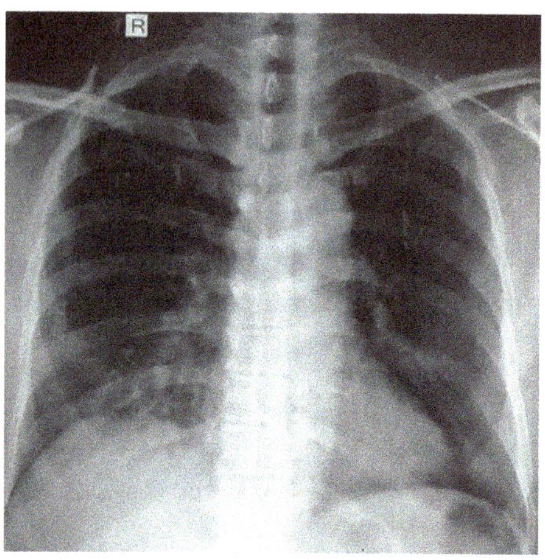

Figure 4: CXR- Patchy opacifications in right mid zone and reticular nodular shadows in mid zones of both lung fields.

exposure to red-vented bulbuls and achieved normal FVC values in spirometry assessment with treatment of oral prednisolone within one-year follow-up period.

3. Discussion

Bird related HP (Bird fancier's lung) is increasingly becoming prevalent around the world and shows worse outcome than other forms [8, 9]. Bird related HP can be caused by high- and

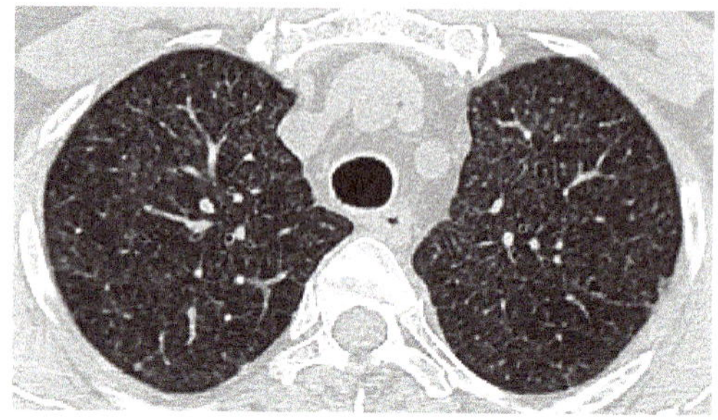

(a)

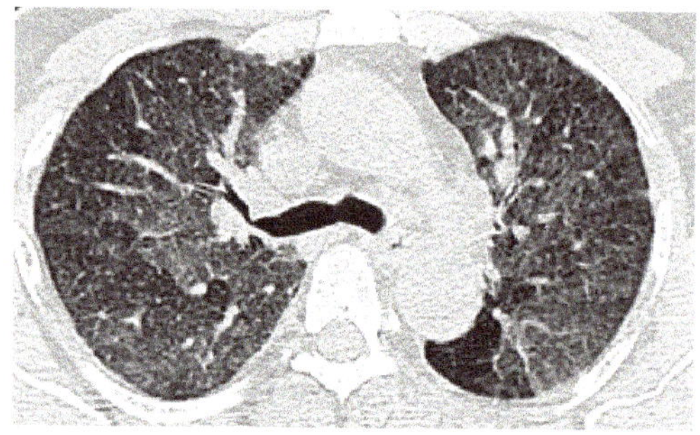

(b)

Figure 5: HRCT demonstrating upper lobe predominant centrilobular nodules of ground glass density (a). Expiratory HRCT slices show air trapping in lobules that had decreased attenuation on inspiratory slices with centrilobular nodules of ground glass density (b).

low-molecular-weight proteins (<5 μm) found in feathers, faeces, and other animal products [10].

Suspicion of an association between symptoms and contact with a provoking antigen is the first step in the diagnostic process of HP, combined with the measurement of serological markers and specific IgG antibody levels, radiological findings, lung function assessment, bronchoalveolar lavage, and lung biopsy for the complete workup [4, 12]. The identification of causal antigen is impossible in about 30–60% of cases [1]. Species specific antibody are commercially available for pigeons, parrots, parakeets, cockatoos, and multiple domestic poultry species at present, and there are emerging avian associations as in this report, to be experimented [1, 11, 13]. However, laboratory measures of exposure, such as precipitin tests, specific inhalation challenge, and lymphocyte proliferation tests have failed to achieve consensus among international experts as important in diagnosing HP according to international modified Delphi survey, possibly due to the limited information on their test characteristics, lack of standardization, or limited availability [14].

Air space involvement of HP in the lung parenchyma presents as patchy ground glass opacities and/or centrilobular nodules in HRCT [15]. Shunting of blood away from poorly ventilated regions manifests as mosaic attenuation. Persistence of hypoattenuated areas in expiratory CT films indicates air-trapping [8]. Spirometry may demonstrate a restrictive lung disease pattern, with moderate to severe reduction of FVC and DLCO [10]. Lung biopsy may show cellular bronchiolitis, diffuse lymphocytic interstitial infiltration, and noncaseating granulomas [10, 16].

Proper history plays a key role in HP as early avoidance of causative associations invariably brings complete or partial recovery whereas delay would cause irreversible lung fibrosis. Multidisciplinary approach is highly recommended when the diagnosis is challenging [6].

The red-vented bulbul (*Pycnonotus cafer*) also known as Kondakurulla in Sinhala, is a resident breeder across the Indian subcontinent including Sri Lanka, and has established itself in several Pacific islands, parts of the United Arab Emirates, United States, and possibly New Zealand, not limiting to a part of the world [17–19]. They build nests in bushes at a height of around 2-3 meters and opportunistically invade houses specially using lamp shades and chandeliers for nesting, leaving an invariable risk exposure to the household [20, 21].

To our knowledge, all published cases of bird related HP are associated with birds raised as pets or for farming. An important fact to be highlighted is that when a clinician questions regarding risk exposure to birds, the patient would give a negative answer initially if they have not raised birds purposefully. The opportunity to remove the exposure would be missed in such instances. Hence, the present observation highlights the importance of specific questioning regarding this kind of casual exposures to visiting birds within living places.

Birds nesting and breeding inside houses is considered to bring prosperity to the household in some cultural beliefs. Hence updating public on harmful aspects of these associations would also be important.

Disclosure

Written informed consent was obtained for publication of this case report and accompanying images from relevant authority.

References

[1] R. Nogueira, N. Melo, H. N. Bastos et al., "Hypersensitivity pneumonitis: antigen diversity and disease implications," *Pulmonology*, vol. 15, no. 2, pp. 97–108, 2019.

[2] A. N. Musa, K. N. Hirmizi, and M. A. Ibrahim, "Hypersensitivity pneumonitis-a case series," *Respirology*, vol. 22, no. S3, pp. 256–256, 2017.

[3] A. Matsuo, T. Horiuchi, K. Sonehara, and Y. Wada, "The first case report of hypersensitivity pneumonitis progressed to pulmonary fibrosis induced by Lyophyllum aggregatum," *Respirology*, vol. 22, no. S3, pp. 266–266, 2017.

[4] T. Ismail, C. Mcsharry, and G. Boyd, "Extrinsic allergic alveolitis," *Respirology*, vol. 11, no. 3, pp. 262–268, 2006.

[5] A. S. Jee, H. E. Jo, and T. J. Corte, "Hypersensitivity pneumonitis: a protean and challenging disease," *Respirology*, vol. 22, no. 8, pp. 1489–1490, 2017.

[6] M. Ueyama, H. Yutani, S. Terada et al., "Usefulness of lymphocyte stimulation test against pigeon serum in management of patients with chronic hypersensitivity pneumonitis," *Respirology*, vol. 22, no. S3, pp. 256–256, 2017.

[7] S. S. S. Aflah, Z. A. Bakar, H. Lockman, G. J. T. John, and A. R. A. Muttalif, "Hypersensitivity pneumonitis case series," *Respirology*, vol. 22, no. S3, pp. 256–257, 2017.

[8] L. Winkler, Z. Patel, and R. Gue, "Pigeon breeder's lung: a case report of hypersensitivity pneumonitis," *West Virginia Medical Journal OA*, 2017.

[9] F. Morell, À. Roger, L. Reyes, M. J. Cruz, C. Murio, and X. Muñoz, "Bird Fancier's Lung," *Medicine*, vol. 87, no. 2, pp. 110–130, 2008.

[10] M. Selman, A. Pardo, and T. E. King, "Hypersensitivity Pneumonitis," *American Journal of Respiratory and Critical Care Medicine*, vol. 186, no. 4, pp. 314-324, 2012.

[11] M. Funke and J. M. Fellrath, "Hypersensitivity pneumonitis secondary to lovebirds: a new cause of bird fancier's disease," *European Respiratory Journal*, vol. 32, no. 2, pp. 517–521, 2008.

[12] S. J. Bourke, J. C. Dalphin, G. Boyd, C. McSharry, C. L. Baldwin, and J. E. Calvert, "Hypersensitivity pneumonitis :current concepts," *European Respiratory Journal*, vol. 18, no. 32 suppl, pp. 81s–92s, 2001.

[13] C. McSharry, G. M. Dye, T. Ismail, K. Anderson, E. M. Spiers, and G. Boyd, "Quantifying serum antibody in bird fanciers' hypersensitivity pneumonitis," *BMC Pulmonary Medicine*, vol. 6, no. 1, 2006.

[14] J. Morisset, K. A. Johannson, K. D. Jones et al., "Identification of diagnostic criteria for chronic hypersensitivity pneumonitis an international modified delphi survey," *American Journal of Respiratory and Critical Care Medicine*, vol. 197, no. 8, pp. 1036-1044, 2018.

[15] M. Remy-Jardin, J. Remy, B. Wallaert, and N. l. Müller, "Subacute and chronic bird breeder hypersensitivity pneumonitis: sequential evaluation with CT and correlation with lung function tests and bronchoalveolar lavage," *Radiology*, vol. 189, no. 1, pp. 111–118, 1993.

[16] Y. Ohtani, S. Saiki, M. Kitaichi et al., "Chronic bird fancier's lung: histopathological and clinical correlation. an application of the 2002 ATS/ERS consensus classification of the idiopathic interstitial pneumonias," *Thorax*, vol. 60, no. 8, pp. 665–671, 2005.

[17] D. Bhatt and A. Kumar, "Foraging ecology of red-vented bulbul in Haridwar India," *Forktail*, vol. 2001, no. 17, pp. 109–110, 2001.

[18] Birdlife international 2018, "Pycnonotus cafer. The IUCN Red list of threatened species," 2018, e.T22712695A132102224. [Cited 13 June 2019.]

[19] Bushana, "Biodiversity of Sri Lanka: Red-vented Bulbul (*Pycnonotus cafer*) [Internet]. Biodiversity of Sri Lanka," 2019, https://biodiversityofsrilanka.blogspot.com/2013/01/kondakurullared-vented-bulbul.html

[20] R. Somasiri, "The Island. The Island," 2012, [cited 2018 Jun 18] http://www.island.lk/index.php?page_cat=article-details&page=article-details&code_title=45008.

[21] C. M. Inglis, "Curious site for nest of the Bengal Redvented Bulbul (Molpastes haemarrhous bengalensis)," *Journal of the Bombay Natural History Society*, vol. 28, no. 3–4, pp. 1135–1136, 1922, 40.

29

High Serum Level of IL-17 in Patients with Chronic Obstructive Pulmonary Disease and the Alpha-1 Antitrypsin PiZ Allele

Margarita Y. Pervakova, Alexandra V. Mazing, Sergey V. Lapin, Olga Y. Tkachenko, Anna I. Budkova, Elena A. Surkova, Vladimir L. Emanuel, and Olga N. Titova

Pavlov First State Medical University of St. Petersburg, 197022 Saint Petersburg, Russia

Correspondence should be addressed to Margarita Y. Pervakova; margaritalerner@gmail.com

Academic Editor: Akio Niimi

Chronic obstructive pulmonary disease (COPD) is multifactorial disease, which is characterized by airflow limitation and can be provoked by genetic factors, including carriage of the PiZ allele of the protease inhibitor (Pi) gene, encoding alpha-1 antitrypsin (A1AT). Both homozygous and heterozygous PiZ allele carriers can develop COPD. It was found recently that normal A1AT regulates cytokine levels, including IL-17, which is involved in COPD progression. The aim of this study was to determine whether homozygous or heterozygous PiZ allele carriage leads to elevated level of IL-17 and other proinflammatory cytokines in COPD patients. *Materials and Methods.* Serum samples and clinical data were obtained from 44 COPD patients, who included 6 PiZZ, 8 PiMZ, and 30 PiMM A1AT phenotype carriers. Serum concentrations of IL-17, IL-6, IL-8, IFN-γ, and TNF-α were measured by the enzyme-linked immunosorbent assay (ELISA). All A1AT phenotypes were verified by narrow pH range isoelectrofocusing with selective A1AT staining. A turbidimetric method was used for quantitative A1AT measurements. *Results.* COPD patients with both PiZZ and PiMZ phenotypes demonstrated elevated IL-17 and decreased IFN-γ levels in comparison to patients with the PiMM phenotype of A1AT. Thereafter, the ratio IL-17/IFN-γ in PiZZ and PiMZ groups greatly exceeded the values of the PiMM group. Homozygous PiZ allele carriers also had significantly higher levels of IL-6 and lower levels of IL-8, and IL-6 values correlated negatively with A1AT concentrations. *Conclusions.* The presence of the PiZ allele in both homozygous and heterozygous states is associated with altered serum cytokine levels, including elevated IL-17, IL-17/IFN-γ ratio, and IL-6 (only PiZZ), but lower IFN-γ and IL-8.

1. Introduction

Chronic obstructive pulmonary disease (COPD) is currently the fourth leading cause of death in the world, a major cause of chronic morbidity and mortality [1]. The current pathophysiologic concept assumes COPD as complex disease with multifactorial background, based on the interaction of environmental and genetic factors [2]. The most well-studied predisposition factor for COPD is alpha-1 antitrypsin deficiency (A1ATD), which occurs as a result of carriage of pathogenic alleles of the Pi gene (SERPINA1, protease inhibitor) [3]. The most common and normally functioning A1AT allelic form is PiM, whereas the most abundant and clinically significant pathological allele is PiZ. About 95% cases of clinically manifested A1ATD occur as a result of the PiZZ phenotype [4]. Meanwhile, the heterozygous PiMZ phenotype leads to the so-called intermediate A1ATD [5] and is associated with increased risk of COPD, but mostly in ever-smokers [6]. The protease/antiprotease hypothesis explains the development of emphysema by the loss of A1AT ability to inhibit neutrophil proteases, mainly neutrophil elastase [7]. Recently, multiple immunomodulatory and anti-inflammatory A1AT functions were described, and several pulmonary and extrapulmonary pathologies, besides COPD, were found to be associated with A1ATD. In particular, A1AT suppresses NF-kβ activation [8], reduces TNF-α expression [9, 10], and regulates TNF-α signaling [11]. Moreover, A1AT is capable of regulating the production of IL-1β, IL-6, and IL-8 [12] and lowering neutrophil chemotaxis by binding and inactivating IL-8 [13].

Neutrophilic inflammation in airways is considered central to the pathogenesis of COPD, regardless of the clinical phenotype, severity of disease, rapidity of lung function decline, and age of onset [14]. It was found that the proinflammatory cytokine IL-17 played a crucial role in COPD progression [15, 16]. This proinflammatory cytokine is essential in the acute phase of COPD, and it mediates COPD exacerbations and provokes bronchial hyperreactivity [17] and corticosteroid resistance [18]. Smoking patients demonstrated higher levels of IL-17 [15].

IL-17 is a key cytokine that is produced by type 17 T helper (Th17) cells and links T cell activation to neutrophil mobilization and activation [19]. IL-17 induces tissue inflammation mainly by stimulating the expression of several proinflammatory cytokines including IL-6, TNF-α, IL-1β, and IL-8 [20]. This leads to the expansion and accumulation of neutrophils in the focus of inflammation, as occurs, for example, in smoke-induced injury [21–23]. The formation of a Th17 cell subset is initiated by transforming growth factor- (TGF-) β together with the obligatory presence of IL-6 [24]. The production of Th17 is suppressed by IFN-γ, which is a proinflammatory cytokine with anti-inflammatory functions, and it possibly participates in resolution of inflammation [24–26]. The IL-17/IFN-γ ratio was suggested as a marker for prognosis and severity of inflammatory diseases [25, 27]. It was confirmed that A1AT also reduces Th17 cell formation, increasing the CD4+FoxP3+ Treg cell population, in contrast to IFN-γ, which stimulates Th1 formation [28].

Thus, both IL-17 and A1AT are very important molecules involved in COPD pathogenesis, and the modulatory A1AT effect on IL-17 secretion was confirmed. But there is still no evidence whether homozygous or heterozygous PiZ allele carriage modifies A1AT immunomodulatory properties and influence on IL-17 level in COPD.

The aim of this study was to evaluate whether homozygous or heterozygous PiZ allele carriage modifies the levels of IL-17 and other proinflammatory cytokines in COPD patients.

2. Materials and Methods

Serum samples and clinical data were collected from 44 male patients, who have suffered COPD exacerbations. The study design was approved by the local university ethics committee. Written informed consent was obtained from all study patients. Those patients included 14 PiZ allele carriers: 6 PiZZ and 8 PiMZ A1AT phenotypes. As far as normal PiMM phenotypes were identified in other 30 patients, their samples were used as a control group. All patients had mean age of 59.42 ± 11.32 years, and most of them were ex-smokers. They all demonstrated an FEV_1 decline lower than 50% of the predicted value.

All A1AT phenotypes were identified by isoelectrofocusing, conducted in ultrathin agarose gels, containing 0.9% agarose IEF (GE Healthcare, USA), 8.7% glycerol (MP Biomedicals, USA), and 7.8% D-sorbitol (Sigma-Aldrich, USA). Narrow pH gradient was generated by adding ampholytes (pH 4.2-4.9) (GE Healthcare, USA) to the gel solution, cooled down to 60°C. Electrophoretic separation was performed with the Multiphor II Electrophoresis System (Pharmacia Biotech, Sweden). Serum samples were applied on gels with 3 μl applicators. The prefocusing step was set at the following parameters: 450 V, 30 mA, 15 W, and 380 V/h. The focusing of A1AT molecules was performed at 1050 V, 28 mA, 21 W, and 1700 V/h. Since the separation was completed, the proteins were transferred to the Hybond-C extra membrane (GE Healthcare, USA) by western blotting under pressure of 2 kg for 10 minutes. The further steps included blocking by membrane incubation in 2.0% BCA solution, washing in saline buffer, and selective staining with horseradish peroxidase-conjugated goat anti-human A1AT antibodies (Bethyl Laboratories, Sweden). The resulting immune complexes were visualized by staining reaction with 3-amino-9-ethylcarbazole as a chromogenic substrate in the presence of hydrogen peroxide.

Quantitative A1AT measurements were performed in the samples with a turbidimetric commercial kit (Sentinel Diagnostics, Italy). Serum concentrations of IL-17, IL-6, IL-8, IFN-γ, and TNF-α were measured by the enzyme-linked immunosorbent assay (ELISA) with commercial kits (OOO «Cytokin», Russia).

The results are presented as median ± 75% interquartile range (IQR). Nonparametric data were compared by Kruskal-Wallis one-way analysis of variance. Dunn's pairwise multiple comparison posttest was used to compare each patient group. Correlations between the parameters were evaluated using Spearman's rank correlation test. Differences between the groups were considered significant at a P value of <0.05. Statistical analyses were performed with GraphPad Prism 6.0 (GraphPad Software, Inc., version for Windows 6.01).

3. Results

The following subgroups of COPD patients were analysed: 6 PiZZ, 8 PiMZ, and 30 PiMM phenotype carriers. Clinical and laboratory parameters of COPD patients with PiZZ, PiMZ, and PiMM phenotypes are presented in Table 1.

The median IL-17 level in patients with the PiZZ phenotype was 57.86 pg/ml (44.76-71.01 pg/ml), which was significantly higher than that in the normal PiMM phenotype: 1.44 pg/ml (1.24-1.81 pg/ml). The IL-17 level in PiMZ individuals was also elevated up to 82.39 pg/ml (37.87-121.8 pg/ml) ($P < 0.01$). The comparison of IL-17 levels in COPD patients with different A1AT phenotypes is presented in Figure 1.

On the contrary, the median level of IFN-γ was lower both in PiZZ (15.52 pg/ml (1.57-62.34 pg/ml)) and in PiMZ (15.98 pg/ml (5.67-22.0 pg/ml)) than in PiMM individuals (62.29 pg/ml (36.29-199.5 pg/ml)).

The comparison of IFN-γ levels in COPD patients with different A1AT phenotypes is presented in Figure 2.

Consequently, the ratio of IL-17/IFN-γ was calculated as an integrative biomarker of disease severity. In both PiZZ and PiMZ groups, the IL-17/IFN-γ ratio exceeded the values of the PiMM group. The median IL-17/IFN-γ ratio value in patients with the PiZZ phenotype was 3.65 (2.38-36.6) and was significantly higher than that in the normal PiMM

Table 1: Clinical and laboratory parameters of groups of COPD patients, divided by the A1AT phenotype.

A1AT phenotype	PiZZ	PiMZ	PiMM	P
A1AT concentration (mg/l)	310.00 (191.50-463.30)	1089.00 (848.00-1464.00)	1209.00 (1084.00-685.00)	ZZ/MZ: $P < 0.05$ ZZ/MM: $P < 0.001$
Age (year)	47.50 (41.25-58.0)	64.50 (57.0-70.25)	64.50 (58.50-65.50)	ZZ/MZ: $P < 0.05$ ZZ/MM: $P < 0.05$
FEV_1 (% predicted)	25.78 (20.35-7.76)	35.64 (24.19-41.62)	27.82 (25.35-38.91)	ns
VLC (% predicted)	61.36 (56.23-6.72)	58.17 (51.66-74.65)	50.12 (40.75-66.55)	ns
FEV_1/FVC (% ratio)	30.20 (23.30-1.59)	42.72 (33.59-45.85)	48.25 (40.58-64.26)	ZZ/MZ: ns ZZ/MM: $P < 0.05$
RBC count ($\times 10^9$/l)	5.36 (5.08-5.79)	4.88 (4.27-5.43)	4.63 (4.36-5.19)	ns
Hemoglobin (g/l)	160.50 (149.80-174.80)	137.50 (128.00-54.80)	151.00 (141.50-158.00)	ZZ/MZ: $P < 0.05$ ZZ/MM: $P < 0.05$
Hematocrit (%)	46.30 (44.0-56.55)	40.40 (38.08-42.55)	42.90 (40.60-45.75)	ZZ/MZ: $P < 0.05$ ZZ/MM: $P < 0.05$
WBC count ($\times 10^9$/l)	7.95 (5.16-12.03)	10.38 (8.60-15.7)	12.97 (8.40-16.94)	ns
Ever-smokers/never-smokers	3/3	8/0	28/2	ns

All quantitative data are presented as median ± 75% interquartile range (IQR). COPD: chronic obstructive pulmonary disease; A1AT: alpha-1 antitrypsin; FEV_1: forced expiratory volume in one second; FVC: forced vital capacity; RBC: red blood cells; WBC: white blood cells.

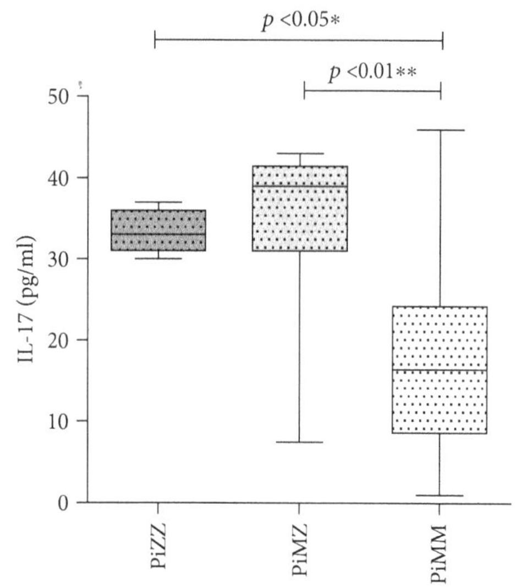

Figure 1: Comparison of IL-17 levels in COPD patients with PiZZ, PiMZ, and PiMM phenotypes of A1AT.

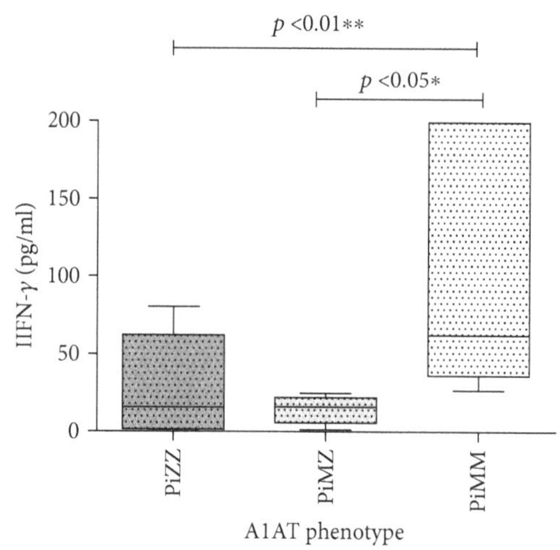

Figure 2: Comparison of IFN-γ levels in COPD patients with PiZZ, PiMZ, and PiMM phenotypes of A1AT.

phenotype (0.026 (0.004-0.53)). The IL-17/IFN-γ ratio in PiMZ individuals was also elevated up to 6.81 (3.68-26.9).

The comparison of IL-17/IFN-γ ratios in COPD patients with different A1AT phenotypes is presented in Figure 3.

The median IL-6 level in PiZZ patients was also elevated up to 74.58 pg/ml (63.15-84.66 pg/ml), in comparison to PiMM (47.0 pg/ml (27.42-73.28 pg/ml)). It was not significantly increased in PiMZ patients (63.38 pg/ml (50.20-82.59 pg/ml)). The comparison of IL-6 levels in COPD patients with different A1AT phenotypes is presented in Figure 4.

On the contrary, the median level of IL-8 was significantly lower in PiZZ (117.5 pg/ml (87.38-143.2 pg/ml)) versus PiMM (319.0 pg/ml (196.9-927.2 pg/ml)). The median level of IL-8 in PiMZ patients was 162.8 pg/ml (142.8-231.7 pg/ml), which was not significantly different. The comparison of IL-8 levels in COPD patients with different A1AT phenotypes is presented in Figure 5.

Both IL-17 and IL-17/IFN-γ ratio did not correlate with A1AT concentrations.

However, IFN-γ level showed a direct correlation with A1AT level, whereas IL-6 level correlated negatively with A1AT concentration. IL-8 showed a weak positive correlation with A1AT. The results of correlation analysis between A1AT concentrations and proinflammatory cytokine levels are presented in Table 2.

Serum TNF-α levels of all individuals except for two PiZZ and PiMM phenotype carriers were below the lower detection limit of assay (1 pg/ml).

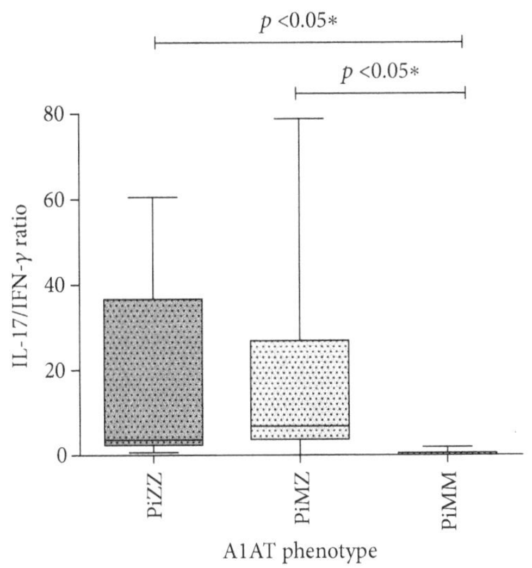

FIGURE 3: Comparison of IL-17/IFN-γ ratios in COPD patients with PiZZ, PiMZ, and PiMM phenotypes of A1AT.

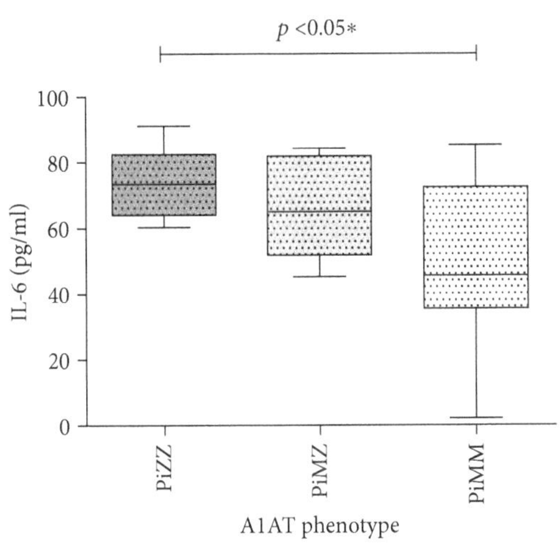

FIGURE 4: Comparison of IL-6 levels in COPD patients with PiZZ, PiMZ, and PiMM phenotypes of A1AT.

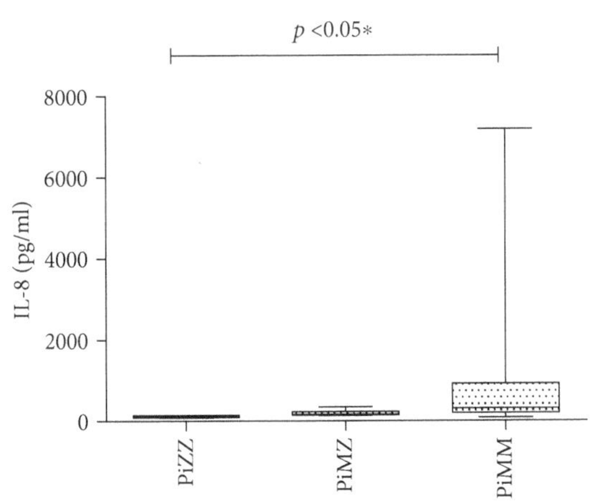

FIGURE 5: Comparison of IL-8 levels in COPD patients with PiZZ, PiMZ, and PiMM phenotypes of A1AT.

TABLE 2: Correlation analysis between A1AT concentrations and proinflammatory cytokine levels in patients with COPD.

	A1AT concentration (mg/l)	
	r	*P*
IL-17 (pg/ml)	-0.029	ns
IFN-γ (pg/ml)	0.5191	<0.05
IL-17/IFN-γ	-0.4262	ns
IL-6 (pg/ml)	-0.5678	<0.01
IL-8 (pg/ml)	0.4534	<0.05

COPD: chronic obstructive pulmonary disease; A1AT: alpha-1 antitrypsin.

4. Discussion

Immunomodulatory and tissue-protective properties of A1AT were described by many researchers during the last decade. It was proven that PiZ allele carriage reduces A1AT adhesion to neutrophil elastase and other proteases, leading to alveolar surfactant, elastin, and extracellular matrix degradation [29]. Regarding immunomodulatory properties, it was also reported that COPD patients with A1ATD had higher TNF-α, IL-6, IL-1β, and IL-8 production in comparison to COPD patients without A1ATD [12, 13, 30]. Meanwhile, we did not find any data about IL-17 and IFN-γ levels in COPD patients with A1ATD in comparison to patients with the PiMM phenotype of A1AT.

This study was aimed at investigating whether PiZ allele carriage influences IL-17 and other proinflammatory cytokine serum levels in COPD. The following COPD patient groups were analysed: 6 PiZZ, 8 PiMZ, and 30 PiMM A1AT phenotype carriers. Patients with the PiZZ phenotype were younger and had a more intensive FEV_1/FVC ratio decline, leading to faster obstruction development. It was also noted that PiZZ patients had higher hemoglobin and hematocrit values ($P < 0.05$), which indicate secondary erythrocytosis because of respiratory failure in COPD. Patients, who were PiMZ carriers, demonstrated slightly lower A1AT level and a lower FEV_1/FVC ratio as compared to controls.

Patients with COPD and also with the PiZZ and PiMZ phenotype of A1AT demonstrated significantly increased IL-17 serum level and decreased IFN-γ level in comparison to PiMM patients. Both IL-17 and IFN-γ are proinflammatory cytokines, but only IFN-γ also exhibits some anti-inflammatory properties [31] and is possibly involved in a resolution of inflammation. This is confirmed by the observation that when inflammation subsides, the expression of IFN-γ remains at relatively high level despite the prominent decrease in the expression of other proinflammatory cytokines [26]. This may be related to Th17 ability to switch the production from IL-17 to IFN-γ [25]. Consequently, we calculated the IL-17/IFN-γ ratio, which was proposed by some researchers as an unfavorable marker of inflammatory disease progression [25, 27]. In this study, the IL-17/IFN-γ ratio was significantly elevated in both homozygous and heterozygous PiZ allele carriers.

In PiZZ patients, the IL-6 level was significantly higher than that in PiMM patients, though in PiMZ patients, it was elevated insignificantly. Moreover, IL-6 showed an invert correlation with A1AT concentrations. This finding confirms a hypothesis that in inflammation A1AT regulates IL-6 expression negatively and low A1AT level results in elevated IL-6 level. IL-6 is a proinflammatory cytokine and an acute phase mediator, which is essential for Th17 differentiation, and IL-17 expression increases further synthesis of IL-6 [24]. Moreover, IL-6 together with TNF-α is considered a mediator of systemic COPD effects (cachexia, skeletal muscle dysfunction, cardiovascular diseases, depression, hypodynamia, and osteoporosis), leading to an unfavorable outcome [32].

Serum IL-8 level in homozygous PiZ allele carriers was lower than that in PiMM phenotype carriers. However, many researchers report an increased IL-8 activity in sputum in both PiZZ and PiMZ phenotype carriers [13, 30]. Such elevation of local, but not systemic, IL-8 concentration can possibly be explained by higher consumption and local airway production of IL-8, stimulated by circulating IL-17 [33].

Undetectable TNF-α levels were found in most study patients. A similar result was reported by Vernooy et al. who have suggested the different regulations of inflammation in the pulmonary and systemic compartment [34].

5. Conclusions

The presence of the PiZ allele in both homozygous and heterozygous states in COPD patients presumably affects A1AT immunomodulatory properties, leading to higher IL-17 and IL-17/IFN-γ ratio and lower IFN-γ. Homozygous PiZ allele carriers also have higher IL-6 levels, but lower IL-8. These changes predict an unfavorable outcome and may identify new potential targets for therapy in COPD patients.

References

[1] D. Singh, A. Agusti, A. Anzueto et al., "Global strategy for the diagnosis, management, and prevention of chronic obstructive lung disease: the GOLD science committee report 2019," *European Respiratory Journal*, vol. 53, no. 5, article 1900164, 2019.

[2] C. Seifart and A. Plagens, "Genetics of chronic obstructive pulmonary disease," *International Journal of Chronic Obstructive Pulmonary Disease*, vol. 2, no. 4, pp. 541–550, 2007.

[3] Organization WWH, "α_1-antitrypsin deficiency: memorandum from a WHO meeting," *Bulletin of the World Health Organization*, vol. 75, pp. 397–415, 1997.

[4] R. Abboud, T. Nelson, B. Jung, and A. Mattman, "Alpha1-antitrypsin deficiency: a clinical-genetic overview," *The Application of Clinical Genetics*, vol. 4, pp. 55–65, 2011.

[5] D. P. Tittensor, C. Mora, W. Jetz et al., "Global patterns and predictors of marine biodiversity across taxa," *The American Review of Respiratory Disease*, vol. 466, no. 7310, pp. 1098–1101, 1979.

[6] K. Molloy, C. P. Hersh, V. B. Morris et al., "Clarification of the risk of chronic obstructive pulmonary disease in α1-antitrypsin deficiency PiMZ heterozygotes," *American Journal of Respiratory and Critical Care Medicine*, vol. 189, no. 4, pp. 419–427, 2014.

[7] P. N. Black, P. S. T. Ching, B. Beaumont, S. Ranasinghe, G. Taylor, and M. J. Merrilees, "Changes in elastic fibres in the small airways and alveoli in COPD," *The European Respiratory Journal*, vol. 31, no. 5, pp. 998–1004, 2008.

[8] G. Ortiz, J. P. Salica, E. H. Chuluyan, and J. E. Gallo, "Diabetic retinopathy: could the alpha-1 antitrypsin be a therapeutic option?," *Biological Research*, vol. 47, p. 58, 2014.

[9] E. C. Lewis, L. Shapiro, O. J. Bowers, and C. A. Dinarello, "Alpha1-antitrypsin monotherapy prolongs islet allograft survival in mice," *Proceedings of the National Academy of Sciences*, vol. 102, no. 34, pp. 12153–12158, 2005.

[10] D. Subramaniyam, R. Virtala, K. Pawłowski et al., "TNF-alpha-induced self expression in human lung endothelial cells is inhibited by native and oxidized alpha1-antitrypsin," *The International Journal of Biochemistry & Cell Biology*, vol. 40, no. 2, pp. 258–271, 2008.

[11] D. A. Bergin, E. P. Reeves, K. Hurley et al., "The circulating proteinase inhibitor α-1 antitrypsin regulates neutrophil degranulation and autoimmunity," *Science Translational Medicine*, vol. 6, no. 217, article 217ra1, 2014.

[12] G. B. Pott, E. D. Chan, C. A. Dinarello, and L. Shapiro, "Alpha-1-antitrypsin is an endogenous inhibitor of proinflammatory cytokine production in whole blood," *Journal of Leukocyte Biology*, vol. 85, no. 5, pp. 886–895, 2009.

[13] H. Stone, G. McNab, A. M. Wood, R. A. Stockley, and E. Sapey, "Variability of sputum inflammatory mediators in COPD and α1-antitrypsin deficiency," *The European Respiratory Journal*, vol. 40, no. 3, pp. 561–569, 2012.

[14] A. Butler, G. M. Walton, and E. Sapey, "Neutrophilic inflammation in the pathogenesis of chronic obstructive pulmonary disease," *COPD: Journal of Chronic Obstructive Pulmonary Disease*, vol. 15, no. 4, pp. 392–404, 2018.

[15] X. Zheng, L. Zhang, J. Chen, Y. Gu, J. Xu, and Y. Ouyang, "Dendritic cells and Th17/Treg ratio play critical roles in pathogenic process of chronic obstructive pulmonary disease," *Biomedicine & Pharmacotherapy*, vol. 108, pp. 1141–1151, 2018.

[16] S. Jiang, F. Shan, Y. Zhang, L. Jiang, and Z. Cheng, "Increased serum IL-17 and decreased serum IL-10 and IL-35 levels correlate with the progression of COPD," *International Journal of Chronic Obstructive Pulmonary Disease*, vol. 13, pp. 2483–2494, 2018.

[17] D. Singh, "Chronic obstructive pulmonary disease, neutrophils and bacterial infection: a complex web involving IL-17 and IL-22 unravels," *eBioMedicine*, vol. 2, no. 11, pp. 1580-1581, 2015.

[18] L. Cosmi, F. Liotta, and F. Annunziato, "Th17 regulating lower airway disease," *Current Opinion in Allergy and Clinical Immunology*, vol. 16, no. 1, pp. 1–6, 2016.

[19] C. Zenobia and G. Hajishengallis, "Basic biology and role of interleukin-17 in immunity and inflammation," *Periodontology 2000*, vol. 69, no. 1, pp. 142–159, 2015.

[20] S. Xu and X. Cao, "Interleukin-17 and its expanding biological functions," *Cellular & Molecular Immunology*, vol. 7, no. 3, pp. 164–174, 2010.

[21] A. R. Zampronio, D. M. Soares, and G. E. P. Souza, "Central mediators involved in the febrile response: effects of antipyretic drugs," *Temperature*, vol. 2, no. 4, pp. 506–521, 2015.

[22] J. B. Koo and J.-S. Han, "Cigarette smoke extract-induced interleukin-6 expression is regulated by phospholipase D1 in human bronchial epithelial cells," *The Journal of Toxicological Sciences*, vol. 41, no. 1, pp. 77–89, 2016.

[23] F. O. de Carvalho, F. A. Felipe, A. C. S. de Melo Costa et al., "Inflammatory mediators and oxidative stress in animals subjected to smoke inhalation: a systematic review," *Lung*, vol. 194, no. 4, pp. 487–499, 2016.

[24] A. C. Parks, "The state of positive psychology in higher education: Introduction to the special issue," *The Journal of Positive Psychology*, vol. 6, no. 6, pp. 429–431, 2011.

[25] E. Kurtenbach and C. G. Martinez, *IFN-γ versus IL-17: a battle during cardiac autoimmunity evolution*, IntechOpen, Rijeka, 2017.

[26] G. Zhang, X. Liu, C. Wang et al., "Resolution of PMA-induced skin inflammation involves interaction of IFN-γ and ALOX15," *Mediators of Inflammation*, vol. 2013, Article ID 930124, 11 pages, 2013.

[27] S. K. Lundy and D. A. Fox, "Reduced Fas ligand-expressing splenic $CD5^{+}B$ lymphocytes in severe collagen-induced arthritis," *Arthritis Research & Therapy*, vol. 11, no. 4, article R128, 2009.

[28] S. Subramanian, G. Shahaf, E. Ozeri et al., "Sustained expression of circulating human alpha-1 antitrypsin reduces inflammation, increases CD4+FoxP3+ Treg cell population and prevents signs of experimental autoimmune encephalomyelitis in mice," *Metabolic Brain Disease*, vol. 26, no. 2, pp. 107–113, 2011.

[29] P. Salahuddin, "Genetic variants of alpha1-antitrypsin," *Current Protein & Peptide Science*, vol. 11, no. 2, pp. 101–117, 2010.

[30] R. Aldonyte, S. Eriksson, E. Piitulainen, A. Wallmark, and S. Janciauskiene, "Analysis of systemic biomarkers in COPD patients," *COPD: Journal of Chronic Obstructive Pulmonary Disease*, vol. 1, no. 2, pp. 155–164, 2004.

[31] H. Mühl and J. Pfeilschifter, "Anti-inflammatory properties of pro-inflammatory interferon-gamma," *International Immunopharmacology*, vol. 3, no. 9, pp. 1247–1255, 2003.

[32] A. Agusti, "Systemic effects of chronic obstructive pulmonary disease: what we know and what we don't know (but should)," *Proceedings of the American Thoracic Society*, vol. 4, no. 7, pp. 522–525, 2007.

[33] K. Honda, H. Wada, M. Nakamura et al., "IL-17A synergistically stimulates TNF-α-induced IL-8 production in human airway epithelial cells: a potential role in amplifying airway inflammation," *Experimental Lung Research*, vol. 42, no. 4, pp. 205–216, 2016.

[34] J. H. Vernooy, M. Küçükaycan, J. A. Jacobs et al., "Local and systemic inflammation in patients with chronic obstructive pulmonary disease: soluble tumor necrosis factor receptors are increased in sputum," *American Journal of Respiratory and Critical Care Medicine*, vol. 166, no. 9, pp. 1218–1224, 2002.

30

Epidemiology of COVID-19 and Predictors of Recovery in the Republic of Korea

Ashis Kumar Das[1] **and Saji Saraswathy Gopalan**[2]

[1]*Research Group, The World Bank, Washington DC, USA*
[2]*Human Development Department, The World Bank, Washington DC, USA*

Correspondence should be addressed to Ashis Kumar Das; drashis@gmail.com

Academic Editor: Stefano Centanni

Background. The recent COVID-19 pandemic has emerged as a threat to global health. Though current evidence on the epidemiology of the disease is emerging, very little is known about the predictors of recovery. *Objectives.* To describe the epidemiology of confirmed COVID-19 patients in the Republic of Korea and identify predictors of recovery. *Materials and Methods.* Using publicly available data for confirmed COVID-19 cases from the Korea Centers for Disease Control and Prevention from January 20, 2020, to April 30, 2020, we undertook descriptive analyses of cases stratified by sex, age group, place of exposure, date of confirmation, and province. Correlation was tested among all predictors (sex, age group, place of exposure, and province) with Pearson's correlation coefficient. Associations between recovery from COVID-19 and predictors were estimated using a multivariable logistic regression model. *Results.* Majority of the confirmed cases were females (56%), 20-29 age group (24.3%), and primarily from three provinces—Gyeongsangbuk-do (36.9%), Gyeonggi-do (20.5%), and Seoul (17.1%). The case fatality ratio was 2.1%, and 41.6% cases recovered. Older patients, patients from provinces such as Daegu, Gyeonggi-do, Gyeongsangbuk-do, Jeju-do, Jeollabuk-do, and Jeollanam-do, and those contracting the disease from healthcare settings had lower recovery. *Conclusions.* Our study adds to the very limited evidence base on potential predictors of recovery among confirmed COVID-19 cases. We call additional research to explore the predictors of recovery and support development of policies to protect the vulnerable patient groups.

1. Introduction

For the first time, a novel coronavirus disease 2019 (COVID-19) originating from Wuhan in China was reported to the World Health Organization in December of 2019 [1]. This novel coronavirus has taken the form of a major pandemic and has affected almost all major nations in the world. There have been more than 3.6 million confirmed cases and about 252,000 deaths as of May 05, 2020 [2]. The very first COVID-19 case was diagnosed in the Republic of Korea (South Korea) on January 20, 2020 [3]. During the first two months of this global epidemic, South Korea had the second highest cases globally following China. According to the Korea Centers for Disease Control and Prevention (KCDC), there have been 10,804 confirmed cases and 254 deaths due to COVID-19 as of May 05, 2020 [4].

We present the epidemiology of COVID-19 in the Republic of Korea using data from the Korea Centers for Disease Control and Prevention and identify the predictors of recovery from the disease.

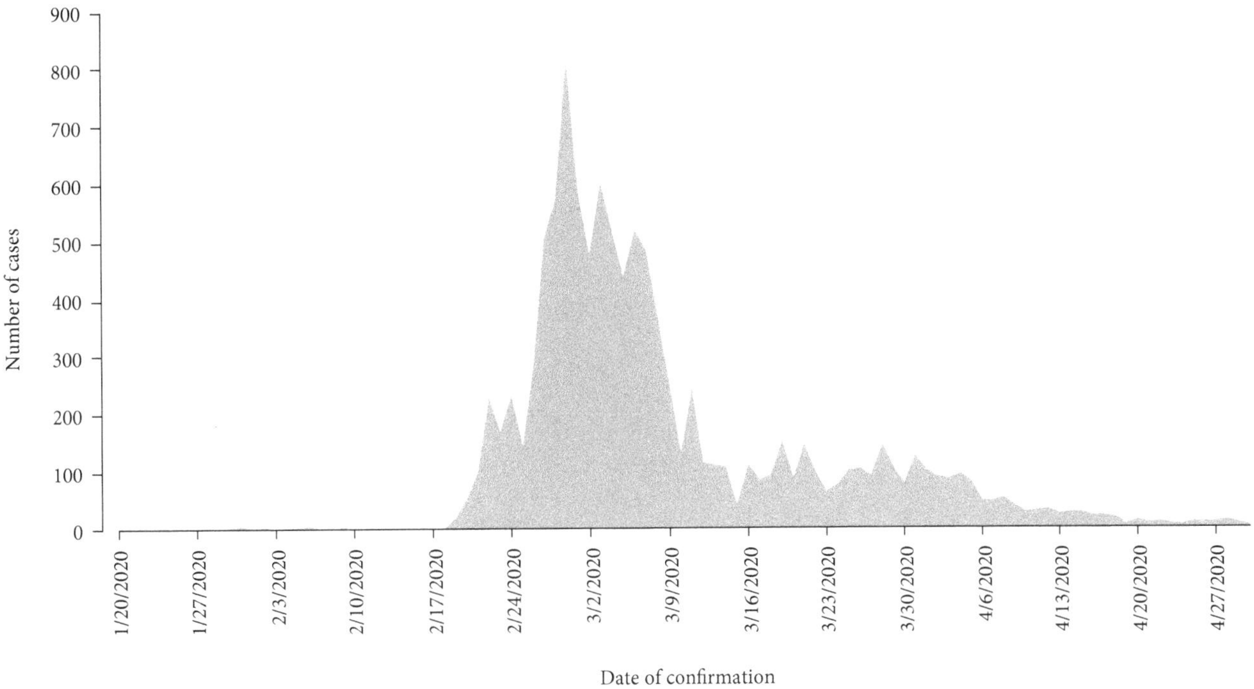

FIGURE 1: Daily new confirmed COVID-19 cases in the Republic of Korea between January 20, 2020, and April 30, 2020.

2. Materials and Methods

2.1. Data Source. The data were obtained from the Korea Centers for Disease Control and Prevention's publicly shared sources. The dataset contains information about 3,388 confirmed COVID-19 cases in the Republic of Korea from January 20, 2020, through April 30, 2020. After excluding cases with missing values, 3,299 cases were included in the analysis.

2.2. Variables. A confirmed case was defined as a person with laboratory-confirmed positive test. The data contained the following patient details: age (in groups), sex, province, date of diagnosis, mode of exposure, and outcome. There were 11 age groups: below10 years, 10-19 years, 20-29 years, 30-39 years, 40-49 years, 50-59 years, 60-69 years, 70-79 years, 80-89 years, 90-99 years, and above 100 years. We combined the last two age groups to create 90 years and above and thus recategorized age to 10 groups. All seventeen provinces of the Republic of Korea were represented: Busan, Chungcheongbuk-do, Chungcheongnam-do, Daegu, Daejeon, Gangwon-do, Gwangju, Gyeonggi-do, Gyeongsangbuk-do, Gyeongsangnam-do, Incheon, Jeju-do, Jeollabuk-do, Jeollanam-do, Sejong, Seoul, and Ulsan. We categorized the dates of diagnosis by weeks, and they were as follows: 20-26 Jan 2020, 27 Jan-02 Feb 2020, 03-09 Feb 2020, 10-16 Feb 2020, 17-23 Feb 2020, 24 Feb-01 Mar 2020, 02-08 Mar 2020, 09-15 Mar 2020, 16-22 Mar 2020, 23-29 Mar 2020, 30 Mar-05 Apr 2020, 06-12 Apr 2020, 13-19 Apr 2020, 20-26 Apr 2020, and 27-30 Apr 2020. Patients were exposed to potential COVID-19 sources in multiple settings. The settings were nursing home, hospital, religious gathering, call center, community center, shelter and apartment, gym facility, overseas inflow, contact with patients, and others. There were three outcomes: death, recovery, and isolation. The confirmed patients after spending some days in isolation were retested. They were considered recovered only after receiving a negative COVID-19 test.

2.3. Statistical Methods. We undertook descriptive analyses for the patient characteristics and presented the results stratified by subgroups for each characteristic. Correlation was tested among all patient characteristics with Pearson's correlation coefficient. Associations between recovery from COVID-19 and predictors (age group, sex, province, and exposure) were estimated using a multivariable logistic regression model. We considered associations statistically significant if the p value was below 0.05. The statistical analyses were performed using Python programming language Version 3.7 (Python Software Foundation, Wilmington, DE, USA) and Stata Version 15 (StataCorp LLC, College Station, TX).

3. Results

3.1. Pattern of the Epidemic. As shown in Figure 1, the first case of COVID-19 was confirmed on January 20, 2020. There were a few daily cases of new infections for about a month. After a month, the curve suddenly rose starting February 19, 2020, to reach the peak around end of February and early March. It reached its peak on the 29th of February with 813 confirmed cases. Though the curve descended after this date, still there were on an average 200 daily new confirmed cases until March 11, 2020. The curve continued its downward

TABLE 1: Sample characteristics ($N = 3,299$).

Variable	Number	Proportion (%)
Sex		
Female	1,848	56.0
Male	1,451	44.0
Age group (years)		
Below 10	53	1.6
10-19	149	4.5
20-29	801	24.3
30-39	438	13.3
40-49	454	13.8
50-59	597	18.1
60-69	401	12.2
70-79	204	6.2
80-89	156	4.7
90 and above	46	1.4
Province		
Busan	134	4.1
Chungcheongbuk-do	44	1.3
Chungcheongnam-do	143	4.3
Daegu	63	1.9
Daejeon	40	1.2
Gangwon-do	49	1.5
Gwangju	30	0.9
Gyeonggi-do	677	20.5
Gyeongsangbuk-do	1,218	36.9
Gyeongsangnam-do	112	3.4
Incheon	92	2.8
Jeju-do	13	0.4
Jeollabuk-do	17	0.5
Jeollanam-do	15	0.5
Sejong	46	1.4
Seoul	563	17.1
Ulsan	43	1.3
Exposure		
Nursing home	46	1.4
Hospital	37	1.1
Religious gathering	160	4.9
Call center	112	3.4
Community center, shelter, and apartment	50	1.5
Gym facility	34	1.0
Overseas inflow	553	16.8
Contact with patients	957	29.0
Others	1,350	40.9
Date of confirmed diagnosis		
20-26 Jan 2020	3	0.1
27 Jan-02 Feb 2020	12	0.4
03-09 Feb 2020	12	0.4
10-16 Feb 2020	3	0.1
17-23 Feb 2020	258	7.8

TABLE 1: Continued.

Variable	Number	Proportion (%)
24 Feb-01 Mar 2020	750	22.7
02-08 Mar 2020	651	19.7
09-15 Mar 2020	356	10.8
16-22 Mar 2020	348	10.6
23-29 Mar 2020	347	10.5
30 Mar-05 Apr 2020	349	10.6
06-12 Apr 2020	102	3.1
13-19 Apr 2020	71	2.2
20-26 Apr 2020	30	0.9
27-30 Apr 2020	7	0.2
Outcome		
Died	69	2.1
Recovered	1,372	41.6
Isolated	1,858	56.3

trend, however, adding at least 100 new daily cases through April 05, 2020. Towards the end of April, daily new confirmed cases were below 10.

3.2. Patient Profile. Table 1 shows the profile of the patients. Out of 3,299 confirmed patients, slightly more than half were females (56%). While there were cases from all age groups, the maximum patients were 20-29 years (24.3%), followed by 50-59 years (18.1%), 40-49 years (13.8%), 30-39 years (13.3%), and 60-69 years (12.2%). Three provinces—Gyeongsangbuk-do (36.9%), Gyeonggi-do (20.5%), and Seoul (17.1%)—together accounted for the maximum patients. With respect to the exposure, it was unknown for the most (44%) followed by direct contact with patients (29%), from overseas (16.8%), and religious gathering (4.9%). According to this available data source, 85% percent of the patients were confirmed of their diagnosis between 24 February and 05 April of 2020. There were 61 deaths accounting for 2.1 percent (case fatality rate) of the patients. More than half were isolated (56.3%), and 41.6% recovered.

3.3. Predictors of Recovery. As shown in Figure 2, there were no correlations between the predictors. Both males and females had similar recovery rates, and their difference was not statistically significant (Table 2). Compared to younger age groups, older patients had lower recovery: 70-79 years (adjusted odds ratio 0.31; p value 0.01), 80-89 years (aOR 0.22; p value 0.001), and 90 years and above (aOR 0.13; p value < 0.001). Provinces such as Daegu, Gyeonggi-do, Gyeongsangbuk-do, Jeju-do, Jeollabuk-do, and Jeollanam-do had statistically significant lower recovery rates than Busan. When compared with exposure from nursing homes, patients who were exposed to COVID-19 infection from religious gatherings, community dwellings, and others had higher recovery rates.

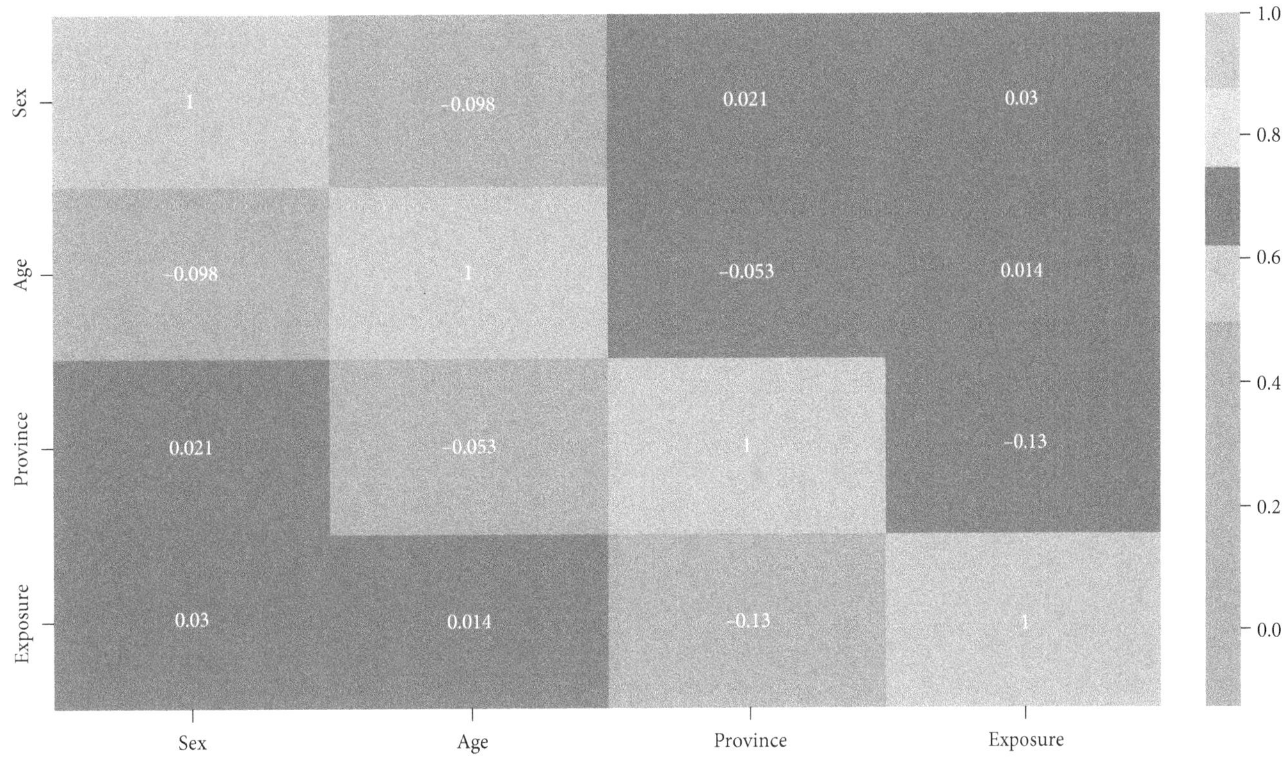

FIGURE 2: Correlation among predictors. Cells show Pearson's correlation coefficient.

4. Discussion

Due to multipronged approaches (proactive surveillance, higher testing, isolation, quarantine, use of technology, masks, and social distancing campaigns) by the government, incidence of new cases came down sharply in South Korea by mid-March and further to less than 10 new cases by mid-April [5].

Our study shows that females constituted the majority of confirmed cases, whereas males accounted for most of the confirmed cases in China and Italy [6–9]. Around a fourth of the cases were from the 20-29 years age group unlike in most other countries where the infected were older [6, 7, 10]. As already pointed out by researchers from South Korea, the possible reason for higher representation of younger population in our sample could also be specific exposure to cluster of cases through participation in religious activities or workplaces [5, 11]. As shown in a study undertaken in Europe, population density might have played a role for the number of higher cases in certain provinces [12]. The case fatality rate was much lower (2.1%) compared to other countries such as Italy (13.3%) and China (4%). Similar to findings from several other countries, we found the elderly to be more vulnerable with lower probabilities of recovery [6, 8, 13]. It is quite possible that the presence of preexisting medical conditions in the elderly predispose them to delayed recovery. We also found that cases contracting the infection in nonhealthcare setting had higher recovery. While there is no such evidence currently, there could be a possibility that the exposure outside nonhealthcare setting might have involved relatively younger and healthier cases. Considering our study findings, we suggest additional measures to protect the vulnerable cases who are less likely to recover from the infection. Thus, the elderly and cases contracting infection from healthcare settings should be given special attention.

Our study has two potential limitations. First, we used publicly available data of only a third of confirmed cases in the country. Thus, we are unable to ascertain the representativeness of the data for all confirmed cases in South Korea. So, the findings will have to be interpreted with caution. Second, the data lacks information of patients' symptoms and clinical features. Inclusion of these potential predictors would have enhanced the relevance of this study further. Despite these limitations, our study adds to the very limited evidence base on potential predictors of recovery among confirmed COVID-19 cases [14]. However, we believe the evidence base can be strengthened with further relevant research as authorities make more data publicly available or through primary hospital-based studies.

5. Conclusions

The COVID-19 pandemic has emerged as a great threat to global health challenging health systems across the world to efficiently deal with this situation. Emerging evidence on vulnerability to COVID-19 and predictors of recovery will inform providers and policy makers to effectively triage and prioritize limited resources. Therefore, we call for additional research to explore the predictors of recovery and support development of policies to protect the vulnerable patient groups.

Table 2: Predictors of recovery.

Variable	Recovery (%)	Odds ratio	95% confidence interval	p value
Sex				
Female	56.6	Reference		
Male	56.0	0.90	0.73-1.10	0.312
Age group (years)				
Below 10	60.4	Reference		
10-19	58.4	1.33	0.55-3.25	0.527
20-29	46.8	1.51	0.68-3.36	0.314
30-39	50.7	1.77	0.78-4.04	0.173
40-49	38.8	1.13	0.50-2.56	0.771
50-59	39.5	1.02	0.45-2.31	0.955
60-69	44.4	0.81	0.35-1.84	0.611
70-79	38.7	0.31	0.13-0.76	0.01
80-89	32.7	0.22	0.09-0.54	0.001
90 and above	32.6	0.13	0.04-0.37	<0.001
Province				
Busan	82.8	Reference		
Chungcheongbuk-do	88.6	1.02	0.35-2.99	0.971
Chungcheongnam-do	88.8	1.38	0.61-3.12	0.432
Daegu	6.4	0.00	0.00-0.01	<0.001
Daejeon	85.0	1.38	0.43-4.44	0.585
Gangwon-do	59.2	0.30	0.12-0.78	0.013
Gwangju	70.0	0.67	0.25-1.79	0.424
Gyeonggi-do	9.0	0.01	0.01-0.02	<0.001
Gyeongsangbuk-do	63.5	0.10	0.05-0.19	<0.001
Gyeongsangnam-do	85.7	0.93	0.40-2.15	0.866
Incheon	59.8	0.55	0.26-1.18	0.125
Jeju-do	53.9	0.29	0.08-1.00	0.05
Jeollabuk-do	23.5	0.03	0.01-0.11	<0.001
Jeollanam-do	20.0	0.03	0.01-0.13	<0.001
Sejong	87.0	1.20	0.25-5.86	0.821
Seoul	74.1	0.70	0.38-1.29	0.257
Ulsan	86.1	1.24	0.32-4.83	0.76
Exposure				
Nursing home	17.4	Reference		
Hospital	43.2	1.14	0.34-3.85	0.833
Religious gathering	80.6	6.29	1.80-21.94	0.004
Call center	84.8	2.68	0.77-9.31	0.122
Community center, shelter, and apartment	82.0	13.34	3.06-58.05	0.001
Gym facility	94.1	6.05	0.63-57.79	0.118
Overseas inflow	40.9	2.71	0.90-8.13	0.075
Contact with patients	41.5	2.80	0.98-8.03	0.055
Others	67.7	7.14	2.58-19.75	<0.001

Disclosure

The views expressed in the paper are that of the authors and do not reflect that of their affiliations.

Acknowledgments

We are grateful to Korea Centers for Disease Control and Prevention for making this data publicly available.

References

[1] WHO, *WHO coronavirus disease (COVID-2019) situation reports*, World Health Organization, 2020.

[2] "COVID-19 dashboard by the Center for Systems Science and Engineering (CSSE) at Johns Hopkins University (JHU)," https://gisanddata.maps.arcgis.com/apps/opsdashboard/index.html#/bda7594740fd40299423467b48e9ecf6.

[3] S. Ryu and B. C. Chun, "An interim review of the epidemiological characteristics of 2019 novel coronavirus," *Epidemiol. Health*, vol. 42, 2020.

[4] KCDC, *Korea Centers for Disease Control and Prevention*, Seoul, Korea, 2020https://www.cdc.go.kr/board/board.es?mid=a30402000000&bid=0030.

[5] COVID-19 National Emergency Response Center, Epidemiology and Case Management Team, Korea Centers for Disease Control and Prevention, "Coronavirus disease-19: the first 7, 755 cases in the Republic of Korea," *Osong Public Health and Research Perspectives*, vol. 11, no. 2, pp. 85–90, 2020.

[6] E. Livingston and K. Bucher, "Coronavirus disease 2019 (COVID-19) in Italy," *JAMA*, vol. 323, no. 14, p. 1335, 2020.

[7] W. Guan, Z. Y. Ni, Y. Hu et al., "Clinical characteristics of coronavirus disease 2019 in China," *The New England Journal of Medicine*, vol. 382, no. 18, pp. 1708–1720, 2020.

[8] Q. Li, X. Guan, P. Wu et al., "Early transmission dynamics in Wuhan, China, of novel coronavirus-infected pneumonia," *New England Journal of Medicine*, vol. 382, no. 13, pp. 1199–1207, 2020.

[9] N. Chen, M. Zhou, X. Dong et al., "Epidemiological and clinical characteristics of 99 cases of 2019 novel coronavirus pneumonia in Wuhan, China: a descriptive study," *Lancet*, vol. 395, no. 10223, pp. 507–513, 2020.

[10] G. Sotgiu, A. G. Gerli, S. Centanni et al., "Advanced forecasting of SARS-CoV-2-related deaths in Italy, Germany, Spain, and New York State," *Allergy: European Journal of Allergy and Clinical Immunology*, vol. 75, no. 7, pp. 1813–1815, 2020.

[11] S. Y. Park, Y. M. Kim, S. Yi et al., "Coronavirus disease outbreak in call center, South Korea," *Emerging Infectious Diseases*, vol. 26, no. 8, pp. 1666–1670, 2020.

[12] A. G. Gerli, S. Centanni, M. R. Miozzo et al., "COVID-19 mortality rates in the European Union, Switzerland, and the UK: effect of timeliness, lockdown rigidity, and population density," *Minerva Medica*, 2020.

[13] M. Nikpouraghdam, A. Jalali Farahani, G. H. Alishiri et al., "Epidemiological characteristics of coronavirus disease 2019 (COVID-19) patients in IRAN: a single center study," *Journal of Clinical Virology*, vol. 127, p. 104378, 2020.

[14] N. Al-Rousan and H. Al-Najjar, "Data analysis of coronavirus CoVID-19 epidemic in South Korea based on recovered and death cases," *Journal of Medical Virology*, vol. 10, 2020.

31

Association of TERT, OGG1 and CHRNA5 Polymorphisms and the Predisposition to Lung Cancer in Eastern Algeria

Asma Mimouni,[1,2] Etienne Rouleau,[3] Patrick Saulnier,[3] Amina Marouani,[4] Med Lamine Abdelali,[5] Taha Filali,[6] Leila Beddar,[7] Abdelhak Lakehal,[8] Ahmed Hireche,[1,2] Asma Boudersa,[9] Mahmoud Aissaoui,[10] Hacene Ramtani,[10] Khalid Bouhedjar,[11] Djamel Abdellouche,[12] Messaouda Oudjehih,[13] Ibtissem Boudokhane,[1,2] Noureddine Abadi,[2] and Dalila Satta[1,2]

[1]*Laboratoire de Biologie Moléculaire et Cellulaire, University Frères Mentouri Constantine 1, Constantine 25000, Algeria*
[2]*Laboratoire de Biologie et Génétique Moléculaire, Univ. Constantine 3, Constantine 25000, Algeria*
[3]*AMMICa/US 23 INSERM / UMS 3655 CNRS, Villejuif Cedex 94805, France*
[4]*Service de Pneumologie, CHU Sétif, 19000, Algeria*
[5]*Physics Department, Univ. Frères Mentouri Constantine 1, Constantine 25000, Algeria*
[6]*Service d'Oncologie CHU Constantine, Faculté de Médecine Univ. Constantine 3, Constantine 25000, Algeria*
[7]*Service d'Anatomie Pathologique, CHU Constantine, Faculté de Médecine Univ. Constantine 3, Constantine 25000, Algeria*
[8]*Registre de Cancer Constantine et Service d'Épidémiologie et Médecine Préventive, CHU Constantine, 25000, Algeria*
[9]*Service d'Oncologie, CHU, Annaba 23000, Algeria*
[10]*Clinique Alfarabi, Annaba 23000, Algeria*
[11]*Centre de Recherche en Biotechnologie, Constantine 25000, Algeria*
[12]*Service D'Anatomie Pathologique, CHU Sétif, Sétif 19000, Algeria*
[13]*Registre de Cancer Batna et Service d'Épidémiologie et Médecine Préventive, CHU Batna, Batna 5000, Algeria*

Correspondence should be addressed to Asma Mimouni; asmamimouni@yahoo.com

Academic Editor: Andrew Sandford

Lung cancer remains the most common cancer in the world. The genetic polymorphisms (rs2853669 in TERT, rs1052133 in OGG1, and rs16969968 in CHRNA5 genes) were shown to be strongly associated with the risk of lung cancer. Our study's aim is to elucidate whether these polymorphisms predispose Eastern Algerian population to non-small-cell lung cancer (NSCLC). To date, no study has considered this association in the Algerian population. This study included 211 healthy individuals and 144 NSCLC cases. Genotyping was performed using TaqMan probes and Sanger sequencing, and the data were analyzed using multivariate logistic regression adjusted for covariates. The minor allele frequencies (MAFs) of TERT rs2853669, CHRNA5 rs16969968, and OGG1 rs1052133 polymorphisms in controls were C: 20%, A: 31%, and G: 29%, respectively. Of the three polymorphisms, none shows a significant association, but stratified analysis rs16969968 showed that persons carrying the AA genotype are significantly associated with adenocarcinoma risk (pAdj = 0.03, ORAdj = 2.55). Smokers with an AA allele have a larger risk of lung cancer than smokers with GG or GA genotype (pAdj = 0.03, ORAdj = 3.91), which is not the case of nonsmokers. Our study suggests that CHRNA5 rs16969968 polymorphism is associated with a significant increase of lung adenocarcinoma risk and with a nicotinic addiction.

1. Introduction

Lung cancer (LC) remains the most common cancer in the world, both in terms of new cases (2 million new cases, 11.6% of all cancers) and deaths each year (1.7 million deaths 18.4%) [1]. As for Algeria, out of a population of some 42 million, 4000 cases of new LC appear every year; it is the first cause of mortality from cancer in men and the seventh in women [1, 2]. Although cigarette consumption accounts for the largest part of this alarming figure, over 80% of LC deaths are tobacco related but only a small fraction of smokers (usually <20%) develops this disease [3, 4]. In addition, a fraction of lifelong nonsmokers will die from LC, suggesting that LC is a multifactorial disease that results from complex interactions with many genetic and environmental factors [5]. Thus, it is of great importance to perform molecular biology studies in order to gain some understanding of susceptibility factors in action in the LC appearance and identify causal variants, which can be useful in the screening, the early diagnosis, and the therapy of LC. Independent Genome-Wide Association Studies (GWAS), which are considered a gold standard for reporting genotype-phenotype associations, and several other studies have been performed with the aim of looking for single-nucleotide polymorphism (SNP) of predisposition to LC [6–8]. Among the important genes which could modify the risk of LC are TERT, CHRNA5, and OGG1, and these are the genes we have been focusing on in this study.

TERT, encoded by the TERT gene, is one of the major components of telomerase; it is a reverse transcriptase that can add a nucleotide sequence (5′-TTAGGG) to telomere end [9]. The promoter region of TERT, located at positions c.124:C>T and c.146:C>T, is considered a regulatory element of telomerase activity [10]. The rs2853669 variant, located at -245 kb upstream (Ets2 binding site) of the TERT gene, prevents Ets/TCF binding, and it has been associated with lower TERT expression and decreased telomerase activity [11]. A growing number of epidemiological studies have been conducted to determine the associations between this polymorphism and cancer risk, particularly for breast cancer and LC; however, the results were inconclusive [12].

The OGG1 gene is located at chromosome 3p26.2. Its protein is a DNA repair enzyme, having both DNA glycosylase and AP lyse (apurinic or apyrimidinic site lyase) activities to remove 8-hydroxyguanine (8-oxoG) lesion produced by reactive oxygen species [13]. The rs1052133 polymorphisms have been identified in the OGG1 gene; it is a substitution at codon 326 (Ser326Cys), located in the promoter region [14]. The Cys326 protein has been shown to have about 7 times weaker 8-hydrox-yguanine-repair capacity than Ser326 protein in a complementation assay using *Escherichia coli* mutant strain deficient in 8-oxoG [15]. It has been suggested that rs1052133 was associated with LC risk; several studies investigated this association [16–18].

CHRNA genes code for proteins that form receptors which bind to nicotine and its metabolites [19]. In a large GWAS study, Hung et al. found a strong association of LC risk and CHRNA5 rs16969968 SNP; it results in the substitution of arginine for aspartic acid at the highly conserved codon 398 (D398N) of the CHRNA5 protein [7]. In vitro studies indicate that rs16969968 decreases CHRNA5 function and favors nicotinic addiction [20]. Numerous studies have been performed to find out whether this association is direct, or whether the rs16969968 SNP is simply a proxy for increased exposure to tobacco carcinogens, which were inconclusive [7, 21–26].

In our study, we were interested in SNPs of three different genes, which were selected based upon GWAS and meta-analyses of multiple populations TERT (promoter region rs2853669, c.-124C>T, and c.-146C>T), OGG1 (rs1052133), and CHRNA5 (rs16969968). The aim of our study is to investigate how these SNPs can modify the risk of LC in the Eastern Algerian population. It is important to mention that our population, to the best of our knowledge, has not been the object of any molecular study concerning the LC till now, and thus this study, as any other pioneering work, had to deal with a relative scarcity of data.

Although this study has been conducted within various population centers in Eastern Algeria which thus encompass several ethnic groups, Arabs and Central Algeria Berbers, yet the population mixing which took place at an accelerated pace after Algeria's independence, the standardization of lifestyles, the rural exodus, all concurred to homogenize the genetic stock to a large extent [27]. Furthermore, the complex processes of admixture and isolation at work has made the genetic heterogeneity found in Algeria not strongly correlated with geography or culture. It would thus be improper to assume that the various population groups to be genetically isolated and immune of gene flow [27, 28].

2. Materials and Methods

2.1. Study Population. We have performed in this work a case control study of 144 LC patients and 211 healthy controls. The patients were first diagnosed with NSCLC between June 2015 and July 2016. They came from a wide zone spanning five Wilayas (territorial units) in Eastern Algeria between governmental University Hospitals (Constantine, Sétif, Batna, and Annaba) and private clinics. There was no restriction on gender, histologic subtype, or stage with the exception of patients who refused to participate in the study. Diagnosis was made by cytological imaging and histopathological examinations. We feel confident as explained previously that our samples are largely homogeneous. In addition to that, the democratization of access to medical treatment, freely provided to all, as shown in the fact that city dwellers and those from rural areas are equally represented in the various patient samples, allowed us to make the claim of genetic homogeneity of the samples with a good degree of confidence.

The control group comprised individuals with no history of cancer and without lung-related disease to avoid possible interference from overlapping genes. They were chosen from a pool of volunteers in the blood transfusion centers during the same period of patients without restriction of age or gender. All subjects were Algerians residing in Eastern Algeria.

We used a standard epidemiological questionnaire submitted to patients and controls, and we used the medical files to collect personal data, including residential region, age, gender, profession, smoking status, symptoms, family history of cancer, histologic subtype, and stage TNM.

2.2. Ethics Statement. Our research has been approved by the local Ethics Committee. The use of human blood sample and the protocol in this study strictly conformed to the principles expressed in the Declaration of Helsinki, and informed consent was obtained from all participants or from their family members.

2.3. DNA Extraction and Genotyping. Genomic DNA was extracted from six to eight milliliters of peripheral venous bloods, which was collected into a tube containing ethylenediamine-tetraacetic acid (EDTA) from each participant. We used standard protocols following the salt extraction procedure. The DNA concentration was measured with NanoDrop One spectrophotometer. For genotyping rs16969968 and rs1052133, we used Polymerase Chain Reaction (PCR) TaqMan; with ViiA 7 (Applied Biosystems) and TaqMan® SNP Genotyping assay kits (Applied Biosystems), we used the standard protocol recommended by the manufacturer.

The promoter TERT was amplified by PCR, and the PCR primers used were as follows: 5′ACCGTTCAGTTA GCGATTTCCCACGTGCGCAGAGGAC3′ (forward), and R: 5′CGGATAGCAAGCTCGTCTCCCAGTGGA TTCG CGGGC3′ (reverse). Then, it was genotyped with Sanger sequencing in both the forward and reverse directions using the Big Dye Terminator Chemistry V.I and an automated fluorescent sequencer, an ABI 48 Capillary Array Sequencer (Applied Biosystems 3730). Data management and analysis were done using SeqScape. For TERT sequencing, we could do sequencing for only 126 cases and 94 controls.

2.4. Statistical Analysis. To estimate sample size, we used functions from the R package "epiCalc" (Version 2.9.0.1) with a minor allele frequency data obtained from NCBI (http://www.ncbi.nlm.nih.gov/SNP/) and a study power fixed at 80%. The Hardy–Weinberg equilibrium of the genotype distributions is evaluated in the control subjects using a function from R package "Hardy–Weinberg" (Version 1.6.1).

The strength of association between the three polymorphisms and LC risk is assessed by calculating odds ratios (ORs) with the corresponding confidence intervals (95% CI). The ORs are also performed for a heterozygote model (AA vs. aa, where A: major allele and a: minor allele), homozygote model (Aa vs. AA), recessive model (AA+Aa vs. aa), and dominant model (AA vs. Aa+aa). We used Pearson's chi-square test to compare distributions of demographic variables, smoking status, and genotypes of the three genes between cases and controls. To calculate ORs and 95% CI, unconditional logistic regression analyses are performed. In addition, multiple unconditional logistic regression analyses with adjustment for possible confounders (age, sex, and smoking) are performed to calculate adjusted ORs and 95% CI. Statistical tests along with ORs and corresponding CIs are done using the publicly available packages of R Project for Statistical Computing (R version 3.5.1) and especially functions from packages MASS and questionr (Version 0.7.0). All statistical analyses are two sided, and the significance level is set at $p = 0.05$.

Table 1: Characteristics of case and control subjects.

Characteristics	Cases (%) ($n = 144$)	Controls (%) ($n = 211$)	p value
Sex			<0.01
Male	119 (83)	134 (63.5)	
Female	25 (17)	77 (36.5)	
Age (years)			<0.01
<60	72 (50)	170 (80.5)	
≥60	72 (50)	41 (19.5)	
Mean age (range)	59.85 (26-80)	52.33 (20-88)	
Smoking status			<0.01
Smokers	104 (73)	61 (38)	
Nonsmokers	38 (27)	100 (62)	
No information	2	50	
Histology			/
Adenocarcinoma	96 (66%)	/	
Squamous cell carcinoma	48 (34%)		

p value based on Pearson's chi-square test.

3. Results

3.1. Subjects Characteristics. To test the association between TERT, OGG1, and CHRNA5 gene polymorphisms and the risk of LC, we conducted a case-control study consisting of 144 NSCLC cases and 211 controls enrolled in four University Hospitals of Eastern Algeria (Constantine, Sétif, Batna, and Annaba). The distributions of age, gender, smoking history, and histology type among the study subjects were summarized in Table 1. The distribution of gender and that of age were statistically significant between the cases and controls ($p < 0.01$). Thus, the cases and controls were incompletely matched in this study population. Among the cases, 66% were diagnosed with adenocarcinoma and 34% with squamous cell carcinoma. Approximately 73% of case subjects and 37% of control subjects were ever smokers. As expected, case subjects had a significantly higher level ($p = <0.01$) of smoking than control subjects.

3.2. Association Analysis of Candidate SNPs with LC Risk. The distribution of TERT, OGG1, and CHRNA5 gene polymorphisms in cases and controls are presented in Table 2. The allele frequencies of the three gene polymorphisms in controls were consistent with the Hardy–Weinberg equilibrium; the p values are as follows: 0.15 for TERT, 0.49 for OGG1, and 0.15 for CHRNA5.

After sequencing the promoter of TERT gene, the two SNPs could not be found in this population (c.124C>T, c.146C>T), but we observed the presence of the rs2853669 polymorphism with a high frequency.

TABLE 2: TERT, OGG1, and CHRNA5 genotypes and lung cancer risk.

Genes	Genotype/mode[a]	Cases (%)	Controls (%)	p	OR* (CI)	p^*
TERT rs2853669		126	94			
	TT	71 (56.3)	57 (61)	Ref	—	—
	TC	49 (38.9)	36 (38)	0.755	0.99 (0.53–1.89)	0.99
	CC	6 (4,8)	1 (1)	0.11	4.15 (0.61–83.73)	0.21
	T	191 (76)	150 (80)	Ref	—	—
	C	61 (24)	38 (20)		1.22 (0.72–2.07)	0.45
	Recessive			0.12	4.72 (0.68–97.04)	0.17
	Dominant			0.52	1.11 (0.59–2.07)	0.75
CHRNA5[b] rs16969968		143	211			
	GG	60 (42)	93 (44.3)	Ref	—	—
	GA	64 (44.8)	105 (49.8)	0.8	0.98 (0.58–1.63)	0.93
	AA	19 (13.2)	13 (6.2)	0.03	1.75 (0.68–4.69)	0.25
	G	184 (64.3)	291 (69)	Ref	—	—
	A	102 (35.7)	131 (31)		1.16 (0.80–1.68)	0.41
	Recessive			0.02	1.83 (0.78–4.48)	0.16
	Dominant			0.69	1.07 (0.65–1.76)	0.78
OGG1[b] rs1052133		144	210			
	CC	79 (54.9)	107 (50.9)	Ref	—	—
	CG	54 (37.5)	83 (39.3)	0.58	0.88 (0.52–1.48)	0.62
	GG	11 (7.6)	20 (9.5)	0.46	1.45 (0.53–4.07)	0.46
	C	212 (73.6)	297 (71)	Ref	—	—
	G	76 (26.4)	123 (29)		1.01 (0.68–1.5)	0.92
	Recessive			0.53	1.44 (0.55–3.83)	0.45
	Dominant			0.46	0.94 (0.57–1.54)	0.79

OR = odds ratio; CI = confidence interval. *OR adjusted for sex age and tobacco consumption. [a]The dominant mode: AA vs Aa+aa, where A is major allele and a is minor allele; the recessive mode: AA+Aa vs aa. [b]Numbers may not add up total number of patients due to genotype failures.

The minor allele frequencies (MAFs) of TERT rs2853669, OGG1 rs1052133, and CHRNA5 rs16969968 and polymorphisms in cases/controls were C: 24%/20%, G: 26.4%/29%, and A: 35.7%/31%, respectively. The genotype distribution of TERT and OGG1 was not significantly different between LC and control groups in all models, although the genotype distribution of CHRNA5 was significantly different in the recessive and homozygote modes ($p = 0.02$ and $p = 0.03$, respectively). After adjustment for the sex and age, the signification becomes marginal (data not shown), and after adjustment for the sex, age, and tobacco consumption factors, we found that the correlation vanished (pAdj = 0.16, OR = 1.83, CI = (0.78 – 4.48), and pAdj = 0.25, OR = 1.75, CI = (0.68 – 4.69), respectively).

3.3. Stratified Analysis for the Three SNPs Studied with LC Risk. We then performed a stratified analysis according to, tobacco consumption, histological type (Table 3), age, and sex (Table 4), in order to investigate associations between genetic polymorphisms and stratified factors in dominant, codominant recessive models. In addition to that, we studied these associations at the level of alleles (Table 5).

For TERT rs2853669, the results showed that the persons having CT or CC genotypes and passed 60 years had a larger risk of suffering from LC than those carrying TT genotype ($p = 0.04$). Among males, the homozygote genotype CC increase the risk of LC than TT or TC genotypes with $p = 0.03$ (Table 3). In addition to that, the patients with CC genotype have a tendency to have a squamous type rather than adenocarcinoma. Yet after adjustment, there was no statistical signification for the three stratified factors.

The OGG1 rs1052133 did not show any signification with stratified factors, except for age (>60 years), which reveals an association with the increase of LC for the persons having a minor allele (GG), in comparison with person with CC genotype ($p = 0.04$). After adjustment for age, sex, and smoking status, the signification become marginally significant ($p = 0.09$, OR = 0.49, CI = (0.21-1.11)).

As for CHRNA5 rs16969968, we observed an increasing risk for LC among males with a recessive genotype (AA) compared with those having GG or GA genotype with $p = 0.02$. However, after adjustment, the signification disappears. Smokers with an AA allele have a larger risk of LC than smokers with GG or GA genotype ($p = 0.02$); after adjustment for age and sex, the signification persists with pAdj = 0.03, ORAdj = 3.91, and CI = (1.24 – 17.34). For the stratified analysis according to the histological type, we observed that the persons with AA allele have preferentially an adenocarcinoma rather than squamous type under the recessive and homozygote models $p = 0.003$ and $p = 0.005$, respectively. This risk

Table 3: Association between TERT, CHRNA5, and OGG1 polymorphisms and lung cancer risk, stratified by histology and tobacco consumption.

Population	Gene	Genotype	Cases/controls[a]	p	OR_{Adj}	CI_{Adj}	P_{Adj}
Smokers*	TERT rs2853669	TT	46/20		Ref		
		TC	40/19	0.81	0.86	(0.39-188)	0.71
		CC	5/0	0.14	—	—	0.99
		Dominant (TC+CC)	46/20	0.93	0.97	(0.44-2.10)	0.94
		Recessive (TC+TT)	86/39	0.13	—	—	0.98
	CHRNA5 rs16969968	GG	42/24		Ref		
		GA	44/34	0.37	0.72	(0.36-1.42)	0.35
		AA	18/3	0.05	3.29	(0.79-15.28)	0.08
		Dominant (GA+AA)	62/37	0.89	0.93	(0.48-1.79)	0.83
		Recessive (GA+GG)	86/58	0.02	3.91	(1.24-17.34)	0.03
	OGG1 rs1052133	CC	59/35		Ref		
		CG	36/23	0.82	0.81	(0.40-1.63)	0.56
		GG	9/3	0.40	2.01	(0.53-9.80)	0.32
		Dominant (CG+GG)	45/26	0.93	0.92	(0.48-1.78)	0.82
		Recessive (CG+CC)	95/58	0.37	2.03	(0.57-9.59)	0.30
Nonsmokers*	TERT rs2853669	TT	23/30		Ref		
		TC	9/9	0.62	1.32	(0.42-4.19)	0.63
		CC	1/1	0.85	1.54	(0.05-41.59)	0.76
		Dominant (TC+CC)	10/10	0.61	1.38	(0.46-4.17)	0.55
		Recessive (TC+TT)	32/39	0.89	1.71	(0.06-47.92)	0.71
	CHRNA5 rs16969968	GG	16/49		Ref		
		GA	22/44	0.4	1.36	(0.61-3.05)	0.44
		AA	1/7	0.44	0.33	(0.01-2.49)	0.36
		Dominant (GA+AA)	21/51	0.54	1.19	(0.54-2.63)	0.65
		Recessive (GA+GG)	36/93	0.34	0.31	(0.01-1.97)	0.29
	OGG1 rs1052133	CC	18/48		Ref		
		CG	18/45	0.86	0.94	(0.42-2.10)	0.89
		GG	2/7	0.74	0.83	(0.10 - 4.23)	0.84
		Dominant	20/52	0.94	0.91	(0.42-1.99)	0.82
		Recessive	36/93	0.71	0.84	(0.11-3.80)	0.83
Adenocarcinoma**	TERT rs2853669	TT	50/57		Ref		
		TC	33/36	0.88	1.01	(0.50-2)	0.97
		CC	3/1	0.26	3.39	(0.39-72.50)	0.31
		Dominant (TC+CC)	36/37	0.73	1.09	(0.55-2.13)	0.79
		Recessive (TC+TT)	83/93	0.27	3.90	(0.43-85.93)	0.26
	CHRNA5 rs16969968	GG	37/93		Ref		
		GA	42/105	0.98	1.01	(0.57-1.79)	0.95
		AA	16/13	0.005	2.54	(0.95-7.07)	0.06
		Dominant (GA+AA)	58/118	0.40	1.18	(0.68-2.06)	0.53
		Recessive (GA+GG)	79/198	0.003	2.55	(1.07-6.35)	0.03
	OGG1 rs1052133	CC	50/107		Ref		
		CG	39/83	0.98	0.95	(0.53-1.67)	0.86
		GG	7/20	0.53	1.61	(0.52-4.80)	0.39
		Dominant (CG+GG)	46/103	0.85	1.00	(0.58-1.73)	0.97
		Recessive (CG+CC)	89/190	0.52	1.49	(0.50-4.24)	0.45

TABLE 3: Continued.

Population	Gene	Genotype	Cases/controls[a]	p	OR_{Adj}	CI_{Adj}	P_{Adj}
		TT	21/57		Ref		
		TC	16/36	0.63	1.10	(0.43-2.77)	0.83
	TERT rs2853669	CC	3/1	0.03	10.87	(0.67-573.04)	0.15
		Dominant (TC+CC)	19/37	0.38	1.26	(0.51-3.12)	0.60
		Recessive (TC+TT)	37/93	0.04	7.60	(0.65-208.01)	0.14
		GG	23/93		Ref		
		GA	22/105	0.61	0.81	(0.37-1.71)	0.58
Squamous**	CHRNA5 rs16969968	AA	3/13	0.91	0.78	(0.13-3.71)	0.76
		Dominant (GA+AA)	25/118	0.62	0.80	(0.38-1.68)	0.56
		Recessive (GA+GG)	45/198	0.98	0.93	(0.18-3.95)	0.93
		CC	29/107		Ref		
		CG	15/83	0.24	0.64	(0.28-1.42)	0.28
	OGG1 rs1052133	GG	4/20	0.60	1.50	(0.31-6.72)	0.59
		Dominant (CG+GG)	19/103	0.23	0.71	(0.33-1.52)	0.39
		Recessive (CG+CC)	44/190	0.79	1.67	(0.38-6.66)	0.46

OR = odds ratio; CI = confidence interval; Adj = adjusted. *OR adjusted for gender and age. **OR adjusted for gender, age, and smoking habit. [a]Numbers may not add up the total number of patients due to genotype failures.

was not affected by adjusting for other factors (age, sex, and smoking) pAdj = 0.03, ORAdj = 2.55, and CI = (1.07 − 6.35).

As for the stratified analysis by sex, smoking, histological type, and age, according to alleles, no significant association was found.

4. Discussion

High incidence and poor prognosis of LC make it a major health problem worldwide. Although the LC is linked to environmental exposure to carcinogens, especially cigarette smoking, only some smokers develop LC, which suggests that there is an interindividual difference in susceptibility to the disease. In this study, polymorphisms in three genes involved in the metabolism of carcinogens or in the repair of damaged DNA in lung cells, TERT (rs2853669), OGG1 (rs1052133), and CHRNA5 (rs16969968), were examined for association with NSCLC risk in a case-control study of 144 patients and 211 control subjects of Eastern Algerian population in an attempt to explain this interindividual difference.

In our population, none of these three genes shows an influence on the LC risk, except the CHRNA5 rs16969968 SNP, which was significantly different between cases and controls, but after adjustment, the signification disappears. These results are in accordance with the findings of numerous studies but contradictory to others [16, 26, 29]. The allelic frequencies were slightly different from those found in other populations and close to those of Caucasian population but differ drastically from Asiatic and African population [30].

For TERT gene, after sequencing its promoter, we identified in our population the rs2853669 polymorphism. The rs2853669 MAFs in our control group is C = 20%. According to literature and HapMap data, there is no big difference between the MAFs of rs2853669 in Caucasian and Asian populations, C: 26%-37% [12, 31]. Overall, in our study, no significant association was found between the rs2853669 and NSCLC. In the stratified analysis, no difference was noticed for all stratified factors. Only two studies were performed in LC which were conducted exclusively on the Asian population, and they found a strong association between rs2853669 and LC risk [32, 33]. A large recent meta-analysis where thirteen studies involving 16 datasets were pooled to evaluate the association between rs2853669 and cancer risk were realized, and researchers demonstrated that rs2853669 alone does not increase or decrease the overall risk and prognosis of cancer. In a stratified analysis by cancer type, a protective effect was found for breast cancer and a significant association was found for LC and glioblastoma; however, the small number of studies limited its credibility [29]. Concurrently, another recent meta-analysis with the same objective of the precedent had the pooled results indicating that the rs2853669 polymorphism was significantly associated with increased cancer risk in a homozygote model. In the stratified analysis, a significantly increased cancer risk was observed for Asians, but not so for Caucasian patients. A subgroup analysis by cancer type also revealed a significant increase in the risk of LC, but not breast cancer [12].

For the OGG1 rs1052133, previous studies have shown that homozygous carriers of the variant appear to have reduced repair capacity toward oxidized DNA lesions, and previous evidence indicated higher levels of 8-oxoG in lung tissue of LC patients than in lung tissue of patients without cancer [34, 35]. Numerous studies have investigated the association between LC and this SNP, and the results are quite diverse [16–18]. In our study, the MAFs in the control group of rs1052133 was G = 29%, which is slightly higher than frequencies previously reported for Caucasians (15% to 25%), and lower than those reported (40% to 62%) for Asian populations, but consistent with those obtained (33%) for the Turkish population, and similar to those found (G = 27%) in a study of the North African population [16, 36, 37]. The

Table 4: Association between TERT, CHRNA5, and OGG1 polymorphisms and lung cancer risk, stratified by gender and age.

Population	Gene	Genotype	Cases/controls[a]	p	OR_{Adj}	CI_{Adj}	P_{Adj}
		TT	55/40		Ref		
		TC	40/32	0.76	0.74	(0.35-1.55)	0.43
	TERT rs2853669	CC	6/0	0.04	—	—	0.99
		Dominant (TC+CC)	46/32	0.88	0.90	(0.43-1.86)	0.78
		Recessive (TC+TT)	95/72	0.03	—	—	0.98
		GG	49/60		Ref		
		GA	51/65	0.88	0.92	(0.50–1.71)	0.80
Male**	CHRNA5 rs16969968	AA	18/9	0.04	1.99	(0.70–6.26)	0.20
		Dominant (GA+AA)	69/74	0.60	1.05	(0.58–1.90)	0.85
		Recessive (GA+GG)	100/125	0.02	2.09	(0.82–5.88)	0.13
		CC	68/67		Ref		
		CG	42/51	0.43	0.80	(0.44-1.48)	0.47
	OGG1 rs1052133	GG	9/15	0.24	1.49	(0.44-5.52)	0.52
		Dominant (CG+GG)	51/66	0.28	0.87	(0.48-1.56)	0.64
		Recessive (CG+CC)	110/118	0.31	1.51	(0.47-5.36)	0.48
		TT	16/17		Ref		
		TC	9/4	0.20	2.49	(0.66-10.91)	0.19
	TERT rs2853669	CC	0/1	0.33	—	—	0.99
		Dominant (TC+CC)	9/5	0.32	2.02	(0.56–7.97)	0.29
		Recessive (TC+TT)	25/21	0.28	—	—	0.99
		GG	11/33		Ref		
		GA	13/40	0.95	1.03	(0.39-2.70)	0.94
Female**	CHRNA5 rs16969968	AA	1/4	0.80	0.75	(0.02-8.22)	0.83
		Dominant (GA+AA)	14/44	0.92	1.01	(0.39-2.62)	0.97
		Recessive (GG+AA)	24/73	0.81	0.85	(0.03-7.46)	0.90
		CC	11/40		Ref		
		CG	12/32	0.51	1.06	(0.39-2.85)	0.89
	OGG1 rs1052133	GG	2/5	0.67	1.23	(0.14–7.25)	0.82
		Dominant	14/37	0.48	1.06	(0.41-2.77)	0.89
		Recessive	23/72	0.79	1.20	(0.16-6.24)	0.83
		TT	32/16		Ref		
		TC	28/5	0.06	2.26	(0.72-7.97)	0.17
	TERT rs2853669	CC	3/0	0.22	—	—	0.99
		Dominant (TC+CC)	31/5	0.04	2.49	(0.80-8.72)	0.12
		Recessive (TC+TT)	60/21	0.30	—	—	0.99
		GG	31/16		Ref		
		GA	29/23	0.30	0.62	(0.26–1.43)	0.27
>60*	CHRNA5 rs16969968	AA	12/2	0.15	2.83	(0.62–20.48)	0.22
		Dominant (GA+AA)	42/93	0.52	1.26	(0.66–2.42)	0.46
		Recessive (GG+AA)	64/159	0.36	1.22	(0.38–3.86)	0.72
		CC	38/15		Ref		
		CG	29/26	0.04	0.49	(0.21-1.11)	0.09
	OGG1 rs1052133	GG	5/0	0.16	—	—	0.99
		Dominant (CG+GG)	34/26	0.09	0.58	(0.25-1.29)	0.18
		Recessive (CG+CC)	67/41	0.08	—	—	0.98

Table 4: Continued.

Population	Gene	Genotype	Cases/controls[a]	p	OR_{Adj}	CI_{Adj}	P_{Adj}
		TT	39/41		Ref		
		TC	21/31	0.34	0.67	(0.30-1.48)	0.33
	TERT rs2853669	CC	3/1	0.30	2.99	(0.33–65.93)	0.37
		Dominant (TC+CC)	24/32	0.49	0.76	(0.34-1.63)	0.48
		Recessive (TC+TT)	60/72	0.24	3.70	(0.41-82.55)	0.28
		GG	29/77		Ref		
		GA	35/82	0.67	1.26	(0.65–2.44)	0.48
<60*	CHRNA5 rs16969968	AA	7/11	0.31	1.27	(0.35–4.48)	0.70
		Dominant (GA+AA)	42/93	0.52	1.26	(0.66–2.42)	0.46
		Recessive (GG+GA)	64/159	0.36	1.22	(0.38–3.86)	0.72
		CC	41/92		Ref		
		CG	25/57	0.95	1.33	(0.76–2.66)	0.41
	OGG1 rs1052133	GG	6/20	0.42	1.01	(0.30–3.20)	0.97
		Dominant (CG+GG)	31/77	0.72	1.27	(0.67–2.44)	0.45
		Recessive (CG+CC)	66/149	0.42	0.90	(0.27–2.75)	0.86

OR = odds ratio; CI = confidence interval; Adj = adjusted. *OR and p adjusted for smoking and gender. **OR adjusted for age and smoking habit. [a]Numbers may not add up the total number of patients due to genotype failures.

frequency of individuals carrying homozygous variant allele GG was slightly higher in the controls (9.5%) than in the cases (7.6%), which suggests a protective effect, but this difference is not statistically significant ($p = 0.46$). Two previous studies found that this SNP could have a protective effect for LC [36, 38]. Overall, the rs1052133 does not have any effect on the risk of NSCLC in our population. These results are in agreement with the finding of three studies but in discordance with evidence from two other studies [13, 36, 39–41]. Duan et al. did a meta-analysis (data from 8 studies), and no association was found between OGG1 rs1052133 and NSCLC risk [16]. It seems that Asians may have a much higher susceptibility to LC than the others due to having a higher frequency for the variant G allele [42, 43].

In our stratified analysis by histological type, gender, age, and smoking habits, only the age showed a marginally significant elevation of risk of NSCLC for persons more than 60 years old and carrying a recessive genotype GG. However, results obtained by Hung et al. were not in agreement with ours [34].

Our findings could not explain the significantly lower capacity to incise 8-oxoG by leukocytes of NSCLC patients in comparison to healthy controls. A possible explication is that OGG1 gene polymorphisms are only one of many parameters that might affect OGG1 activity. Another explanation as suggested by Lee et al. is that the GG genotype is deficient in the repair of oxidatively generated DNA damage only under conditions of cellular oxidative stress [44]. However, both of these hypotheses need to be confirmed in future studies.

The rs16969968 CHRNA5 polymorphism was the subject of a large number of investigations [21, 23, 26, 45]. Different gene expression and disease association studies provided evidence that both nicotine-dependence risk and LC risk are influenced by this polymorphism. This variant is common in populations of European and Middle Eastern origin, (MAFs = 37%–43%) but uncommon in African, East Asian, and Native American populations (<5%) [20]. For the Algerian population, the MAFs of the rs16969968 in the control group is A = 31%, which is in disagreement with the result found for the Mozabit ethnic group (MAFs = 18%) [46]. This result can be explained because the Mozabit ethnicity stands out genetically from the remaining population due to their practice of endogamy [46]. Our results show a decrease of the variant allele in cases and not in controls, but after adjustment for sex, age, and smoking, the signification disappears ($p = 0.16$). Thus, our data do not support an important role for the SNP in NSCLC risk. However, previous studies on different ethnic groups, predominantly Caucasian, showed a rather important association between rs16969968 and LC risk.

When stratified according to histologic subtype, rs16969968 was associated with LC risk in ADK but not in SCC ($p = 0.03$) under the recessive model. Falvella et al. reported that CHRNA5 mRNA levels are upregulated 30-fold in ADK compared with normal lung tissue in individuals carrying AA genotype compared with those having GG genotype [47]. Nevertheless, Jaworoska et al. showed that this locus is implicated in all histopathologic subtypes of LC [48]. In spite of ADK and SCC being categorized as NSCLC, they have as molecular pattern, and for that reason, the rs16969968 may influence LC susceptibility differently according to histologic subtype. Additional studies are needed to confirm this hypothesis.

The stratified study on the smoking factor showed that smokers with AA genotype exhibit a four-fold higher risk of NSCLC compared with those carrying GA and GG genotypes. Results reported by Le Marchand et al. could explain our results; the authors found that smokers with the AA genotype smoke more cigarettes, but also smoke more intensely, extracting a greater amount of nicotine and carcinogens per cigarette, compared with noncarriers [49]. On the

TABLE 5: Association between TERT, CHRNA5, and OGG1 polymorphisms and lung cancer risk, stratified by gender, age, smoking, and histological at the level of alleles.

Population	Gene	Allele	Case/control[a]	p	OR_{Adj}	CI_{Adj}	P_{Adj}
Smokers[§]	TERT	T	132/59				
		C	50/19	0.60	1.15	0.62–2.18	0.66
	CHRNA5	G	128/82				
		A	80/40	0.30	1.25	0.78–2.03	0.34
	OGG1	C	154/93				
		G	54/29	0.65	1.07	0.64–1.83	0.79
Nonsmokers[§]	TERT	T	55/69				
		C	11/11	0.62	1.36	0.52–3.54	0.52
	CHRNA5	G	52/142				
		A	22/58	0.91	0.98	0.53–1.78	0.95
	OGG1	C	54/141				
		G	22/59	0.93	0.92	0.50–1.67	0.81
Adenocarcinoma[§§]	TERT	T	131/128				
		C	39/30	0.38	1.16	0.66–2.04	0.57
	CHRNA5	G	114/224				
		A	74/98	0.04	1.33	0.89–1.98	0.15
	OGG1	C	137/234				
		G	53/88	0.88	1.07	0.69–1.63	0.75
Squamous[§§]	TERT	T	56/128				
		C	22/30	0.11	1.48	0.71–3.08	0.28
	CHRNA5	G	66/224				
		A	28/98	0.90	0.87	0.49–1.52	0.64
	OGG1	C	71/234				
		G	23/88	0.58	0.88	0.48–1.60	0.70
Male[**]	TERT	T	146/90				
		C	52/24	0.30	1.15	0.64–2.11	0.63
	CHRNA5	G	145/123				
		A	87/57	0.21	1.21	0.78–1.87	0.38
	OGG1	C	175/133				
		G	60/47	0.91	0.98	0.61–1.57	0.93
Female[**]	TERT	T	41/38				
		C	9/6	0.56	1.45	0.47–4.76	0.51
	CHRNA5	G	35/101				
		A	15/41	0.88	0.99	0.47–2.02	0.98
	OGG1	C	34/101				
		G	16/41	0.68	1.07	0.51–2.16	0.85
>60[*]	TERT	T	92/37				
		C	34/5	0.04	2.21	0.84–6.96	0.13
	CHRNA5	G	91/53				
		A	53/27	0.65	1.12	0.63–2.03	0.69
	OGG1	C	105/55				
		G	39/25	0.51	0.86	0.47–1.61	0.64

TABLE 5: Continued.

Population	Gene	Allele	Case/control[a]	p	OR_{Adj}	CI_{Adj}	P_{Adj}
<60*	TERT	T	95/91				
		C	27/25	0.91	0.94	0.49–1.79	0.86
	CHRNA5	G	89/171				
		A	49/71	0.21	1.18	0.73–1.90	0.48
	OGG1	C	103/179				
		G	37/63	0.93	1.14	0.68–1.89	0.60

OR = odds ratio; CI = confidence interval; Adj = adjusted. *OR and p adjusted for smoking and gender. **OR adjusted for age and smoking habit. [a]Numbers may not add up total number of patients due to genotype failures. [§]OR adjusted for gender and age. [§§]OR adjusted for gender, age and smoking habit.

other hand, another plausible explanation is that the variant of rs16969968 leads to reduced receptor activity and that individuals carrying the A allele may require larger amounts of nicotine to achieve the same level of dopamine release [20]. On the other hand, a meta-analysis concluded that the rs16969968-A predicts delayed smoking cessation and an earlier age of LC diagnosis [50]. It was confirmed by a recent study realized by Forget et al. showing that transgenic rats expressing a human nicotinic receptor polymorphism self-administer more nicotine at high doses and exhibit higher nicotine-induced reinstatement of nicotine seeking than wild type. This relapse is associated with reduced neuronal activity in the interpeduncular nucleus [51]. All these studies show the importance of the rs16969968, especially for early diagnosis of LC, and may provide potential targets for new therapies for smoking cessation interventions. Especially, prospective studies indicate that in 2030, tobacco use will be responsible for 10 million deaths, making it the leading cause of preventable deaths [52].

It is important to mention that the Algerian population—which belongs to Africa's largest country—is a very specific population genetically wise due to both historical and cultural reasons with the Berbers being the native population of the region [53]. History of the region bears witness to many invasions, conquests, and migrations by Phoenicians, Romans, Vandals, Byzantines, Arabs, Jews, Spanish, and French, making it a true admixture which could explain why the MAFs of the Algerian population is close to the Caucasian and Middle Eastern ones and that no significant association was found. In addition, it was shown that some Berber populations (Tuareg, Mozabite) are different compared to the genetic North African ones, having gone through long periods of genetic isolation [27]. This can explain the remarkable difference between the rs16969968 CHRNA5 MAFs of Mozabite that were found (A = 18%) and ours (A = 31%) [46]. Another characteristic of our population, related to cultural factors connected with smoking, is that Algerian women do not smoke except in rare cases, which could explain the lack of significance between rs16969968, (strongly associated with the risk of LC) in Caucasian population.

5. Conclusions

In conclusion, our study, which is the first of its kind related to the molecular of LC for the East Algerian population, has considered the association of the polymorphisms of three genes TERT (rs2853669), CHRNA5 (rs16969968), and OGG1 (rs1052133) in Eastern Algerian population, and has shown that the rs16969968 CHRNA5 has a significant association with adenocarcinoma LC, and interestingly that the risk is important for smoking patients carrying the AA genotype.

These significant and novel results of our study have however some limitations. First, there is the limited sample size used in the study and the mismatch of our population in sex, age, and smoking, which could result in some bias in the results (although the unconditional logistic regression we used with adjustment for confounding variables, such as sex, age, and smoking, mostly neutralized this effect). Secondly, as the sample was not too large, the statistical power to detect the modest effect of three potential functional SNPs in stratified analyses is relatively low. Besides this, there were some missing information on the smoking status for some people and the duration and intensity of the nicotinic addiction tests. In any case, to fully apprehend the difference in the genetic background of the various North African populations will require more studies, and some of the results reported here may help bring new perspectives on the topic.

Authors' Contributions

A.M. is responsible for writing the manuscript and study design. A.M., A.Ma, A.B., H.R., M.A., T.F., L.B., D.A., I.B., and N.A. are responsible for sample collection and data. A.M. and P.S. are responsible for the experiments. A.M., P.S., and E.R. are responsible for the data analysis. ML.A., A.L., K.B., and M.O. are responsible for the statistical analysis. A.M., E.R., D.S., and A.H. are responsible for the participants in the discussion. D.S. and E.R. are responsible for the validation and supervision. All authors have read and agreed to the published version of the manuscript.

Acknowledgments

We would like to extend our gratitude to all who contributed to this work, especially: Pr. Vialard François, Dr. Lacroix Ludovic, Boumechoune Saliha, Dadsi Yasmina, Ghalem Habiba, Pr. Moumeni Abdelhak, Pr. Djebbar Abdelmadjid, Dr. Tayeb Abderahmane, Dr. Kherbache Tarek, Dr. Rebahi

Faycel, Dr. Kassah Laouar Chouaib, Pr. Messaadi Med Salah, Pr. Djeddi Hanane, Pr. Hamidechi Hafid, Pr. Benbrahim Wassila, Haddad Bahria, and all patients and control subjects for their participation. This study was financially supported by the Ministry of Higher Education and Scientific Research of Algeria.

References

[1] J. Ferlay, M. Colombet, I. Soerjomataram et al., "Estimating the global cancer incidence and mortality in 2018: GLOBOCAN sources and methods," *International Journal of Cancer*, vol. 144, no. 8, pp. 1941–1953, 2018.

[2] M. Hamdi-Cherif, E. Bidoli, S. Birri et al., "Le cancer à Sétif, Algérie, 1986–2010," *Journal Africain du Cancer/African Journal of Cancer*, vol. 6, no. 3, pp. 166–173, 2014.

[3] D. M. Parkin, P. Pisani, A. D. Lopez, and E. Masuyer, "At least one in seven cases of cancer is caused by smoking. Global estimates for 1985," *International Journal of Cancer*, vol. 59, no. 4, pp. 494–504, 1994.

[4] M. Furrukh, "Tobacco smoking and lung cancer: perception-changing facts," *Sultan Qaboos University Medical Journal*, vol. 13, no. 3, pp. 345–358, 2013.

[5] P. D. P. Pharoah, A. M. Dunning, B. A. J. Ponder, and D. F. Easton, "Association studies for finding cancer-susceptibility genetic variants," *Nature Reviews Cancer*, vol. 4, no. 11, pp. 850–860, 2004.

[6] C. I. Amos, X. Wu, P. Broderick et al., "Genome-wide association scan of tag SNPs identifies a susceptibility locus for lung cancer at 15q25.1," *Nature Genetics*, vol. 40, no. 5, pp. 616–622, 2008.

[7] R. J. Hung, J. D. McKay, V. Gaborieau et al., "A susceptibility locus for lung cancer maps to nicotinic acetylcholine receptor subunit genes on 15q25," *Nature*, vol. 452, no. 7187, pp. 633–637, 2008.

[8] T. E. Thorgeirsson, F. Geller, P. Sulem et al., "A variant associated with nicotine dependence, lung cancer and peripheral arterial disease," *Nature*, vol. 452, no. 7187, pp. 638–642, 2008.

[9] D. Wu, H. Yu, J. Sun et al., "Association of genetic polymorphisms in the telomerase reverse transcriptase gene with prostate cancer aggressiveness," *Molecular Medicine Reports*, vol. 12, no. 1, pp. 489–497, 2015.

[10] S. Borah, L. Xi, A. J. Zaug et al., "TERT promoter mutations and telomerase reactivation in urothelial cancer," *Science*, vol. 347, no. 6225, pp. 1006–1010, 2015.

[11] U. Nencha, A. Rahimian, M. Giry et al., "TERT promoter mutations and rs2853669 polymorphism: prognostic impact and interactions with common alterations in glioblastomas," *Journal of Neuro-Oncology*, vol. 126, no. 3, pp. 441–446, 2016.

[12] Z. Liu, T. Wang, Z. Wu et al., "Association between TERT rs2853669 polymorphism and cancer risk: a meta-analysis of 9,157 cases and 11,073 controls," *PLoS One*, vol. 13, no. 3, e0191560, 2018.

[13] H. Wikman, A. Risch, F. Klimek et al., "hOGG1 polymorphism and loss of heterozygosity (LOH): significance for lung cancer susceptibility in a caucasian population," *International Journal of Cancer*, vol. 88, no. 6, pp. 932–937, 2000.

[14] H. Ito, N. Hamajima, T. Takezaki et al., "A limited association of OGG1 Ser326Cys polymorphism for adenocarcinoma of the lung," *Journal of Epidemiology*, vol. 12, no. 3, pp. 258–265, 2002.

[15] T. Kohno, K. Shinmura, M. Tosaka et al., "Genetic polymorphisms and alternative splicing of the hOGG1 gene, that is involved in the repair of 8-hydroxyguanine in damaged DNA," *Oncogene*, vol. 16, no. 25, pp. 3219–3225, 1998.

[16] W.-X. Duan, R. X. Hua, W. Yi et al., "The association between OGG1 Ser326Cys polymorphism and lung cancer susceptibility: a meta-analysis of 27 studies," *PLoS One*, vol. 7, no. 4, p. e35970, 2012.

[17] Z. Xu, L. Yu, and X. Zhang, "Association between the hOGG1 Ser326Cys polymorphism and lung cancer susceptibility: a meta-analysis based on 22,475 subjects," *Diagnostic Pathology*, vol. 8, no. 1, 2013.

[18] P.-T. Zhou, B. Li, J. Ji, M. M. Wang, and C. F. Gao, "A systematic review and meta-analysis of the association between OGG1 Ser326Cys polymorphism and cancers," *Medical Oncology*, vol. 32, no. 2, 2015.

[19] H. M. Schuller, "Nitrosamines as nicotinic receptor ligands," *Life Sciences*, vol. 80, no. 24-25, pp. 2274–2280, 2007.

[20] L. J. Bierut, J. A. Stitzel, J. C. Wang et al., "Variants in nicotinic receptors and risk for nicotine dependence," *American Journal of Psychiatry*, vol. 165, no. 9, pp. 1163–1171, 2008.

[21] B. M. Ayesh, R. al-Masri, and A. A. Abed, "CHRNA5 and CHRNA3 polymorphism and lung cancer susceptibility in Palestinian population," *BMC Research Notes*, vol. 11, no. 1, p. 218, 2018.

[22] E. H. Lips, V. Gaborieau, J. D. McKay et al., "Association between a 15q25 gene variant, smoking quantity and tobacco-related cancers among 17 000 individuals," *International Journal of Epidemiology*, vol. 39, no. 2, pp. 563–577, 2010.

[23] N. Pandey, S. Pal, L. K. Sharma, R. Guleria, A. Mohan, and T. Srivastava, "SNP rs16969968 as a strong predictor of nicotine dependence and lung cancer risk in a North Indian population," *Asian Pacific Journal of Cancer Prevention*, vol. 18, no. 11, pp. 3073–3079, 2017.

[24] R. Pérez-Morales, A. González-Zamora, M. F. González-Delgado et al., "*CHRNA3* rs1051730 and *CHRNA5* rs16969968 polymorphisms are associated with heavy smoking, lung cancer, and chronic obstructive pulmonary disease in a mexican population," *Annals of Human Genetics*, vol. 82, no. 6, pp. 415–424, 2018.

[25] T. Truong, R. J. Hung, C. I. Amos et al., "Replication of lung cancer susceptibility loci at chromosomes 15q25, 5p15, and 6p21: a pooled analysis from the International Lung Cancer Consortium," *JNCI: Journal of the National Cancer Institute*, vol. 102, no. 13, pp. 959–971, 2010.

[26] Z.-W. Xu, G.-N. Wang, Z.-Z. Dong, T.-H. Li, C. Cao, and Y.-H. Jin, "CHRNA5 rs16969968 polymorphism association with risk of lung cancer - evidence from 17,962 lung cancer cases and 77,216 control subjects," *Asian Pacific Journal of Cancer Prevention*, vol. 16, no. 15, pp. 6685–6690, 2015.

[27] A. Bekada, L. R. Arauna, T. Deba, F. Calafell, S. Benhamamouch, and D. Comas, "Genetic heterogeneity in Algerian human populations," *PLoS One*, vol. 10, no. 9, 2015.

[28] A. Bekada, R. Fregel, V. M. Cabrera et al., "Introducing the Algerian mitochondrial DNA and Y-chromosome profiles into the North African landscape," *PLoS One*, vol. 8, no. 2, 2013.

[29] N. Shen, Y. Lu, X. Wang, J. Peng, Y. Zhu, and L. Cheng, "Asso-

ciation between rs2853669 in TERT gene and the risk and prognosis of human cancer: a systematic review and meta-analysis," *Oncotarget*, vol. 8, no. 31, p. 50864, 2017.

[30] *rs16969968 RefSNP Report - dbSNP - NCBI*September 2019 https://www.ncbi.nlm.nih.gov/snp/rs16969968#frequency_tab.

[31] NCBIMarch 2019 https://www.ncbi.nlm.nih.gov/variation/news/NCBI_retiring_HapMap/.

[32] S. S. Yoo, S. K. Do, J. E. Choi et al., "*TERT* polymorphism rs2853669 influences on lung cancer risk in the Korean population," *Journal of Korean Medical Science*, vol. 30, no. 10, pp. 1423–1428, 2015.

[33] R. Zhong, L. Liu, L. Zou et al., "Genetic variations inTERT-CLPTM1Llocus are associated with risk of lung cancer in chinese population," *Molecular Carcinogenesis*, vol. 52, no. S1, pp. 118–126, 2013.

[34] R. J. Hung, P. Brennan, F. Canzian et al., "Large-scale investigation of base excision repair genetic polymorphisms and lung cancer risk in a multicenter study," *JNCI: Journal of the National Cancer Institute*, vol. 97, no. 8, pp. 567–576, 2005.

[35] M. Inoue, T. Osaki, M. Noguchi, S. Hirohashi, K. Yasumoto, and H. Kasai, "Lung cancer patients have increased 8-hydroxydeoxyguanosine levels in peripheral lung tissue DNA," *Japanese Journal of Cancer Research*, vol. 89, no. 7, pp. 691–695, 1998.

[36] B. Karahalil, E. Emerce, B. Koçer, S. Han, N. Alkiş, and A. Karakaya, "The association of OGG1 Ser326Cys polymorphism and urinary 8-OHdG levels with lung cancer susceptibility: a hospital-based case-control study in Turkey," *Archives of Industrial Hygiene and Toxicology*, vol. 59, no. 4, pp. 241–250, 2008.

[37] N. Laantri, M. Jalbout, M. Khyatti et al., "XRCC1 and hOGG1 genes and risk of nasopharyngeal carcinoma in North African countries," *Molecular Carcinogenesis*, vol. 50, no. 9, pp. 732–737, 2011.

[38] K. De Ruyck, M. Szaumkessel, I. De Rudder et al., "Polymorphisms in base-excision repair and nucleotide-excision repair genes in relation to lung cancer risk," *Mutation Research/Genetic Toxicology and Environmental Mutagenesis*, vol. 631, no. 2, pp. 101–110, 2007.

[39] B. Qian, H. Zhang, L. Zhang, X. Zhou, H. Yu, and K. Chen, "Association of genetic polymorphisms in DNA repair pathway genes with non-small cell lung cancer risk," *Lung Cancer*, vol. 73, no. 2, pp. 138–146, 2011.

[40] J. Janik, M. Swoboda, B. Janowska et al., "8-Oxoguanine incision activity is impaired in lung tissues of NSCLC patients with the polymorphism of *OGG1* and *XRCC1* genes," *Mutation Research/Fundamental and Molecular Mechanisms of Mutagenesis*, vol. 709-710, pp. 21–31, 2011.

[41] S. Zienolddiny, D. Campa, H. Lind et al., "Polymorphisms of DNA repair genes and risk of non-small cell lung cancer," *Carcinogenesis*, vol. 27, no. 3, pp. 560–567, 2006.

[42] P. Guan, D. Huang, Z. Yin, and B. Zhou, "Association of the hOGG1 Ser326Cys polymorphism with increased lung cancer susceptibility in Asians: a meta-analysis of 18 studies including 7592 cases and 8129 controls," *Asian Pacific Journal of Cancer Prevention*, vol. 12, no. 4, pp. 1067–1072, 2011.

[43] W. Wei, X. F. He, J. B. Qin et al., "Association between the OGG1 Ser326Cys and APEX1 Asp148Glu polymorphisms and lung cancer risk: a meta-analysis," *Molecular Biology Reports*, vol. 39, no. 12, pp. 11249–11262, 2012.

[44] A. J. Lee, "Interindividual variability in response to sodium dichromate-induced oxidative DNA damage: role of the Ser326Cys polymorphism in the DNA-repair protein of 8-oxo-7,8-dihydro-2'-deoxyguanosine DNA glycosylase 1," *Cancer Epidemiology Biomarkers & Prevention*, vol. 14, no. 2, pp. 497–505, 2005.

[45] M. E. Gabrielsen, P. Romundstad, A. Langhammer, H. E. Krokan, and F. Skorpen, "Association between a 15q25 gene variant, nicotine-related habits, lung cancer and COPD among 56 307 individuals from the HUNT study in Norway," *European Journal of Human Genetics*, vol. 21, no. 11, pp. 1293–1299, 2013.

[46] N. A. Rosenberg, J. K. Pritchard, J. L. Weber et al., "Genetic structure of human populations," *Science*, vol. 298, no. 5602, pp. 2381–2385, 2002.

[47] F. S. Falvella, A. Galvan, E. Frullanti et al., "Transcription deregulation at the15q25Locus in association with lung adenocarcinoma risk," *Clinical Cancer Research*, vol. 15, pp. 1837–1842, 2009.

[48] E. Jaworowska, J. Trubicka, M. R. Lener et al., "Smoking related cancers and loci at chromosomes 15q25, 5p15, 6p22.1 and 6p21.33 in the Polish population," *PLoS One*, vol. 6, no. 9, 2011.

[49] L. Le Marchand, K. S. Derby, S. E. Murphy et al., "Smokers with the CHRNA lung cancer-associated variants are exposed to higher levels of nicotine equivalents and a carcinogenic tobacco-specific nitrosamine," *Cancer Research*, vol. 68, no. 22, pp. 9137–9140, 2008.

[50] L.-S. Chen, R. J. Hung, T. Baker et al., "CHRNA5 risk variant predicts delayed smoking cessation and earlier lung cancer diagnosis—a meta-analysis," *JNCI: Journal of the National Cancer Institute*, vol. 107, no. 5, 2015.

[51] B. Forget, P. Scholze, F. Langa et al., "A human polymorphism in CHRNA5 is linked to relapse to nicotine seeking in transgenic rats," *Current Biology*, vol. 28, no. 20, pp. 3244–3253.e7, 2018.

[52] P. Jha and R. Peto, "Global effects of smoking, of quitting, and of taxing tobacco," *New England Journal of Medicine*, vol. 370, no. 1, pp. 60–68, 2014.

[53] M. Brett and E. Fentress, *The Berbers*, Wiley-Blackwell, 1997, ISBN 0-631-20767-8.

32

A Case Report of Steroid-Resistant Cryptogenic Organizing Pneumonia Managed with Intravenous Immunoglobulins

Christian Akem Dimala[1] **Urvi Patel,**[1] **Benjamin Lloyd,**[1] **Anthony Donato**[1] **William B. Kimmel,**[2] **Robert Hallowell,**[3] **and Caitlyn Moss**[1]

[1]*Department of Medicine, Reading Hospital-Tower Health, West Reading, PA, USA*
[2]*Department of Pathology, Reading Hospital-Tower Health, West Reading, PA, USA*
[3]*Department of Pulmonary & Critical Care Medicine, Massachusetts General Hospital, Boston, MA, USA*

Correspondence should be addressed to Christian Akem Dimala; christian.akem.dimala1@alumni.lshtm.ac.uk

Academic Editor: Tun-Chieh Chen

Fewer than ten reported cases of cryptogenic organizing pneumonia (COP) have been managed with intravenous immunoglobulins (IVIg). We report a case of a 72-year-old man who presented with a worsening cough and diffuse opacities on chest radiograph. Following no improvement with antibiotics and negative complementary investigations for infectious, malignant, and autoimmune etiologies, COP was confirmed on lung biopsy. Due to continued clinical deterioration despite high-dose steroids and new severe steroid-induced hallucinations, the patient was placed on intravenous immunoglobulins (IVIg) and mycophenolate mofetil and made a satisfactory recovery. IVIg should be considered as an important steroid-sparing alternative in patients with COP.

1. Introduction

Cryptogenic organizing pneumonia (COP) is a rare respiratory condition characterized by the filling of alveolar airspaces and alveolar ducts with fibrin and granulation tissue, and for which there is no identifiable cause [1, 2]. COP often presents with respiratory symptoms including cough, fever, shortness of breath, and fatigue; however, its clinical presentation could span through a wide spectrum [1–3]. Lung examination is usually remarkable for focal or widespread crackles. Radiologic changes often observed are unilateral or bilateral lung opacities on chest radiographs and ground glass shadowing on computed tomography (CT) scans [4, 5]. Typical histopathologic features are patchy cellular airspace fibrosis involving alveoli and alveolar ducts, foamy alveolar macrophages, and fibroblasts embedded in a myxoid matrix [4]. The mainstay of management of COP involves corticosteroids. Improvement in symptoms and oxygen requirements is seen in more than half of the cases [3] and clinical improvement over several months [1]. There have been reports of corticosteroid-resistant and refractory cases of COP requiring alternate management options including macrolides and cytotoxic agents [6, 7]. Steroid pulse therapy with high doses of methylprednisolone has also been reported [8–10]. However, intolerance to high-dose steroids in some patients warrants alternative treatment options. We report a case of corticosteroid-resistant COP in a patient who developed steroid psychosis, requiring treatment with intravenous immunoglobulins (IVIg).

2. Case Presentation

A 72-year-old man with atrial fibrillation on apixaban and a left total knee replacement four weeks prior, complicated by hemarthrosis and joint infection requiring arthrocentesis and currently receiving a 6-week course of intravenous

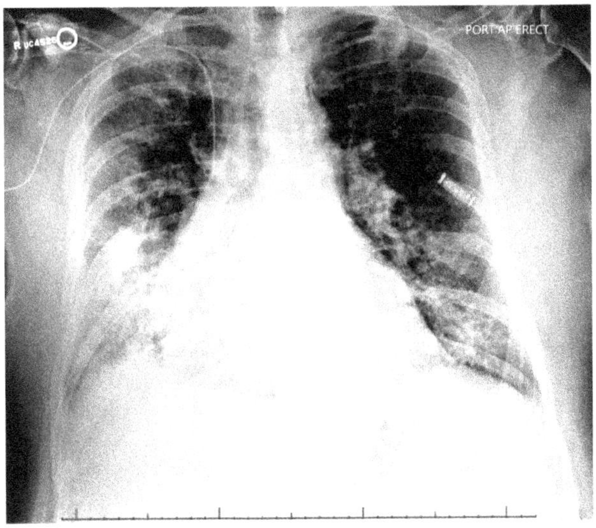

FIGURE 1: Anteroposterior erect chest radiograph at presentation. Frontal view of chest radiograph showing bilateral patchy infiltrates most pronounced in the right lower lobe concerning for multifocal pneumonia. Right PICC line and cardiac recorder device noted in the left anterior chest wall.

daptomycin presented to the hospital from a rehabilitation facility due to worsening cough for over one week. Chest radiograph showed patchy infiltrates, most pronounced in right lower lobe suggestive of multifocal pneumonia (Figure 1). He complained of intermittent productive cough with one episode of hemoptysis, as well as dyspnea and chills. On presentation, the patient appeared comfortable. However, he was febrile to 100.4 degrees Fahrenheit and tachypneic. On examination, heart rhythm was irregularly irregular, there was no jugular venous distension, and the patient had bilateral rales from lung bases up to mid-lung zones. No lower extremity edema was noted. His left knee surgical incision site was intact and clean, with minimal sanguineous drainage and minor surrounding erythema. Laboratory studies were notable for white blood cell count of 10,900 cells/μL with 4.7% eosinophils and 69.7% neutrophils, hemoglobin of 11.0 g/dL, sedimentation rate of 22 mm/hour (normal < 15 mm/hr), and c-reactive protein of 7.23 mg/dL (normal < 1.00 mg/dL). Chemistries were significant for a sodium of 129 mmol/L. The patient was admitted for presumed sepsis secondary to multifocal pneumonia and treated with cefepime and metronidazole for pneumonia, and he continued with daptomycin for septic arthritis. Cefepime and metronidazole were subsequently switched to levofloxacin for seven days to treat community-acquired pneumonia. Despite antimicrobial therapy, the patient gradually deteriorated with worsening respiratory failure. On day four of his hospital stay, a computed tomography (CT) scan of the chest demonstrated ground glass opacities involving all lobes bilaterally with consolidation at bilateral lung bases (Figure 2). Due to concern for daptomycin-induced eosinophilic pneumonitis, the patient was switched to intravenous vancomycin for septic arthritis antimicrobial coverage. Seven days after admission, the patient had increasing oxygen requirements, requiring four liters of oxygen. Transthoracic echocardiogram from the current admission demonstrated an ejection fraction of 55% with no regional wall motion abnormalities. B-type natriuretic peptide was initially raised at 486 pg/mL, but subsequently declined to 179 pg/mL on day seven of admission and 111 pg/mL on day 15 of admission. Multiple trials of diuresis were attempted due to suspicions of volume overload with a net negative fluid balance of 12.4 liters over 17 days. Despite attempted diuresis, there was no change in oxygen requirements, and his repeat chest X-ray still demonstrated bilateral patchy infiltrates. A repeat CT of the chest demonstrated worsening ground glass opacities and small bilateral pleural effusions. All investigations including two coronavirus-19 nucleic acid amplification (NAA) tests and respiratory pathogen panel were negative. Blood cultures were negative. Urine *Legionella* and *Streptococcal pneumoniae* antigens, as well as serum mycoplasma IgM antibody were negative. HIV antibody/antigen testing was negative. Procalcitonin was 0.07 ng/mL (normal < 0.5 ng/mL). Patient's inflammatory markers were, however, increasing with C-reactive protein at 20.8 mg/L, erythrocyte sedimentation rate of 38 mm/hr, and white blood cell count to 14,700/μL with 4.2% eosinophils and 76.9% neutrophils on day seven of admission. Rheumatic and autoimmune laboratories were negative including anti neutrophilic cytoplasmic antibody, rheumatoid factor, myeloperoxidase antibody IgG, serine proteinase antibody, dsDNA antibody, and autoantibodies to SSA and SSB. Antinuclear antibody was positive at 1:80, speckled. The workup for hypersensitivity pneumonitis was negative for antibodies to *Aspergillus*, *Thermoactinomyces vulgaris*, and *Micropolyspora faeni*. The patient was transferred to an intermediate care unit due to worsening respiratory failure. Pulmonology was consulted and recommended initiation of prednisone 1 mg/kg per day for potential cryptogenic organizing pneumonia. Despite steroid therapy, the patient's respiratory status continued to decline, requiring up to 10 liters of oxygen via oxi-mask to maintain oxygen saturations above 92%. A limited bronchoscopy with bronchoalveolar lavage was completed on day 11 but biopsies could not be obtained due to respiratory distress. Fluid studies from bronchoalveolar lavage showed white blood cell count of 355 c/mm^3 with 36% segmented cells, 8% lymphocytes, 16% monocytes, and 3% eosinophils. Bronchial culture was suggestive of oral flora and negative for acid fast bacilli. Bronchial fungal culture was positive for *Candida albicans* but was thought to be a contaminant. Cytology from the bronchial washing was negative for malignancy. On day 14, the patient underwent video-assisted thoracoscopic surgery for lung biopsy that was complicated by pneumothorax requiring chest tube placement. His respiratory status worsened with arterial blood gas demonstrating hypercapnia despite continuing 1 mg/kg of steroids (80 mg prednisone orally). Oxygen requirements escalated to 60 liters O_2 via high flow nasal canula at 55% FiO_2. His hospital course was further complicated by steroid-associated psychosis and delirium requiring physical and chemical restraints, and the patient was hence deemed unsafe for BiPAP. On hospital day 18, lung biopsy result was consistent

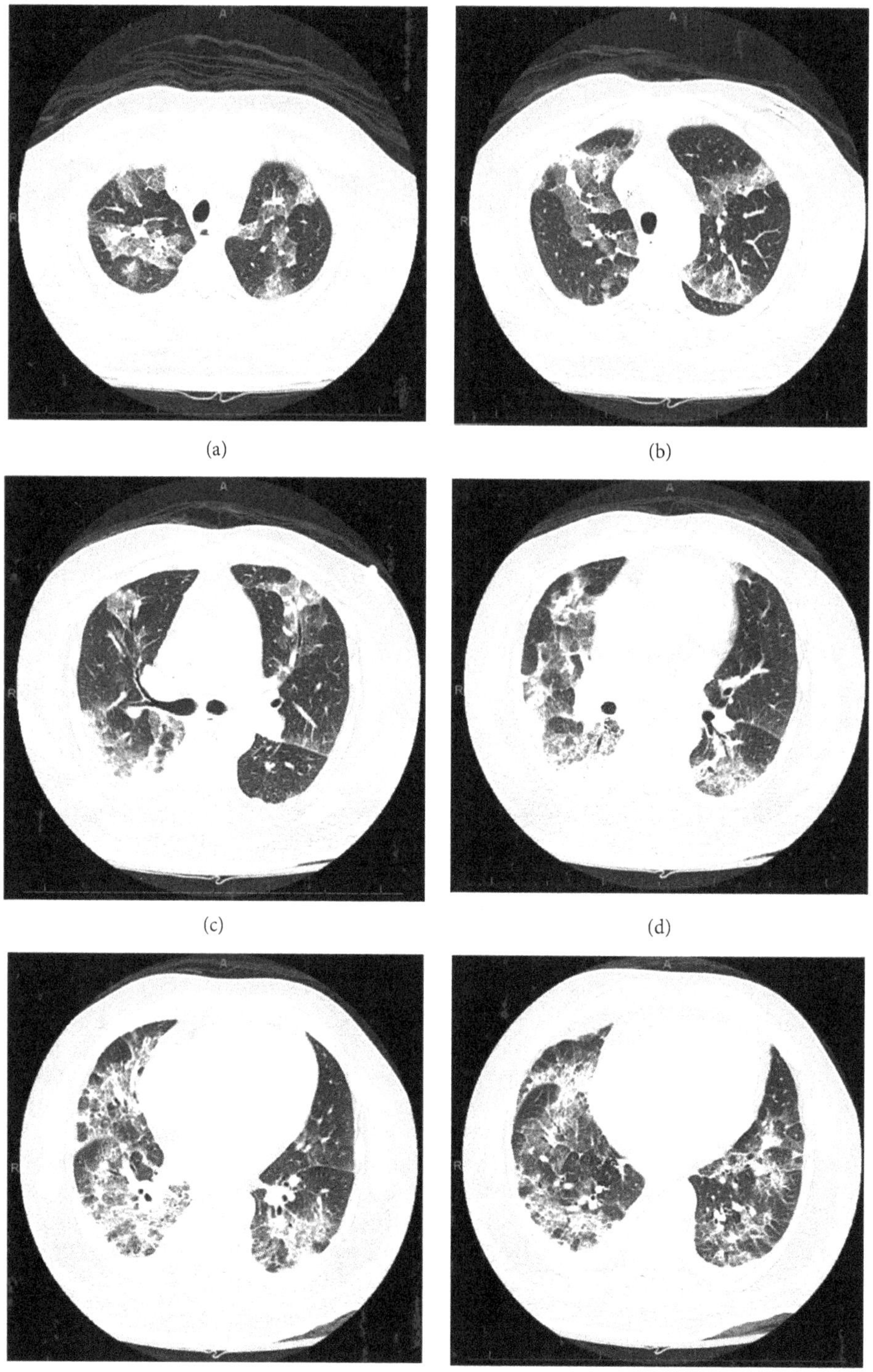

FIGURE 2: CT scan of the chest with intravenous contrast at day four of admission. CT chest images (a)–(f) showing patchy opacities of both lungs involving all lobes bilaterally (right greater than left) with some consolidation changes and mild bilateral pleural effusions.

with cryptogenic organizing pneumonia (Figure 3). Given worsening respiratory status, medications to induce remission were discussed. Given severe delirium and psychosis from steroids, intravenous immunoglobulin (IVIg) 0.4 g/kg/dose was initiated on day 23 and continued for five days as an alternative to pulse steroids based on multiple case reports. Mycophenolate mofetil 500 mg twice daily was also initiated to wean down prednisone, which was decreased to 0.4 mg/kg after a one-time dose of methylprednisolone 125 mg on day 23. Trimethoprim-sulfamethoxazole was initiated for *Pneumocystis jirovecii* pneumonia prophylaxis. The patient made a significant improvement after initiation of IVIg with complete resolution of acute hypoxic respiratory failure and ended his oxygen dependence by day 4 of

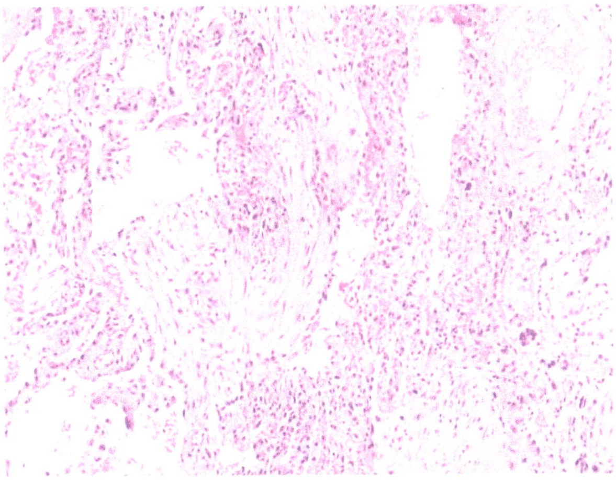

FIGURE 3: Surgical biopsy obtained from right lung. Pathology with hematoxylin-eosin stain at 200× magnification shows organizing pneumonia in a background of diffuse alveolar damage.

IVIg (hospital day 27). The patient was discharged on an eight-week prednisone taper, vitamin D and calcium supplementation, mycophenolate mofetil, and trimethoprim sulfamethoxazole. A follow-up chest CT scan of the patient at 6 months showed significant interval improvement of the ground glass opacities and interstitial infiltrates in the lungs with just a few markings remaining in the lung bases (Figure 4), suggesting interval resolution of the inflammatory process. A summary of the patient's hospital course is presented on Figure 5.

3. Discussion

Cryptogenic organizing pneumonia (COP) was first described in 1983 by Davison et al. in eight patients who presented with respiratory symptoms, bilateral radiographic changes, elevated inflammatory markers, and intra-alveolar organization but no identifiable etiology [11]. The disease is believed to be caused by injury to the alveolar epithelium with subsequent deposition of fibrin [1, 2]. COP classically presents with nonspecific symptoms, including a subacute cough lasting weeks to months associated with fever, shortness of breath, malaise, fatigue, and sparse crackles on auscultation with multifocal alveolar infiltrates on chest imaging [1, 5]. Typical radiological findings on chest CT scan include multifocal airspace opacities or peripheral consolidations with by ground glass opacities [12]. Atypical radiological patterns include infiltrative opacities, multiple nodular opacities, crazy-paving patterns, and linear and band-like opacities among others [12]. Symptoms with similar clinical and histologic features include infections, autoimmune diseases, connective tissue diseases, and drug injury among others. It is important to exclude all these causes to be able to arrive at the diagnosis of COP. Untreated typical COP has a good prognosis with spontaneous recovery in up to half of the cases [3]. Treated COP has an even better long-term outcome in most cases with significant improvement in symptoms within days [1, 3]. Cases with interstitial fibrosis as opposed to those with airspace opacities on chest imaging, however, have persistence of the disease even with treatment [1, 3]. Current treatment guidelines for COP are based on the severity of the disease at presentation and include observation for mild disease with minimal symptoms or oral glucocorticoids for patients with worsening symptoms, moderately decreased pulmonary functions tests, and diffuse radiographic changes. After initial loading doses of 500-1000 mg of intravenous methylprednisolone for three days, the recommended maintenance doses of steroids are 0.75-1.5 mg/kg prednisone for up to three months with gradual weaning over several months and potentially up to a year, if there is satisfactory clinical improvement [2, 3]. The side effects of steroids should always be kept in mind when used on a long-term basis, and these patients should be followed-up regularly with repeat radiographic imaging to ensure nonprogression or relapse of the disease that will require steroid dose adjustment or an alternative treatment.

Although steroids are the main treatment modality for moderate to severe COP[2], complete response to steroids has been observed in only 60% of cases, with nonresponse noted in up to 14% of cases [3]. Likewise, relapses are not infrequent, especially when the steroid dose is rapidly tapered. Unfortunately, the side-effect profile of steroids makes them unsuitable in some individuals such as those with steroid-induced psychosis as was the case in this patient. In these cases, alternative treatment options should be sought. Antibiotics with anti-inflammatory properties such as macrolides have been increasingly used for the treatment of patients with COP usually administered over a period of several months or up to a year [7, 13]. Other treatment modalities which have been used previously include adjunctive immunosuppression therapy with cyclophosphamide [14], cyclosporine [15], azathioprine [16], and mycophenolate mofetil [17]. In our case, macrolide therapy was not attempted.

Another important etiology considered in this patient was daptomycin-induced lung injury as he had been on daptomycin. A case of organizing pneumonia with pulmonary eosinophilic infiltrates following prolonged use of daptomycin in a very similar context has previously been reported [18]. In the former case report, clinical improvement was achieved within a couple of weeks, following discontinuation of daptomycin. However, there was rather a persistent clinical deterioration in our patient after discontinuation of daptomycin, and there was no eosinophilia on differential blood count or evidence of eosinophilic inflammation on bronchoalveolar lavage and lung biopsy. He was started on high-dose prednisone when COP became a likely diagnosis but showed no improvement on steroids, and a decision was made to start the patient on intravenous immunoglobulins to which he responded within 24 hours and experienced complete recovery and discharge over the following days. Although mycophenolate mofetil was also started at the same time as IVIg, we believe IVIg to be responsible for his improvement given that the effects of antimetabolites such as mycophenolate mofetil are generally not seen for several weeks. To date, we found only seven published cases that used intravenous

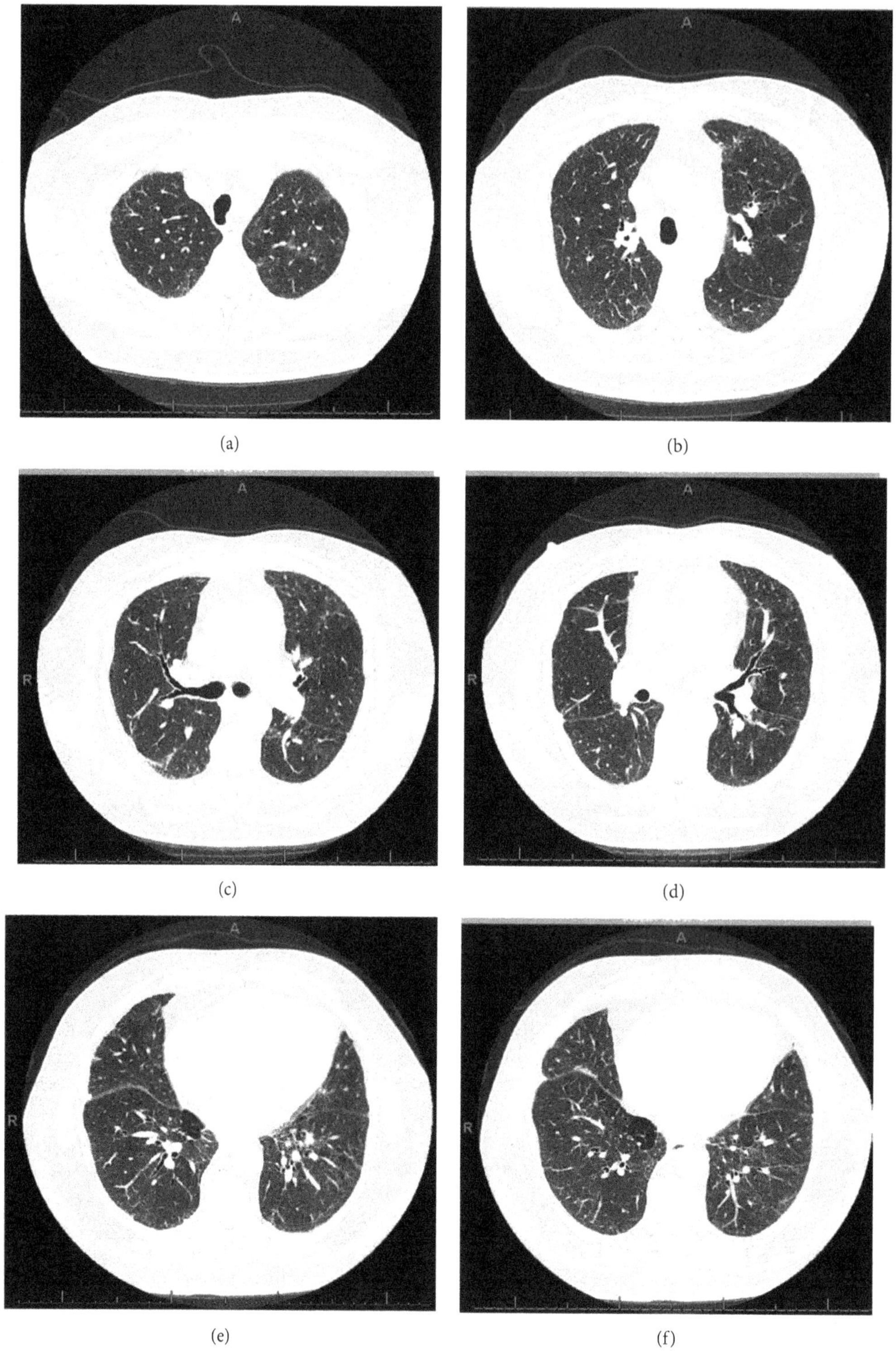

FIGURE 4: CT scan of the chest with intravenous contrast at 6-month follow-up visit. CT chest images (a)–(f) showing significant interval improvement of ground glass opacities and interstitial infiltrates in the lungs with just a few markings remaining in the lung bases, suggesting interval resolution of the inflammatory process.

immunoglobulins (IVIg) for the treatment of organizing pneumonia, often in the context of underlying selective immunodeficiency or hypogammaglobulinemia and/or non-response to steroid [19–25]. These cases suggest that a normal and functional humoral immune response is not an absolute requirement for the development of COP and also raise the possibility of an association of COP to hypogammaglobulinemia in the setting of repeated infections.

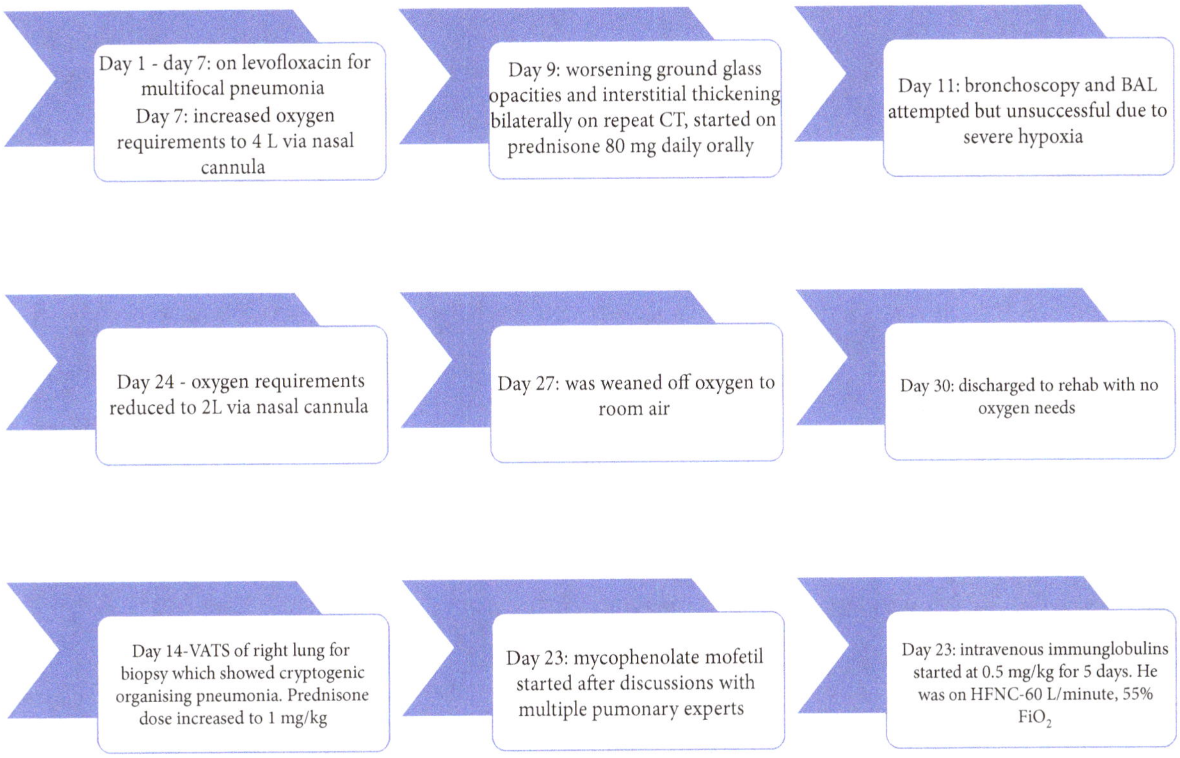

FIGURE 5: Flow chart summarizing hospital course of patient.

However, further research is needed in this area. Our patient did not have features suggestive of underlying immunodeficiency such as recurrent or opportunistic infections. This patient was discharged with scheduled outpatient follow-up visits given the high relapse rates of COP especially in cases presenting with multifocal opacities on radiologic test [26].

4. Conclusion

(1) Cryptogenic organizing pneumonia remains a rare respiratory entity, typically managed with corticosteroids

(2) Intravenous immunoglobulins should be considered as an important steroid-sparing alternative treatment even in patients without underlying immunodeficiencies or hypogammaglobulinemia

Abbreviations

COP: Cryptogenic organizing pneumonia
CT: Computed tomography
IVIg: Intravenous immunoglobulins
NAA: Nucleic acid amplification.

Authors' Contributions

CAD, UP, BL, AD, WBK, RH, and CM were involved in the care and management of the patient and drafted the manuscript. All authors read and approved the final manuscript.

Acknowledgments

Special thanks are due to the Tower Heath Research Day for giving us a platform to present a poster of the case report.

References

[1] V. Cottin and J.-F. Cordier, "Cryptogenic organizing pneumonia," *Seminars in Respiratory and Critical Care Medicine*, vol. 33, no. 5, pp. 462–475, 2012.

[2] J.-F. Cordier, "Cryptogenic organising pneumonia," *The European Respiratory Journal*, vol. 28, no. 2, pp. 422–446, 2006.

[3] A. U. Wells, N. Hirani, and on behalf of the BTS Interstitial Lung Disease Guideline Group, a subgroup of the British Thoracic Society Standards of Care Committee, in collaboration with the Thoracic Society of Australia and New Zealand and the Irish Thoracic Society, "Interstitial lung disease guideline," *Thorax*, vol. 63, Supplement 5, pp. v1–58, 2008.

[4] J. F. Cordier, R. Loire, and J. Brune, "Idiopathic bronchiolitis obliterans organizing pneumonia: definition of characteristic clinical profiles in a series of 16 patients," *Chest*, vol. 96, no. 5, pp. 999–1004, 1989.

[5] D. Chandra, R. Maini, and D. M. Hershberger, "Cryptogenic organizing pneumonia," in *StatPearls*, StatPearls Publishing, Treasure Island, FL, 2020.

[6] V. Pathak, J. M. Kuhn, C. Durham, W. K. Funkhouser, and D. C. Henke, "Macrolide use leads to clinical and radiological improvement in patients with cryptogenic organizing pneumonia," *Annals of the American Thoracic Society*, vol. 11, no. 1, pp. 87–91, 2014.

[7] J. Lee, S. I. Cha, T. I. Park, J. Y. Park, T. H. Jung, and C. H. Kim, "Adjunctive effects of cyclosporine and macrolide in rapidly progressive cryptogenic organizing pneumonia with no

prompt response to steroid," *Internal Medicine*, vol. 50, no. 5, pp. 475–479, 2011.

[8] S. J. Husain, M. Irfan, A. S. Zubairi, and N. Salahuddin, "Rapidly-progressive bronchiolitis obliterans organising pneumonia," *Singapore Medical Journal*, vol. 45, no. 6, pp. 283–285, 2004.

[9] S. Xie, C. Shen, Y. Zhang et al., "Cryptogenic organizing pneumonia associated with invasive pulmonary aspergillosis: a case report and review of the literature," *International Journal of Clinical and Experimental Pathology*, vol. 7, no. 12, pp. 8637–8646, 2014.

[10] A. J. Cohen, T. E. King, and G. P. Downey, "Rapidly progressive bronchiolitis obliterans with organizing pneumonia," *American Journal of Respiratory and Critical Care Medicine*, vol. 149, no. 6, pp. 1670–1675, 1994.

[11] A. G. Davison, B. E. Heard, W. A. McAllister, and M. E. Turner-Warwick, "Cryptogenic organizing pneumonitis," *The Quarterly Journal of Medicine*, vol. 52, no. 207, pp. 382–394, 1983.

[12] F. Tiralongo, M. Palermo, G. Distefano et al., "Cryptogenic organizing pneumonia: evolution of morphological patterns assessed by HRCT," *Diagnostics*, vol. 10, no. 5, p. 262, 2020.

[13] J. A. Kastelik, M. Greenstone, D. V. McGivern, and A. H. Morice, "Cryptogenic organising pneumonia," *European Respiratory Journal*, vol. 28, no. 6, pp. 1291-1291, 2006.

[14] I. F. Purcell, S. J. Bourke, and S. M. Marshall, "Cyclophosphamide in severe steroid-resistant bronchiolitis obliterans organizing pneumonia," *Respiratory Medicine*, vol. 91, no. 3, pp. 175–177, 1997.

[15] D. Koinuma, M. Miki, M. Ebina et al., "Successful treatment of a case with rapidly progressive bronchiolitis obliterans organizing pneumonia (BOOP) using cyclosporin A and corticosteroid," *Internal Medicine*, vol. 41, no. 1, pp. 26–29, 2002.

[16] A. Laszlo, Y. Espolio, A. Auckenthaler, J.-P. Michel, and J.-P. Janssens, "Azathioprine and low-dose corticosteroids for the treatment of cryptogenic organizing pneumonia in an older patient," *Journal of the American Geriatrics Society*, vol. 51, no. 3, pp. 433-434, 2003.

[17] S. Bhatti, A. Hakeem, J. Torrealba, J. P. McMahon, and K. C. Meyer, "Severe acute fibrinous and organizing pneumonia (AFOP) causing ventilatory failure: successful treatment with mycophenolate mofetil and corticosteroids," *Respiratory Medicine*, vol. 103, no. 11, pp. 1764–1767, 2009.

[18] E. Cobb, R. C. Kimbrough, K. M. Nugent, and M. P. Phy, "Organizing pneumonia and pulmonary eosinophilic infiltration associated with daptomycin," *The Annals of Pharmacotherapy*, vol. 41, no. 4, pp. 696–701, 2007.

[19] I. Gueta, Y. Shoenfeld, and H. Orbach, "Intravenous immune globulins (IVIg) treatment for organizing pneumonia in a selective IgG immune deficiency state," *Immunologic Research*, vol. 60, no. 2-3, pp. 165–169, 2014.

[20] D. A. Dibbern, H. N. Claman, and S. C. Dreskin, "Dyspnea and pulmonary infiltrates in a 53-year-old woman with common variable immunodeficiency," *Annals of Allergy, Asthma & Immunology*, vol. 87, no. 1, pp. 18–21, 2001.

[21] R. C. Oriel and B. Kaplan, "Decreased IgG and suboptimal pneumococcal response: remission of cryptogenic organizing pneumonia (COP) with subcutaneous immunoglobulin (SCIG) and mycophenolate mofetil (MMF)," in *American College of Allergy, Asthma & Immunology 2015 Annual Scientific Meeting*, San Antonio, Texas, 2015.

[22] D. H. Lee, J. H. Yeo, Y. I. Kim, S. J. Gim, J. W. Sohn, and J. Y. Yhi, "Successful immunoglobulin treatment in severe cryptogenic organizing pneumonia caused by dermatomyositis," *The Korean Journal of Critical Care Medicine*, vol. 30, no. 3, pp. 212–217, 2015.

[23] A. L. Vieira, A. Vale, N. Melo et al., "Organizing pneumonia revisited: insights and uncertainties from a series of 67 patients," *Sarcoidosis, Vasculitis, and Diffuse Lung Diseases*, vol. 35, no. 2, pp. 129–138, 2018.

[24] J. A. Miskoff, R. Ali, and M. Chaudhri, "A case of dermatomyositis causing cryptogenic organizing pneumonia," *Cureus*, vol. 11, no. 12, 2019.

[25] N. Arish, R. Eldor, Y. Fellig et al., "Lymphocytic interstitial pneumonia associated with common variable immunodeficiency resolved with intravenous immunoglobulins," *Thorax*, vol. 61, no. 12, pp. 1096-1097, 2006.

[26] E. Barroso, L. Hernandez, J. Gil, R. Garcia, I. Aranda, and S. Romero, "Idiopathic organizing pneumonia: a relapsing disease," *Respiration*, vol. 74, no. 6, pp. 624–631, 2007.

33

Large Spontaneous Right Catamenial Pneumothorax with Diaphragmatic Defect and Liver Herniation

Venkata Kishore Mukku ,[1] Emily Cassidy,[2] Catalina Negulescu,[1] Tonya Jagneaux,[3] and John Godke[3]

[1] *Department of Internal Medicine, Baton Rouge General Internal Medicine Residency Program, an affiliate of Tulane University School of Medicine, Baton Rouge, Louisiana, USA*
[2] *Cardiovascular Thoracic Surgery, CVT Surgical Center, Baton Rouge, Louisiana, USA*
[3] *Pulmonary Critical Care, Louisiana State University Health Sciences Center, Baton Rouge Campus, Louisiana, USA*

Correspondence should be addressed to Venkata Kishore Mukku; vkmukku@gmail.com

Academic Editor: Inger F. Oey

Catamenial pneumothorax is a spontaneous pneumothorax that occurs predominantly women of child bearing age. We describe a case of a 40-year-old nulliparous woman with medical history significant for endometriosis who presented with severe chest tightness of one-day duration. Chest radiography (CXR) showed a large right spontaneous pneumothorax, what was thought to be a 5.6 cm pleural mass at the right lung base. Following pneumothorax diagnosis, the patient underwent emergent right thoracostomy with pigtail catheter placement. A repeat CXR revealed marked re-expansion of the lung but persistence of a right pleural mass. Follow up computed tomography scan of the chest showed a 33 mm diaphragmatic defect with 5.8 x 4.6 x 3.9 cm area of herniated liver corresponding to the presumed pleural mass. Following complete thoracic imaging, patient underwent video-assisted thoracoscopic surgery, mechanical pleurodesis, and open repair of the right diaphragmatic defect. Intraoperatively, an endometrial implant was noted on the chest wall. On postoperative day three, she began her menstrual cycle and was evaluated by gynecologist who recommended hormonal therapy to reduce risk of recurrent pneumothorax. Due to a persistent air leak, the chest tube was transitioned to a Heimlich valve to facilitate home discharge. The patient was discharged on postoperative day eight, seen as outpatient with resolution of air leak and removal of chest tube.

1. Introduction

Catamenial pneumothorax is a rare cause of spontaneous pneumothorax that affects predominantly women of child bearing age [1]. In the literature, only a few cases of catamenial pneumothorax with diaphragmatic defect and liver herniation are reported [2–7]. In some of these cases, liver herniation was only diagnosed intraoperatively [2–6]. In a case report by Tomescot et al., a chest X-ray (CXR) showed numerous diaphragmatic defects with liver herniation prior to surgical exploration [7]. However, in all these cases liver herniation occurred after recurrence of the pneumothorax. In our case, liver herniation occurred during the first episode of pneumothorax. A computed tomography scan (CT) confirmed liver herniation of what originally appeared to be a pleural based mass on CXR.

Catamenial pneumothorax is most common in premenopausal women aged 30–50 years, with a peak incidence between 30 and 35 years [8]. Catamenial pneumothorax usually occurs within 72-96 hours of onset of menstruation [9]. Catamenial pneumothorax is associated with pelvic endometriosis in 30-50% of cases [10] and almost always involves the right thorax [11]. The etiology of catamenial pneumothorax is poorly understood but several proposed theories exists: migration of air from peritoneal cavity into the pleural space through pre-existing diaphragmatic defects, retrograde implantation of endometrial tissue through diaphragmatic defects, lymphatic or hematogenous spread of endometrial tissue to visceral pleura, and spontaneous rupture of blebs during hormonal changes [12]. Diaphragmatic defects are correlated with endometriosis and have been seen in 29-66% of catamenial pneumothorax patients [11, 13].

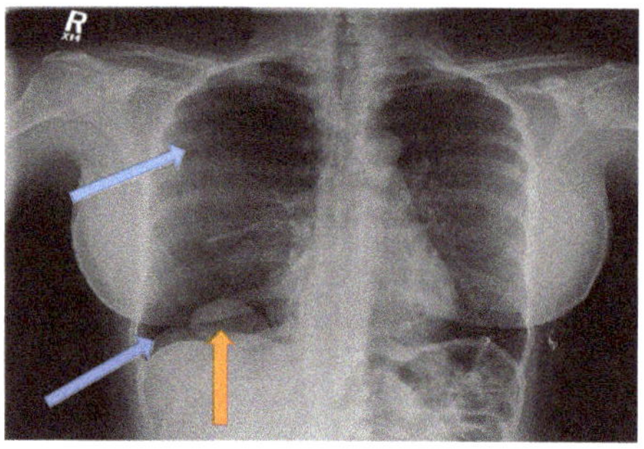

FIGURE 1: The blue arrows show the visceral pleural line indicating the presence of pneumothorax and diaphragmatic free air. The orange arrow reveals a large 56 mm mass at the base of the lung (confirmed as liver on computed tomography).

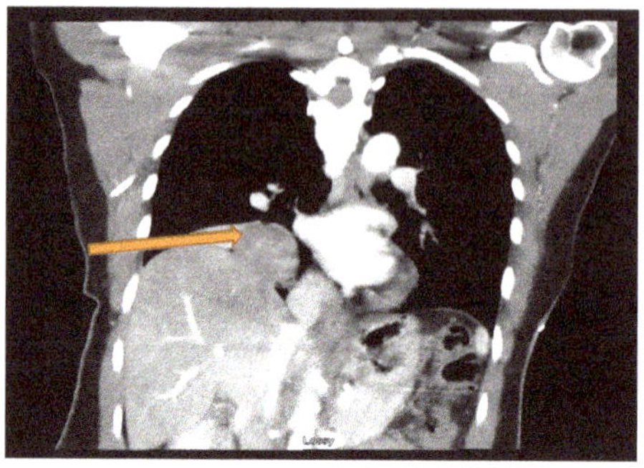

FIGURE 2: Coronal view of CT scan with orange arrow showing a 33 mm diaphragmatic defect with liver herniation, 5.8 x 4.6 x 3.9cm.

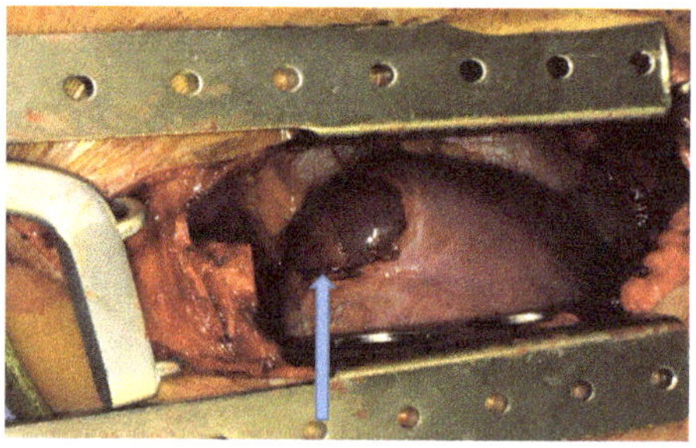

FIGURE 3: Blue arrow showing large diaphragmatic defect with herniation of liver before repair.

2. Case Report

A 40-year-old nulliparous woman with no past medical history, other than endometriosis, presented to the emergency room with severe chest tightness of one day duration. She described chest tightness while exercising on a bicycle after 10 minutes. The next day she developed a severe hacking cough at work during a conference call. The cough was associated with disorientation and severe chest tightness. This prompted her to present to the emergency department in February 2018. The patient is a pharmacist, nonsmoker, and denies illicit drug use or recent travel. She had endometrial laser ablation with myomectomy in 2006. Hormonal contraceptives have been used since 2004 and were stopped three months before presentation in hopes of conception. Her last menstrual period was four days before the onset of symptoms. On physical examination, she had chest tightness localizing to the right side and decreased right sided breath sounds. All the routine laboratory work and vital signs were normal. The CXR showed a large right spontaneous pneumothorax with what approved to be a 5.6 cm pleural mass at the right lung base (Figure 1).

Following the pneumothorax diagnosis, the patient underwent emergent right thoracostomy with pigtail catheter placement. A repeat CXR revealed marked re-expansion of the lung but persistence of the right cardiophrenic opacity of unclear etiology. A follow-up CTof chest showed a 33 mm diaphragmatic defect with a 5.8 x 4.6 x 3.9 cm area of herniated liver corresponding to the presumed pleural mass (Figure 2).

Following complete thoracic imaging the patient underwent video-assisted thoracoscopic surgery (VATS), mechanical pleurodesis, and open repair of the right diaphragmatic defect by Dr. Emily Cassidy (Figures 3 and 4). Intraoperatively, the lungs appeared grossly normal. An obvious diaphragmatic defect was noted in the posteromedial portion of the central tendon of the diaphragm with a sizable protrusion of liver in to the chest cavity. There was an attempt to dissect liver adhesions from the diaphragm. Extensive liver adhesions forced conversion of the right VATS to a posterior lateral muscle sparing thoracotomy. Electrocautery and blunt dissection were used to separate the liver and diaphragm. Once the liver hernia was completely reduced, the diaphragm was repaired using multiple interrupted prolene pledgeted horizontal mattress sutures. Later, right parietal pleurectomy was performed by scoring the pleura posteriorly, anteriorly throughout the entire chest cavity. At the apex as well as the base, where pleurectomy was difficult, mechanical pleurodesis using a Bovie scratch pad was perfomred. A 24-french chest tube was placed at the apex of the chest cavity and 24-french blake was placed at the level of diaphragm.

Intraoperatively, an endometrial implant (blue berry spot) was noted on the chest wall (Figure 5), but the endometrial implant was not successfully biopsied for pathology evaluation due to the extent of liver adhesions and due to conversion of procedure from VATS to open thoracotomy.

On postoperative day three, the patient began her menstrual cycle. She was evaluated by a gynecologist consultant who recommended hormonal therapy, leuprolide a Gonadotropin releasing hormone (GnRH) analogue, to begin 2-3 weeks postoperatively for a period of 6-12 months for hormonal suppression to reduce the risk of recurrent pneumothorax. GnRH analogs are highly effective at suppressing ovarian hormone production and inhibition of growth of endometrial tissue. Due to a persistent air leak, the patient's chest tube was transitioned to a Heimlich valve to facilitate home discharge. We believed that the persistent air leak indicated there was some minor defect in the visceral pleura that was too small to identify intraoperatively. The patient was discharged on postoperative day eight and was seen as an outpatient by the cardiothoracic surgeon. At this time, there was resolution of air leak and removal of the chest tube.

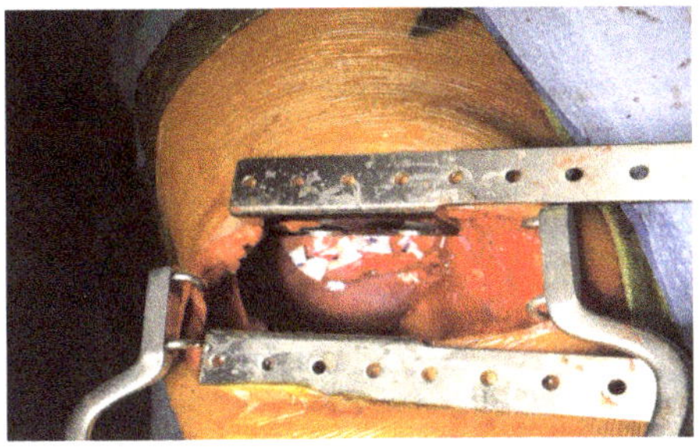

FIGURE 4: Suture repair of the diaphragmatic defect.

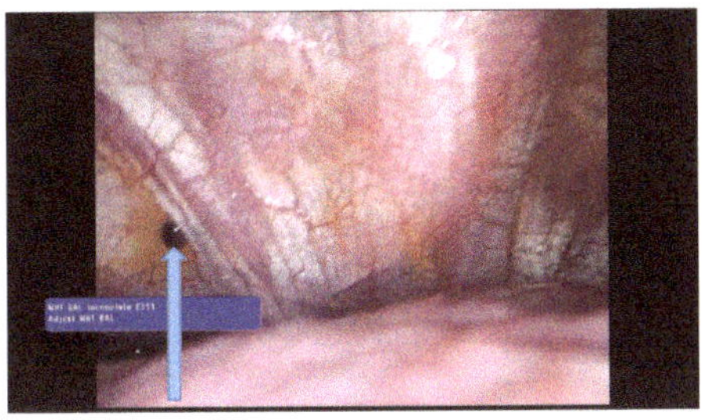

FIGURE 5: Blue arrow showing an endometrial implant on the chest wall.

Patient was also seen after two months in a primary care clinic for follow-up visit with no issues.

3. Discussion

Though uncommon, this case describes a young woman with endometriosis who presented with pneumothorax and a large diaphragmatic defect. Even though histologic confirmation is lacking, her clinical course, intraoperative finding of endometrial implant, and diaphragmatic defect with liver herniation are consistent with catamenial pneumothorax. She underwent VATS and mechanical pleurodesis with open diaphragmatic repair followed by hormonal therapy. VATS should be timed around beginning of menstrual flow to allow maximum visibility of endometriosis implants. Diaphragm, visceral and parietal pleura needs to be explored for endometriosis implants and all accessible lesions need to be excised [10]. We suspect catamenial pneumothorax in our case could be likely lymphatic or hematogenous spread of endometrial tissue to visceral pleura through pre-existing diaphragmatic defects and spontaneous rupture of blebs during hormonal changes. In our patient, she had an episode of pneumothorax seven days after menstruation and also had menstruation on postoperative day three. So, it is important to block the hormonal support from the ovary to the existing endometrial tissue, to prevent further seeding. Hormonal therapy such as a Gonadotropin-releasing hormone (GnRH) analogue, oral contraceptive pills, progestational drugs, and danazol will help to induce endometrial hypotrophy. Combination of surgery and hormonal treatment reduces recurrence [1, 11, 12].

4. Conclusion

Catamenial pneumothorax has a high rate of recurrence, nearly 30 to 40% [13]. Due to high rate of recurrence, these patients require a more aggressive approach of pleurodesis followed by hormonal treatment. Therefore, in an effort to prevent morbidity/mortality, it is important to consider catamenial pneumothorax in any young female presenting with pneumothorax during menses.

Consent

The authors would like to state that informed verbal consent was obtained from the patient to allow presentation of this case report.

Disclosure

The authors would like to state that the case report was presented as an e-poster at the 10th Annual Congress on Pulmonology & Respiratory Medicine, Feb 27th, 2019 at Paris, France.

Acknowledgments

The authors thank Dr. Vasudev Tati, Program Director, Department of Internal Medicine and Dr. Aaron Dewitt, Internal Medicine Faculty for reviewing the manuscript.

References

[1] A. N. Visouli, K. Darwiche, A. Mpakas et al., "Catamenial pneumothorax: A rare entity? Report of 5 cases and review of the literature," *Journal of Thoracic Disease*, vol. 4, Supplement 1, pp. 17–31, 2012.

[2] A. Bobbio, P. Carbognani, L. Ampollini, and M. Rusca, "Diaphragmatic laceration, partial liver herniation and catamenial pneumothorax," *Asian Cardiovascular and Thoracic Annals*, vol. 15, no. 3, pp. 249–251, 2007.

[3] A. Afzal, I. Wong, A. T. Reyes, I. Gulkarov, and B. Worku, "Catamenial Pneumothorax With Hepatic Herniation," *The Annals of Thoracic Surgery*, vol. 102, no. 5, p. e455, 2016.

[4] P. S. Y. Yu and A. D. L. Sihoe, "Beware the 'raised right hemidiaphragm' in a female patient with previous pneumothorax surgery: Liver herniation through a massive endometrosis-related diaphragmatic fenestration," *Journal of Thoracic Disease*, vol. 7, no. 5, pp. E112–E116, 2015.

[5] S. Sanna, M. Taurchini, M. Monteverde, V. Agnoletti, and G. L. Casoni, "Catamenially recurring pneumothorax with partial liver herniation: A particular view," *Respiration*, vol. 82, no. 5, pp. 476-477, 2011.

[6] M. Pryshchepau, D. Gossot, and P. Magdeleinat, "Unusual presentation of catamenial pneumothorax," *European Journal of Cardio-Thoracic Surgery*, vol. 37, no. 5, p. 1221, 2010.

[7] A. Tomescot and D. Fabre, "Catamenial pneumothorax with multiple transdiaphragmatic hepatic herniations," *Asian Cardiovascular and Thoracic Annals*, vol. 20, no. 2, p. 205, 2012.

[8] S. Attaran, A. Bille, W. Karenovics, and L. Lang-Lazdunski, "Videothoracoscopic repair of diaphragm and pleurectomy/abrasion in patients with catamenial pneumothorax: A 9-year experience," *CHEST*, vol. 143, no. 4, pp. 1066–1069, 2013.

[9] M. Alifano, R. Trisolini, A. Cancellieri, and J. F. Regnard, "Thoracic endometriosis: Current knowledge," *The Annals of Thoracic Surgery*, vol. 81, no. 2, pp. 761–769, 2006.

[10] S. Aissa, W. Benzarti, F. Alimi et al., "Catamenial pneumothorax revealing diaphragmatic endometriosis: A case report and revue of literature," *Pan African Medical Journal*, vol. 27, p. 112, 2017.

[11] J. Joseph and S. A. Sahn, "Thoracic endometriosis syndrome: New observations from an analysis of 110 cases," *American Journal of Medicine*, vol. 100, no. 2, pp. 164–170, 1996.

[12] T. Peikert, D. J. Gillespie, and S. D. Cassivi, "Catamenial pneumothorax," *Mayo Clinic Proceedings*, vol. 80, no. 5, pp. 677–680, 2005.

[13] P. Bagan, F. L. P. Barthes, J. Assouad, R. Souilamas, and M. Riquet, "Catamenial pneumothorax: Retrospective study of surgical treatment," *The Annals of Thoracic Surgery*, vol. 75, no. 2, pp. 378–381, 2003.

34

The Effect of Smoking on COVID-19 Symptom Severity

Askin Gülsen,[1] **Burcu Arpinar Yigitbas**,[2] **Berat Uslu**,[2] **Daniel Drömann**,[1] **and Oguz Kilinc**[3]

[1]*Department of Pneumology, Airway Research Center North (ARCN), Member of the German Center for Lung Research (DZL), University of Luebeck, Germany*
[2]*Department of Pneumology, Yedikule Chest Disease and Thoracic Surgery Hospital, Istanbul, Turkey*
[3]*Department of Pneumology, Dokuz Eylül University, Izmir, Turkey*

Correspondence should be addressed to Askin Gülsen; askingulsen@hotmail.com

Academic Editor: Roberto Walter Dal Negro

Background. Coronavirus disease 2019 (COVID-19) is caused by severe acute respiratory syndrome coronavirus 2 (SAR2-COV-2) and was first identified in Wuhan, China, in December of 2019, but quickly spread to the rest of the world, causing a pandemic. While some studies have found no link between smoking status and severe COVID-19, others demonstrated a significant one. The present study aimed to determine the relationship between smoking and clinical COVID-19 severity via a systematic meta-analysis approach. *Methods.* We searched the Google Scholar, PubMed, Scopus, Web of Science, and Embase databases to identify clinical studies suitable for inclusion in this meta-analysis. Studies reporting smoking status and comparing nonsevere and severe patients were included. Nonsevere cases were described as mild, common type, nonintensive care unit (ICU) treatment, survivors, and severe cases as critical, need for ICU, refractory, and nonsurvivors. *Results.* A total of 16 articles detailing 11322 COVID-19 patients were included. Our meta-analysis revealed a relationship between a history of smoking and severe COVID-19 cases ($OR = 2.17$; 95% CI: 1.37–3.46; $P < .001$). Additionally, we found an association between the current smoking status and severe COVID-19 ($OR = 1.51$; 95% CI: 1.12–2.05; $P < .008$). In 10.7% (978/9067) of nonsmokers, COVID-19 was severe, while in active smokers, severe COVID-19 occurred in 21.2% (65/305) of cases. *Conclusion.* Active smoking and a history of smoking are clearly associated with severe COVID-19. The SARS-COV-2 epidemic should serve as an impetus for patients and those at risk to maintain good health practices and discontinue smoking. The trial is registered with the International Prospective Register of Systematic Reviews (PROSPERO) CRD42020180173.

1. Introduction

Coronavirus disease 2019 (COVID-19), which is caused by severe acute respiratory syndrome coronavirus 2 (SAR2-COV-2), was first identified in Wuhan, China, in December of 2019. It has subsequently spread across the world, causing a global pandemic. This highly contagious disease has thus far infected 23.4 million people worldwide and killed approximately 808000 patients, yielding a case fatality rate (CFR) that varies between 0.7 and 12.7% (average: 3.4%) [1, 2].

COVID-19 primarily targets lung epithelial cells, causing viral pneumonia and acute respiratory distress syndrome (ARDS), especially in elderly patients. Therefore, mortality is higher in the elderly and in patients with at least one accompanying comorbid disease [3]. In the last report issued by the Centers for Disease Control and Prevention Institute, the incidence of respiratory disease was 9.2% in patients diagnosed with a severe COVID-19 clinical course [4]. Chronic obstructive pulmonary disease (COPD) and asthma are also common comorbidities in severe cases and are reported in

10.8% and 17.0%, respectively, of hospitalized patients aged ≥18 years with COVİD-19 [5].

However, it has been reported that COVID-19 progresses more severely in COPD patients [6]. Given that smoking plays an important role in the etiopathogenesis of COPD, it may have a similar effect on symptoms. In a recent meta-analysis of smoking and COVID-19 severity, smoking was found to not increase the severity of COVID-19 (odds ratio [OR], 1.69; 95% Cl: 0.41-6.92). However, only five studies were included in this meta-analysis, and heterogeneity among the studies was low ($I^2 = 38\%$) [7].

In another meta-analysis involving more studies, COVID-19 severity was found to increase with smoking (OR, 1.97; 95% Cl: 0.95-4.10) [6]. To increase the statistical power of this analysis, case reports and series were also included, not just case-control studies. As previously, the heterogeneity of the studies included here was also low ($I^2 = 44\%$) [6]. The different results of both meta-analyses create confusion about the issue of smoking status.

Given diverging findings in the existing literature, we systematically reviewed English-language studies to investigate whether smoking was associated with a more severe clinical course of COVID-19.

2. Material and Methods

All guidelines listed in the Preferred Reporting Items for Systematic Reviews and Meta Analyses (PRISMA) statement were followed in conducting this meta-analysis [8]. Our methodological systematic review and meta-analysis of pooled case-control studies were recorded in the International Prospective Register of Systematic Reviews (https://www.crd.york.ac.uk/prospero; registration number: CRD42020180173).

2.1. Study Search Strategy. We searched the Google Scholar, PubMed, Scopus, Web of Science, and Embase databases to identify clinical studies suitable for inclusion here. Only English-language articles published between December 2019 and April 15, 2020, were included. Case series/reports, commentaries, reviews, and editorial letters were excluded. Unpublished articles were not searched, but "ahead of print" and "first only" articles with a DOI link in the given database were included. The following search terms were used: "COVID-19," OR "SARS-COV-2," OR "novel coronavirus (nCOV)," AND "smoking," OR "tobacco," AND "clinical features," OR "characteristic," AND "severity," OR "severe".

2.2. Inclusion and Exclusion Criteria. Inclusion criteria were as follows: (i) studies that examined COVID-19 patients older than 18 years and diagnosed COVID-19 according to WHO criteria; (ii) observational, cross-sectional, prospective, or retrospective studies; (iii) studies which compared smokers with mild and severe COVID-19; (iv) studies comparing smokers with survivors and nonsurvivors of COVID-19; and (v) studies comparing smokers who developed COVID-19 that required intensive-care unit (ICU) and non-ICU treatment.

Exclusion criteria were as follows: (i) studies from the same medical center that did not contribute to meta-analysis, (ii) non-English-language studies, (iii) case reports/series, (iv) reviews, (v) editorial letters, (vi) studies lacking a full-text (unavailable or not yet published), (vii) studies without a DOI, and (viii) studies with small sample sizes (<50 patients) because of low statistical power.

2.3. Data Extraction. A researcher (AG) scanned study titles and abstracts obtained via an initial database search and included relevant ones in a secondary pool. Next, two independent researchers (AG and BU) evaluated the full text of these articles to determine whether they met study inclusion criteria. Any disputes were resolved by discussion and negotiation with a third investigator (BAY). Agreed-upon studies were included in the final meta-analysis.

The following data were obtained from all studies: title, first author, publication year, location, sample size, age (median), history of smoking (former or current), and distribution of nonsevere or severe COVID-19 status. Given these groups, we were able to compare nonsevere (mild, common type, non-ICU, survivors) and severe (critical, severe, ICU, nonsurvivors) COVID-19 cases.

2.4. Risk of Bias (Quality) Assessment. Two researchers (BAY and BU) evaluated the collected articles using the Newcastle-Ottawa scale (NOS) for study quality and risk of bias [9]. This scale evaluates three aspects of each study: (i) selection (0 to 4 points), (ii) comparability (0 to 2 points), and (iii) detection of the outcome of interest (0 to 3 points). According to the obtained total score, study quality was rated as follows: 0-3 points (poor), 4-6 points (intermediate), and 7-9 points (high). Studies with a high risk of bias were excluded during the meta-analysis phase.

2.5. Statistical Analyses. OpenMeta Analyst version 10.10 (https://www.cebm.brown.edu/open_meta) was used to calculate odds ratios with 95% confidence intervals, which are depicted using forest plots. Quantitative numbers were measured in terms of total numbers and percentages (*n*, %). The odds ratio of smokers among nonsevere COVID-19 and severe COVID-19 cases, as well as survivors and nonsurvivors, was calculated. Heterogeneity was evaluated with Cochran's Q, χ^2, and the Higgins I^2 test. The Higgins I^2 test uses a fixed effect model when $I^2 <50\%$, and a random effects model when $I^2 >50\%$. When heterogeneity was detected, a sensitivity adjustment was made to determine its source. This procedure was performed by leaving one study out of the analysis at a time, with a fixed effect model used after excluding heterogeneity. Publication bias was evaluated with Statsdirect version 3.2.10 (StatsDirect Ltd, Cambridge, UK) and visualized using Begg's funnel plots and Egger's test. P values (two-sided) were considered statistically significant if $P < .05$.

3. Results

Our initial search of international databases using the keywords described above yielded 265 articles. After duplicate articles were excluded, 197 articles remained. After article titles and abstracts were evaluated for appropriateness, a final 34 articles were found to meet study inclusion criteria. In

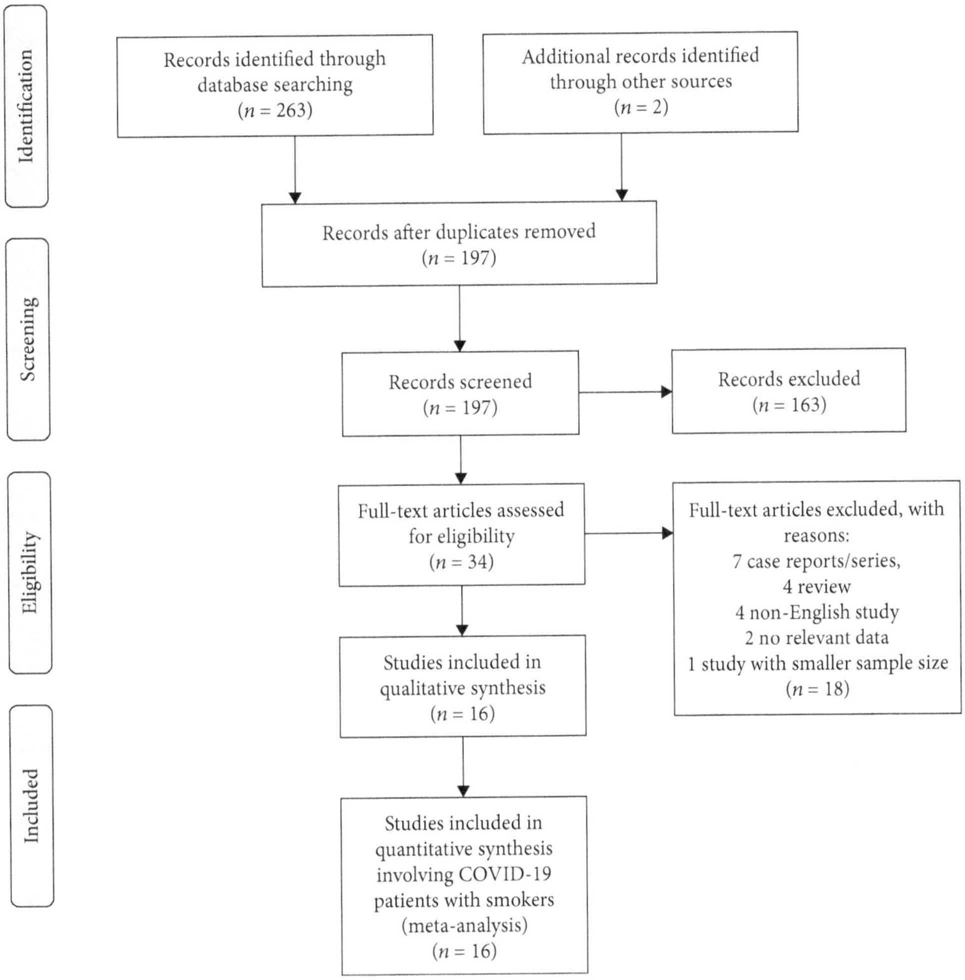

FIGURE 1: PRISMA flow diagram of study selection procedures.

addition, 18 of the studies for which full texts were obtained were excluded because they met exclusion criteria. A total of 16 articles met all our criteria. The relevant PRISMA study flow chart is shown in Figure 1. A quality analysis of the pooled articles included in this meta-analysis was done by applying NOS. As a result, overall quality was found to be moderate (NOS score min: 5, max: 8). Results of a quality analysis of the pooled articles are available in Table 1.

3.1. Features of the Included Studies. In the initial meta-analysis pool, 11322 patients with COVID-19 from 16 studies [4, 10–24] were included. However, given CDC reporting guidelines [4], 525 patients whose hospitalization statuses were reported as "unknown" were excluded from the final analysis, yielding a final 10797 patients. Of these, 9414 (87.2%) were nonsevere COVID-19 patients, while 1383 (12.8%) were severe or critical COVID-19 patients who required intensive care. Among the severe or critical patients, smoking prevalence ranged from 3.6 to 19.9% (average: 8.4%). While nine studies provided current smoker information, three provided both current smoker and former smoker information, and seven provided only historical smoking information. All of the included studies were retrospective (six multicenter and 10 single-center). A summary of the studies included in this meta-analysis is available in Table 2.

3.2. History of Smoking and COVID-19 Severity. The prevalence of smoking among patients with mild to moderate COVID-19 was 493/9414 (5.2%), while among severe and critical cases, it was 173/1383 (12.5%). A meta-analysis revealed a significant relationship between smoking history and severe COVID-19 (random effect model, OR = 2.17; 95% CI:1.37–3.46; $P < .001$) (Table 3) (Figure 2(a)). A funnel plot was used to evaluate publication bias and revealed substantial heterogeneity between the pooled studies (I^2 = 71.4%; $P < .001$) (Figure 2(b)). A sensitivity analysis conducted after removing two studies (Qi et al. [16] and Zhang et al. [23]), which were primary causes of heterogeneity, revealed that smoking was significantly related to COVID-19 severity (fixed effect model, OR = 1.85; 95% CI:1.50–2.29; $P < .001$) (Figure 2(c)). Furthermore, this updated analysis had low heterogeneity (I^2 = 40.6%; $P = .06$), while a funnel plot and Egger's test revealed no publication bias ($tau^2 = -0.87$, $P = .16$) (Figure 2(d)).

3.3. Smoking Status and COVID-19 Severity. Only 10 of the pooled studies provide information about current

Table 1: Newcastle-Ottawa scale for quality assessment and risk of bias.

Study	Year	Case selection (max. 4)	Comparability (max. 2)	Exposure/outcome (max. 3)	Total score
CDC report [4]	2020	****	*	**	7
Chen Q [10]	2020	***	*	**	6
Feng Y [11]	2020	**	*	***	6
Goyal P [12]	2020	**	—	***	5
Guan WJ [13]	2020	**	**	**	6
Liu W [14]	2020	**	*	*	7
Mo P [15]	2020	**	*	***	6
Qi D [16]	2020	***	*	***	7
Shi Y [17]	2020	**	*	**	5
Wang R [18]	2020	***	*	**	6
Wan S [19]	2020	***	*	***	7
Yang X [20]	2020	***	**	***	8
Yu X [21]	2020	***	**	**	7
Zhang JJ [22]	2020	***	**	**	7
Zhang R [23]	2020	***	*	**	6
Zhou F [24]	2020	***	*	***	7

Table 2: Features of the studies included in the meta-analysis.

First author	Location of patients	Study design	Comparison	n	Age, year	Prevalence of smoking	Former smokers	Current smokers
CDC report [4]	—	R, MC	Non-ICU vs. ICU	7162	—	261 (3.6)	165 (2.3)	96 (1.3)
Chen Q [10]	Taizhou, China	R, O, SC	Nonsevere vs. severe	145	47.5	15 (10.3)	—	—
Feng Y [11]	Wuhan, Anhui, Shanghai	R, O, MC	Moderate vs. severe, critical	454	53.0	44 (9.7)	—	—
Goyal P [12]	Newyork, USA	R, MC	Non-IMV vs. IMV	393	62.2	20 (5.1)	—	20 (5.1)
Guan WJ [13]	552 hospitals in China	R, MC	Nonsevere vs. severe	1085	47.0	158 (12.6)	21 (1.9)	137 (12.6)
Liu W [14]	Wuhan, China	R, SC	Stabilization vs. progression	78	38.0	5 (6.4)	—	—
Mo P [15]	Wuhan, China	R, SC	General vs. refractory	155	54.0	6 (3.9)	—	6 (3.9)
Qi D [16]	Chongqing, China	R, MC	Nonsevere vs. severe	267	48.0	53 (19.9)	—	—
Shi Y [17]	Zhejiang, China	R	Mild vs. severe	487	46.0	40 (8.2)	—	—
Wang R [18]	Fuyang, China	R, SC	Noncritical vs. ritical	125	49.4	16 (12.8)	—	16 (12.8)
Wan S [19]	Chongqing, China	R, SC	Mild vs. severe	135	47.0	9 (6.7)	—	9 (6.7)
Yang X [20]	Wuhan, China	R, O, SC	Survivors vs. nonsurvivors	52	51.9	2 (10.0)	—	—
Yu X [21]	Shanghai, China	R, SC	Nonsevere vs. severe	333	50.0	26 (7.8)	—	—
Zhang JJ [22]	Wuhan, China	R, SC	Nonsevere vs. severe	140	57.0	9 (6.4)	7 (5.0)	2 (1.4)
Zhang R [23]	Wuhan, China	R, SC	Common type vs. severe	120	45.4	6 (5.0)	—	6 (5.0)
Zhou F [24]	Wuhan, China	R, O, MC	Nonsurvivor vs. survivor	191	56.0	11 (6.0)	—	11 (6.0)

Data are presented as "n" or "n (%)." Age-related data are given as "median year." n: population; R: retrospective; CS: cross-sectional; O: observational; IMV: invasive mechanic ventilation; ICU: intensive care unit; SC: single-center; MC: multicenter.

smoking, specifically ($n = 305$). Current smoking prevalence in patients with mild to moderate COVID-19 was 229/7850 (2.9%), while in severe or critical cases, it was 66/1134 (5.8%). However, in 10.7% (978/9067) of nonsmokers, COVID-19 disease was severe, while in active smokers, it was severe in 21.2% (65/305) of cases (Table 4). This clearly demonstrates a significant relationship between current smoking and severe COVID-19 patients (fixed effect model, OR = 1.51; 95% CI: 1.12–2.05; $z = 2.65$; $P = .008$), with an approximate 1.5-fold increased risk of ICU admission, symptom, severity, and mortality in smokers (Figure 3(a)). In this analysis, we used a fixed effect model due to the low level

TABLE 3: The relationship between history of smoking and the severity of COVID-19.

Studies Authors	Severe COVID-19 with history of smoking Event	Total	%	Nonsevere COVID-19 with history of smoking Event	Total	%
CDC report [4]	38	457	8.3	208	6180	3.3
Chen et al. [10]	3	43	7.0	12	102	11.0
Feng et al. [11]	17	121	14.0	27	333	8.1
Goyal et al. [12]	6	130	4.6	14	263	5.3
Guan et al. [13]	38	172	22.0	120	913	13.0
Liu et al. [14]	3	11	27.3	2	67	2.0
Mo et al. [15]	4	85	4.7	2	70	2.9
Qi et al. [16]	31	50	62.0	22	217	10.1
Shi et al. [17]	6	49	12.2	34	438	7.8
Wang et al. [18]	7	25	28.0	9	100	9.0
Wan et al. [19]	1	40	2.5	8	95	8.4
Yang et al. [20]	0	32	0	2	20	10.0
Yu et al. [21]	2	26	8.0	24	307	8.9
Zhang et al. [22]	6	58	10.3	3	82	3.6
Zhang et al. [23]	6	30	20.0	0	90	0
Zhou et al. [24]	5	54	9.0	6	137	4.0
Total	173	1383	12.5	493	9414	5.2

of heterogeneity ($I^2 = 48.9\%$; $P = .40$). A funnel pilot and Egger's test revealed no publication bias ($tau^2 = 0.22$, $P = .77$) (Figure 3(b)).

A sensitivity analysis conducted after removing one study (Zhang et al. [23]) revealed a similar relationship with severe COVID-19 (fixed effect model; OR = 1.36; 95% CI: 1.00–1.87; $P = 0.05$) and low heterogeneity ($I^2 = 34.0\%$; $P = .14$) (Figure 3(c)). A funnel plot and Egger's test further revealed no publication bias ($tau^2 = -0.31$, $P = .67$) (Figure 3(d)).

4. Discussion

The present meta-analysis contained 16 studies and revealed that those with a history of smoking and active smokers had significantly increased risk for severe COVID-19. Previous studies have reported a similar result [14, 18, 23]. In addition, one prior meta-analysis reported that disease severity increased given a history of smoking (OR: 1.98) [6]. Our analysis adds to this growing consensus in the literature, invoking more studies and examining both a history of smoking and current smoking status in risk for increased COVID-19 severity.

Five prior studies have reported results which disagree with those presented here—namely, no significant difference between patients with and without a smoking history in terms of COVID-19 severity [10, 15, 21, 22, 24]. In addition, a meta-analysis performed by Lippi et al. [7] failed to find a relationship between active smoking and severe COVID-19 on Chinese patients, and another meta-analysis indicates that active smoking is not a predisposing factor for hospitalization [25]. First of all, both meta-analysis [7, 25] was not systematic and included no assessment of publication bias or study quality. As such, it should be considered only preliminary. Hence, the present systematic meta-analysis offers a more detailed view as it covers 16 studies. The heterogeneity was low to moderate, and after sensitivity adjustments, the prevalence of a history of smoking was found to be 5.2% in nonsevere COVID-19 cases and 12.5% in severe cases. Furthermore, the prevalence of active smoking was 2.9% in nonsevere COVID-19 cases and 5.8% in severe cases. Therefore, severe COVID-19 was observed almost 1.5 to 2 times more frequently in history of smoking and current smoking groups. There are studies [4, 11, 14, 16, 18, 23] and meta-analysis [6, 26–34] results supporting this finding.

In addition, a recent meta-analysis revealed that active smokers are at higher risk of mortality and serious complications [27]. Interestingly, this meta-analysis indicated that serious complications were observed in 48% of former smokers and 24% of current smokers during COVID-19 course [27]. This appears to be because former smokers have longer exposure times or accompanying diseases such as COPD due to smoking. This issue was explained recently in a rapid nonsystematic meta-analysis conducted by Guo FR, which showed that COPD increased the development of severe COVID-19 by 4.38 times [28]. These findings are supported by another rapid nonsystematic meta-analysis, suggesting that smoking increases the severity and mortality of COVID-19 in hospitalized patients [29]. In addition, a history of smoking has been reported to increase the progression of COVID-19 disease [30]. There is growing evidence to support WHO's statements that smokers are at a higher risk of developing severe COVID-19 and consequent death [31]. It seems very clear that the pandemic period is an opportunity to quit smoking due to the possibility of encountering worse clinical outcomes and complications in patients with smoking history [32].

The relationship between smoking and illness severity due to other respiratory viruses has been investigated

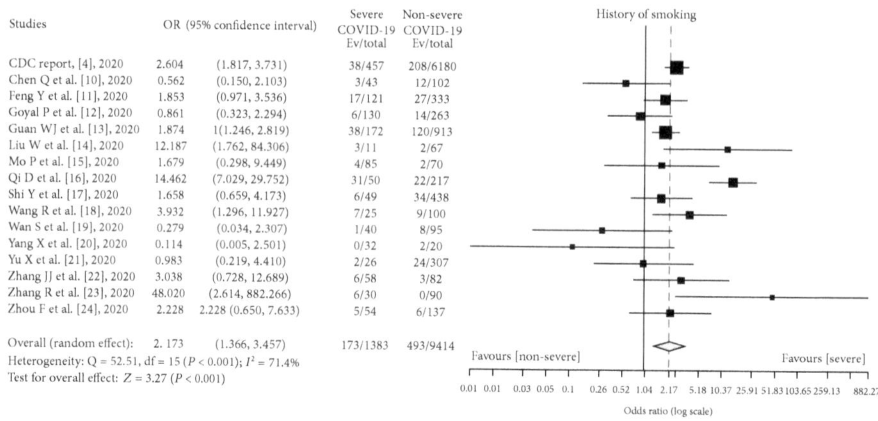

(a)

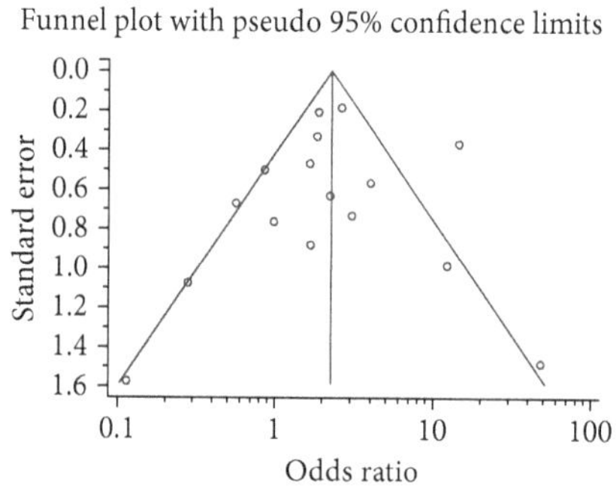

(b)

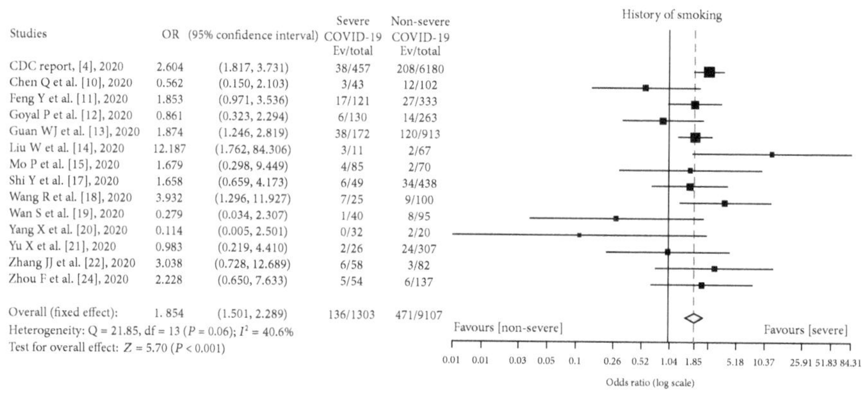

(c)

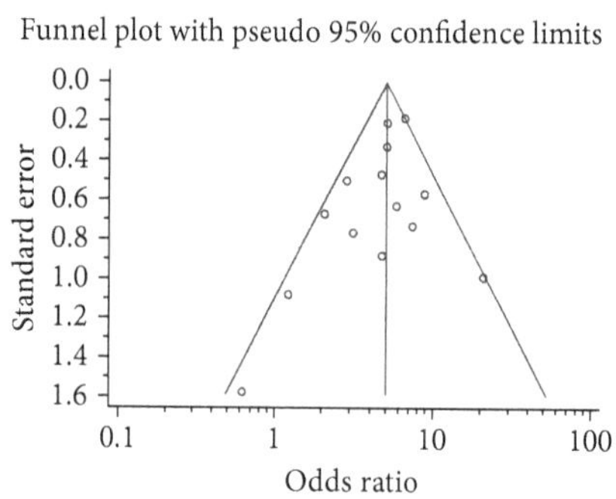

(d)

Figure 2: (a) Prevalence of smoking in severe COVID-19 patients. (b) Funnel plot for meta-analysis of the prevalence of smoking in severe COVID-19 patients. (c) Prevalence of smoking among severe COVID-19 patients after the exclusion of studies by Qi et al. [16] and Zhang et al. [23]. (d) Funnel plot for the meta-analysis of smoking among severe COVID-19 patients after the exclusion of studies by Qi D et al. [16] and Zhang R et al. [23].

Table 4: The relationship between smoking status and the severe COVID-19.

Studies Authors	Current smokers with severe COVID-19 Event	Total	%	Nonsmokers with severe COVID-19 Event	Total	%
CDC report [4]	5	96	8.3	419	6901	60.7
Goyal et al. [12]	6	20	30.0	124	373	33.2
Guan et al. [13]	29	137	21.1	134	927	14.4
Mo et al. [15]	4	6	66.6	81	149	54.3
Wang et al. [18]	7	16	43.7	18	109	16.5
Wan et al. [19]	1	9	11.1	39	126	30.9
Yang et al. [20]	0	2	0	32	50	64.0
Zhang et al. [22]	2	2	100	58	138	42.0
Zhang et al. [23]	6	6	100	24	114	21.0
Zhou et al. [24]	5	11	45.4	49	180	27.2
Total	65	305	21.3	978	9067	10.7

previously. In one recent study, COPD patients who smoked had decreased leukemia inhibitory factor levels during respiratory syncytial viral infection, particularly during exacerbations, which may have contributed to lung tissue injury [35]. In addition, smoking may reduce the protective effect of influenza vaccines in elderly patients and increase the risk of hospitalization [36]. As a result, adverse effects on the lungs in smokers may aggravate the symptom severity of viral infections.

Furthermore, novel SARS-CoV-2 uses an angiotensin-converting enzyme (ACE)-2 in the lungs to enter cells and cause infection. In patients using ACE inhibitors or angiotensin II receptor blockers (ARBs) for hypertension, upregulated ACE2 expression impacts on disease course remains unclear. However, the Council on Hypertension of the European Society of Cardiology does not recommend discontinuation of ACEI and ARB medications for all patients [37]. The ACE-2 upregulation may increase infectiousness and therefore infection risk, as the SARS-COV-2 virus uses this receptor for host entry. Paradoxically, it is stated that it may be useful in protecting people from acute lung injury [38].

In one recent study, ACE-2 gene expression was upregulated in the airway epithelium of COPD patients and active smokers, thereby suggesting a mechanism by which risk for severe COVID-19 increases in smokers [39]. This upregulation may occur through the α7 subtype of nicotine acetylcholine receptors (α7-nAChR) in people who smoke and consequently consume nicotine [40]. Therefore, α7-nAChR antagonists (e.g., α-conotoxin, methyllycaconitine), which may be used to assist with smoking cessation, should be investigated for their potential impact on ACE-2 expression and thus SARS-COV-2 entry into the host [41, 42]. Furthermore, α7-nAChR and ACE-2 may be potential therapeutic targets, a topic which requires further investigation.

Common comorbidities including cardiovascular disease, chronic kidney disease, diabetes, and hypertension are associated with increased risk for severe COVID-19 [43]. Similarly, COPD is also associated with a poor clinical progression and poor outcomes despite treatment, and it was reported that the risk of severe COVID-19 was observed 4 times higher in patients with preexisting COPD than in patients without COPD [6]. This may be explained by systemic and chronic inflammation, diminished respiratory function and capacity, and COPD-related respiratory failure in some patients. The prevalence of COPD was previously reported to be 2.8% in nonsmokers, 7.6% in former smokers, and 15.2% in active smokers [44]. Given this, smoking and COPD comorbidity should be considered together as a single risk factor for severe COVID-19.

Another important point for consideration is that acute respiratory distress syndrome and cytokine storms, which are seen in some severe COVID-19 patients, are key causes of mortality in COVID-19. In these patients, proinflammatory cytokines such as interleukin (IL)-1, IL-2, IL-6, IL-8, IL-17, interferon-γ, and TNF-α are elevated, which affect patients clinical symptoms and severity [45]. Nicotine is a cholinergic agonist that acts via the a7-nAChR pathway and also inhibits proinflammatory cytokines such as IL-1, IL-6, and TNF, but has no effect on IL-10, an anti-inflammatory cytokine [46]. Therefore, nicotine may be beneficial for the treatment of severe COVID-19 when delivered via chewing gum, inhaler/aerosol, or patch [47, 48]. This potential therapeutic application should be clarified with future clinical research, however.

Several factors limit the interpretation of the present study. First, the vast majority of studies included here were retrospective epidemiological studies conducted in China. Second, some included studies did not distinguish between former or current smoking status. Third, studies classified COVID-19 cases broadly as follows: (i) mild to moderate: mild, nonsevere, common type, did not require ICU care, and COVID-19 survivors and (ii) severe: severe, critical, required ICU care, and nonsurvivors. Given these limitations, caution should be exercised while interpreting our results. Future studies may respond to these issues by defining disease severity more clearly and by obtaining more detailed information about smoking habit.

In addition to classical tobacco smoking behavior, water pipe and electronic cigarette use should not be overlooked, as these modes of consumption may increase contamination risk due to repetitive hand interactions with the mouth,

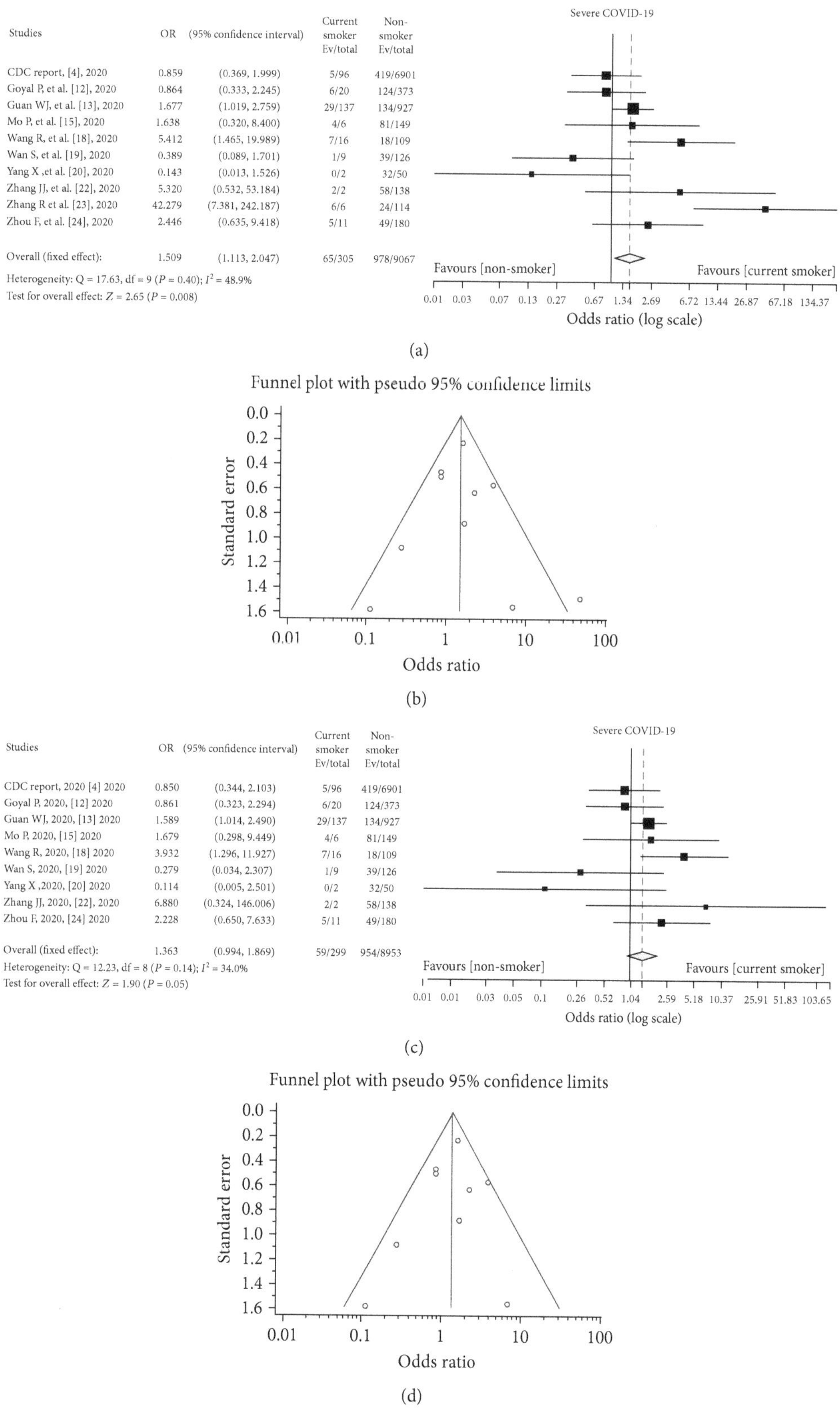

FIGURE 3: (a) Comparison of smoking status in severe COVID-19 patients. (b) Funnel plot for the meta-analysis of smoking among severe COVID-19 patients. (c) Comparison of smoking status among severe COVID-19 patients after the exclusion of a study by Zhang et al. [23]. (d) Funnel plot for the meta-analysis of smoking among severe COVID-19 patients after the exclusion of a study by Zhang et al. [23].

carrying cigarette packets in the pockets, and blowing of smoke. Similarly, exposure to passive smoke can alter ACE-2 gene expression and cause immune system changes. Naturally, these patients also have the potential to have severe COVID-19 symptoms, and smoke exposure is a potential risk factor for those around the patient, including their friends and family.

Future studies should continue to collect nicotine consumption information, including the number of cigarettes smoked per day, passive exposure, and degree of COPD, and should evaluate the dynamics of interactions between cigarette smoking and COVID-19. In addition, the effects of various smoking habits (e.g., mild versus heavy consumption, water pipe use, and electronic cigarettes use) on the transmission of SARS-COV-2, the clinical severity of COVID-19, and the clinical progression of COVID-19 should be investigated. Finally, the relationship between COPD severity and COVID-19, and the potential therapeutic effect of nicotine on severe COVID patients should also be examined and clarified. In addition, clinicians can pay more attention to the history of smoking of COVID-19 patients, and more further research may aim to determine mechanisms that drive or decrease this risk.

5. Conclusion

The present meta-analysis revealed that active smoking and a history of smoking are significantly associated with increased COVID-19 symptom severity. The SARS-COV-2 epidemic should serve as an impetus for patients and those at risk to maintain good health practices and discontinue smoking.

Authors' Contributions

AG performed the concept of the manuscript, data collection, design of tables and figures, analysis and interpretation of data, and writing and drafting of the manuscript; BU performed the data collection and quality analysis; BAY performed the acquisition of data, quality analysis, and writing and revising the manuscript; DD and OK performed the major role in reviewing and revising the manuscript.

Acknowledgments

Funding of the Federal Ministry for Science and Education (BMBF), German Center for Lung Research, is gratefully acknowledged.

References

[1] World Health Organisation, "Coronavirus disease (COVID-2019) situation reports," https://www.who.int/docs/default-source/coronaviruse/situation-reports/20200824-weekly-epi-update.pdf?sfvrsn=806986d1_4.

[2] Coronavirus Worldometer, "Country-specific case fatality rates (CFR) of COVID-19 patients," August 2020 https://www.worldometers.info/coronavirus/.

[3] J. Yang, Y. Zheng, X. Gou et al., Prevalence of comorbidities and its effects in patients infected with SARS-CoV-2: a systematic review and meta-analysis," *International Journal of Infectious Diseases*, vol. 94, pp. 91–95, 2020.

[4] CDC COVID-19 Response Team, CDC COVID-19 Response Team, N. Chow et al., "Preliminary Estimates of the Prevalence of Selected Underlying Health Conditions Among Patients with Coronavirus Disease 2019- United States, February 12-March 28, 2020," *MMWR. Morbidity and Mortality Weekly Report*, vol. 69, no. 13, pp. 382–386, 2020.

[5] S. Garg, L. Kim, M. Whitaker et al., "Hospitalization Rates and Characteristics of Patients Hospitalized with Laboratory-Confirmed Coronavirus Disease 2019 — COVID-NET, 14 States, March 1–30, 2020," *MMWR. Morbidity and Mortality Weekly Report*, vol. 69, no. 15, pp. 458–464, 2020.

[6] Q. Zhao, M. Meng, R. Kumar et al., "The impact of COPD and smoking history on the severity of COVID-19: A systemic review and meta-analysis," *Journal of Medical Virology*, 2020.

[7] G. Lippi and B. M. Henry, "Active smoking is not associated with severity of coronavirus disease 2019 (COVID-19)," *European Journal of Internal Medicine*, vol. 75, pp. 107-108, 2020.

[8] D. Moher, A. Liberati, J. Tetzlaff, D. G. Altman, and for the PRISMA Group, "Preferred reporting items for systematic reviews and meta-analyses: the PRISMA statement," *BMJ*, vol. 339, article b2535, 2009.

[9] G. A. Wells, B. Shea, D. O'Connell et al., *The Newcastle-Ottawa Scale (NOS) for assessing the quality of nonrandomised studies in meta-analyses*Ottawa Hospital Research InstituteMay 2020 http://www.ohri.ca/programs/clinical_epidemiology/oxford.asp.

[10] Q. Chen, Z. Zheng, C. Zhang et al., "Clinical characteristics of 145 patients with corona virus disease 2019 (COVID-19) in Taizhou, Zhejiang, China," *Infection*, vol. 48, no. 4, pp. 543–551, 2020.

[11] Y. Feng, Y. Ling, T. Bai et al., "COVID-19 with Different Severities: A Multicenter Study of Clinical Features," *American Journal of Respiratory and Critical Care Medicine*, vol. 201, no. 11, pp. 1380–1388, 2020.

[12] P. Goyal, J. J. Choi, L. C. Pinheiro et al., "Clinical Characteristics of Covid-19 in New York City," *The New England Journal of Medicine*, vol. 382, no. 24, pp. 2372–2374, 2020.

[13] W. J. Guan, Z. Y. Ni, Y. Hu et al., "Clinical Characteristics of Coronavirus Disease 2019 in China," *New England Journal of Medicine*, vol. 382, no. 18, pp. 1708–1720, 2020.

[14] W. Liu, Z. W. Tao, L. Wang et al., "Analysis of factors associated with disease outcomes in hospitalized patients with 2019 novel coronavirus disease," *Chinese Medical Journal*, vol. 133, no. 9, pp. 1032–1038, 2020.

[15] P. Mo, Y. Xing, Y. Xiao et al., "Clinical characteristics of refractory COVID-19 pneumonia in Wuhan, China," *Clinical Infectious Diseases*, 2020.

[16] Q. Di, X. Yan, X. Tang et al., "Epidemiological and clinical features of 2019-nCoV acute respiratory disease cases in

Chongqing municipality, China: a retrospective, descriptive, multiple-center study," *medRxiv*, 2020.

[17] Y. Shi, X. Yu, H. Zhao, H. Wang, R. Zhao, and J. Sheng, "Host susceptibility to severe COVID-19 and establishment of a host risk score: findings of 487 cases outside Wuhan," *Critical Care*, vol. 24, no. 1, 2020.

[18] R. Wang, M. Pan, X. Zhang et al., "Epidemiological and clinical features of 125 Hospitalized Patients with COVID-19 in Fuyang, Anhui, China," *International Journal of Infectious Diseases*, vol. 95, pp. 421–428, 2020.

[19] S. Wan, Y. Xiang, W. Fang et al., "Clinical features and treatment of COVID-19 patients in northeast Chongqing," *Journal of Medical Virology*, vol. 92, no. 7, pp. 797–806, 2020.

[20] X. Yang, Y. Yu, J. Xu et al., "Clinical course and outcomes of critically ill patients with SARS-CoV-2 pneumonia in Wuhan, China: a single-centered, retrospective, observational study," *The Lancet Respiratory Medicine*, vol. 8, no. 5, pp. 475–481, 2020.

[21] X. Yu, X. Sun, P. Cui et al., "Epidemiological and clinical characteristics of 333 confirmed cases with coronavirus disease 2019 in Shanghai, China," *Transboundary and Emerging Diseases*, vol. 67, no. 4, pp. 1697–1707, 2020.

[22] J. J. Zhang, X. Dong, Y. Y. Cao et al., "Clinical characteristics of 140 patients infected with SARS-CoV-2 in Wuhan, China," *Allergy*, vol. 75, no. 7, pp. 1730–1741, 2020.

[23] R. Zhang, H. Ouyang, L. Fu et al., "CT features of SARS-CoV-2 pneumonia according to clinical presentation: a retrospective analysis of 120 consecutive patients from Wuhan city," *European Radiology*, vol. 30, no. 8, pp. 4417–4426, 2020.

[24] F. Zhou, T. Yu, R. Du et al., "Clinical course and risk factors for mortality of adult inpatients with COVID-19 in Wuhan, China: a retrospective cohort study," *Lancet*, vol. 395, no. 10229, pp. 1054–1062, 2020.

[25] K. Farsalinos, A. Barbouni, and R. Niaura, "Systematic review of the prevalence of current smoking among hospitalized COVID-19 patients in China: could nicotine be a therapeutic option?," *Internal and Emergency Medicine*, vol. 15, no. 5, pp. 845–852, 2020.

[26] A. Emami, F. Javanmardi, N. Pirbonyeh, and A. Akbari, "Prevalence of Underlying Diseases in Hospitalized Patients with COVID-19: a Systematic Review and Meta-Analysis," *Archives of Academic Emergency Medicine*, vol. 8, no. 1, article e35, 2020.

[27] J. S. Alqahtani, T. Oyelade, A. M. Aldhahir et al., "Prevalence, Severity and Mortality associated with COPD and Smoking in patients with COVID-19: A Rapid Systematic Review and Meta-Analysis," *PLOS ONE*, vol. 15, no. 5, article e0233147, 2020.

[28] F. R. Guo, "Smoking links to the severity of COVID-19: An update of a meta-analysis," *Journal of Medical Virology*, 2020.

[29] A. Karanasos, K. Aznaouridis, G. Latsios et al., "Impact of Smoking Status on Disease Severity and Mortality of Hospitalized Patients With COVID-19 Infection: A Systematic Review and Meta-analysis," *Nicotine & Tobacco Research*, 2020.

[30] R. Patanavanich and S. A. Glantz, "Smoking is Associated with COVID-19 Progression: A Meta-Analysis,," *Nicotine & Tobacco Research*, 2020.

[31] E. Grundy, T. Suddek, F. T. Filippidis, A. Majeed, and S. Coronini-Cronberg, "Smoking, SARS-CoV-2 and COVID-19: A review of reviews considering implications for public health policy and practice," *Tobacco Induced Diseases*, vol. 18, 2020.

[32] R. K. Reddy, W. N. Charles, A. Sklavounos, A. Dutt, P. T. Seed, and A. Khajuria, "The effect of smoking on COVID-19 severity: A systematic review and meta-analysis," *Journal of Medical Virology*, 2020.

[33] K. Farsalinos, A. Barbouni, K. Poulas, R. Polosa, P. Caponnetto, and R. Niaura, "Current smoking, former smoking, and adverse outcome among hospitalized COVID-19 patients: a systematic review and meta-analysis," *Therapeutic Advances in Chronic Disease*, vol. 11, 2020.

[34] D. C. Sanchez-Ramirez and D. Mackey, "Underlying respiratory diseases, specifically COPD, and smoking are associated with severe COVID-19 outcomes: A systematic review and meta-analysis," *Respiratory Medicine*, vol. 171, article 106096, 2020.

[35] J. Poon, M. Campos, R. F. Foronjy et al., "Cigarette smoke exposure reduces leukemia inhibitory factor levels during respiratory syncytial viral infection," *International Journal of Chronic Obstructive Pulmonary Disease*, vol. 14, pp. 1305–1315, 2019.

[36] P. Godoy, J. Castilla, N. Soldevila et al., "Smoking may increase the risk of influenza hospitalization and reduce influenza vaccine effectiveness in the elderly," *European Journal of Public Health*, vol. 28, no. 1, pp. 150–155, 2018.

[37] European Society of Cardiology, "Position Statement of the ESC Council on Hypertension on ACE-Inhibitors and Angiotensin Receptor Blockers," March 2020 https://www.escardio.org/Councils/Council-on-Hypertension-(CHT)/News/position-statement-of-the-esc-council-on-hypertension-on-ace-inhibitors-and-ang.

[38] S. H. Javanmard, K. Heshmat-Ghahdarijani, and G. Vaseghi, "Angiotensin-converting-enzyme inhibitors (ACE inhibitors) and angiotensin II receptor blocker (ARB) use in COVID-19 prevention or treatment: A paradox," *Infection Control and Hospital Epidemiology*, pp. 1-2, 2020.

[39] J. M. Leung, C. X. Yang, A. Tam et al., "ACE-2 expression in the small airway epithelia of smokers and COPD patients: implications for COVID-19," *European Respiratory Journal*, vol. 55, no. 5, article 2000688, 2020.

[40] P. Russo, S. Bonassi, R. Giacconi, M. Malavolta, C. Tomino, and F. Maggi, "COVID-19 and smoking: is nicotine the hidden link?," *European Respiratory Journal*, vol. 55, no. 6, article 2001116, 2020.

[41] J. M. Leung, C. X. Yang, and D. D. Sin, "COVID-19 and nicotine as a mediator of ACE-2," *European Respiratory Journal*, vol. 55, no. 6, article 2001261, 2020.

[42] L. Ramachandran Nair and X. Liu, "Targeting the $\alpha 4\beta 2$- and $\alpha 7$-Subtypes of Nicotinic Acetylcholine Receptors for Smoking Cessation Medication Development," *Journal of Addiction Research & Therapy*, vol. 10, no. 2, p. 381, 2019.

[43] X. Wang, X. Fang, Z. Cai et al., "Comorbid Chronic Diseases and Acute Organ Injuries Are Strongly Correlated with Disease Severity and Mortality among COVID-19 Patients: A Systemic Review and Meta-Analysis," *Research*, vol. 2020, pp. 1–17, 2020.

[44] A. G. Wheaton, Y. Liu, J. B. Croft et al., "Chronic Obstructive Pulmonary Disease and Smoking Status — United States, 2017," *MMWR. Morbidity and Mortality Weekly Report*, vol. 68, no. 24, pp. 533–538, 2019.

[45] D. McGonagle, K. Sharif, A. O'Regan, and C. Bridgewood, "The Role of Cytokines including Interleukin-6 in COVID-19 induced Pneumonia and Macrophage Activation Syndrome-

Like Disease," *Autoimmunity Reviews*, vol. 19, no. 6, article 102537, 2020.

[46] L. Ulloa, "The vagus nerve and the nicotinic anti-inflammatory pathway," *Nature Reviews. Drug Discovery*, vol. 4, no. 8, pp. 673–684, 2005.

[47] S. Zi, J. Li, L. Liu, and F. Liu, "Cholinergic anti-inflammatory pathway and its role in treatment of sepsis," *Journal of Central South University. Medical Sciences*, vol. 45, no. 1, pp. 68–73, 2020.

[48] K. Farsalinos, R. Niaura, J. Le Houezec et al., "Editorial: Nicotine and SARS-CoV-2: COVID-19 may be a disease of the nicotinic cholinergic system," *Toxicology Reports*, vol. 7, pp. 658–663, 2020.

35

Safety and Feasibility of a Novel Protocol for Percutaneous Dilatational Tracheostomy in Patients with Respiratory Failure due to COVID-19 Infection: A Single Center Experience

Ziad Boujaoude,[1] **Nagendra Madisi**,[1] **Bhavi Patel**,[1] **Jean-Sebastien Rachoin**,[2] **R. Phillip Dellinger**,[2] and **Wissam Abouzgheib**[1]

[1]*Division of Pulmonary and Interventional Pulmonary Medicine, Department of Medicine, Cooper University Health Care, Cooper Medical School of Rowan University, Camden, NJ, USA*
[2]*Division of Critical Care Medicine, Department of Medicine, Cooper University Health Care, Cooper Medical School of Rowan University, Camden, NJ, USA*

Correspondence should be addressed to Ziad Boujaoude; boujaoude-ziad@cooperhealth.edu

Academic Editor: Stefano Centanni

Introduction. The rapidly spreading Novel Coronavirus 2019 (COVID-19) appeared to be a highly transmissible pathogen in healthcare environments and had resulted in a significant number of patients with respiratory failure requiring tracheostomy, an aerosol-generating procedure that places healthcare workers at high risk of contracting the infection. Instead of deferring or delaying the procedure, we developed and implemented a novel percutaneous dilatational tracheostomy (PDT) protocol aimed at minimizing the risk of transmission while maintaining favorable procedural outcome. *Patients and Methods.* All patients who underwent PDT per novel protocol were included in the study. The key element of the protocol was the use of apnea during the critical part of the insertion and upon any opening of the ventilator circuit. This was coupled with the use of enhanced personnel protection equipment (PPE) with a powered air-purifying respirator (PAPR). The operators underwent antibody serology testing and were evaluated for COVID-19 symptoms two weeks from the last procedure included in the study. *Results.* Between March 12th and June 30th, 2020, a total of 32 patients underwent PDT per novel protocol. The majority (80%) were positive for COVID-19 at the time of the procedure. The success rate was 94%. Only one patient developed minor self-limited bleeding. None of the proceduralists developed positive serology or any symptoms compatible with COVID-19 infection. *Conclusion.* A novel protocol that uses periods of apnea during opening of the ventilator circuit along with PAPR-enhanced PPE for PDT on COVID-19 patients appears to be effective and safe for patients and healthcare providers.

1. Introduction

Since it was first identified in Wuhan City, Hubei Province, China, on December 30th, 2019, the Novel Coronavirus 2019 (COVID-19) has spread rapidly and widely resulting in a worldwide pandemic, affecting over 22 million persons worldwide and causing over 700 thousand deaths to date [1]. While the majority of infected patients do not develop severe disease, around 15% may develop significant dyspnea and hypoxemia and 5% may evolve to respiratory failure, acute respiratory distress syndrome (ARDS), and/or multiorgan failure that require invasive ventilatory support for an extended period of time [2, 3]. Tracheostomy is a common procedure for those critically ill patients, but it is an aerosol-generating procedure that places healthcare workers (HCW) at risk of infection during insertion and subsequent care. Similar to the severe acute respiratory syndrome (SARS) pandemic in 2003, COVID-19 appeared to be a highly transmissible pathogen in healthcare environments [4].

At the beginning of the current pandemic, medical societies and experts have recommended to delay or avoid tracheostomies in this population. The American Academy of Otolaryngology and the Ears, Nose, and Throat Surgery in the United Kingdom, have stated that providers should "avoid tracheotomy in COVID-19 positive or suspected patients" due to the risks to healthcare providers. They recommended that tracheostomies should not be performed before 2-3 weeks after intubation, preferably after negative COVID-19 testing, and favored open tracheostomy placement in these circumstances as opposed to percutaneous dilatational tracheostomy (PDT) [5, 6]. Earlier tracheostomy, however, would assist in resource preservation by facilitating weaning from mechanical ventilation as well as throughput to a lower level of care [7]. PDT is routinely performed in our medical ICU by the interventional pulmonary service. This emerging situation presented us with a new challenge of maintaining a balance between providing medical care to those in need while limiting disease spread and exposure to patients and staff. The decision was made at our institution to not delay tracheostomy based on the presence of COVID-19 but instead to establish a protocol that would facilitate safe PDT. We developed and implemented a novel protocol that introduced several modifications to the standard technique designed to minimize the risk of aerosolization of the virus while maintaining a low risk of complications. We report in this study the feasibility of this novel protocol and its safety for the patients and the providers.

2. Patients and Methods

2.1. Patient Population. We collected data on all patients admitted to the intensive care unit (ICU) at Cooper University Hospital (CUH), from March 12th to June 30th, 2020, who had confirmed COVID-19 by nasal pharyngeal swab for reverse transcriptase polymerase chain reaction (rtPCR) assay, who required mechanical ventilation for severe respiratory failure, and who underwent PDT per novel protocol by the interventional pulmonary service. The CUH institutional review board approved this study (IRB #120-00475).

2.2. Novel Percutaneous Tracheostomy Protocol. PDT was performed at the bedside in the patient's ICU room. Timing of the procedure should be at least 2 weeks from time of intubation in line with our standard procedure. A negative PCR was preferable but not necessary. The team participants were limited to only essential personnel—this included one of the two hospital interventional pulmonologist, one of the two interventional pulmonary fellows in training, a registered nurse, and a respiratory therapist. A technician and nearby nurses were available outside the room to obtain equipment or medications as needed. All equipment and medications were checked prior to entering the room and then were taken into the room, including an extra supply of medication that potentially may be used. Backup equipment was left immediately outside the room with a technologist to be readily available if needed. A powered air-purifying respirator (PAPR) with standard donning (per CDC guidelines) was utilized by all four members of the team along with an N95 mask under the PAPR hood as a backup in case of an unexpected malfunction [8]. Full sedation and analgesia were used as well as neuromuscular blockade, to prevent cough and minimize aerosolization.

Mechanical ventilation setting thresholds recommended to proceed with PDT were a positive end expiratory pressure (PEEP) ≤ 12 mmHg and a fraction of inspired oxygen (FIO_2) ≤ 60%. A 60-second apnea test on 100% FIO_2 was performed to assess the patient's ability to tolerate apnea during the critical part of the procedure. The ventilator was placed on standby while the patient's oxygen saturations and hemodynamics were monitored for 60 seconds. If at any point during the apnea the patient experienced oxygen desaturation below 90% and or hemodynamic instability, the apnea test was aborted, and the procedure deferred. After passing the apnea test, the patient was fully draped in sterile fashion to avoid any contamination of equipment and bed. Ventilation was paused for the introduction of a bronchoscope into the endotracheal tube (ETT).

A single-use flexible Ambu® aScope™ (Ambu A/S, Ballerup, Denmark) was used. Once the bronchoscope was introduced, ventilation was resumed. The bronchoscopist and the respiratory therapist retracted the endotracheal tube (ETT) in harmony, while maintaining an adequate intraluminal view of the trachea until ETT was just proximal to the 1st tracheal ring. The cuff of the ETT remained inflated to minimize any aerosolization. Then, the main operator proceeded with incision and needle insertion between the first and second tracheal ring under direct visualization via bronchoscope. Of note, the syringe attached to the needle was not removed immediately. Ventilation was then paused, at which point the rest of the procedure was performed under the standard PDT technique. Once tracheostomy was inserted and visualized with the bronchoscope from above through the ETT, the cuff was inflated, the inner cannula was immediately inserted, the ventilator was attached via flexible tubing, and ventilation was resumed. $EtCO_2$ was not checked, but inspiratory and expiratory volumes were observed on the ventilator. (Table 1).

2.3. End Points. The endpoints for this study were the safety and feasibility of our PDT protocol, the healthcare providers' contraction of COVID-19 virus (development of COVID-19 symptoms and/or positive serology testing), and posttracheostomy early patients' outcome. The constant members of the tracheostomy team included the four physicians. They all agreed to testing with COVID-19 antibody serology (IgG and IgM against SARS-CoV-2) and an evaluation for COVID-19 symptoms fourteen days from the last procedure included in the study. The other members were variable and included different nurses and respiratory therapists working in the ICU. Individual evaluation for the variable members was not possible.

3. Results (Table 2)

Between March 12th and June 30th, 2020, a total of 32 patients underwent PDT using the novel protocol. The majority (80%) were PCR positive at the time of procedure. The mean age was 54 ± 12 years; 50% were male; the mean body mass index (BMI) was 33 ± 10. At the time of tracheostomy, all patients had FIO_2 and PEEP less than 60% and 12, respectively, with mean FIO_2 of 44 ± 8 and PEEP of 8 ± 3.

Table 1: Novel PDT protocol.

(1) Equipment and medication checklist prior to entering room
Disposable bronchoscope function check
Tracheostomy kit verification
Sedative and neuromuscular blocker drawing
(2) Universal protocol and time out outside the room followed by donning of augmented PPE (N95 and PAPR)
(3) Apnea trial before start to mimic apnea
100% FIO_2 and current PEEP
Place ventilator on standby for 60 seconds
Pass test if able to tolerate without desaturations
(4) Administer sedatives and paralytics to minimize cough and movement
(5) Short apnea to add adaptor to circuit and insert bronchoscope in the ETT
(6) Pull back ETT while keeping cuff inflated
(7) Local anesthesia, incision, and insertion of introducer needle and angiocatheter by most experienced operator
(8)Place ventilator on standby and complete dilation and insertion of tracheostomy tube
(9) Connect ventilator to tracheostomy, inflate tracheostomy cuff, and resume ventilation. Verify inspiratory and expiratory volumes
(10) Remove the ETT and bronchoscope en bloc from oropharynx directly in a bag

PDT=percutaneous dilatational tracheostomy; PPE=personnel protective equipment; PAPR=powered air-purifying respirator; ETT=endotracheal tube.

Table 2: Clinical characteristics of COVID-19 patients undergoing PDT.

Variable	PDT patients ($n = 32$)
Age (y)	54 ± 12
Gender (male/female)	16/16
Body mass index (kg/m^2)	33 ± 10 (min 17-max 66) 17 > 30
PCR positive at the time of PDT	20, 5 false negative
FIO_2	44 ± 8 (min 30-max 70)
PEEP	8 ± 3 (min 5-max 14)
Anticoagulation at the time of PDT	24
ECMO at any time/ECMO at time of PDT	7/0
Days on ventilator before PDT	22 ± 8 (min 14-max 39)
Follow-up after PDT (d)	17 ± 10 (min 4-max 45)
Follow-up after initial intubation	40 ± 14 (min 22-max 72)
Outcome	
Weaned from MV	18 (56%)
Remain on MV	5 (16%)
Death	9 (28%)

The procedure was successful in 30 of 32 patients (94%). All patients passed the apnea test. In two patients, there was variation from the set protocol. In one patient, desaturation occurred after needle insertion; the ET tube was then advanced and positioned above the carina with dilation and insertion performed next to the ETT. In another patient, the flow was restarted after needle insertion due to severe desaturation. There were no direct complications related to the tracheostomy procedure. Only an early onset minor bleeding was present in one patient and self-resolved.

3.1. Healthcare Providers' Outcome. None of the four proceduralists developed symptoms suggestive of COVID-19 infection and none tested positive for COVID-19 antibodies. None have missed any days of work and to this date all continue to perform their usual clinical duties.

3.2. Early Patients' Outcome. The mean time from the start of invasive mechanical ventilation to PDT was 22 ± 8 days. The mean follow-up for all the patients after starting mechanical ventilation was 40 ± 14 days, and after PDT, it was 17 ± 10 days. Of the 32 patients who underwent a PDT, 18 patients were weaned from MV (56%), 5 remained on full ventilator support (16%), and 9 died as a result of respiratory and/or multiorgan failure (28%).

4. Discussion

We describe in this retrospective study a novel protocol for percutaneous placement of tracheostomy in patients with respiratory failure due to COVID-19 infection. It was designed to minimize the risk of healthcare workers' aerosol exposure while maintaining optimal procedural safety and outcome. To our knowledge, this study is the first to report on operator's safe outcome for COVID-19 contraction during tracheostomy. We have demonstrated the protocol to be safe and effective with no negative impact on patients or staff.

Tracheostomy is a major aerosol-generating procedure that was identified as a leading cause of viral transmission and superspreading events during the SARS outbreak in 2003 [5]. A systematic review of 10 studies from the 2003 SARS outbreak suggests that tracheostomy has an OR of 4.2 for risk of transmission to healthcare workers (HCWs) [9]. While severe acute respiratory syndrome coronavirus 2 (SARS-CoV-2) is associated with lower mortality than the related viruses that cause severe acute SARS and Middle East respiratory syndrome (MERS), it appears to have a higher infectivity and rates of transmission [10]. An early report of infections related to aerosol-generating procedures has already emerged in the current pandemic [11].

When the influx of COVID-19 critically ill patients admitted to our ICUs began to accelerate in early March, the available data regarding guidance on how to mitigate the risk of transmission was very limited [10, 12–14]. We were faced with the need to rapidly develop and implement a PDT protocol aimed at minimizing the risk of aerosol exposure to the staff while maintaining safe and effective care to the patients in need.

Tracheostomy procedures are performed at bedside in the ICU to minimize the risk of transmission during transport. Since not all rooms are negative pressure flow rooms, enhanced PPE with PAPR was used by all members of the team.

The main focus of the protocol was on maintaining a closed ventilator circuit at all times and opening only during periods of apnea. A major advantage of our protocol compared with a standard bedside PDT is the avoidance of an open-air system that leads to active ventilation/aerosolization through most of the procedure. Equally important was the use of standard timing for the procedure, a short procedural time, adequate sedation and paralytics, and the use of a disposable scope.

The protocol allows the cuff to remain inflated during the ETT retraction into the subglottic area and the ability to place the ventilator on standby when adding the adapter to the circuit, inserting the scope in the ETT and during the insertion of tracheostomy. The protocol required patient qualification characteristics of a PEEP lower than 12 cm H_2O and an FIO_2 lower than 60%. A negative apnea test (absence of desaturations or hemodynamic instability while ventilator is placed on standby for one minute) was also required in order to consider if the patient is able to tolerate the apnea during the procedure. The cut-offs for PEEP and FIO_2 are similar to those that we use for non-COVID patients in our practice. The duration of the apnea test was arbitrary. Based on our experience, it does not take more than 60 seconds for an experienced operator to insert the tracheostomy from the time of successful needle insertion between the tracheal rings. The combination of PEEP/FIO_2 cut-off of 12 cm H_2O/60% and a negative apnea test appears to be a good predictor of apnea tolerance.

In order to minimize apnea time, all steps up to the insertion of the needle in the airway were performed before scope insertion. Identifying the landmarks, skin incision, and insertion of the needle were performed by the most experienced operator, and the apnea was not initiated until precise insertion of needle was confirmed.

A conventional timing for tracheostomy of 2 weeks from time of intubation for patients with ongoing mechanical ventilation was adopted for the protocol. Although early tracheostomy has clear benefits, including lower sedation requirements and increased patient comfort [15], the data regarding the optimum timing of tracheostomy is conflicting [16, 17] and published literature does not clearly support a mortality benefit or reduction of ventilator-associated pneumonia with earlier tracheostomy [18]. Our standard ICU general criteria based on days of mechanical ventilation is 14 days with the caveat that the patient is not improving as to weaning capability. Given that published reports from China and Italy demonstrated that COVID-19 has a high ICU mortality [19], it seemed prudent to wait until the course of disease is declared before committing patients to earlier tracheostomy and leading to procedures in patients who may not need it altogether during the course of their illness. Two weeks seemed an appropriate timing in that light.

A negative PCR test was not required as the results of the test would not impact the decision on protective measures. The test has variable sensitivity in clinical practice ranging from 37% to 71% [20]. The immune response (antiviral antibody) is more reliable in predicting infectivity, but serology testing was not available. Recent data also shows that patients may remain PCR positive despite no longer having viable virus and capability to transmit [21].

Guidance with bronchoscopy is routinely used by interventional pulmonologists during PDT, and the procedure has been demonstrated to be safe and effective. We restricted the use to disposable bronchoscopes. It allows a lower number of support staff and does not require reprocessing. This minimizes both the staff exposed and the surfaces needed to be disinfected post procedure in addition to preservation of critical PPE. Of note, bronchoscopy has been commonly required in critically ill patients with COVID-19 to manage complications like atelectasis and hemoptysis, particularly for patients on ECMO, and to obtain samples for microbiological cultures [22, 23]. We favor the use of a disposable bronchoscope for these indications.

A key finding of this study is that all four physicians providing the procedure were COVID-19 negative by symptoms and/or by serology 14 days after the last procedure included in the study. The sensitivity of serologic testing since the time of infection is very high, and the rate of positive IgG approaches 100 percent at 19 days [24]. All physicians wore enhanced PPE during the procedure. Although the use of PPE and PAPR has been reported to limit communication (hearing) among members of the team, no issues were reported as a consequence of wearing PPE [25]. While the availability of PAPR may represent a potential limitation to implementing our protocol, given the limited number of PAPR used and the nonurgent nature of the procedure, we believe that this will not be an issue for most intensive care units.

The use of apnea during tracheostomy is not new. A recent report by Niroula et al. described the use of apnea during tracheostomy on COVID patients [26]. They concluded that the technique is safe, but they did not report on healthcare workers' safety. To our knowledge, our study is the first to report on operators' safe outcome for COVID-19 contraction. Furthermore, their apnea duration was significantly longer with an average of 3.96 min versus less than one minute in our study. This is due to a major difference between protocols. We did not initiate apnea until we confirmed adequate insertion of the needle. A shorter time of ventilation disruption provide a major advantage for patients with limited respiratory reserve in terms of ability to tolerate the procedure.

The main limitation of this study is that not all healthcare workers involved in the procedure were tested or evaluated for COVID-19 contraction, but this was not possible due to the large number of nurses and respiratory therapists providing care to ICU patients and the inability to have a dedicated group for the procedures.

In summary, this novel protocol is associated with a high success rate and appears to be safe for patients and healthcare providers. It is described in detail and is easy to implement.

Future larger and controlled studies to confirm these findings will be valuable.

References

[1] *Coronavirus COVID-19 global cases by the Center for Systems Science and Engineering (CSSE) at Johns Hopkins University*August 2020, https://coronavirus.jhu.edu/map.html.

[2] C. M. Petrilli, S. A. Jones, J. Yang et al., "Factors associated with hospital admission and critical illness among 5279 people with coronavirus disease 2019 in New York City: prospective cohort study," *BMJ*, vol. 369, 2020.

[3] Z. Wu and J. M. McGoogan, "Characteristics of and important lessons from the coronavirus disease 2019 (COVID-19) outbreak in China: summary of a report of 72 314 cases from the Chinese Center for Disease Control and Prevention," *Journal of the American Medical Association*, vol. 323, no. 13, pp. 1239–1242, 2020.

[4] K. Tran, K. Cimon, M. Severn, C. L. Pessoa-Silva, and J. Conly, "Aerosol generating procedures and risk of transmission of acute respiratory infections to healthcare workers: a systematic review," *PLoS One*, vol. 7, no. 4, article e35797, 2012.

[5] N. P. Parker, B. A. Schiff, M. A. Fritz et al., *Tracheotomy recommendations during the COVID-19 pandemic. Airway and Swallowing Committee of the American Academy of Otolaryngology-Head and Neck Surgery*April 2020, https://www.entnet.org/content/tracheotomy-recommendations-during-covid-19-pandemic.

[6] *Guidance for surgical tracheostomy and tracheostomy tube change during the COVID-19 pandemic*April 2020, https://www.entuk.org/tracheostomy-guidance-during-covid-19-pandemic.

[7] C. C. Tong, A. J. Kleinberger, J. Paolino, and K. W. Altman, "Tracheotomy timing and outcomes in the critically ill," *Otolaryngology and Head and Neck Surgery*, vol. 147, no. 1, pp. 44–51, 2012.

[8] *Using personal protective equipment (PPE). How to put on (don) PPE gear. How to take off (doff) PPE gear*https://www.cdc.gov/coronavirus/2019-ncov/hcp/using-ppe.html.

[9] W. Q. Chen, W. H. Ling, C. Y. Lu et al., "Which preventive measures might protect health care workers from SARS?," *BMC Public Health*, vol. 9, no. 1, p. 81, 2009.

[10] J. K. Tay, M. L. Khoo, and W. S. Loh, "Surgical considerations for tracheostomy during the COVID-19 pandemic: lessons learned from the severe acute respiratory syndrome outbreak," *JAMA Otolaryngology–Head & Neck Surgery*, vol. 146, 2020.

[11] J. Chu, N. Yang, Y. Wei et al., "Clinical characteristics of 54 medical staff with COVID-19: a retrospective study in a single center in Wuhan, China," *Journal of Medical Virology*, vol. 92, no. 7, pp. 807–813, 2020.

[12] UK ENT, "Guidance for surgical tracheostomy and tracheostomy tube change during the COVID-19 pandemic," 2020, https://www.entuk.org/tracheostomy-guidance-during-covid-19-pandemic.

[13] B. Givi, B. A. Schiff, S. B. Chinn et al., "Safety recommendations for evaluation and surgery of the head and neck during the COVID-19 pandemic," *JAMA Otolaryngology-Head and Neck Surgery*, vol. 146, no. 6, pp. 579–584, 2020.

[14] B. Pichi, F. Mazzola, A. Bonsembiante et al., "CORONA-steps for tracheotomy in COVID-19 patients: a staff-safe method for airway management," *Oral Oncology*, vol. 105, p. 104682, 2020.

[15] J.-L. Trouillet, C.-E. Luyt, M. Guiguet et al., "Early percutaneous tracheotomy versus prolonged intubation of mechanically ventilated patients after cardiac Surgery," *Annals of internal medicine*, vol. 154, no. 6, pp. 373–383, 2011.

[16] J. Griffiths, V. S. Barber, L. Morgan, and J. D. Young, "Systematic review and meta-analysis of studies of the timing of tracheostomy in adult patients undergoing artificial ventilation," *BMJ*, vol. 330, no. 7502, p. 1243, 2005.

[17] F. Wang, Y. Wu, L. Bo et al., "The timing of tracheotomy in critically ill patients undergoing mechanical ventilation: a systematic review and meta-analysis of randomized controlled trials," *Chest*, vol. 140, no. 6, pp. 1456–1465, 2011.

[18] T. Szakmany, P. Russell, A. R. Wilkes, and J. E. Hall, "Effect of early tracheostomy on resource utilization and clinical outcomes in critically ill patients: meta-analysis of randomized controlled trials," *British Journal of Anaesthesia*, vol. 114, no. 3, pp. 396–405, 2015.

[19] F. Zhou, T. Yu, R. Du et al., "Clinical course and risk factors for mortality of adult inpatients with COVID-19 in Wuhan, China: a retrospective cohort study," *The Lancet*, vol. 395, no. 10229, pp. 1054–1062, 2020.

[20] T. Ai, Z. Yang, H. Hou et al., "Correlation of chest CT and RT-PCR testing for coronavirus disease 2019 (COVID-19) in China: a report of 1014 cases," *Radiology*, vol. 296, no. 2, pp. E32–E40, 2020.

[21] J. Zhao, Q. Yuan, and H. Wang, "Antibody responses to SARS-CoV-2 in patients of novel coronavirus disease 2019," *Clinical Infectious Diseases*, vol. 71, no. 16, pp. 2027–2034, 2020.

[22] A. Torrego, V. Pajares, C. Fernández-Arias, P. Vera, and J. Mancebo, "Bronchoscopy in patients with COVID-19 with invasive mechanical ventilation: a single-center experience," *American Journal of Respiratory and Critical Care Medicine*, vol. 202, no. 2, pp. 284–287, 2020.

[23] M. Mondoni, G. F. Sferrazza Papa, R. Rinaldo et al., "Utility and safety of bronchoscopy during the SARS-CoV-2 outbreak in Italy: a retrospective, multicentre study," *The European Respiratory Journal*, vol. 56, no. 4, p. 2002767, 2020.

[24] Q. X. Long, B. Z. Liu, H. J. Deng et al., "Antibody responses to SARS-CoV-2 in patients with COVID-19," *Nature Medicine*, vol. 26, no. 6, pp. 845–848, 2020.

[25] W. I. Wei, H. H. Tuen, R. W. M. Ng, and L. K. Lam, "Safe tracheostomy for patients with severe acute respiratory syndrome," *Laryngoscope*, vol. 113, no. 10, pp. 1777–1779, 2003.

[26] A. Niroula, K. M. Van Nostrand, O. V. Khullar et al., "Percutaneous tracheostomy with apnea during coronavirus disease 2019 era: a protocol and brief report of cases," *Critical Care Explorations*, vol. 2, no. 5, article e0134, 2020.

Permissions

All chapters in this book were first published by Hindawi Publishing Corporation; hereby published with permission under the Creative Commons Attribution License or equivalent. Every chapter published in this book has been scrutinized by our experts. Their significance has been extensively debated. The topics covered herein carry significant findings which will fuel the growth of the discipline. They may even be implemented as practical applications or may be referred to as a beginning point for another development.

The contributors of this book come from diverse backgrounds, making this book a truly international effort. This book will bring forth new frontiers with its revolutionizing research information and detailed analysis of the nascent developments around the world.

We would like to thank all the contributing authors for lending their expertise to make the book truly unique. They have played a crucial role in the development of this book. Without their invaluable contributions this book wouldn't have been possible. They have made vital efforts to compile up to date information on the varied aspects of this subject to make this book a valuable addition to the collection of many professionals and students.

This book was conceptualized with the vision of imparting up-to-date information and advanced data in this field. To ensure the same, a matchless editorial board was set up. Every individual on the board went through rigorous rounds of assessment to prove their worth. After which they invested a large part of their time researching and compiling the most relevant data for our readers.

The editorial board has been involved in producing this book since its inception. They have spent rigorous hours researching and exploring the diverse topics which have resulted in the successful publishing of this book. They have passed on their knowledge of decades through this book. To expedite this challenging task, the publisher supported the team at every step. A small team of assistant editors was also appointed to further simplify the editing procedure and attain best results for the readers.

Apart from the editorial board, the designing team has also invested a significant amount of their time in understanding the subject and creating the most relevant covers. They scrutinized every image to scout for the most suitable representation of the subject and create an appropriate cover for the book.

The publishing team has been an ardent support to the editorial, designing and production team. Their endless efforts to recruit the best for this project, has resulted in the accomplishment of this book. They are a veteran in the field of academics and their pool of knowledge is as vast as their experience in printing. Their expertise and guidance has proved useful at every step. Their uncompromising quality standards have made this book an exceptional effort. Their encouragement from time to time has been an inspiration for everyone.

The publisher and the editorial board hope that this book will prove to be a valuable piece of knowledge for researchers, students, practitioners and scholars across the globe.

List of Contributors

Raju Reddy
Division of Pulmonary, Critical Care and Sleep Medicine, Department of Internal Medicine, University of Florida, 1600 SW Archer Rd, Gainesville, FL, USA

Nupur Verma and Tan-Lucien Mohammed
Department of Radiology, University of Florida, 1600 SW Archer Rd, Gainesville, FL, USA

Marie Sylvie Kouassi, Fabien A. Gounongbe, Ibrahim Cisse and Spero H. R. Hounkpatin
Faculty of Medicine, University of Parakou, Parakou, Benin

Serge Ade
Faculty of Medicine, University of Parakou, Parakou, Benin
International Union Against Tuberculosis and Lung Diseases, Paris, France

Mênonli Adjobimey and Gildas Agodokpessi
Faculty of Health Sciences, University of Abomey-Calavi, Cotonou, Benin
National and Teaching Hospital of Respiratory Diseases, Cotonou, Benin

Mnahi Bin Saeedan and Ruchi Yadav
Section of Thoracic Imaging, Imaging Institute, Cleveland Clinic, Cleveland, OH, USA

Carol Farver
Department of Pathology, University of Michigan, Ann Arbor, MI, USA

Atul C. Mehta
Department of Pulmonary and Critical Care Medicine, Cleveland Clinic, Cleveland, OH, USA

Pardeep Masuta
Pulmonary & Critical Care, SUNY Upstate Medical University, Syracuse, USA

Ioana Amzuta
Assistant Professor of Medicine, Pulmonary & Critical Care, SUNY Upstate Medical University, Syracuse, USA

Daniel Melese Desalegn, Kumera Terfa Kitila, Boja Dufera Taddese, Tariku Takle Dinku, Kassahun Demisse Asferie, Hanna Mekonnen Balcha and Chalachew Sisay Gebeyehu
Ethiopian Public Health Institute (EPHI), Addis Ababa, Ethiopia
Addis Ababa Public Health Research and Emergency Management Core Process, Addis Ababa City Administration Health Bureau, Addis Ababa, Ethiopia

Tinsae Kidanemariam Hailu
Addis Ababa Public Health Research and Emergency Management Core Process, Addis Ababa City Administration Health Bureau, Addis Ababa, Ethiopia

Girmay Medhin
Aklilu Lemma Institute of Pathobiology Addis Ababa University, Addis Ababa, Ethiopia

Vilen Molotov-Luchanskiy, Larissa Muravlyova, Ryszhan Bakirova, Aruna Kossybayeva, Dmitry Klyuyev, Ludmila Demidchik and Irina Beinikova
"Karaganda Medical University" Non-commercial Joint-Stock Company, Kazakhstan

Altynbek Nukhuly
Pavlodar State Pedagogical University, Kazakhstan

Carlos Metz, Torben Rixecker, Sebastian Mang, André Becker, Frederik Seiler, Guy Danziger, Robert Bals and Philipp M. Lepper
Department of Pneumology, Allergology and Critical Care Medicine, Saarland University, Homburg/Saar, Germany

Alexander Maßmann
Department for Diagnostic and Interventional Radiology, Saarland University Medical Center, Homburg/Saar, Germany

Sören L. Becker, Cihan Papan and Barbara Gärtner
Center for Infectious Diseases, Institute of Medical Microbiology and Hygiene, Saarland University, Homburg/Saar, Germany

Fernando Figueroa Rodriguez and Justine Nasr
Department of Internal Medicine, Beaumont Health, Royal Oak, MI, USA

Ahsan Uddin
Department of Internal Medicine-Pediatrics, Beaumont Health, Royal Oak, MI, USA

Srinivas R. Mummadi and Peter Y. Hahn
Department of Pulmonary and Critical Care Medicine, Metro Health-University of Michigan Health, Suite 220, 2122 Health Dr. SW, Wyoming, MI 49519, USA

A. Burkett, P. Bajpai, A. Elkholy, U. Manne and P. Benson
Department of Pathology, Division of Anatomic Pathology, University of Alabama at Birmingham, Birmingham, Alabama, USA

S. McElwee
Department of Medicine, Division of Cardiovascular Disease, University of Alabama at Birmingham, Birmingham, Alabama, USA

C. Margaroli and K. Wille
Department of Medicine, Division of Pulmonary, Allergy & Critical Care Medicine, University of Alabama at Birmingham, Birmingham, Alabama, USA

Vijay Jaimni, Barkur Ananthakrishna Shasty, Sharath P. Madhyastha, Ganesh V. Shetty, Raviraja V. Acharya and Ragini Bekur
Department of Medicine, Kasturba Medical College, Manipal Academy of Higher Education, 576104, Manipal, Karnataka, India

Akhila Doddamani
Department of Community Medicine, Kasturba Medical College, Manipal Academy of Higher Education, 576104, Manipal, Karnataka, India

Hiromi Ide, Kazunori Tobino, Masanobu Okahisa, Kojin Murakami, Yuki Goto, Takuto Sueyasu, Saori Nishizawa, Kohei Yoshimine and Miyuki Munechika
Department of Respiratory Medicine, Iizuka Hospital, Japan

Yoshikazu Yamaji
Department of Respiratory Medicine and Infectious Disease, Graduate School of Medicine, Yamaguchi University, Japan

Masafumi Oya and Yuka Hiraki
Department of Pathology, Iizuka Hospital, Japan

Yvette Farrugia, Bernard Paul Spiteri Meilak, Neil Grech, Rachelle Asciak, Liberato Camilleri, Stephen Montefort and Christopher Zammit
Mater Dei Hospital, Triq id-Donaturi tad-Demm, Msida MSD2090, Malta

Zsófia Lázár, Lilla Tamási and Veronika Müller
Dept. Pulmonology, Semmelweis University, 25-29 Tömő Str. 1083 Budapest, Hungary

Alpár Horváth and Gábor Tomisa
Dept. Pulmonology, Semmelweis University, 25-29 Tömő Str. 1083 Budapest, Hungary
Chiesi Hungary Ltd., Dunavirág u. 2, 1138 Budapest, Hungary

Zeeshan Sattar, Alnardo Lora, Bakr Jundi and Christopher Railwah
Division of Pulmonary and Critical Care Medicine, Department of Medicine, State University of New York Downstate Health Sciences University, 450 Clarkson Avenue, Brooklyn, NY 11203, USA

Patrick Geraghty
Division of Pulmonary and Critical Care Medicine, Department of Medicine, State University of New York Downstate Health Sciences University, 450 Clarkson Avenue, Brooklyn, NY 11203, USA
Department of Cell Biology, State University of New York Downstate Health Sciences University, 450 Clarkson Avenue, Brooklyn, NY 11203, USA

Aishwarya Nair, Gopala Krishna Alaparthi and Shyam Krishnan
Department of Physiotherapy, Kasturba Medical College, Manipal Academy of Higher Education, Bejai, Mangalore-575004, India

Santhosh Rai
Department of Radiodiagnosis, Kasturba Medical College Mangalore, Manipal Academy of Higher Education, Mangalore-575004, India

R. Anand, Vishak Acharya and Preetam Acharya
Department of Pulmonary Medicine, Kasturba Medical College, Manipal Academy of Higher Education, Mangalore-575004, India

Muhammed Abdu, Eshetu Girma and Wondwosen Mebratu
Wollo University, Ethiopia

Awraris Balchut
Debre Birhan University, Ethiopia

Kritika Krishnamurthy and Pukhraz Basra
AM Rywlin Department of Pathology and Laboratory Medicine, Mount Sinai Medical Centre, Miami Beach, FL, USA

John Alexis and Ana Maria Medina
AM Rywlin Department of Pathology and Laboratory Medicine, Mount Sinai Medical Centre, Miami Beach, FL, USA
Florida International University Herbert Wertheim College of Medicine, Miami, FL, USA

Mazin Barry
Department of Internal Medicine, Division of Infectious Diseases, College of Medicine, King Saud University, Riyadh, Saudi Arabia

Adam Purdy, Firas Ido and Deborah Stahlnecker
Division of Pulmonary and Critical Care, St. Luke's University Health Network, Bethlehem, PA, USA

Zoheir Bshouty
Section of Pulmonary Medicine, Department of Medicine, University of Manitoba, Winnipeg, MB, Canada

Hassan Alfraidi
Section of Pulmonary Medicine, Department of Medicine, University of Manitoba, Winnipeg, MB, Canada
Division of Cardiology, Department of Medicine, McGill University, Montreal, QC, Canada

Sultan Qanash
King Saud Bin Abdulaziz University for Health Sciences, King Abdulaziz Medical City, Jeddah, Saudi Arabia

Saad Ullah and Mingchen Song
Division of Pulmonary and Critical Care Medicine, Southern Illinois University, Springfield, IL, USA

Mirza Ali
Department of Internal Medicine, Southern Illinois University, Springfield, IL, USA

Tomohiko Asakawa, Mea Asou, Eri Nohara, Tomoyuki Seki and Makoto Araki
Department of Internal Medicine, Suwa Central Hospital, Chino, Nagano 391-8503, Japan

Eri Nakano
Department of Internal Medicine, Suwa Central Hospital, Chino, Nagano 391-8503, Japan
National Hospital Organization, Tokyo National Hospital, Takeoka, Kiyose, Tokyo 204-8585, Japan

Divya R, Rajesh Venkitakrishnan, Jolsana Augustine and Melcy Cleetus
Department of Pulmonary Medicine, Rajagiri Hospital Chunangamvely, Aluva, 683112, Kochi, Kerala, India

Pravesh Vishwakarma, Rishi Sethi and Akshyaya Pradhan
Department of Cardiology, King George's Medical University, Lucknow, Uttar Pradesh 226003, India

Kauser Usman
Department of Internal Medicine, King George's Medical University, Lucknow, Uttar Pradesh 226003, India

Rajiv Garg and Jyoti Bajpai
Department of Respiratory Medicine, King George's Medical University, Lucknow, Uttar Pradesh 226003, India

Cory Primaturia, Lelani Reniarti and Heda M. N. Nataprawira
Department of Child Health, Faculty of Medicine Universitas Padjadjaran/Dr. Hasan Sadikin General Hospital, Jl. Pasteur No. 38 Bandung 40161, Indonesia

Mahmood Mubasher, Amir Hanafi, Tausif Syed, Abir Zinal, Ibrahim Y. Abubeker, Mohan Rao and Ryan Hoefen
Rochester Regional Health-Unity Hospital, Rochester, NY, USA

Mouhand F. H. Mohamed and Mohammed Danjuma
Internal Medicine Department, Hamad General Hospital, Hamad Medical, Corporation, Doha, Qatar

W. D. N. L. Amarasinghe, R. Jayasekara and A. Fernando
Central Chest Clinic, Colombo, Sri Lanka

B. D. W. Jayamanne
Department of Public Health, Faculty of Medicine, University of Kelaniya, Sri Lanka

T. D. K. Nalaka
Department of Radiology, National Hospital of Sri Lanka, Sri Lanka

W. A. D. L. Amarasiri
Department of Physiology, Faculty of Medicine, University of Colombo, Sri Lanka

R. Punchihewa
Department of Pathology, National Hospital for Respiratory Diseases, Welisara, Sri Lanka

Margarita Y. Pervakova, Alexandra V. Mazing, Sergey V. Lapin, Olga Y. Tkachenko, Anna I. Budkova, Elena A. Surkova, Vladimir L. Emanuel and Olga N. Titova
Pavlov First State Medical University of St. Petersburg, 197022 Saint Petersburg, Russia

Ashis Kumar Das
Research Group, The World Bank, Washington DC, USA

Saji Saraswathy Gopalan
Human Development Department, The World Bank, Washington DC, USA

Asma Mimouni, Ahmed Hireche, Ibtissem Boudokhane and Dalila Satta
Laboratoire de Biologie Moléculaire et Cellulaire, University Frères Mentouri Constantine 1, Constantine 25000, Algeria
Laboratoire de Biologie et Génétique Moléculaire, Univ. Constantine 3, Constantine 25000, Algeria

Noureddine Abadi
Laboratoire de Biologie et Génétique Moléculaire, Univ. Constantine 3, Constantine 25000, Algeria

Etienne Rouleau and Patrick Saulnier
AMMICa/US 23 INSERM / UMS 3655 CNRS, Villejuif Cedex 94805, France

Amina Marouani
Service de Pneumologie, CHU Sétif, 19000, Algeria

Med Lamine Abdelali
Physics Department, Univ. Frères Mentouri Constantine 1, Constantine 25000, Algeria

Taha Filali
Service d'Oncologie CHU Constantine, Faculté de Médecine Univ. Constantine 3, Constantine 25000, Algeria

Leila Beddar
Service d'Anatomie Pathologique, CHU Constantine, Faculté de Médecine Univ. Constantine 3, Constantine 25000, Algeria

Abdelhak Lakehal
Registre de Cancer Constantine et Service d'Épidémiologie et Médecine Préventive, CHU Constantine, 25000, Algeria

Asma Boudersa
Service d'Oncologie, CHU, Annaba 23000, Algeria

Mahmoud Aissaoui and Hacene Ramtani
Clinique Alfarabi, Annaba 23000, Algeria

Khalid Bouhedjar
Centre de Recherche en Biotechnologie, Constantine 25000, Algeria

Djamel Abdellouche
Service D'Anatomie Pathologique, CHU Sétif, Sétif 19000, Algeria

Messaouda Oudjehih
Registre de Cancer Batna et Service d'Épidémiologie et Médecine Préventive, CHU Batna, Batna 5000, Algeria

Christian Akem Dimala, Urvi Patel, Benjamin Lloyd, Anthony Donato and Caitlyn Moss
Department of Medicine, Reading Hospital-Tower Health, West Reading, PA, USA

William B. Kimmel
Department of Pathology, Reading Hospital-Tower Health, West Reading, PA, USA

Robert Hallowell
Department of Pulmonary & Critical Care Medicine, Massachusetts General Hospital, Boston, MA, USA

Venkata Kishore Mukku and Catalina Negulescu
Department of Internal Medicine, Baton Rouge General Internal Medicine Residency Program, an affiliate of Tulane University School of Medicine, Baton Rouge, Louisiana, USA

Emily Cassidy
Cardiovascular Thoracic Surgery, CVT Surgical Center, Baton Rouge, Louisiana, USA

Tonya Jagneaux and John Godke
Pulmonary Critical Care, Louisiana State University Health Sciences Center, Baton Rouge Campus, Louisiana, USA

Askin Gülsen and Daniel Drömann
Department of Pneumology, Airway Research Center North (ARCN), Member of the German Center for Lung Research (DZL), University of Luebeck, Germany

Burcu Arpinar Yigitbas and Berat Uslu
Department of Pneumology, Yedikule Chest Disease and Thoracic Surgery Hospital, Istanbul, Turkey

Oguz Kilinc
Department of Pneumology, Dokuz Eylül University, Izmir, Turkey

Ziad Boujaoude, Nagendra Madisi, Bhavi Patel and Wissam Abouzgheib
Division of Pulmonary and Interventional Pulmonary Medicine, Department of Medicine, Cooper University Health Care, Cooper Medical School of Rowan University, Camden, NJ, USA

Jean-Sebastien Rachoin and R. Phillip Dellinger
Division of Pulmonary and Interventional Pulmonary Medicine, Department of Medicine, Cooper University Health Care, Cooper Medical School of Rowan University, Camden, NJ, USA
Division of Critical Care Medicine, Department of Medicine, Cooper University Health Care, Cooper Medical School of Rowan University, Camden, NJ, USA

Index